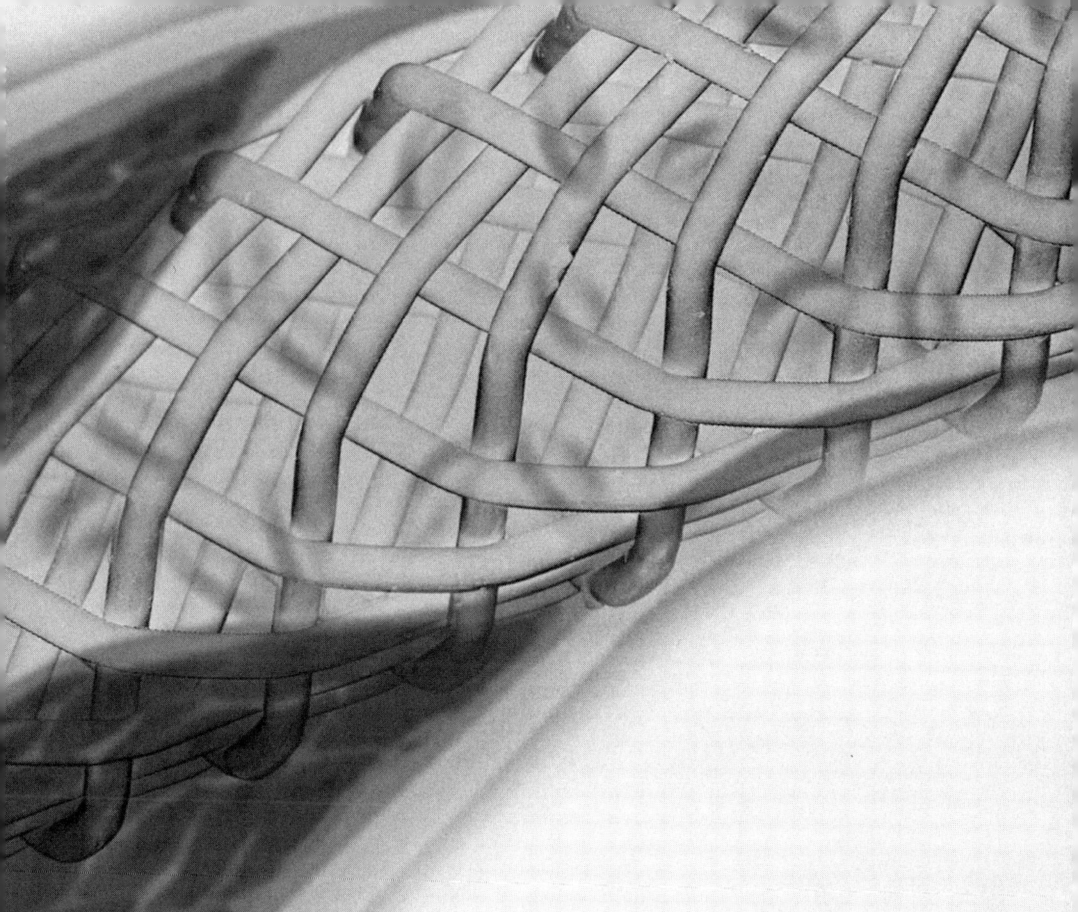

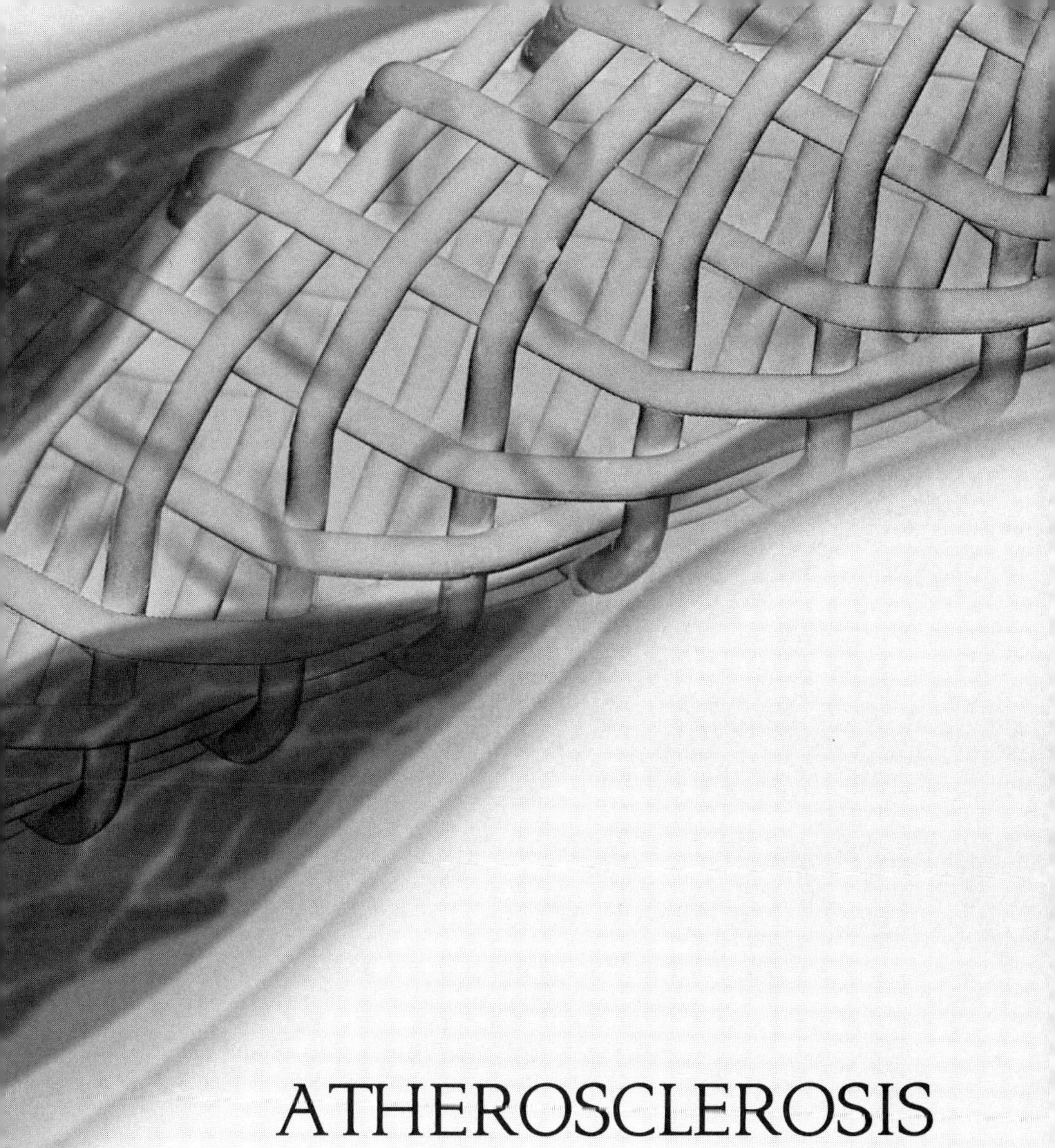

ATHEROSCLEROSIS

edited by
Christian Weber
Oliver Soehnlein

ATHEROSCLEROSIS
Treatment and Prevention

PAN STANFORD PUBLISHING

Published by

Pan Stanford Publishing Pte. Ltd.
Penthouse Level, Suntec Tower 3
8 Temasek Boulevard
Singapore 038988

Email: editorial@panstanford.com
Web: www.panstanford.com

British Library Cataloguing-in-Publication Data
A catalogue record for this book is available from the British Library.

Atherosclerosis: Treatment and Prevention

ISBN 978-981-4316-26-2 (Hardcover)
ISBN 978-981-4364-26-3 (eBook)

Printed in the USA

Contents

Preface

Despite all innovations in prevention, diagnosis, and treatment, cardiovascular diseases as a consequence of atherosclerosis remain the leading cause for mortality and morbidity in industrial countries. Traditionally, atherosclerosis was attributed to progressive narrowing of the artery lumen owing to hyperlipidemia. It is now clear that the vascular wall is a site of chronic inflammation, resulting from complex interactions between the environment and the genetic make-up of the host. Over the past years, a tremendous number of preclinical studies have revealed novel aspects of the disease pathophysiology, and the feasibility of translating such knowledge to novel therapeutic approaches is currently being explored at various levels. This volume builds a bridge between the various aspects of recent advances of our understanding of the disease mechanisms underlying atherosclerosis and atherothrombosis and possible clinical applications that might derive from there.

Christian Weber

Oliver Soehnlein

Winter 2012

Chapter 1

Chemokines and Their Receptors as Therapeutic Targets in Atherosclerosis

Rory R. Koenen[a] **and Christian Weber**[a,b,c]
[a] *Cardiovascular Research Institute Maastricht, Maastricht University, Maastricht, The Netherlands*
[b] *Institute for Preventive Cardiology, University Clinic of the Ludwig-Maximilians-University Munich, Munich, Germany*
[c] *Munich Heart Alliance*
rory.koenen@med.uni-muenchen.de, christian.weber@med.uni-muenchen.de

1.1 Introduction

Cardiovascular disease is a major cause of mortality and morbidity in Western countries and is expected to become the predominant cause of death worldwide. In developed countries, the incidence is still rising due to the increasing prevalence of risk factors such as diabetes mellitus and obesity. The main underlying pathology of cardiovascular disease is atherosclerosis, a chronic inflammation elicited by hyperlipidemia and perpetuated by a dysbalanced immune response, which is characterized by the development of lipid-rich lesions, called plaques, in the larger arteries of the body [1]. These plaques originate from an initial localized dysfunction of the endothelial lining of blood vessels, causing an infiltration of

Atherosclerosis: Treatment and Prevention
Edited by Christian Weber and Oliver Soehnlein

ISBN 978-981-4316-26-2 (Hardcover), ISBN 978-981-4364-26-3 (eBook)
www.panstanford.com

inflammatory blood cells and increased uptake and retention of lipid-rich plasma proteins, such as low-density lipoprotein (LDL), in the vessel wall [2, 3]. Subsequently modified LDL species (such as oxidized LDL) cause activation of smooth muscle cells (SMC) and endothelial cells (EC) leading to an increased expression and presentation of adhesion molecules and chemokines on the vessel wall, which in turn enhances the harmful influx of leukocytes. The resulting subendothelial accumulation of white blood cells and lipids is known as a fatty streak, which can progress into more complex atherosclerotic lesions. Due to mechanisms which are still largely unknown, advanced plaques can destabilize and eventually rupture, exposing the highly thrombotic interior and leading to massive platelet aggregation and occlusive thrombosis. In the major arteries, an interruption of the blood and oxygen supply to downstream tissue is the precipitating event for clinically manifest *angina pectoris*, myocardial infarction, or ischemic stroke. The result of such ischemic episodes is often massive tissue damage and organ dysfunction, owing to which patients are often subject to long-term medical care. Along with the high incidence of cardiovascular disease, this imposes a huge burden on the social and health care systems. In both non-profit and profit sectors, major investments are being made in a search for means to prevent the occurrence of cardiovascular disease and for its treatment in patients. Even though the currently available therapeutics against atherosclerosis represent a multi-billion dollar market, their modes of action are largely restricted to the modulation of lipid metabolism to alleviate hyperlipidemia and the control of hemostasis to prevent thrombotic complications. However, these therapeutic strategies do not directly address the actual mechanisms that drive the progression of atherosclerosis, namely the influx of inflammatory cells into plaques. Since chemokines play an important role in directing the egress, migration, and infiltration of leukocytes [4, 5], they represent an attractive target for therapeutic intervention. In this chapter, an overview of the many options for pharmacologic intervention and of the current status of the development of chemokine-related therapeutics in atherosclerotic vascular disease is provided. In addition to the potential advantages, also drawbacks of the therapeutic targeting of the chemokine system are highlighted.

1.2 Chemokines: Crucial Regulators of Leukocyte Trafficking

1.2.1 Structure and Function of Chemokines

1.2.1.1 Chemokine classification

Chemokines, small chemotactic cytokines, can be categorized into a family with two major CC and CXC classes, depending on the spacing of their conserved cysteine residues, with XC and CX_3C chemokines as exceptions. They activate specific chemokine receptors, which are members of the seven-transmembrane G protein-coupled receptor superfamily and are classified analogously to the chemokine class that binds to the receptor. At present, the chemokine system consists of more than 50 chemokines and 19 G protein-coupled chemokine receptors. The tertiary structure of chemokines is characterized by the so-called "chemokine fold", a structure consisting of a more or less unfolded N-terminus and a central β-sheet constituted by three antiparallel β-strands and by a C-terminal α-helix, which is conserved among all members of the chemokine family. Whereas all chemokines share a high homology on the tertiary structure level, the CC- and CXC-chemokine subgroups form defined quaternary structures. CC chemokines preferentially form elongated N-terminal dimers, while CXC-chemokines rather dimerize to a compact globular structure with an extended central β-sheet. Particular regions within the global chemokine structure can be defined which serve specific purposes. For example, patches of basic residues at molecular surfaces and/or C-terminal α-helices are present in most chemokines and are involved in binding to glycosaminoglycans (GAGs), allowing chemokines to be immobilized and presented on cell surfaces thereby creating two-dimensional "haptotactic gradients" [6]. Beyond dimerization, particular members of the chemokine family are also able to form higher order structures such as tetramers and high molecular weight aggregates, and many chemokines exist in dimeric or multimeric forms in free solution. This so-called oligomerization, along with binding to GAGs, is essential for their *in vivo* function and supports the correct presentation of chemokines on cell surfaces for cell guidance and receptor activation [7, 8]. It is believed that the globular part of chemokines is involved in binding to their receptors, while the disordered and flexible N-terminus enters a defined pocket between the transmembrane helices of the chemokine receptor, leading to its activation.

1.2.1.2 Chemokine oligomerization and binding to glycosaminoglycans

During the past decades, the relationship between the primary and the quaternary structures of chemokines has been subject to precise characterization. Having a relatively short and conserved amino acid sequence and a defined three-dimensional structure, chemokines are well amenable to structure-function studies. Here, it was often observed that single amino acid substitutions had a high impact on chemokine structure and activity. Particularly N-terminal modifications are functionally poorly tolerated, and the potential of chemokines to oligomerize can be strongly reduced by mutations in single amino acids. Interestingly, monomeric variants of the chemokines CCL2, CXCL8, and CCL5 were fully competent in receptor activation *in vitro* [8–10], indicating that a monomer is the minimally required form for receptor activation. In fact, obligate dimeric chemokine mutants may show reduced receptor binding and only partial agonist activity [11, 12], but retain activity *in vivo.* However, while retaining receptor agonist and chemotactic activities *in vitro,* monomeric mutants of several chemokines virtually lost their ability to recruit leukocytes in various mouse models of inflammation [8, 13]. This strongly indicates that oligomerization of chemokines is an essential feature for their correct function. Interestingly, there appears to be a connection between the potential of chemokines to oligomerize and their binding to GAGs. The GAGs present on the surface of vascular and blood cells could facilitate the oligomerization of chemokines [14, 15]. On the other hand, monomeric chemokine variants of CCL5 and CXCL8 did not oligomerize on heparin, implying that the ability of chemokines to form higher order structures is required for oligomerization on GAGs. In analogy with oligomerization mutants, most chemokine variants with impaired GAG binding are devoid of chemoattractant activity *in vivo*, highlighting the importance of chemokine presentation for the efficient recruitment of leukocytes. This presentation on the surface of vascular cells is facilitated by the ability of chemokines to oligomerize and interact with GAGs.

1.2.1.3 Formation of heteromeric chemokine complexes

Besides the formation of homo-oligomeric complexes, chemokines are also able to engage in heterophilic interactions with other chemokines. To date, 10 different heterophilic complexes have been identified that are constituted by 13 chemokines (reviewed in [16]). This is energetically feasible in many cases, because of the high structural homology between chemokines. Molecular dynamics simulation studies have predicted the possibility of several heteromeric combination of CC and CXC chemokines [17], but experimental studies are needed to confirm their existence. The first chemokine heteromer described was a complex of CCL3 and CCL4 which was secreted by monocytes under physiological conditions [18]. Unfortunately, this study did not include further functional characterization of this heterodimer. It did not take very long, however, before functional consequences could be linked to the occurrence of chemokine heterodimers: the activation of hematopoietic cells by CXCL8 was inhibited by CXCL4, an effect attributable to the binding of CXCL8 by CXCL4 in solution [19]. Further structural characterization confirmed these chemokines formed CXC-type heterodimers and that their interaction could potentiate the biologic responses typical for CXCL4 and CXCL8, such as the inhibition of endothelial cell proliferation and chemotaxis of CXCR2-transfected cells, respectively [20]. Since CXCL4 and CXCL8 share considerable structural homology, the existence of a heterodimer of the CXC type was within the line of expectation. Likewise, the structurally-related CCL2 and CCL8 have also been shown to form heterodimers of the CC type [21]. In contrast, predictions concerning the structure of mixed heterodimers between CC and CXC chemokines, such as CCL5 and CXCL4, are accompanied by difficulties because of the structural diversity of CC- and CXC-chemokine oligomers. Molecular dynamics simulations and NMR studies revealed that these chemokines were likely to form CC-type heterodimers through an involvement of the N-terminal region of CCL5 in the interaction with CXCL4 [17, 22] and studies are currently being performed to refine the heteromeric structure between CCL5 and CXCL4. Given the massive amount of combinations of chemokines that could theoretically form heteromeric complexes, a so-called "chemokine interactome" has been postulated [23]. This interactome constitutes the collective of existing chemokine interactions for a finely-tuned leukocyte regulation. Acting in concert with presentation on GAGs, chemokine heteromerization might assist to create a context-dependent and tailor-made repertoire of cues in order to direct the actions of specific leukocyte subsets in a particular microenvironment during health and disease.

1.2.2 Mechanisms of Chemokine Action

1.2.2.1 Regulation of leukocyte trafficking by chemokines

Since the discovery of chemokines more than 20 years ago, researchers have been puzzled about the successive identification of ever new chemokines and chemokine receptors. This apparent redundancy in the chemokine system became even more astounding when it turned out that several chemokines can bind to multiple receptors and vice versa. Furthermore, some chemokines can act as natural antagonists for certain chemokine receptors, and post-translational modifications can render a chemokine more or less active [24, 25]. It has to be noted that much of the redundancy is based on results obtained with isolated chemokines and cells *in vitro* and does not reflect the actual situation in a living organism, where a given cell type might never encounter a particular chemokine. Considering the large number of leukocyte subsets and the vast diversity of physiologic situations in which leukocytes act, the redundancy in the chemokine system should rather be perceived as robust and sophisticated. At a particular site of inflammation, one can envision a specific palette of presented chemokines tailored to attract particular subsets of leukocytes. A context-specific chemokine presentation might be facilitated by a locally-defined repertoire of GAGs with differential binding affinities for chemokines [7]. Accordingly, chemokines have specific leukocyte-recruiting activities, depending on the situation in a certain microenvironment [26, 27]. For example, CXCL1 is secreted by activated EC and stays immobilized on their surface, where it induces stable arrest of monocytes under flow, whereas CCL2 secreted in a polarized fashion rather triggers transendothelial migration of adherent monocytes [26, 28]. Such a "division of labor" of chemokines also appears to apply for chemokine receptors. Stable arrest of CD45RO$^+$ memory T cells under flow has been found to be induced through activation of CCR1, whereas CCR5 activation mediated spreading and transmigration [29]. Because

CCL5 is a functional ligand for both receptors, this observation provides a good example how the presence of a single chemokine can elicit complementary leukocyte responses. Further, this might argue against a functional redundancy, since the expression of both receptors could be a prerequisite for recruiting that particular T-cell type. An interesting aspect of chemokine biology is the variety of processes regulated by chemokines, beyond leukocyte migration. It is well established that chemokines with the N-terminal ELR motive such as CXCL1 and CXCL8 have pro-angiogenic activity, whereas CXC-type chemokines lacking this motive generally act angiostatic [30]. An exception of an angiogenic non-ELR chemokine is CXCL12, which attracts hematopoietic progenitor cells and is implicated in the promotion of tumor angiogenesis [31, 32]. Moreover, CXCL12 is essential in embryogenesis, where it regulates the formation of large vessels and parts of the nervous system [33, 34]. The chemokine receptor CXCR4 has long been considered to be the only receptor for CXCL12, a notion that was supported by the observation that CXCR4 knockout mice showed a similar lethal phenotype as mice lacking CXCL12. However, a novel chemokine receptor, CXCR7, has been identified as a high-affinity receptor for CXCL12. Although CXCR7 does not mediate classical chemokine receptor responses such as chemotaxis or calcium mobilization [35], it has been shown to be important for the formation of functional heart valves during embryonic development in mice [36]. Thus, CXCR7 may not be linked to G-proteins in an ordinary manner, but might rather act as silent chemokine receptor, similar to the scavenger receptor Duffy antigen receptor for chemokines (DARC) [37]. Some of the effects of CXCR7 might be caused by its modulation of CXCR4, which is mediated by heterodimerization of the two receptors [36, 38].

1.2.2.2 Transportation and clearance of chemokines in tissues

Recent studies have highlighted an importance for the presentation of chemokines during inflammation, e.g., through the manipulation of enzymes involved in the synthesis of GAGs. Endothelium-specific gene deletion of *N*-deacetylase–*N*-sulfotransferase-1 (ndst-1), an enzyme essential for the sulfation of heparan sulfate, in mice reduced inflammation in various models [39]. Interestingly, the ability of exogenously administered CXCL1 and CXCL2 to recruit leukocytes into subcutaneous air pouches was also impaired in these mice.

Since hyposulfated GAGs have a lower affinity for chemokines, the aforementioned observation might be explained by a decreased potential of ndst-1–deficient EC to capture and immobilize these chemokines on their surface. In addition, ndst-1–deficient EC transported CXCL8 less efficiently from their basal to apical surface than wild-type cells, corroborating a previously identified role for heparan sulfate in the directional transcytosis of CXCL8 [40]. Receptors other than GAGs can also mediate the transport, immobilization, and presentation of chemokines. The promiscuous scavenger DARC, in particular, a non-signaling chemokine receptor that binds to a diversity of chemokines, has been implicated in the transport and presentation of chemokines for more than a decade [40, 41]. A recent study further elucidated the importance of DARC in the transport of chemokines [42]. Cell monolayers expressing DARC effectively transported basally administered CCL2 or CXCL8 and eventually presented these chemokines on the apical surface. Notably, overexpression of the related non-signaling scavenger receptor D6 in EC entailed degradation of chemokines, instead of their presentation, underscoring the functional distinction of DARC. Transgenic mice overexpressing DARC displayed an increased responsiveness to injected CXCL1 and signs of increased contact hypersensitivity, findings that provided strong support for the concept of DARC as chemokine transporter through tissues *in vivo* [42].

1.3 The Chemokine System in Atherogenesis

1.3.1 Platelet Chemokines

Apart from being transported through the endothelium, chemokines can also be deposited on the vessel lumen by activated platelets. Platelets have been found to exert important functions in driving atherosclerosis and will be discussed more extensively in Chapter 15. Activated platelets might initiate the development of early plaques at atherosclerotic predilection sites by inducing an inflammatory reaction of EC through ligation of platelet CD40 ligand with CD40 present on EC [43]. In addition, activated platelets have been shown to deposit CCL5 onto inflamed endothelium during transient rolling interactions [44]. This deposition of platelet-derived CCL5 onto the surface of arterial EC required P-selectin on platelets, induced the recruitment of monocytes, and was shown to promote neointima formation after wire-induced injury in apolipoprotein E (Apoe) knockout mice [45]. Video microscopic observations in the carotid arteries of hyperlipidemic Apoe$^{-/-}$ knockout mice revealed notable amounts of adherent platelets preferentially at sites that would later develop into plaques [46]. Since the majority of platelet–endothelial interactions were transient in nature and preceded leukocyte arrest and infiltration, the subsequent recruitment of leukocytes might be explained by the vascular deposition of CCL5 and CXCL4. A concomitant study in mice indeed linked the deposition of CCL5 and CXCL4 to an exacerbation of atherosclerotic lesion formation after repeated injection of activated platelets [47]. In a recent study, a role of neutrophils in the development of early atherosclerosis was characterized [48]. Here, it was shown that CCL5 deposited by activated platelets could specifically be utilized by neutrophils to enter early atherosclerotic plaques [48]. Upon activation and during prolonged storage, platelets shed considerable amounts of procoagulant and proinflammatory microparticles, small membrane-enclosed cell fragments [49], which contain several chemokines [50] and can actively deposit CCL5 during transient interactions with the endothelium. Thus, microparticles from platelets might be conceived as a transport mechanism for chemokines with potential relevance in atherogenesis [51]. In a follow-up study, microparticles have also been shown to modulate the responsiveness and regenerative potential of early outgrowth cells through the transfer of the chemokine receptor CXCR4 to these angiogenic cells [52].

1.3.2 Chemokines in the Progression and Regression of Atherosclerosis

1.3.2.1 Phase and cell type-specific function of chemokines

The important role of chemokines in atherosclerosis is currently well established. During the past years, research has focused on the functions of individual chemokines in the diverse phases of atherosclerotic lesion development. Interestingly, it was found that chemokines display distinct temporal patterns of expression and cell-recruiting function during atherogenesis. In a pioneering work, genetic deletion of CCR2 did not prevent the formation of early atherosclerotic lesions in the abdominal aorta [53]. This was corroborated by later findings, revealing an effect of CCR2-deficiency specifically in later stages of plaque formation, which was ascribed to a reduction of monocyte infiltration [54]. In contrast, absence of CXCR3 primarily retarded lesion formation in early atherosclerosis, due reduced recruitment of T cells of the Th1 subtype into developing plaques, while leaving the influx of beneficial $CD4^{+}CD25^{+}$ regulatory T cells (Treg), which down-regulate inflammatory T-cell responses, unaffected [54]. Surprisingly, combined deficiency of CCR2 and CXCR3 did not further reduce plaque burden. This could be attributed to a decreased recruitment of Treg in the additional absence of CCR2, since these Treg might rather use CCR2 for extravasation. Manipulation of T-cell responses in favor of Treg is an intriguing approach to reduce atherosclerosis and has successfully been exploited through interruption of the CXCR3–CXCL10 axis or the administration of exogenous immune modulators [55–57]. The proatherogenic function of CCR2 may also be influenced by the actions of cytokines, such as growth differentiation factor 15 (GDF-15), which has been shown to stimulate CCR2-driven macrophage migration [58]. Deficiency of GDF-15 reduced macrophage infiltration and necrosis in Low Density Lipoprotein Receptor-deficient ($Ldlr^{-/-}$) mice, which could be explained by a reduction of CCR2 expression and function in GDF-15–deficient macrophages [58]. Thus, the proatherogenic activity of chemokines might also be attenuated by a pharmacologic intervention of specific cytokines. On the other hand, the function of GDF-15 might be specialized to particular leukocyte subtypes and chemokines, since GDF-15 inhibited integrin activation in neutrophils and reduced CXCL1-induced adhesion of leukocytes to immobilized adhesion molecules [59]. In a mouse model of myocardial infarction, GDF-15–deficiency was accompanied with increased neutrophil infiltration, cardiac rupture and mortality, indicating that GDF-15 acts cell type- and context-dependent [59].

A peculiar role is reserved for CCR1 and CCR5, the major receptors for CCL5. Whereas both receptors have been involved in CCL5-induced atherogenic mononuclear cell recruitment [29, 60], no reduction in early lesion formation was observed in an initial study with $CCR5^{-/-}$ mice crossed to an Apoe-deficient background [61]. Subsequent work, however, identified an importance of CCR5 in later stages of plaque development [62, 63]. Interestingly, absence of CCR5 in somatic or blood cells was accompanied by a difference in cytokine expression compared to wild-type controls. Particularly the anti-inflammatory cytokine interleukin (IL)-10 was up-regulated, whereas interferon-γ was down-regulated, reflecting a decreased Th1-type lymphocyte response and a general reduction of systemic inflammation. This suggests that CCR5 deficiency does not protect against atherosclerosis by directly reducing CCL5-induced mononuclear cell infiltration but rather through a beneficial modulation of the immune balance. Genetic deletion of CCR1 yielded an even more surprising result, as it was found to increase atherosclerosis, likely by tipping the balance towards a proinflammatory lymphocyte response [63, 64].

1.3.2.2 Combined blockade of chemokines

The combined blockade or deletion of chemokines or their receptors has become increasingly interesting for the prevention and treatment of atherosclerosis. This approach can be particularly advantageous when chemokine functions are complementary, and its feasibility has been probed and illustrated in the recent literature. Especially in the light of the recent advances in our understanding about the role of monocyte subsets in the development of atherosclerosis, combined chemokine blockade might be a suitable method to influence the behavior of these monocyte subsets to minimize their migration into developing lesions. In general, two major monocyte subsets exist, the inflammatory Ly6C^{hi} and the "resident" Ly6C^{low} monocytes [65]. In Apoe$^{-/-}$ mice, the Ly6C^{hi} subset is strongly increased during high-fat diet-induced monocytosis and entered plaques more abundantly than Ly6C^{low} monocytes, where they differentiated into macrophages [66]. This might be explained by their differential use of chemokines to invade lesions. Notably, whereas extravasation of the Ly6C^{low} subset rather depends on CCR5 [67], the atherogenic recruitment of inflammatory Ly6C^{hi} monocytes is predominantly regulated through the CCL2–CCR2 and CX_3CL1–CX_3CR1 axes, giving rise to the question whether these chemokine-receptor pairs act in concert or independently. The latter appears to be the case, because combined genetic deficiency of both CCL2 and either CX_3CR1 or CX_3CL1 in Apoe$^{-/-}$ mice [68, 69] decreased atherosclerosis compared with control mice that had single deficiencies of either chemokine-receptor couples. These findings were explained by a reduction of macrophage accumulation in plaques on one hand and an attenuation of hyperlidipemia-associated blood monocytosis by deficiencies of CXC_3L1 and of CCL2 on the other hand [68, 69]. However, the combined knockdown of CCL2 and CX_3CR1 still did not fully abolish atherosclerotic lesion formation. Since monocyte (e.g., Ly6C^{low}) infiltration into plaques can also occur through use of CCR5 [67], pharmacologic blockade of CCR5 was superimposed on combined CCL2/CX_3CR1 deficiency [68]. Notably, the inhibition of CCR5 functions further decreased circulating monocyte counts and almost fully protected the mice against atherosclerosis. Besides monocytes, a proatherogenic role for neutrophils has recently been described [48, 70, 71]. Neutrophils appear to play a detrimental role particularly in early phases of atherosclerosis [48]. During hyperlipidemia, increased counts of neutrophils were observed due to stimulated proliferation in and enhanced egress from the bone marrow, facilitated by elevated plasma levels of CXCL1. Experiments with genetically deficient animals and blocking antibodies revealed that neutrophils use CCR1, CCR2, CCR5, and CXCR2 to enter atherosclerotic plaques. Interestingly, blockade or genetic deletion of CXCR4 increased atherosclerosis, due to a decreased retention of neutrophils in the bone marrow, leading to neutrophilia [48, 70]. The reports discussed above indicate that chemokines have differential actions in the recruitment of pro- and anti-atherogenic leukocyte subtypes and in the progression of atherosclerosis and more importantly that combined blockade of chemokine functions might achieve a cell-specific and time-dependent attenuation of inflammatory leukocyte recruitment and might be a more effective approach than blocking a single chemokine.

1.3.2.3 Role of chemokines in plaque regression

Although chemokines play an important role in plaque progression, their function in plaque regression is less well characterized. One reason might be that plaque regression models are not very straightforward in mice. In an explorative study by the group of van Berkel, Apoe$^{-/-}$ mice with established lesions were transplanted with wild type bone marrow or bone marrow deficient in CCR2 [72]. Surprisingly, no differences were found in the lesion size 9 weeks after transplantation. Thus, the authors concluded that the CCL2–CCR2 axis does not influence plaque progression in later stages of atherosclerosis and does not induce plaque regression. However, in an aortic transplantation model, where plaque-containing aortic segments from hyperlipidemic Apoe$^{-/-}$ mice were transplanted into normolipidemic wild-type mice, rapid regression of plaques was observed [73]. Gene expression analysis of the regressing plaques revealed an up-regulation of CCR7, and regression of plaques was inhibited by blocking antibodies against CCR7 ligands CCL19 and CCL21, indicating that CCR7-driven egress of mononuclear cells from the plaque might be the mechanism behind plaque regression. However, in a recent study implementing a novel mouse model of gene therapy-induced plaque regression, no involvement of CCR7 in the decrease of plaque size could be observed [74]. Instead, it was hypothesized that a reduction of mononuclear cell influx after viral transfer of the Apoe-gene was the mechanism driving plaque regression rather than the efflux of inflammatory cells from the plaque. It would be of exceptional interest to identify the mediators that drive the influx of inflammatory cells in advanced stages of atherosclerotic lesions, since this would open the perspective for a causative treatment of atherosclerosis.

1.4 Therapeutic Targeting of the Chemokine System

The chemokine system offers various opportunities for pharmacological manipulation. Chemokine receptors have well-defined binding pockets that are amenable to the design of small molecular inhibitors, and chemokines have distinct domains that can be modified in such way that receptor binding capabilities are preserved while abolishing receptor activation. Newer approaches aim to compromise the ability of chemokines to form higher order aggregates or aim to reduce their binding to GAGs. For example, in a recent study, the N-terminus of CX_3CL1 was modified using a phage display library, which yielded a particularly potent antagonist of CX_3CR1 termed F1 [75]. The implementation of this new CX_3CR1 antagonist in atherosclerosis models is still pending. Similarly, N-terminal truncation of CCL2 yielded mutants that bound to CCR2 but failed to activate the receptor, thereby competing with natural CCL2 [76] and a monomeric mutant of CCL2, which retained *in vitro* activity towards CCR2 but, nevertheless, acted as an antagonist *in vivo*, possibly by displacing endogenous CCL2 from GAGs on the vessel wall [77]. A new class of chemokine blockers might encompass modified chemokines with increased potential to bind to GAGs but without affinity for their cognate receptors, such as the recently described PA508 [78]. This novel chemokine antagonist is a modified form of CCL2, which displays strongly increased binding to GAGs, yet decreased affinity for CCR2. In mice, administration of PA508 resulted in reduced neointima formation after arterial injury due to a reduced infiltration of monocytes in the neointimal lesions [79]. In a model of heart ischemia and reperfusion, PA508 reduced myocardial damage and improved heart function by decreasing the immigration of monocytes and beneficially altering scar composition. Thus, by competing with endogenous CCL2, PA508 attenuates the inflammatory response after arterial and myocardial injury and is able to reduce inflammatory cell influx. Similar results were achieved with proteins derived from pox or herpes virus that are able to inhibit the binding of chemokines to GAGs on the vessel wall [80]. In an allogeneic vascular transplant remodeling model in mice, a single injection of pox virus M-T7 protein, which inhibited chemokine binding to GAGs, strongly reduced transplant neointima formation in wild type and $CCL2^{-/-}$ transplants, but not in ndst-$1^{-/-}$ transplants, indicating that the inhibitory effects of M-T7 were specific for chemokine-GAG interactions. The above studies indicate that interference with chemokine binding to GAGs might present an attractive approach for the treatment of vascular inflammatory disease. Direct blockade of CCR2 has also been investigated in the context of cardiovascular disease with variable success. Recently, the CCR2 antibody MLN1202 (Millenium), which is in phase II clinical trial, has been shown to reduce serum C-reactive protein (CRP) levels in patients at risk for cardiovascular disease [81], suggesting that CCR2 blockade reduces inflammation and might supplement existing therapeutic approaches, such as statin therapy. The small molecular antagonist CCX140 (ChemoCentryx) might show similar effects in patients, but clinical trials are still ongoing. In mice, pharmacologic blockade of the CCL2–CCR2 axis has shown variable success. A blocking antibody against CCL2 and CCL12 reduced plaque formation and inflammatory leukocyte infiltration in $Apoe^{-/-}$ mice [82], whereas no reduction in atherosclerosis was observed in mice treated with INCB-3344, a potent CCR2 antagonist, although this antagonist effectively reduced the number of circulating inflammatory Ly6C^{hi} monocytes [83].

Modification of the N-terminus of chemokines often results in antagonists, with the CCL5-variants Met-RANTES and AOP-RANTES blocking CCR1, CCR3, and CCR5 as their most prominent representatives [84–86]. Although initially developed as entry inhibitors against anti-human immunodeficiency virus (HIV), it did not take long before these CCL5 antagonists were successfully tested in animal models of inflammatory disease [87, 88], including atherosclerosis. Treatment of Apoe$^{-/-}$ mice with Met-RANTES after wire-induced denudation injury reduced *neointimal hyperplasia* and macrophage content [45]. Administration of Met-RANTES was also effective in diminishing plaque formation and decreasing T-cell and monocyte infiltration during diet-induced atherosclerosis [68, 89]. Similarly, the GAG binding-defective [^{44}AANA^{47}] mutant of CCL5, which besides being inactive *in vivo*, antagonized the biologic activity of CCL5 [90]. The antagonism could be explained by the formation of mixed dimers of murine CCL5 with this [^{44}AANA^{47}] mutant, which would consequently be devoid of GAG-binding. A potential benefit of this dominant-negative [^{44}AANA^{47}] variant for atherosclerosis was revealed by its administration in LDLr-deficient mice, which inhibited inflammatory cell recruitment and progression of established atherosclerotic lesions [91]. In addition, application of [^{44}AANA^{47}]-CCL5 was also effective in reducing myocardial injury in a model of heart ischemia and reperfusion in atherosclerotic mice by decreasing leukocyte infiltration and chemokine expression in ischemic hearts [92]. Likewise, antibody blockade of CCL5 during ischemia-reperfusion or chronic ischemia in atherosclerotic Apoe$^{-/-}$ mice resulted in a significantly decreased infarct size, accompanied by reduced troponin I levels and reduced infiltration of neutrophils and macrophages as well as the plasma levels of chemokines specific for these cell types [93]. Correspondingly, cardiac function was improved after CCL5 antibody treatment. These results indicate that CCL5 is a central mediator in the inflammatory response after cardiac ischemia.

For chemokine receptors, numerous small-molecular inhibitors have been designed. One of the first described was TAK779 (Takeda Pharmaceuticals), which potently blocks CCR5 in humans and, additionally, inhibits CXCR3 in mice [94]. Administration of TAK779 in mice effectively reduced atherosclerotic lesion formation due to a reduction of T helper type 1 cells in the lesions [95]. In a later study, the reduction of atherosclerosis with the CXCR3 antagonist NBI-74330 (Amgen) was ascribed to an increased amount of Treg in plaques [56]. In addition, the CXCR2 antagonist SB-517785-M (GlaxoSmithKline) was found to reduce ATII-induced leukocyte recruitment in rat arterioles and may thereby limit vascular damage that precedes atherogenesis, suggesting that blocking CXCR2 might exert benefits for the prevention of atherosclerotic disease in patients at risk [96]. Although this collective of results indicates that small-molecular antagonists of chemokine receptors hold promise for the prevention and treatment of atherosclerosis in principle, some caution should be exercised as well. Whereas blockade of CXCR4, which is crucial for maintaining the homeostasis of hematopoietic cells, with the small-molecule antagonist AMD3465 (AnorMED) limited neointima formation after arterial injury in mice [97], chronic treatment with AMD3465 clearly exacerbated diet-induced atherosclerosis by mobilizing neutrophils and increasing their recruitment to the plaques [70].

Generally, clinical trials with chemokine inhibitors returned rather disappointing results. The poor oral bioavailability of TAK779 prevented its entry into clinical trials as anti-HIV agent and this compound has been replaced with improved derivatives, which have not been tested in models of atherosclerosis [98]. In addition, unexpected side effects such as liver toxicity or cardiac arrhythmias were encountered during clinical trials of potential antiviral CCR5 or CXCR4 antagonists [99], possibly due to unspecific drug interactions or toxic metabolites. The fact that among the large amount of chemokine receptor antagonists tested as therapeutics for various inflammatory diseases to date only two chemokine receptor antagonists against CCR5 (Maraviroc, Pfizer) and CXCR4 (AMD3100, AnorMed) have achieved Food and Drug Administration (FDA) approval as anti-HIV agent and hematopoietic stem cell-mobilizer, respectively, emphasizes the challenge of discovering, developing, and refining suitable antagonists against the chemokine system [100]. Another issue to take into account is the fact that the chemokine system is an integral part of the immune system. Therefore, completely shutting down its constituents might be accompanied by an increased risk of unwanted immunologic side effects, such as impairment of host defense. In this respect, one should keep in mind that animals used for validating antagonists are usually maintained in a pathogen-free environment, a situation that is poorly related to daily human life. Even the blockade of a single chemokine could result in impaired immune responses. This appears, at least, to be the case for CCL2 and CCL5. Inhibition of CCL2-CCR2 resulted in an impairment of host defense against bacterial infection [101, 102]. Similarly, administration of Met-RANTES compromises immune responses against herpes simplex virus type 2 (HSV-2), causing increased viral titers in multiple organs due to impaired clearance of virus particles [103].

A potential solution to this dilemma might be an attenuation of the chemokine system, instead of a full blockade, which might be sufficient to favorably shift the immune balance, while leaving normal physiologic functions intact. In line with this notion, the manipulation of heterophilic chemokine interactions could represent a novel and promising approach for the treatment of inflammatory disease without immunologic side effects. Recent work aimed at unraveling the importance of CCL5 and CXCL4 heteromerization for atherosclerosis [22]. Based on structural predictions, cyclic peptides that could interfere with the complex formation of CCL5 and CXCL4 were designed. Validation of the peptides CKEY2 (human) and MKEY (mouse) revealed strong binding to CCL5 (and CXCL4) and effective inhibition of the CXCL4-mediated synergistic enhancement of CCL5-induced monocyte recruitment to inflamed endothelium, while leaving CCL5-related functions unaffected. Administration of MKEY but not control peptides in hyperlipidemic mice during a high-fat diet resulted in a marked reduction of atherosclerotic lesion formation. As opposed to the full CCL5 inhibitor Met-RANTES, MKEY did not compromise host defense against HSV-2 infection, suggesting that disruption of heterophilic chemokine interactions may not be accompanied by immunologic side effects [22]. Beyond revealing the *in vivo* relevance of chemokine heteromerization, this study highlights the therapeutic feasibility of disrupting functional interactions between chemokines. Newly identified chemokine-scavenging proteins derived from ticks or viruses might similarly hold therapeutic potential [104–106]. However, the occurrence of side effects with these antagonists remains yet to be determined. The chemokine and chemokine receptor antagonists with potential relevance for the prevention and treatment of atherosclerosis are summarized in Table 1.1.

1.5 Concluding Remarks

With its diversity, its versatility, and its relevance in many inflammatory diseases, the chemokine system offers many options for therapeutic intervention. Especially in the light of the rather limited availability of causative pharmacologic treatments for atherosclerosis, the targeting of chemokines and their receptors would harbor perspectives for the identification and introduction of novel drugs. However, although results in animal models have shown promising results, the transfer of therapeutics directed against the chemokine system to the clinic has been hampered by several setbacks. This is reflected by the fact that after over 10 years of intensive research in this field, only two chemokine receptor antagonists have reached FDA approval, namely Maraviroc (Celsentri®) and AMD3100 (Plerixafor®). Of note, neither of these drugs has been approved for the treatment of atherosclerosis. Thus, the search for suitable compounds against the chemokine system continues. The humanized anti-CCR2 antibody MLN1202 has achieved phase II clinical testing and booked success in reducing CRP levels in patients (Table 1.1). Yet, the question remains whether parenterally administered drugs (such as antibodies) are optimally suitable for the treatment of chronic diseases like atherosclerosis, particularly when orally applicable therapeutics, like statins, are already available. Apart from the route of administration, the potential safety issues that may be accompanied with full blockade of a chemokine receptor have to be carefully investigated. Notably in elderly people representing the majority of cardiovascular patients and who may be naturally immune compromised, chemokine blockade might impose an additional burden on the immune system, increasing the risk for infections. Thus, novel innovative approaches are still needed to tackle the diverse problems that have arisen during the development of chemokine system-based therapeutics. The disruption of chemokine heteromers and chemokine-GAG interactions or the use of newly identified chemokine binding proteins from ticks or viruses might create new viewpoints and open novel perspectives for the therapeutic targeting of the chemokine system in atherosclerosis and other inflammatory diseases.

Table 1.1 Chemokine-receptor antagonists with therapeutic potential for atherosclerosis

Compound	Target	Study outcome	Company	Refs
F1	CX_3CR1	Not	N/A	[75]
Met-RANTES	CCR1/CCR5	Reduction	Merck Serono	[68,89]
$[^{44}AANA^{47}]$-CCL5	CCL5	Reduction	Merck Serono	[91,92]
TAK779	CCR5/CXCR3	Reduction	Takeda	[95]
Maraviroc	CCR5	Not	Pfizer	[100]
NBI-74330	CXCR3	Reduction	Amgen	[56]
SB-517785-M	CXCR2	Reduced	GSK	[96]
CKEY2	CCL5/CXCL4[b]	Reduction	Carolus	[22]
MLN1202	CCR2	Reduction	Milennium	[81]
CCX140	CCR2	Phase	CCX	[100]
INCB-3344	CCR2	No	Incyte Corp.	[83]

[a]Maraviroc achieved US and EU approval as anti-HIV agent.
[b]CKEY2 targets heterophilic interaction of CCL5 and CXCL4.
[c]Results from animal models not disclosed by company.
GSK: GlaxoSmithKline, CCX: ChemoCentryx.

References

1. Hansson, G. K., and Hermansson, A. (2011). The immune system in atherosclerosis, *Nat. Immunol.* **12**, pp. 204–212.
2. Sima, A. V., Stancu, C. S., and Simionescu, M. (2009). Vascular endothelium in atherosclerosis, *Cell Tissue Res.* **335**, pp. 191–203.
3. Simionescu, N., Vasile, E., Lupu, F., Popescu, G., and Simionescu, M. (1986). Prelesional events in atherogenesis. Accumulation of extracellular cholesterol-rich liposomes in the arterial intima and cardiac valves of the hyperlipidemic rabbit, *Am. J. Pathol.* **123**, pp. 109–125.
4. Charo, I. F., and Taub, R. (2011). Anti-inflammatory therapeutics for the treatment of atherosclerosis, *Nat. Rev. Drug Discov.* **10**, pp. 365–376.
5. Zernecke, A., and Weber, C. (2010). Chemokines in the vascular inflammatory response of atherosclerosis, *Cardiovasc. Res.* **86**, pp. 192–201.

6. Rot, A. (2010). Chemokine patterning by glycosaminoglycans and interceptors, *Front. biosc.* **15**, pp. 645–660.
7. Salanga, C. L., and Handel, T. M. (2011). Chemokine oligomerization and interactions with receptors and glycosaminoglycans: The role of structural dynamics in function, *Exp. Cell Res.* **317**, pp. 590–601.
8. Proudfoot, A. E., Handel, T. M., Johnson, Z., Lau, E. K., LiWang, P., Clark-Lewis, I., Borlat, F., Wells, T. N., and Kosco-Vilbois, M. H. (2003). Glycosaminoglycan binding and oligomerization are essential for the in vivo activity of certain chemokines, *Proc. Natl. Acad. Sci. U. S. A.* **100**, pp. 1885–1890.
9. Paavola, C. D., Hemmerich, S., Grunberger, D., Polsky, I., Bloom, A., Freedman, R., Mulkins, M., Bhakta, S., McCarley, D., Wiesent, L., Wong, B., Jarnagin, K., and Handel, T. M. (1998). Monomeric monocyte chemoattractant protein-1 (MCP-1) binds and activates the MCP-1 receptor CCR2B, *J. Biol. Chem.* **273**, pp. 33157–33165.
10. Rajarathnam, K., Sykes, B. D., Kay, C. M., Dewald, B., Geiser, T., Baggiolini, M., and Clark-Lewis, I. (1994). Neutrophil activation by monomeric interleukin-8, *Science* **264**, pp. 90–92.
11. Rajarathnam, K., Prado, G. N., Fernando, H., Clark-Lewis, I., and Navarro, J. (2006). Probing receptor binding activity of interleukin-8 dimer using a disulfide trap, *Biochemistry (Mosc.)* **45**, pp. 7882–7888.
12. Veldkamp, C. T., Seibert, C., Peterson, F. C., De la Cruz, N. B., Haugner, J. C., 3rd, Basnet, H., Sakmar, T. P., and Volkman, B. F. (2008). Structural basis of CXCR4 sulfotyrosine recognition by the chemokine SDF-1/CXCL12, *Sci. Signal.* **1**, pp. ra4.
13. Campanella, G. S., Grimm, J., Manice, L. A., Colvin, R. A., Medoff, B. D., Wojtkiewicz, G. R., Weissleder, R., and Luster, A. D. (2006). Oligomerization of CXCL10 is necessary for endothelial cell presentation and in vivo activity, *J. Immunol.* **177**, pp. 6991–6998.
14. Hoogewerf, A. J., Kuschert, G. S., Proudfoot, A. E., Borlat, F., Clark-Lewis, I., Power, C. A., and Wells, T. N. (1997). Glycosaminoglycans mediate cell surface oligomerization of chemokines, *Biochemistry (Mosc.)* **36**, pp. 13570–13578.
15. Vives, R. R., Sadir, R., Imberty, A., Rencurosi, A., and Lortat-Jacob, H. (2002). A kinetics and modeling study of RANTES(9-68) binding to heparin reveals a mechanism of cooperative oligomerization, *Biochemistry (Mosc.)* **41**, pp. 14779–14789.
16. Koenen, R. R., and Weber, C. (2010). Therapeutic targeting of chemokine interactions in atherosclerosis, *Nat. Rev. Drug Discov.* **9**, pp. 141–153.

17. Nesmelova, I. V., Sham, Y., Gao, J., and Mayo, K. H. (2008). CXC and CC chemokines form mixed heterodimers: Association free energies from molecular dynamics simulations and experimental correlations, *J. Biol. Chem.* **283**, pp. 24155–24166.

18. Guan, E., Wang, J., and Norcross, M. A. (2001). Identification of human macrophage inflammatory proteins 1alpha and 1beta as a native secreted heterodimer, *J. Biol. Chem.* **276**, pp. 12404–12409.

19. Dudek, A. Z., Nesmelova, I., Mayo, K., Verfaillie, C. M., Pitchford, S., and Slungaard, A. (2003). Platelet factor 4 promotes adhesion of hematopoietic progenitor cells and binds IL-8: Novel mechanisms for modulation of hematopoiesis, *Blood* **101**, pp. 4687–4694.

20. Nesmelova, I. V., Sham, Y., Dudek, A. Z., van Eijk, L. I., Wu, G., Slungaard, A., Mortari, F., Griffioen, A. W., and Mayo, K. H. (2005). Platelet factor 4 and interleukin-8 CXC chemokine heterodimer formation modulates function at the quaternary structural level, *J. Biol. Chem.* **280**, pp. 4948–4958.

21. Crown, S. E., Yu, Y., Sweeney, M. D., Leary, J. A., and Handel, T. M. (2006). Heterodimerization of CCR2 chemokines and regulation by glycosaminoglycan binding, *J. Biol. Chem.* **281**, pp. 25438–25446.

22. Koenen, R. R., von Hundelshausen, P., Nesmelova, I. V., Zernecke, A., Liehn, E. A., Sarabi, A., Kramp, B. K., Piccinini, A. M., Paludan, S. R., Kowalska, M. A., Kungl, A. J., Hackeng, T. M., Mayo, K. H., and Weber, C. (2009). Disrupting functional interactions between platelet chemokines inhibits atherosclerosis in hyperlipidemic mice, *Nat. Med.* **15**, pp. 97–103.

23. Weber, C., and Koenen, R. R. (2006). Fine-tuning leukocyte responses: Towards a chemokine 'interactome', *Trends Immunol.* **27**, pp. 268–273.

24. Loetscher, P., Pellegrino, A., Gong, J. H., Mattioli, I., Loetscher, M., Bardi, G., Baggiolini, M., and Clark-Lewis, I. (2001). The ligands of CXC chemokine receptor 3, I-TAC, Mig, and IP10, are natural antagonists for CCR3, *J. Biol. Chem.* **276**, pp. 2986–2991.

25. Mortier, A., Gouwy, M., van Damme, J., and Proost, P. (2011). Effect of posttranslational processing on the in vitro and in vivo activity of chemokines, *Exp. Cell Res.* **317**, pp. 642–654.

26. Weber, K. S., von Hundelshausen, P., Clark-Lewis, I., Weber, P. C., and Weber, C. (1999). Differential immobilization and hierarchical involvement of chemokines in monocyte arrest and transmigration on inflamed endothelium in shear flow, *Eur. J. Immunol.* **29**, pp. 700–712.

27. Shamri, R., Grabovsky, V., Gauguet, J. M., Feigelson, S., Manevich, E., Kolanus, W., Robinson, M. K., Staunton, D. E., von Andrian, U. H., and Alon, R. (2005). Lymphocyte arrest requires instantaneous induction of an extended LFA-1 conformation mediated by endothelium-bound chemokines, *Nat. Immunol.* **6**, pp. 497–506.

28. Huo, Y., Weber, C., Forlow, S. B., Sperandio, M., Thatte, J., Mack, M., Jung, S., Littman, D. R., and Ley, K. (2001). The chemokine KC, but not monocyte chemoattractant protein-1, triggers monocyte arrest on early atherosclerotic endothelium, *J. Clin. Invest.* **108**, pp. 1307–1314.

29. Weber, C., Weber, K. S., Klier, C., Gu, S., Wank, R., Horuk, R., and Nelson, P. J. (2001). Specialized roles of the chemokine receptors CCR1 and CCR5 in the recruitment of monocytes and T(H)1-like/CD45RO(+) T cells, *Blood* **97**, pp. 1144–1146.

30. Mehrad, B., Keane, M. P., and Strieter, R. M. (2007). Chemokines as mediators of angiogenesis, *Thromb. Haemost.* **97**, pp. 755–762.

31. Jin, D. K., Shido, K., Kopp, H. G., Petit, I., Shmelkov, S. V., Young, L. M., Hooper, A. T., Amano, H., Avecilla, S. T., Heissig, B., Hattori, K., Zhang, F., Hicklin, D. J., Wu, Y., Zhu, Z., Dunn, A., Salari, H., Werb, Z., Hackett, N. R., Crystal, R. G., Lyden, D., and Rafii, S. (2006). Cytokine-mediated deployment of SDF-1 induces revascularization through recruitment of CXCR4+ hemangiocytes, *Nat. Med.* **12**, pp. 557–567.

32. Kryczek, I., Lange, A., Mottram, P., Alvarez, X., Cheng, P., Hogan, M., Moons, L., Wei, S., Zou, L., Machelon, V., Emilie, D., Terrassa, M., Lackner, A., Curiel, T. J., Carmeliet, P., and Zou, W. (2005). CXCL12 and vascular endothelial growth factor synergistically induce neoangiogenesis in human ovarian cancers, *Cancer Res.* **65**, pp. 465–472.

33. Ma, Q., Jones, D., Borghesani, P. R., Segal, R. A., Nagasawa, T., Kishimoto, T., Bronson, R. T., and Springer, T. A. (1998). Impaired B-lymphopoiesis, myelopoiesis, and derailed cerebellar neuron migration in CXCR4- and SDF-1-deficient mice, *Proc. Natl. Acad. Sci. U. S. A.* **95**, pp. 9448–9453.

34. Tachibana, K., Hirota, S., Iizasa, H., Yoshida, H., Kawabata, K., Kataoka, Y., Kitamura, Y., Matsushima, K., Yoshida, N., Nishikawa, S., Kishimoto, T., and Nagasawa, T. (1998). The chemokine receptor CXCR4 is essential for vascularization of the gastrointestinal tract, *Nature* **393**, pp. 591–594.

35. Balabanian, K., Lagane, B., Infantino, S., Chow, K. Y., Harriague, J., Moepps, B., Arenzana-Seisdedos, F., Thelen, M., and Bachelerie, F. (2005). The chemokine SDF-1/CXCL12 binds to and signals through the orphan receptor RDC1 in T lymphocytes, *J. Biol. Chem.* **280**, pp. 35760–35766.

36. Sierro, F., Biben, C., Martinez-Munoz, L., Mellado, M., Ransohoff, R. M., Li, M., Woehl, B., Leung, H., Groom, J., Batten, M., Harvey, R. P., Martinez, A. C., Mackay, C. R., and Mackay, F. (2007). Disrupted cardiac development but normal hematopoiesis in mice deficient in the second CXCL12/SDF-1 receptor, CXCR7, *Proc. Natl. Acad. Sci. U. S. A.* **104**, pp. 14759–14764.

37. Naumann, U., Cameroni, E., Pruenster, M., Mahabaleshwar, H., Raz, E., Zerwes, H. G., Rot, A., and Thelen, M. (2010). CXCR7 functions as a scavenger for CXCL12 and CXCL11, *Plos One* **5**, pp. e9175.

38. Levoye, A., Balabanian, K., Baleux, F., Bachelerie, F., and Lagane, B. (2009). CXCR7 heterodimerizes with CXCR4 and regulates CXCL12-mediated G protein signaling, *Blood* **113**, pp. 6085–6093.

39. Wang, L., Fuster, M., Sriramarao, P., and Esko, J. D. (2005). Endothelial heparan sulfate deficiency impairs L-selectin- and chemokine-mediated neutrophil trafficking during inflammatory responses, *Nat. Immunol.* **6**, pp. 902–910.

40. Middleton, J., Neil, S., Wintle, J., Clark-Lewis, I., Moore, H., Lam, C., Auer, M., Hub, E., and Rot, A. (1997). Transcytosis and surface presentation of IL-8 by venular endothelial cells, *Cell* **91**, pp. 385–395.

41. Colditz, I. G., Schneider, M. A., Pruenster, M., and Rot, A. (2007). Chemokines at large: In-vivo mechanisms of their transport, presentation and clearance, *Thromb. Haemost.* **97**, pp. 688–693.

42. Pruenster, M., Mudde, L., Bombosi, P., Dimitrova, S., Zsak, M., Middleton, J., Richmond, A., Graham, G. J., Segerer, S., Nibbs, R. J., and Rot, A. (2009). The duffy antigen receptor for chemokines transports chemokines and supports their promigratory activity, *Nat. Immunol.* **10**, pp. 101–108.

43. Henn, V., Slupsky, J. R., Grafe, M., Anagnostopoulos, I., Forster, R., Muller-Berghaus, G., and Kroczek, R. A. (1998). CD40 ligand on activated platelets triggers an inflammatory reaction of endothelial cells, *Nature* **391**, pp. 591–594.

44. von Hundelshausen, P., Weber, K. S., Huo, Y., Proudfoot, A. E., Nelson, P. J., Ley, K., and Weber, C. (2001). RANTES deposition by platelets triggers monocyte arrest on inflamed and atherosclerotic endothelium, *Circulation* **103**, pp. 1772–1777.

45. Schober, A., Manka, D., Von Hundelshausen, P., Huo, Y., Hanrath, P., Sarembock, I. J., Ley, K., and Weber, C. (2002). Deposition of platelet RANTES triggering monocyte recruitment requires P-selectin and is involved in neointima formation after arterial injury, *Circulation* **106**, pp. 1523–1529.

46. Massberg, S., Brand, K., Gruner, S., Page, S., Muller, E., Muller, I., Bergmeier, W., Richter, T., Lorenz, M., Konrad, I., Nieswandt, B., and Gawaz, M. (2002). A critical role of platelet adhesion in the initiation of atherosclerotic lesion formation, *J. Exp. Med.* **196**, pp. 887–896.

47. Huo, Y., Schober, A., Forlow, S. B., Smith, D. F., Hyman, M. C., Jung, S., Littman, D. R., Weber, C., and Ley, K. (2003). Circulating activated platelets exacerbate atherosclerosis in mice deficient in apolipoprotein E, *Nat. Med.* **9**, pp. 61–67.

48. Drechsler, M., Megens, R. T., van Zandvoort, M., Weber, C., and Soehnlein, O. (2010). Hyperlipidemia-triggered neutrophilia promotes early atherosclerosis, *Circulation* **122**, pp. 1837–1845.

49. Vasina, E., Heemskerk, J. W., Weber, C., and Koenen, R. R. (2010). Platelets and platelet-derived microparticles in vascular inflammatory disease, *Inflamm. Allergy Drug Targets* **9**, pp. 346–354.

50. Garcia, B. A., Smalley, D. M., Cho, H., Shabanowitz, J., Ley, K., and Hunt, D. F. (2005). The platelet microparticle proteome, *J. Proteome Res.* **4**, pp. 1516–1521.

51. Mause, S. F., von Hundelshausen, P., Zernecke, A., Koenen, R. R., and Weber, C. (2005). Platelet microparticles: A transcellular delivery system for RANTES promoting monocyte recruitment on endothelium, *Arterioscler. Thromb. Vasc. Biol.* **25**, pp. 1512–1518.

52. Mause, S. F., Ritzel, E., Liehn, E. A., Hristov, M., Bidzhekov, K., Muller-Newen, G., Soehnlein, O., and Weber, C. (2010). Platelet microparticles enhance the vasoregenerative potential of angiogenic early outgrowth cells after vascular injury, *Circulation* **122**, pp. 495–506.

53. Boring, L., Gosling, J., Cleary, M., and Charo, I. F. (1998). Decreased lesion formation in CCR2-/- mice reveals a role for chemokines in the initiation of atherosclerosis, *Nature* **394**, pp. 894–897.

54. Veillard, N. R., Steffens, S., Pelli, G., Lu, B., Kwak, B. R., Gerard, C., Charo, I. F., and Mach, F. (2005). Differential influence of chemokine receptors CCR2 and CXCR3 in development of atherosclerosis in vivo, *Circulation* **112**, pp. 870–878.

55. Heller, E. A., Liu, E., Tager, A. M., Yuan, Q., Lin, A. Y., Ahluwalia, N., Jones, K., Koehn, S. L., Lok, V. M., Aikawa, E., Moore, K. J., Luster, A. D., and Gerszten, R. E. (2006). Chemokine CXCL10 promotes atherogenesis by modulating the local balance of effector and regulatory T cells, *Circulation* **113**, pp. 2301–2312.

56. van Wanrooij, E. J., de Jager, S. C., van Es, T., de Vos, P., Birch, H. L., Owen, D. A., Watson, R. J., Biessen, E. A., Chapman, G. A., van Berkel,

T. J., and Kuiper, J. (2008). CXCR3 antagonist NBI-74330 attenuates atherosclerotic plaque formation in LDL receptor-deficient mice, *Arterioscler. Thromb. Vasc. Biol.* **28**, pp. 251–257.

57. Ait-Oufella, H., Horvat, B., Kerdiles, Y., Herbin, O., Gourdy, P., Khallou-Laschet, J., Merval, R., Esposito, B., Tedgui, A., and Mallat, Z. (2007). Measles virus nucleoprotein induces a regulatory immune response and reduces atherosclerosis in mice, *Circulation* **116**, pp. 1707–1713.

58. de Jager, S. C., Bermudez, B., Bot, I., Koenen, R. R., Bot, M., Kavelaars, A., de Waard, V., Heijnen, C. J., Muriana, F. J., Weber, C., van Berkel, T. J., Kuiper, J., Lee, S. J., Abia, R., and Biessen, E. A. (2011). Growth differentiation factor 15 deficiency protects against atherosclerosis by attenuating CCR2-mediated macrophage chemotaxis, *J. Exp. Med.* **208**, pp. 217–225.

59. Kempf, T., Zarbock, A., Widera, C., Butz, S., Stadtmann, A., Rossaint, J., Bolomini-Vittori, M., Korf-Klingebiel, M., Napp, L. C., Hansen, B., Kanwischer, A., Bavendiek, U., Beutel, G., Hapke, M., Sauer, M. G., Laudanna, C., Hogg, N., Vestweber, D., and Wollert, K. C. (2011). GDF-15 is an inhibitor of leukocyte integrin activation required for survival after myocardial infarction in mice, *Nat. Med.* **17**, pp. 581–588.

60. Baltus, T., Weber, K. S., Johnson, Z., Proudfoot, A. E., and Weber, C. (2003). Oligomerization of RANTES is required for CCR1-mediated arrest but not CCR5-mediated transmigration of leukocytes on inflamed endothelium, *Blood* **102**, pp. 1985–1988.

61. Kuziel, W. A., Dawson, T. C., Quinones, M., Garavito, E., Chenaux, G., Ahuja, S. S., Reddick, R. L., and Maeda, N. (2003). CCR5 deficiency is not protective in the early stages of atherogenesis in apoE knockout mice, *Atherosclerosis* **167**, pp. 25–32.

62. Potteaux, S., Combadiere, C., Esposito, B., Lecureuil, C., Ait-Oufella, H., Merval, R., Ardouin, P., Tedgui, A., and Mallat, Z. (2006). Role of bone marrow-derived CC-chemokine receptor 5 in the development of atherosclerosis of low-density lipoprotein receptor knockout mice, *Arterioscler. Thromb. Vasc. Biol.* **26** pp. 1858–1863.

63. Braunersreuther, V., Zernecke, A., Arnaud, C., Liehn, E. A., Steffens, S., Shagdarsuren, E., Bidzhekov, K., Burger, F., Pelli, G., Luckow, B., Mach, F., and Weber, C. (2007). Ccr5 but not Ccr1 deficiency reduces development of diet-induced atherosclerosis in mice, *Arterioscler. Thromb. Vasc. Biol.* **27**, pp. 373–379.

64. Potteaux, S., Combadiere, C., Esposito, B., Casanova, S., Merval, R., Ardouin, P., Gao, J. L., Murphy, P. M., Tedgui, A., and Mallat, Z. (2005).

Chemokine receptor CCR1 disruption in bone marrow cells enhances atherosclerotic lesion development and inflammation in mice, *Mol. Med.* **11**, pp. 16–20.

65. Geissmann, F., Jung, S., and Littman, D. R. (2003). Blood monocytes consist of two principal subsets with distinct migratory properties, *Immunity* **19**, pp. 71–82.

66. Swirski, F. K., Libby, P., Aikawa, E., Alcaide, P., Luscinskas, F. W., Weissleder, R., and Pittet, M. J. (2007). Ly-6Chi monocytes dominate hypercholesterolemia-associated monocytosis and give rise to macrophages in atheromata, *J. Clin. Invest.* **117**, pp. 195–205.

67. Tacke, F., Alvarez, D., Kaplan, T. J., Jakubzick, C., Spanbroek, R., Llodra, J., Garin, A., Liu, J., Mack, M., van Rooijen, N., Lira, S. A., Habenicht, A. J., and Randolph, G. J. (2007). Monocyte subsets differentially employ CCR2, CCR5, and CX3CR1 to accumulate within atherosclerotic plaques, *J. Clin. Invest.* **117**, pp. 185–194.

68. Combadiere, C., Potteaux, S., Rodero, M., Simon, T., Pezard, A., Esposito, B., Merval, R., Proudfoot, A., Tedgui, A., and Mallat, Z. (2008). Combined inhibition of CCL2, CX3CR1, and CCR5 abrogates Ly6C(hi) and Ly6C(lo) monocytosis and almost abolishes atherosclerosis in hypercholesterolemic mice, *Circulation* **117**, pp. 1649–1657.

69. Saederup, N., Chan, L., Lira, S. A., and Charo, I. F. (2008). Fractalkine deficiency markedly reduces macrophage accumulation and atherosclerotic lesion formation in CCR2-/- mice: Evidence for independent chemokine functions in atherogenesis, *Circulation* **117**, pp. 1642–1648.

70. Zernecke, A., Bot, I., Djalali-Talab, Y., Shagdarsuren, E., Bidzhekov, K., Meiler, S., Krohn, R., Schober, A., Sperandio, M., Soehnlein, O., Bornemann, J., Tacke, F., Biessen, E. A., and Weber, C. (2008). Protective role of CXC receptor 4/CXC ligand 12 unveils the importance of neutrophils in atherosclerosis, *Circ. Res.* **102**, pp. 209–217.

71. van Leeuwen, M., Gijbels, M. J., Duijvestijn, A., Smook, M., van de Gaar, M. J., Heeringa, P., de Winther, M. P., and Tervaert, J. W. (2008). Accumulation of myeloperoxidase-positive neutrophils in atherosclerotic lesions in LDLR-/- mice, *Arterioscler. Thromb. Vasc. Biol.* **28**, pp. 84–89.

72. Guo, J., de Waard, V., Van Eck, M., Hildebrand, R. B., van Wanrooij, E. J., Kuiper, J., Maeda, N., Benson, G. M., Groot, P. H., and Van Berkel, T. J. (2005). Repopulation of apolipoprotein E knockout mice with CCR2-deficient bone marrow progenitor cells does not inhibit ongoing atherosclerotic lesion development, *Arterioscler. Thromb. Vasc. Biol.* **25**, pp. 1014–1019.

73. Trogan, E., Feig, J. E., Dogan, S., Rothblat, G. H., Angeli, V., Tacke, F., Randolph, G. J., and Fisher, E. A. (2006). Gene expression changes in foam cells and the role of chemokine receptor CCR7 during atherosclerosis regression in ApoE-deficient mice, *Proc. Natl. Acad. Sci. U. S. A.* **103**, pp. 3781–3786.

74. Potteaux, S., Gautier, E. L., Hutchison, S. B., van Rooijen, N., Rader, D. J., Thomas, M. J., Sorci-Thomas, M. G., and Randolph, G. J. (2011). Suppressed monocyte recruitment drives macrophage removal from atherosclerotic plaques of Apoe-/- mice during disease regression, *J. clin. investig.* **121**, pp. 2025–2036.

75. Dorgham, K., Ghadiri, A., Hermand, P., Rodero, M., Poupel, L., Iga, M., Hartley, O., Gorochov, G., Combadiere, C., and Deterre, P. (2009). An engineered CX3CR1 antagonist endowed with anti-inflammatory activity, *J. Leukoc. Biol.* **86**, pp. 903–911.

76. Gong, J. H., and Clark-Lewis, I. (1995). Antagonists of monocyte chemoattractant protein 1 identified by modification of functionally critical NH2-terminal residues, *J. Exp. Med.* **181**, pp. 631–640.

77. Handel, T. M., Johnson, Z., Rodrigues, D. H., Dos Santos, A. C., Cirillo, R., Muzio, V., Riva, S., Mack, M., Deruaz, M., Borlat, F., Vitte, P. A., Wells, T. N., Teixeira, M. M., and Proudfoot, A. E. (2008). An engineered monomer of CCL2 has anti-inflammatory properties emphasizing the importance of oligomerization for chemokine activity in vivo, *J. Leukoc. Biol.* **84**, pp. 1101–1108.

78. Piccinini, A. M., Knebl, K., Rek, A., Wildner, G., Diedrichs-Moehring, M., and Kungl, A. J. (2010). Rationally evolving MCP-1/CCL2 into a decoy protein with potent anti-inflammatory activity in vivo, *J. Biol. Chem.* **285**, pp. 8782–8792.

79. Liehn, E. A., Piccinini, A. M., Koenen, R. R., Soehnlein, O., Adage, T., Fatu, R., Curaj, A., Popescu, A., Zernecke, A., Kungl, A. J., and Weber, C. (2010). A new monocyte chemotactic protein-1/chemokine CC motif ligand-2 competitor limiting neointima formation and myocardial ischemia/reperfusion injury in mice, *J. Am. Coll. Cardiol.* **56**, pp. 1847–1857.

80. Dai, E., Liu, L. Y., Wang, H., McIvor, D., Sun, Y. M., Macaulay, C., King, E., Munuswamy-Ramanujam, G., Bartee, M. Y., Williams, J., Davids, J., Charo, I., McFadden, G., Esko, J. D., and Lucas, A. R. (2010). Inhibition of chemokine-glycosaminoglycan interactions in donor tissue reduces mouse allograft vasculopathy and transplant rejection, *Plos One* **5**, pp. e10510.

81. Gilbert, J., Lekstrom-Himes, J., Donaldson, D., Lee, Y., Hu, M., Xu, J., Wyant, T., and Davidson, M. (2011). Effect of CC chemokine receptor

2 CCR2 blockade on serum C-reactive protein in individuals at atherosclerotic risk and with a single nucleotide polymorphism of the monocyte chemoattractant protein-1 promoter region, *Am. J. Cardiol.* **107**, pp. 906–911.

82. Lutgens, E., Faber, B., Schapira, K., Evelo, C. T., van Haaften, R., Heeneman, S., Cleutjens, K. B., Bijnens, A. P., Beckers, L., Porter, J. G., Mackay, C. R., Rennert, P., Bailly, V., Jarpe, M., Dolinski, B., Koteliansky, V., de Fougerolles, T., and Daemen, M. J. (2005). Gene profiling in atherosclerosis reveals a key role for small inducible cytokines: Validation using a novel monocyte chemoattractant protein monoclonal antibody, *Circulation* **111**, pp. 3443–3452.

83. Aiello, R. J., Perry, B. D., Bourassa, P. A., Robertson, A., Weng, W., Knight, D. R., Smith, A. H., Frederick, K. S., Kalgutkar, A., and Gladue, R. P. (2010). CCR2 receptor blockade alters blood monocyte subpopulations but does not affect atherosclerotic lesions in apoE(-/-) mice, *Atherosclerosis* **208**, pp. 370–375.

84. Proudfoot, A. E., Power, C. A., Hoogewerf, A. J., Montjovent, M. O., Borlat, F., Offord, R. E., and Wells, T. N. (1996). Extension of recombinant human RANTES by the retention of the initiating methionine produces a potent antagonist, *J. Biol. Chem.* **271**, pp. 2599–2603.

85. Simmons, G., Clapham, P. R., Picard, L., Offord, R. E., Rosenkilde, M. M., Schwartz, T. W., Buser, R., Wells, T. N., and Proudfoot, A. E. (1997). Potent inhibition of HIV-1 infectivity in macrophages and lymphocytes by a novel CCR5 antagonist, *Science* **276**, pp. 276–279.

86. Proudfoot, A. E., Buser, R., Borlat, F., Alouani, S., Soler, D., Offord, R. E., Schroder, J. M., Power, C. A., and Wells, T. N. (1999). Amino-terminally modified RANTES analogues demonstrate differential effects on RANTES receptors, *J. Biol. Chem.* **274**, pp. 32478–32485.

87. Grone, H. J., Weber, C., Weber, K. S., Grone, E. F., Rabelink, T., Klier, C. M., Wells, T. N., Proudfood, A. E., Schlondorff, D., and Nelson, P. J. (1999). Met-RANTES reduces vascular and tubular damage during acute renal transplant rejection: Blocking monocyte arrest and recruitment, *Faseb J.* **13**, pp. 1371–1383.

88. Panzer, U., Schneider, A., Wilken, J., Thompson, D. A., Kent, S. B., and Stahl, R. A. (1999). The chemokine receptor antagonist AOP-RANTES reduces monocyte infiltration in experimental glomerulonephritis, *Kidney Int.* **56**, pp. 2107–2115.

89. Veillard, N. R., Kwak, B., Pelli, G., Mulhaupt, F., James, R. W., Proudfoot, A. E., and Mach, F. (2004). Antagonism of RANTES receptors reduces atherosclerotic plaque formation in mice, *Circ. Res.* **94**, pp. 253–261.

90. Johnson, Z., Kosco-Vilbois, M. H., Herren, S., Cirillo, R., Muzio, V., Zaratin, P., Carbonatto, M., Mack, M., Smailbegovic, A., Rose, M., Lever, R., Page, C., Wells, T. N., and Proudfoot, A. E. (2004). Interference with heparin binding and oligomerization creates a novel anti-inflammatory strategy targeting the chemokine system, *J. Immunol.* **173**, pp. 5776–5785.

91. Braunersreuther, V., Steffens, S., Arnaud, C., Pelli, G., Burger, F., Proudfoot, A., and Mach, F. (2008). A novel RANTES antagonist prevents progression of established atherosclerotic lesions in mice, *Arterioscler. Thromb. Vasc. Biol.* **28**, pp. 1090–1096.

92. Braunersreuther, V., Pellieux, C., Pelli, G., Burger, F., Steffens, S., Montessuit, C., Weber, C., Proudfoot, A., Mach, F., and Arnaud, C. (2010). Chemokine CCL5/RANTES inhibition reduces myocardial reperfusion injury in atherosclerotic mice, *J. Mol. Cell. Cardiol.* **48**, pp. 789–798.

93. Montecucco, F., Braunersreuther, V., Lenglet, S., Delattre, B. M., Pelli, G., Buatois, V., Guilhot, F., Galan, K., Vuilleumier, N., Ferlin, W., Fischer, N., Vallee, J. P., Kosco-Vilbois, M., and Mach, F. (2011). CC chemokine CCL5 plays a central role impacting infarct size and post-infarction heart failure in mice, *Eur. Heart J.* doi:10.1093/eurheartj/ehr127.

94. Gao, P., Zhou, X. Y., Yashiro-Ohtani, Y., Yang, Y. F., Sugimoto, N., Ono, S., Nakanishi, T., Obika, S., Imanishi, T., Egawa, T., Nagasawa, T., Fujiwara, H., and Hamaoka, T. (2003). The unique target specificity of a nonpeptide chemokine receptor antagonist: Selective blockade of two Th1 chemokine receptors CCR5 and CXCR3, *J. Leukoc. Biol.* **73**, pp. 273–280.

95. van Wanrooij, E. J., Happe, H., Hauer, A. D., de Vos, P., Imanishi, T., Fujiwara, H., van Berkel, T. J., and Kuiper, J. (2005). HIV entry inhibitor TAK-779 attenuates atherogenesis in low-density lipoprotein receptor-deficient mice, *Arterioscler. Thromb. Vasc. Biol.* **25**, pp. 2642–2647.

96. Nabah, Y. N. A., Losada, M., Estelles, R., Mateo, T., Company, C., Piqueras, L., Lopez Gines, C., Sarau, H., Cortijo, J., Morcillo, E. J., Jose, P. J., and Sanz, M.-J. (2007). CXCR2 Blockade impairs angiotensin II induced CC chemokine synthesis and mononuclear leukocyte infiltration, *Arterioscler. Thromb. Vasc. Biol.* **27**, pp. 2370–2376.

97. Karshovska, E., Zagorac, D., Zernecke, A., Weber, C., and Schober, A. (2008). A small molecule CXCR4 antagonist inhibits neointima formation and smooth muscle progenitor cell mobilization after arterial injury, *J. Thromb. Haemost.* **6**, pp. 1812–1815.

98. Imamura, S., Ichikawa, T., Nishikawa, Y., Kanzaki, N., Takashima, K., Niwa, S., Iizawa, Y., Baba, M., and Sugihara, Y. (2006). Discovery of a

piperidine-4-carboxamide CCR5 antagonist (TAK-220) with highly potent Anti-HIV-1 activity, *J. Med. Chem.* **49**, pp. 2784–2793.

99. Koenen, R. R., von Hundelshausen, P., and Weber, C. (2007). Antagonism of chemokine receptors as a novel therapeutic approach in the combined treatment of viral and atherosclerotic disease, *J. Viral Entry* **3**, pp. 18–23.

100. Horuk, R. (2009). Chemokine receptor antagonists: Overcoming developmental hurdles, *Nat. Rev. Drug Discov.* **8**, pp. 23–33.

101. Matsukawa, A., Hogaboam, C. M., Lukacs, N. W., Lincoln, P. M., Strieter, R. M., and Kunkel, S. L. (1999). Endogenous monocyte chemoattractant protein-1 (MCP-1) protects mice in a model of acute septic peritonitis: Cross-talk between MCP-1 and leukotriene B4, *J. Immunol.* **163**, pp. 6148–6154.

102. Serbina, N. V., and Pamer, E. G. (2006). Monocyte emigration from bone marrow during bacterial infection requires signals mediated by chemokine receptor CCR2, *Nat. Immunol.* **7**, pp. 311–317.

103. Sorensen, L. N., and Paludan, S. R. (2004). Blocking CC chemokine receptor (CCR) 1 and CCR5 during herpes simplex virus type 2 infection in vivo impairs host defence and perturbs the cytokine response, *Scand. J. Immunol.* **59**, pp. 321–333.

104. Bursill, C. A., Cash, J. L., Channon, K. M., and Greaves, D. R. (2006). Membrane-bound CC chemokine inhibitor 35K provides localized inhibition of CC chemokine activity in vitro and in vivo, *J. Immunol.* **177**, pp. 5567–5573.

105. Deruaz, M., Frauenschuh, A., Alessandri, A. L., Dias, J. M., Coelho, F. M., Russo, R. C., Ferreira, B. R., Graham, G. J., Shaw, J. P., Wells, T. N., Teixeira, M. M., Power, C. A., and Proudfoot, A. E. (2008). Ticks produce highly selective chemokine binding proteins with antiinflammatory activity, *J. Exp. Med.* **205**, pp. 2019–2031.

106. Martin, A. P., Canasto-Chibuque, C., Shang, L., Rollins, B. J., and Lira, S. A. (2006). The chemokine decoy receptor M3 blocks CC chemokine ligand 2 and CXC chemokine ligand 13 function in vivo, *J. Immunol.* **177**, pp. 7296–7302.

Chapter 2

MIF Antagonism as a Therapeutic Approach to Atherosclerosis

J. Bernhagen and A. Schober
[a] *Institute of Biochemistry and Molecular Cell Biology, RWTH Aachen University, Pauwelstrasse 30, D-52074 Aachen, Germany*
[b] *Institute of Molecular Cardiovascular Research (IMCAR), RWTH Aachen University, Pauwelstrasse 30, D-52074 Aachen, Germany*
jbernhagen@ukaachen.de, aschober@ukaachen.de

Macrophage migration inhibitory factor (MIF) is a structurally unique cytokine that plays a crucial role in inflammation, cancer, and cardiovascular diseases. Chronic inflammation of the arterial wall is a hallmark in the pathogenesis of atherosclerosis and is characterized by chemokine-mediated influx of leukocytes. The investigation of MIF in atherosclerotic vascular disease has established a chemokine-like function (CLF) of MIF, which is primarily based on its non-cognate interaction with the chemokine receptors CXCR2 and CXCR4. Through this activity, MIF contributes decisively to atherogenic leukocyte recruitment and, thus, affects lesion progression and plaque stability.

Atherosclerosis: Treatment and Prevention
Edited by Christian Weber and Oliver Soehnlein

ISBN 978-981-4316-26-2 (Hardcover), ISBN 978-981-4364-26-3 (eBook)
www.panstanford.com

2.1 Introduction

Atherosclerotic plaques are the pathologic basis for coronary heart disease (CHD) and consist of a subintimal accumulation of leukocytes, characteristically lipid-laden macrophages and foam cells, smooth muscle cells (SMCs), and deposited extracellular matrix proteins. In advanced stages, a necrotic core with cell debris and cholesterol crystals is detected. Monocyte adhesion and subsequent transendothelial migration are the first morphological features of early lesion formation. Therefore, the mechanisms of atherogenic leukocyte recruitment into the vessel wall are of great interest for the development of therapeutic strategies against atherosclerosis. The different steps such as rolling, firm adhesion, and transmigration are controlled by functionally specialized chemokines, which act in a sequential and cooperative manner [1, 2]. Whereas soluble chemokines induce directed chemotaxis of leukocytes, chemokines immobilized on the endothelial cell surface trigger the integrin-mediated arrest of rolling leukocytes [3, 4]. In atherogenesis, the arrest function has been established for platelet-derived CCL5 and the CXCR2 ligands CXCL1 and CXCL8 [2]. However, the genetic or functional deletion of these chemokines, e.g., that of KC, the murine ortholog of CXCL8, has suggested that additional mediators must be involved in atherogenic leukocyte recruitment processes [5]. MIF has recently emerged as a previously unrecognized arrest factor.

Originally discovered as a protein mediator that inhibited the random migration of macrophages out of capillary tubes [6], MIF later on was redefined as a pleiotropic inflammatory cytokine that is involved in the pathogenesis of a number of acute and chronic inflammatory diseases [7] such as septic shock [8, 9], colitis [10], delayed-type hypersensitivity [11], glomerulonephritis [12], inflammatory lung disease [13], and rheumatoid arthritis [14]. In all these conditions, the proinflammatory recruitment of mononuclear cells plays a critical role and, in fact, MIF has been demonstrated to potently support inflammatory leukocyte recruitment [15–18]. MIF is an upstream regulator of innate immunity and inflammation and triggers inflammatory signal transduction pathways to promote macrophage survival and TNF or interleukin (IL) expression [7]. Its proinflammatory activity also is based on its unique property to counter-regulate the immunosuppressive and anti-inflammatory activity of endogenous glucocorticoids [7, 19, 20].

Strikingly, MIF shares many functional features with chemokines and has, therefore, been classified as a "chemokine-like function (CLF)" chemokine [18, 21, 22]. This functional "chemokinism" of MIF has emerged to be pivotal for its contribution to the pathogenesis of atherosclerosis.

In this chapter, we have updated the available evidence for the various links between MIF and atherogenesis, discussed the underlying mechanisms, and outlined therapeutic strategies that may be pursued in cardiovascular disease by targeting MIF.

2.2 Biochemical and Structural Properties of MIF

MIF is an evolutionarily-conserved protein that is abundantly expressed in humans and non-primate mammals. MIF orthologs also are found in unicellular parasites such as *Leishmania major* or *Plasmodium falsiparum*. The cloning of human and mouse MIF and the elucidation of the three-dimensional (3D) structure of human MIF by x-ray crystallography and NMR revealed that the sequence and structure of MIF are unique within the family of cytokines [8, 23–25]. MIF consists of 114 amino acids and has a molecular weight of 12.5 kDa. The 3D structure of human MIF shows that MIF crystallizes as a trimer of three identical subunits. Each monomer consists of a four-stranded β-sheet placed above two antiparallel α-helices. Two remaining β-strands are part of intertwining loops and contribute to the stabilization of the trimer by forming interactions with β-sheets of adjacent subunits [24]. In contrast to the trimer determined by crystallography, biochemical studies relying on solute MIF led to the conclusion that monomers, dimers, and trimers exist in an equilibrium with monomers and dimers representing the major species at physiological concentrations in the ng/ml range, whereas the trimer is the predominant species at higher MIF concentrations >10 μg/ml [7, 26, 27]. The structural folds of MIF show a remote similarity to the cytokine interleukin-1β, but this does not allow for a classification of MIF into any of the known structural cytokine families. However, the 3D architecture of MIF is highly similar to that of a family of bacterial isomerases/tautomerases as well as to human D-dopachrome tautomerase, indicating that these proteins may have evolved from a joint ancestral gene [7]. In fact, uniquely among cytokines, the MIF trimer shares with these enzymes a catalytic pocket that is formed by the N-terminal proline residue of one subunit and several residues of the same and a second subunit and that enables MIF to catalyze certain isomerization/tautomerization reactions. So far, only non-natural and synthetic substrates have been identified for this catalytic activity and it is controversial whether the catalytic isomerase activity of MIF is functionally related to its numerous inflammatory properties. Notwithstanding, the identification of a catalytic site in MIF has triggered several studies to develop small-molecular-weight (SMW)-based inhibitors that could target this site, and it has been hoped that, for the first time, this would make a cytokine amenable to targeting by SMW drugs [14] (see Section 2.11). In addition, the MIF protein features a second conserved catalytic site. This is a Cys-Xaa-Xaa-Cys motif, and MIF shares this motif with thiol-protein oxidoreductases (TPORs). Accordingly, MIF has been demonstrated to have redox activity *in vitro* [28].

2.3 MIF Expression and Secretion: Mechanism and Occurrence in Disease

Redox regulation by MIF has been observed in cells, suggesting that intracellular MIF protein has a role in cellular redox homeostasis [29]. In fact, there are preformed stores of MIF in the cytosol, where it engages in interactions with several proteins [30]. MIF was originally discovered as T cell-derived cytokine, but today it is clear that rather mononuclear phagocytes constitute the main MIF-producing cell type in inflammation. However, several other inflammatory cells such as eosinophils and endothelial cells as well as numerous epithelial, parenchymal, and tumor cells can express MIF in substantive amounts [7]. Whereas the expression of MIF is fairly ubiquitous, its secretion is tightly regulated and only occurs upon inflammatory, immune, or stress stimulation of a MIF-producing cell. For example, MIF secretion from monocytes/macrophages is triggered by endotoxin and inflammatory cytokines such as tumor necrosis factor-α (TNF-α) [7]. Endothelial cells secrete MIF upon stimulation with oxidized low-density lipoprotein (LDL) or hypoxia. Cardiomyocytes secrete MIF upon ischemia/reperfusion (I/R) challenge, i.e., following combined hypoxic and hyperoxic stress. These latter conditions are of particular relevance to the release of MIF in atherogenic tissues and, thus, to its contribution to atherogenic leukocyte recruitment, but also to endothelial progenitor cell (EPC) recruitment during repair and angiogenesis [31, 32], as well as to MIF's cardioprotective functions during myocardial I/R injury [33]. In spite of recent progress, the precise mechanism of MIF secretion has not been fully clarified. MIF secretion follows a so-called non-classical ER/Golgi-independent pathway, but we have only begun to uncover the molecular components of this pathway, which also is likely to be heterogeneous over different MIF-secreting cell types. First evidence for a non-conventional secretion pathway of MIF arose when the molecular cloning of MIF revealed that the N-terminus was lacking a signal sequence, suggesting that during secretion, MIF would not enter the ER/Golgi compartment [8, 25]. This notion was indeed confirmed in a mechanistic study, which also offered pharmacological inhibitor-based evidence that the endotoxin-triggered secretion of MIF from monocytes/macrophages encompassed ATP-binding cassette (ABC) transporter-mediated membrane translocation at some stage during the secretion process [34]. Hypoxia-induced secretion of MIF from endothelial cells also appears to involve ABC transporter activity [32]. In addition, at least two of the known cytosolic interaction partners of MIF are functionally involved in MIF secretion. Silencer RNA-mediated knock-down of the Golgi-associated protein p115 leads to a drastic reduction of MIF secretion in endotoxin-stimulated monocytes/macrophages, suggesting that p115, which is situated on the cytosolic side of the cis-Golgi and which is involved in Golgi vesicle trafficking, is a component of the MIF secretion pathway [35]. In contrast, protein-protein interaction between MIF and JAB1/CSN5 appears to convey inhibitory signals within the MIF secretion pathway. This has been implied by JAB1-siRNA knock down experiments in fibroblasts and tumor cells [36].

2.4 MIF Receptors and Molecular Determinants of MIF Action

MIF differs from classical cytokines in that it has both intra- and extracellular functions. Notwithstanding, its secretion is tightly regulated and is strongly up-regulated in several disease conditions. It was, therefore, suggested to exert specific cytokine functions in the extracellular space. Because MIF does not belong to any of the known structural cytokine families, homology-based receptor cloning strategies could not be applied. Not unexpectedly, it, thus, took more than a decade after MIF cloning until CD74 was identified as the first MIF plasma membrane receptor [37]. CD74 is the membrane-expressed form of invariant chain (Ii), a MHC class II chaperone that plays a critical role in class II trafficking and peptide antigen loading in the endolysosomal compartment [38]. CD74 expression is typically restricted to class II-positive cells such as B cells, monocytes/macrophages, and dendritic cells, but under inflammatory conditions as well as in several tumor cell types, CD74 can be up-regulated and expressed in the absence of measurable class II expression. Receptor activities of membrane-expressed Ii/CD74 were first recognized on B cells, in which CD74 promotes proliferation and survival by triggering a nuclear factor kappa-B (NFκB)/TAp63/CXCL8-dependent pathway [39–41]. MIF binds to CD74 by high affinity interaction in the nanomolar range, but signaling requires the recruitment of signalling-competent co-receptors such as CD44 [42] or the chemokine receptors CXCR2 and CXCR4 (see below), because CD74 only contains a short cytoplasmic domain that is devoid of any signalling-transducing motif [38]. This latter observation as well as the fact that CD74 is not expressed on key MIF-responsive cells, such as neutrophils, triggered efforts to identify additional MIF receptors. MIF does not directly interact with CD44, which, therefore, solely serves as a signal-transducing co-receptor. However, a gross architectural similarity between the MIF monomer and the CXCL8 dimer elicited biochemical investigations to probe potential interactions between MIF and the *bona fide* CXCL8 receptor CXCR2. Receptor binding studies by tracer competition and internalization experiments, coimmunoprecipitation, and flow cytometry revealed that MIF engages in a non-cognate, high affinity (K_D 1.5 nM) interaction with CXCR2 [15]. CXCR2 is the main chemokine receptor mediating the inflammatory and angiogenic activities of CXCL8; however, CXCR2 is highly promiscuous as it also is the receptor for 6 other ELR+ CXC chemokines such as CXCL7 and CXCL1. These findings as well as functional data demonstrating chemokine-like activities for MIF (see below) suggested that MIF belongs to the heterogeneous family of CLF chemokines. Mediators belonging to this family exhibit chemotactic activities on immune cells and despite a lack of sequence and structural homology with chemokines of the CC-, CXC-, C-, or CX3C- families, bind to and utilize chemokine receptors for target cell activation [21]. Non-cognate binding of MIF to CXCR2, thus, expands the ligand spectrum of CXCR2 and adds a CLF chemokine to the ligand list of this important inflammatory receptor. The signal transduction pathways triggered by MIF/CXCR2 but have not been studied systematically, but initial evidence shows that in monocytes and neutrophils MIF binding to CXCR2 leads to canonical G_i coupling and can elicit calcium transients. A limited screen of other chemokine receptors that may potentially interact with MIF as well as observed pro-chemotactic effects of MIF on T cells, which do not express CXCR2 and only low levels of CD74, led to the discovery that MIF also serves as a non-cognate ligand of CXCR4 but not CXCR1, CXCR3, or CCR5 [15]. The MIF/CXCR4 interaction is less affine than that between MIF and CXCR2 but still in the nanomolar range (K_D 19 nM).

Chemokine receptor activation leads to variety of G_i-coupled signalling responses that can trigger numerous cellular responses, most prominently chemotactic cell movements. Chemokine receptor signalling is further complicated and fine-tuned by receptor homo- and heterodimerization, which can serve to activate or inhibit, accelerate or attenuate, sensitize or desensitize the response. Identified chemokine receptor heterodimers for which a functional role has been demonstrated encompass heterodimers from both the CC- and CXC families as well as cross-family heterodimers, i.e., CXCR4/CXCR7, CXCR1/CXCR2, CCR2/CCR5, and CXCR4/CCR5 [43–46]. Of note, further research into the receptors of MIF revealed that CD74 forms heteromeric complexes with either CXCR2 or CXCR4 [15, 47]. This is intriguing because such complexes represent receptor complexes between a single helix-spanning type II membrane protein (CD74) and a seven helix-spanning G protein-coupled receptor (GPCR) (CXCR). Yet, such cross-receptor family complexes are not unique to CD74/CXCR, as a dopamine receptor/CXCR4 complex was also observed [45]. Also, heterologous desensitization of CCL2/CCR2-mediated monocyte chemotaxis by MIF has been observed, suggesting that MIF receptor complexes functionally interact with other chemokine receptor complexes to control leukocyte migration.

2.5 MIF Expression in Atherosclerotic Plaque

Expression of MIF in atherosclerosis was first characterized in hypercholesterolemic rabbits. Endothelial cells in such animals express increased MIF mRNA and protein [48] in early fatty streaks and advanced lesions. In contrast, MIF was only found in medial SMCs next to subendothelial macrophage accumulation in early lesions [48]. Since macrophages activated by lipopolysaccharide, tumor necrosis factor (TNF)-α, and interferon (IFN)-γ have been shown to secrete substantial amounts of preformed MIF [7, 49] (see Section 2.3), it is reasonable to assume that macrophage-derived MIF plays a role in atherogenesis. Indeed, in early fatty streak lesions monocytes adhering to the endothelium and subendothelial monocytes express MIF. However, in lesional macrophage-derived foam cells and macrophages in advanced plaques, MIF was barely detectable [48]. It was concluded from these data that MIF is predominantly involved in early lesion development presumably by supporting monocyte recruitment. In *Apoe*$^{-/-}$ mice on a regular diet, MIF is expressed in the cytoplasm and nuclei of all cell types of the atherosclerotic lesions, including endothelial cells, lymphocytes, SMCs, but predominantly in foam cells [50]. In addition, up-regulation of MIF has been described following accelerated plaque formation after endothelial denudation of the carotid artery of hyperlipidemic mice [51, 52]. Prominent expression of MIF was found especially in endothelial cells and macrophage-derived foam cells [52].

In contrast to the rabbit model, the expression of MIF increases during plaque progression in human atherosclerosis [31]. Whereas in arteries without atherosclerotic findings or with type I (initial) lesions without macrophage infiltration, MIF was only detected in a small number of endothelial cells and SMCs, the number of MIF-expressing cells was significantly higher in fatty-streak (type II) and advanced inflammatory lesions [31]. MIF expression was most prominent in vicinity to the acellular lipid core, especially in macrophages. Similar findings were obtained in human carotid endatherectomy samples, where MIF expression is progressively increased during plaque progression, particularly in CD40 ligand- and angiotensin II-positive macrophages in complicated atherosclerotic plaques [53]. *In vitro,* MIF was up-regulated in monocytes through CD40 ligand, angiotensin II, hyperglycemia, and hypoxia, as well as in endothelial cells through hypoxia and oxidized LDL [31, 53]. Kong *et al.* found considerably higher MIF expression in human vulnerable than in fibrous plaques, primarily in macrophages and SMCs, concomitantly with an overexpression of matrix metalloproteinase (MMP)-1 and -9 [54, 55]. Along the same line, Kleemann and colleagues found a MIF and MMP upregulation in human abdominal aortic aneurysms [56].

Taken together, MIF is predominantly expressed in chronic advanced human plaques with features of high inflammatory activity. Furthermore, important cardiovascular risk factors may contribute to enhanced MIF expression in atherosclerotic lesions.

2.6 Role of MIF in Atherogenesis

The functional involvement of MIF in atherosclerotic plaque progression was first interrogated in animal studies using *Mif*$^{-/-}$/*Ldlr*$^{-/-}$ mice on an atherogenic diet [57]. Genetic MIF deficiency greatly reduced the lesion area and intimal thickness after 26 weeks of a high fat diet [57]. Interestingly, the absence of MIF in this model resulted in the formation of macrophage-rich fatty streaks with fewer SMCs and less collagen content, thus impairing the progression of atherosclerotic lesions [57]. This finding may be explained by a diminished proliferation rate of neointimal cells in MIF-deficient mice. Of note, total serum cholesterol and LDL cholesterol were reduced in MIF-deficient mice [57]. A similar reduction of the aortic plaque formation was observed in *Mif*$^{-/-}$/*Ldlr*$^{-/-}$ mice on a regular diet for 52 weeks [58]. In this model, however, the lesional macrophage content was greatly diminished in the absence of MIF [58].

The blockade of primarily circulating Mif in *Apoe*$^{-/-}$ mice on a regular diet by treatment with a Mif antibody tended to reduce the plaque volumes without reaching statistical significance [50]. The macrophage accumulation in the plaques, however, was inhibited in Mif antibody-treated mice [50]. In contrast to *Mif*$^{-/-}$/*Ldlr*$^{-/-}$ mice on a high fat diet, treatment with the Mif antibody did not significantly affect the lipid levels [50, 57]. These data indicate that MIF exposed to the blood stream is involved in atherogenic monocyte recruitment but does not regulate lipid metabolism. The effect of MIF on atherosclerotic plaque progression has been studied in more detail in *Apoe*$^{-/-}$ mice. After 12 weeks of a high fat diet, a 4 week treatment course with a blocking Mif antibody almost completely prevented further plaque development and, strikingly, led to plaque regression

[15]. This was associated with a marked reduction of the macrophage and T cell content in the lesions [15].

Accelerated plaque formation by endothelial denudation of the carotid artery in *Ldlr*$^{-/-}$ mice was reduced through treatment with a blocking MIF antibody. This was associated with a reduced influx of inflammatory cells into the injured vascular wall in the early stage of neointima formation. Furthermore, blocking MIF increased the injury-induced apoptosis and diminished the proliferation rate of neointimal cells [51]. In a model of wire-induced carotid artery injury in hypercholesterolemic *Apoe*$^{-/-}$ mice, blocking MIF did not significantly reduce the plaque size but shifted the composition of the lesion towards a more stable phenotype with less macrophages and an increased content of SMCs and collagen [52]. The susceptibility to low flow-induced intimal thickening of the carotid artery appears to be mediated by enhanced expression of MIF as revealed in mouse model microarray profiling [59].

2.7 Epidemiologic Correlations Between MIF and Cardiovascular Disease

A role for MIF in atherogenesis is further supported by several epidemiologic studies that correlate MIF expression with atherosclerotic disease severity. In humans, a large case-cohort study showed that the -173G/C polymorphism in the MIF promoter region, but not the MIF serum level, correlates with an increased risk for CHD [60]. The G-to-C transition at position -173 of the MIF gene has been reported to increase the susceptibility to various inflammatory diseases [61]. Another study indicates that the GG genotype of the MIF SNP rs1007888 was associated with myocardial infarction (MI) in female patients [62]. In patients with rheumatic arthritis, however, the MIF -173 G/C SNP was not associated with increased cardiovascular risk [63]. Moreover, elevated circulating MIF levels were predictive for an increased rate of major coronary events in patients with CHD and impaired glucose tolerance or diabetes mellitus [64].

Taken together, there is substantial evidence – both functional and epidemiologic – for a proatherogenic role of MIF in mouse models and in humans through inhibition of inflammatory cell accumulation, especially of macrophages and T cells, in the lesions and, thus, the progression of atherosclerosis.

2.8 Pro-Atherogenic MIF Mechanisms

Diverse pro-atherogenic functions of MIF that may be instrumental in atherogenesis have been described. In human plaques, MIF forms a complex with the transcriptional co-activator c-Jun activation domain-binding protein (JAB)-1/CSN5 [31]. The functional role of this interaction in atherogenesis, however, remains to be determined. Interestingly, CSN5 and the COP9 signalosome (CSN) have been shown to control the IKK/NFκB pathway and to regulate β2 integrin signalling-mediated activator protein (AP)-1 activity [65–67]. NFκB pathway is central in the induction of inflammatory chemokine and adhesion molecule expression in endothelial cells and monocytes/macrophages. Thus, co-regulation of the NFκB pathway by MIF/JAB1 might represent a yet uncharacterized regulatory element in atherogenesis. Independent of any potential JAB1-mediated mechanisms, MIF was found to induce intercellular adhesion molecule-1 (ICAM-1) expression on endothelial cells *in vitro* [48] and blocking MIF in *Apoe*$^{-/-}$ mice inhibits ICAM-1 expression in the aortic wall [50]. ICAM-1 mediates the immune cell trafficking into the arterial wall; MIF-induced ICAM-1 expression might, therefore, contribute to increased adhesion of monocytes to activated endothelial cells and promote atherogenesis.

In addition, blood levels of inflammatory proteins and local expression of TNF-α and CD40 ligand in the aortic wall were reduced in Mif antibody-treated *Apoe*$^{-/-}$ mice, whereas matrix metalloprotease (MMP)-2 and interleukin-12-p40 mRNA levels were up-regulated [50]. Possible transcriptional regulators of plaque development and inflammation, such as phospho-c-Jun and C-EBP-β, were suppressed by the MIF antibody treatment [50]. A possible contribution to plaque inflammation may result from the inhibition of p53 activity through MIF [68, 69]. In *Mif*$^{-/-}$ mice, endotoxin-treated macrophages showed decreased viability, reduced proinflammatory function, and increased apoptosis mediated by increased p53 activity [68]. This may partially explain the athero-protective effects of MIF inhibition, since p53 deficiency promotes native atherosclerosis [70].

Other reports indicate that MIF stimulates the uptake of oxidized LDL by macrophages [71] and foam cell formation was reduced in the neointimal lesions of Mif antibody-treated mice [52]. Since oxidized LDL induces the expression and secretion of MIF in a NFκB-dependent manner, a positive feedback loop might be initiated that promotes intracellular cholesterol accumulation [31, 72].

In vitro, a mitogenic effect of MIF on serum- or platelet-derived-growth-factor (PDGF)-stimulated vascular SMCs has been reported through an autocrine feedback loop [51]. Moreover, MIF stimulates the migration of SMCs either directly or after treatment with PDGF [73]. Both mechanisms may contribute to the reduced neointimal accumulation of SMCs after vascular injury and in diet-induced plaques [52, 57].

In addition to the promotion of plaque growth, *in vitro* results indicate that MIF also initiates mechanisms involved in plaque destabilization. In the absence of MIF, SMC proliferation and SMC-dependent proteolytic activity as evident by reduced elastin and collagen degradation is reduced [57]. Although the expression of MMPs was not reduced in *Mif*$^{-/-}$ SMCs, MIF can induce MMP-1 and MMP-9 expression in SMCs resulting in enhanced collagenase activity [54, 55]. In conjunction, the data infer that blocking MIF in manifest atherosclerosis may serve to mediate a conversion of vulnerable plaques into a more stable condition less susceptible to rupture.

2.9 MIF Acts as a Functional Chemokine in Atherosclerosis

Interestingly, *in vitro* adhesion assays revealed that monocyte adhesion on oxidized LDL-treated human aortic endothelial cells depends almost completely on endothelial MIF and stimulation of aortic endothelial cells with MIF for two hours induced monocyte adhesion under flow conditions, providing preliminary hints to a CLF of MIF in leukocyte recruitment [52]. As discussed above, the mechanism of MIF-induced leukocyte adhesion has recently been further established by the finding that the chemokine receptors CXCR2 and CXCR4, which have been amply implicated in atherogenesis [5, 74], are functional MIF receptors [15]. Binding of MIF to CXCR2 or CXCR4 induces calcium influx and rapid integrin activation in conjunction with monocyte and T cell adhesion on endothelial monolayers, respectively [15]. Thus, MIF-induced monocyte adhesion on human aortic endothelial cells under flow conditions could be prevented by a blocking MIF or CXCR2 antibody and pertussis toxin, whereas the neutralization of the CXCR2 ligands CXCL1 and CXCL8 was not effective, indicating that MIF effect on leukocyte adhesion was not indirectly mediated via these bona fide CXCR2 ligands. Similar to CXCL1, MIF was found to be immobilized and presented on the endothelial surface. The MIF-induced adhesion of monocytes is mediated by β_2-integrin. In addition to CXCR2, CD74 is required for efficient MIF-induced monocyte adhesion on CHO cells, engineered to express adhesion molecules [15]. Since co-expression of CXCR2 and CD74 results in the formation of heteromeric CXCR2/CD74 complexes [15], MIF signalling in leukocyte recruitment processes may be mediated by this receptor complex. Although MIF can bind to CXCR2 in the absence of CD74 and vice versa, adjunctive binding to CD74 may facilitate GPCR activation and formation of a receptor signalling complex, including SRC kinases, similar to the role of CD44 as an auxiliary receptor for CCL5 [75]. As reported for CXCL8 [4], MIF-induced monocyte adhesion *in vitro* was triggered by rapid activation of $\alpha_L\beta_2$- or $\alpha_4\beta_1$-integrin [15]. This mechanism of MIF-induced monocyte arrest has been confirmed in atherogenic leukocyte recruitment. In *ex vivo*-perfused carotid arteries of hyperlipdemic *Apoe*$^{-/-}$ mice, blockade of CXCR2, CD74, or MIF significantly reduced monocyte adhesion, suggesting that MIF induces atherogenic leukocyte arrest through CXCR2/CD74 [15]. A similar arrest chemokine function on early atherosclerotic endothelium has been previously described for the CXCR2 ligand CXCL1 [76]. In carotid arteries from *Mif*$^{-/-}$/*Ldlr*$^{-/-}$ mice, monocyte adhesion under flow conditions was clearly reduced compared with *Mif*$^{+/+}$/*Ldlr*$^{-/-}$ mice. In *Mif*$^{-/-}$/*Ldlr*$^{-/-}$ mice, inhibition of CXCR2 did not further impair monocyte adhesion. After loading exogenous MIF, the inhibitory effect of the CXCR2 antibody was fully restored in *Mif*$^{-/-}$/*Ldlr*$^{-/-}$ mice [15]. Furthermore, impaired leukocyte recruitment has also been observed in acute vascular inflammation after TNF-α treatment in irradiated *Mif*$^{-/-}$ mice supplemented with Cxcr2-deficient bone marrow cells (from *Il8rb*$^{-/-}$ *mice).*

In addition to integrin-dependent leukocyte adhesion, directed migration of leukocytes along a soluble gradient is another principal chemokine/chemokine receptor-mediated effect [3]. As discussed, MIF, in contrast to its eponymous name, was found to induce rather than inhibit monocyte migration [15, 17]. Similar to monocyte migration processes triggered by CCL2 and CXCL8, MIF-mediated migration of monocytes occurs through $G_{\alpha i}$ protein and phosphoinositide-3 kinase (PI3K) activation compatible with the activation of a GPCR [15]. Moreover, blocking CXCR2 and CD74 antibodies clearly impaired MIF-induced monocyte transmigration indicating a crucial role of both receptors in MIF-induced leukocyte chemotaxis [15].

Highly specialized functions have been ascribed to different chemokines in atherogenic monocyte and T cell recruitment [2]. In addition to monocyte recruitment, MIF induces $\alpha_L\beta_2$-dependent T cell adhesion and transmigration through interaction with CXCR4, but not CXCR1 or CXCR3 [15]. This mechanism of T cell recruitment may be responsible for the reduced T cell content in advanced atherosclerotic plaques after MIF blockade. Thus, MIF is involved in atherogenic leukocyte recruitment in a more universal sense: It has slightly reduced efficacy as compared with the cognate ligand chemokines, but through interaction with both CXCR4 and CXCR2, MIF promotes the recruitment of both monocytes and T cells [15]. This contrasts the more cell-restricted action of CXCL8 and CXCL12. Given the atherogenic function of MIF as a dual agonist of CXCR2 and CXCR4, the striking effects of MIF inhibition on limiting atheroprogression and even mediating plaque regression can be explained by blocking MIF actions on both CXCR2 and CXCR4 [15]. Thus, MIF would be expected to retain a potent and predominant CXCR2 activity in atherogenesis, when the CXCR4/CXCL12 axis is blocked [15]. This would be in line with the CXCR2-mediated recruitment of neutrophils, incriminated to underly the exacerbation of atherosclerosis caused by interference with CXCR4 and a dysbalance in neutrophil homeostasis [15, 77]. The data also comply with a more pronounced inhibition of atherosclerosis by genetic deficiency in bone marrow CXCR2 as compared to deletion of its cognate ligand CXCL1, supporting an activity of additional CXCR2 ligands, namely MIF, in atherogenesis [5, 15].

Besides these chemokines-like functions, MIF-induced macrophage recruitment may also partly rely on enhanced expression of other inflammatory mediators, such as adhesion molecules or cytokines [12], which could further sustain the mononuclear cell influx. In postcapillary venules, MIF-induced monocyte recruitment critically depends on the CCL2/CCR2 axis, possibly due to enhanced endothelial release of CCL2 by MIF [17]. In fact, MIF might regulate macrophage recruitment sequentially; first a rapid activation of integrin-dependent monocyte adhesion may occur through direct interaction with CXCR2 (or CXCR2/CD74 complexes), while MIF-induced CCL2 might subsequently promote monocyte transmigration.

2.10 CLF Chemokines in Atherosclerosis

MIF cannot be grouped into any of the four classical chemokine subfamilies [78] and has instead been classified as a CLF chemokine [21, 77]. Structural analysis indeed revealed a pseudo-(E)LR-motif in MIF, represented by two non-adjacent amino acids in exposed neighboring loops with a spacing identical to that in the ELR-motif present in canonical CXCR2 ligands. In addition, MIF features an N-like loop that is functionally similar to the N-loop of the ELR+ CXC chemokines [79–81]. Thus, despite lack of the conserved N-terminal chemokine fold containing the CC or CXC cysteine motif, MIF carries critical structural chemokine elements and has chemokine-like functions in leukocyte recruitment [15]. This is the structural basis for non-cognate binding of MIF to its chemokine receptors. Like MIF, an N-terminal cleavage fragment of tyrosyl-tRNA synthetase (TyrRS) has been shown to act as a non-canonical CXCR1 ligand via the presence of an ELR-motif [82]. Although aminoacyl-tRNA synthetases (aminoacyl-RS) normally exhibit intracellular functions, their cleavage, i.e., by the extracellular protease leukocyte elastin upon its secretion under apoptotic conditions generates fragments with chemokine activities. Whereas the endothelial monocyte-activating polypeptide II-like C-terminal domain functions as a potent monocyte and neutrophil chemoattractant and induces the production of myeloperoxidase, TNF-α, and tissue factor, the N-terminal "mini-TyrRS" containing both the catalytic and anticodon-recognition domain is proangiogenic and induces neutrophil chemotaxis [82]. These functions of mini-TyrRS are manifested through its interaction with CXCR1 but not CXCR2 and depend on an ELR-motif [83]. Furthermore, the human antimicrobial peptides β-defensin-1 and -2 (HBD-1 and -2) were identified as non-cognate ligands for CCR6, mediating CCR6-dependent chemotaxis of immature dendritic cells and memory T cells [84]. By recruiting these cell types to sites of microbial infection, HBD-1 and -2 may, thus, promote adaptive immune responses in addition to their prominent role in innate immunity. Conversely, the CCR6-ligand CCL20 has been shown to display remarkable antimicrobial activity [85]. Similarly, specific autoantigenic aminoacyl-RS, released under apoptotic conditions, exerts leukocyte recruitment by triggering CC receptors. Both histidyl-RS and its N-terminal fragment are chemoattractants for T cells, activated monocytes, and immature dendritic cells via stimulation of the CCR5 receptor, whereas the same cell types are recruited by asparaginyl-RS via its interaction with CCR3 [85].

Thus, despite the absence of typical structural chemokine motifs, an increasing number of host proteins involved in inflammatory and immune processes seem to act via direct *non-cognate* interaction with chemokine receptors, that leads to chemokine receptor triggering via a mechanism of molecular mimicry. It should be mentioned at this point that viruses and other parasites also prominently capitalize on this principle of "molecular hijacking", e.g., to facilitate their dissemination and evasion from the host system. Examples are: Toxoplasma gondii-derived cyclophilin-18, which potently stimulates IL-12 production by DCs through triggering CCR5 [86] or HIV-1 gp120, which interacts with host CXCR4 (and CCR5) to infect leukocytes [87]. It is currently unknown, whether these other CLF chemokines can also modulate atherogenic responses through chemokine-like mechanisms.

However, given that MIF potently promotes leukocyte chemotaxis and recruitment in atherogenesis in a CLF manner via direct binding to CXCR2 and CXCR4 [15], it may be speculated that other CLF chemokines may also play causal roles in the pathogenesis of atherosclerosis.

2.11 Therapeutic Approaches to Target MIF in Inflammation and Atherosclerosis

MIF is distinct from classical chemokines/cytokines in that (i) it is secreted by a non-conventional pathway, (ii) it does not structurally belong to any of the known cytokine or chemokine families, (iii) it interacts by non-cognate binding with two distinct CXC chemokine receptors and a type II membrane receptor, and (iv) it has two evolutionarily conserved catalytic activities that are linked to distinct amino acid motifs. MIF should, thus, be amenable to a number of specifically-tailored therapeutic approaches. These could include SMW drug approaches to target the MIF secretion pathway, specific antibodies or soluble receptor fusions proteins to target circulating MIF but not other cytokines/chemokines, peptide- or SMW drug-based antagonists or antibodies targeting the MIF/CXCR interface, and SMW drugs to target the conserved catalytic site(s) of MIF.

2.11.1 Targeting the Non-Conventional Secretion of MIF

MIF differs from most cytokines/chemokines in that it is secreted by an ER/Golgi-independent secretion pathway. Specific components of this pathway have been identified; p115 and an ABC transporter, likely of the subtype ABC-A1, are involved in MIF secretion from monocytes, promoting or at least facilitating the release of MIF [34, 35]. In principle, these and other, yet to be identified components of the pathway, would represent attractive targets for SMW drug-based approaches. For example, the channel function of ABC-A1 could be tackled by an SMW drug. However, IL-1β, a pivotal inflammatory cytokine and pyrogen necessary for host defense also, is secreted by a non-classical, ABC-A1-mediated, pathway [88]. Also, non-classical protein secretion, also called LLS (*leaderless secretion*) protein secretion, is an emerging secretion route that evidently is utilized by a number of critical inflammatory mediators to support the host defense response [89–91]. Up to 20 structurally heterogeneous proteins may follow this pathway. Although it appears that there are at least four different non-classical secretion routes [89–91], targeting the secretion of MIF would need to account for potential other LLS proteins and would need to make sure that homeostatic functions of such proteins would not be affected. Targeting ABC-A1 as an anti-MIF approach (Fig. 2.1) also seems pre-mature, because the ABC transporter subtype that promotes MIF secretion has so far only been profiled by pharmacological inhibitors and not been confirmed by genetic deletion or RNA silencing studies. More importantly, ABC-A1 is a multi-functional transporter that transports cholesterol. ABC-A1 plays a critical role in high-density lipoprotein (HDL) generation, maintaining cholesterol homeostasis. Moreover, it was recently shown that deletion of ABC-A1 (and ABC-G1) causes a redistribution of cholesterol into the inner leaflet of the plasma membrane an effect that modulates leukocyte migration [92]; this has been suggested to promote regression of atherosclerosis. Similarly, p115 is centrally involved in Golgi vesicle trafficking and is, thus, of broad significance for cellular membrane maintenance. Marked knock down of p115 in monocytes/macrophages leads to a massive breakdown in Golgi integrity [35]. Accordingly, targeting p115 as a means to interfere with the MIF secretion pathway is unlikely to be a practical strategy to block MIF in the near future. In conclusion, approaches targeting the secretion pathway of MIF are still at an early stage.

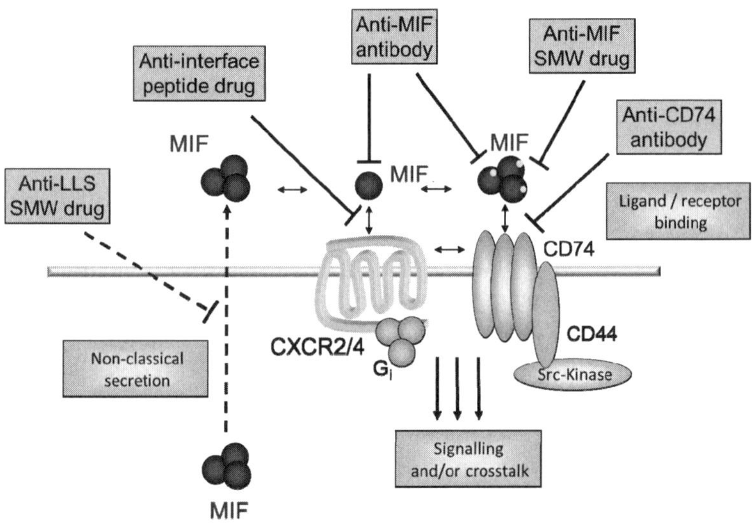

Figure 2.1 Schematic depicting potential anti-MIF approaches to antagonize inflammation and atherosclerosis. A schematic cell expressing MIF receptors and/or secreting MIF is shown. MIF/MIF receptor binding events and MIF receptor-driven signaling responses are also depicted. MIF itself can be targeted by antibody or SMW drug approaches. The MIF/CXCR interface can be targeted by peptidomimetic drugs tailored to interfere with MIF/CXCR binding. MIF/CD74 interactions can be targeted by anti-CD74 antibodies or anti-MIF antibodies or anti-MIF SMW drugs, which — likely due to the induction of conformational changes — can interfere with the tautomerase site of MIF and MIF binding to CD74. Strategies targeted at the MIF secretion pathway (a non-classical), or leaderless protein secretion (LLS) pathway are less likely to be specific (dashed lines).

2.11.2 Targeting the Unique Structural Characteristics and MIF/MIF Receptor Interactions

Cytokines and their receptors are interesting drug targets for the treatment of inflammatory and immune diseases and atherosclerosis, especially given their role in leukocyte recruitment and activation. In this context, the identification of MIF as a crucial chemokine-like protein turns MIF and its receptor interactions into an appealing target for the development of new drugs (Fig. 2.1). Anti-MIF antibodies have been shown to exhibit protection from atherogenesis [15, 93], septic shock [9], lethal endotoxemia [8], glomerulonephritis [12], and adjuvant arthritis [94] in corresponding animal models. In fact, neutralizing anti-MIF antibodies are being developed by several pharmaceutical companies and are in the pre-clinical or early clinical trial stage. Another option to interfere with MIF activity would be the use of soluble MIF receptors. Among the MIF receptors, it seems that only CD74 would be amenable to such a strategy, as it is the only MIF receptor that possesses an extended extracellular domain (ECD). Targeting CD74 appears attractive at first sight, because CD74 is already a target to which antibodies are being developed by pharmaceutical companies for application in cancer. However, CD74 has recently been reported to mediate important cardioprotective effects of MIF in myocardial ischemia/reperfusion (I/R) injury [33, 95], whereas others have observed that MIF exacerbates myocardial I/R damage [96].

Overall, the high production costs of such protein-based therapeutics render their application for the treatment of high-incidence diseases, such as atherosclerosis, not very appealing. An alternative is provided by non-protein-based anti-cytokine therapeutics. In the case of MIF, such approaches would encompass SMW drugs, peptide antagonists, and peptidomimetics. Both MIF and its receptors could be targeted. Synthesis strategies and production costs for peptide-based anti-MIF drugs would be straight forward and reasonable, respectively. Therapeutic peptides frequently lack complex 3D structures compared, but interaction surface areas are considerably larger than those of SMW drugs, enabling for higher specificities. Indeed, the identification of the pseudo-(E)LR and the N-like-loop motifs in MIF as being critical for MIF-CXCR2 interaction [80, 81] could offer such a target site for the design of peptide-based inhibitors obstructing the chemokine-like functions of MIF (Fig. 2.1).

Numerous SMW drugs have been developed against chemokine receptors, including some directed against CXCR2 and CXCR4, for a number of inflamematory and immune diseases as well as cancer. However, several of these drugs have already failed in clinical studies [97]. While the expression of CXCR2 is limited to neutrophils, mast cells, and activated monocytes and endothelial cells, CXCR4 is broadly expressed not only on all leukocyte subsets but also on essentially all other cell types in the body. This will render it difficult to identify sufficiently specific drug strategies. In order for such a compound to target MIF-driven diseases, such a compound would need to interfere with the MIF/CXCR2 interface, but should ideally not affect MIF/CXCR4 and/or CXCL12/CXCR4 interactions. While again the identified pseudo-(E)LR and N-like-loop motifs in MIF [80, 81] could be exploited as a structural basis for designing and optimizing such drugs, it remains unclear whether the limited interaction surface of an SMW drug would be sufficient to specifically target these motifs, which also, at least in the case of the N-like loop regions, have conformational flexibility. In fact, it is well known that the SMW drugs normally lack high-affinity binding to the chemokine ligand or receptor [14]. By comparison, chemokine-based peptide drugs are advantageous in that they feature higher binding activities [98]. Yet, SMW drugs can be orally administrated, show no or low antigenicity, and are associated with affordable production costs.

2.11.3 Targeting the Evolutionarily Conserved Catalytic Sites of MIF

The identification of the unusual catalytic tautomerase and redox motifs of MIF [29, 99] offers the possibility to design small-molecule inhibitors inhibiting certain MIF functions [14]. In fact, directly targeting a cytokine/chemokine by an SMW drug is novel as cytokines/chemokines normally solely act by interaction with a receptor. The tautomerase site of is evolutionary-conserved and has, otherwise, only been identified in bacterial enzymes. Interestingly, SMW inhibitors such as ISO-1 targeting the tautomerase pocket of MIF have been shown to inhibit MIF cell surface binding and inflammatory cytokine functions of MIF [100–102]. However, other studies have shed doubt on the notion that inhibiting MIF tautomerase activity would cross-interfere with the biologic and inflammatory actions of MIF [14]. In essence, it has remained unclear whether the catalytic tautomerase activity of MIF, which so far was only observed *in vitro*, is directly linked to MIF's inflammatory actions, whether inhibition of the tautomerase pocket (thus, affecting several residues distributed over the 3D structure of MIF) induces a conformational change in the MIF structure, or whether the residues in the pocket directly participate in receptor binding of MIF. Of note, a tautomerase-null MIF gene knock-in mouse recently revealed that protein interactions and not enzymatic activity per se mediate MIF-dependent growth regulation, arguing that also the inflammatory activities of MIF would not be targeted directly by tautomerase site inhibitors [103]. It would be interesting to examine whether these inhibitors also interfere with CXCL2-mediated MIF signalling and function. However, such studies have not been undertaken. In addition, the development of membrane-permeable SMW inhibitors of MIF could allow to interfere with intracellular MIF functions. On the other hand, one might argue that interference with intracellular MIF activities, which have been suggested to promote cell homeostasis [29], should be explicitly avoided by an anti-MIF drug.

Although it is still unknown whether inhibition of MIF could induce immunosuppression in treated patients, studies of *Mif*$^{-/-}$ mice have not shown a high-infection risk under normal conditions in the absence of MIF. Therefore, anti-MIF-based strategies could be highly attractive for a number of inflammatory diseases, including atherosclerosis. As to the latter, anti-MIF strategies could represent an interesting novel approach. In particular, given that MIF neutralization even induces regression of established atherosclerotic lesions in a mouse model [15], targeting MIF may represent an interesting therapeutic option for treating and stabilizing advanced atherosclerosis.

Substantial evidence from both animal models and the study of human atherosclerotic lesions supports a key role for MIF in the progression of atherosclerosis. As discussed, MIF functions via several mechanisms, including triggering atherogenic leukocyte recruitment and arrest via its chemokine-like functions, production of proinflammatory cytokines, foam cell formation, and processes of cell proliferation and apoptosis inhibition. Given the disappointing results concerning the use of the acyl-coenzyme A/cholesterol acyltransferase inhibitor pactimibe or the cholesteryl ester transfer protein inhibitor torcetrapib in the treatment of atherosclerosis [104, 105], the design of new inhibitors, e.g., targeting MIF, and the study of their effects on the diverse biologic functions of this cytokine will be extremely valuable and promising for treatment options of instable atherosclerosis in the future.

2.12 Concluding Remarks

A substantial body of evidence has been gathered for a pivotal role of MIF in the pathogenesis of atherosclerosis. Inborn MIF deficiency in *Ldlr*$^{-/-}$ mice and short term inhibition of MIF in *Apoe*$^{-/-}$ mice reduced atherosclerotic plaque burden and lesion progression. MIF affects various aspects of lesion development, such as neointimal SMC homeostasis, transformation of macrophages into foam cells, and degradation of extracellular matrix proteins. Moreover, MIF induces atherogenic leukocyte recruitment through binding to the chemokine receptors CXCR2 and CXCR4. For MIF-induced monocyte adhesion and transmigration, both CD74 and CXCR2 are required, whereas T cell recruitment by MIF is mediated through CXCR4. The identification of heteromeric receptor complexes likely further diversifies regulation of atherogenic inflammatory processes by MIF. The discovery that MIF is a non-canonical chemokine receptor ligand that induces inflammatory cell recruitment through binding to CXCR2 and CXCR4 sheds new light on the complex interplay of chemokines in atherogenesis and vascular remodelling and offers novel options for the treatment of atherosclerosis. Although it is currently unknown how MIF affects plaque burden via individual chemokine-receptor subtypes, experimental results suggest that targeting MIF is a promising treatment strategy in established atherosclerosis and vulnerable plaques, whereat the unique structural properties of MIF make it possible in principle to pursue SMW, peptide-based, and antibody-based anti-MIF strategies.

Acknowledgement

This work was supported by Deutsche Forschungsgemeinschaft (DFG) grant BE1977/4-2.

References

1. Libby, P. (2002) Inflammation in atherosclerosis. *Nature* **420**, pp. 868–874.

2. Weber, C., Schober, A., and Zernecke, A. (2004) Chemokines: Key regulators of mononuclear cell recruitment in atherosclerotic vascular disease. *Arterioscler Thromb Vasc Biol* **24**, pp. 1997–2008.
3. Weber, C. (2003) Novel mechanistic concepts for the control of leukocyte transmigration: Specialization of integrins, chemokines, and junctional molecules. *J Mol Med* **81**, pp. 4–19.
4. Laudanna, C., and Alon, R. (2006) Right on the spot. Chemokine triggering of integrin-mediated arrest of rolling leukocytes. *Thromb Haemost* **95**, pp. 5–11.
5. Boisvert, W.A., Rose, D.M., Johnson, K.A., Fuentes, M.E., Lira, S.A., Curtiss, L.K., and Terkeltaub, R.A. (2006) Up-regulated expression of the CXCR2 ligand KC/GRO-alpha in atherosclerotic lesions plays a central role in macrophage accumulation and lesion progression. *Am J Pathol* **168**, pp. 1385–1395.
6. David, J.R. (1966) Delayed hypersensitivity in vitro: Its mediation by cell-free substances formed by lymphoid cell-antigen interaction. *Proc Natl Acad Sci U S A* **56**, pp. 72–77.
7. Calandra, T., and Roger, T. (2003) Macrophage migration inhibitory factor: A regulator of innate immunity. *Nat Rev Immunol* **3**, pp. 791–800.
8. Bernhagen, J., Calandra, T., Mitchell, R.A., Martin, S.B., Tracey, K.J., Voelter, W., Manogue, K.R., Cerami, A., and Bucala, R. (1993) MIF is a pituitary-derived cytokine that potentiates lethal endotoxaemia. *Nature* **365**, pp. 756–759.
9. Calandra, T., Echtenacher, B., Le Roy, D., Pugin, J., Metz, C.N., Hültner, L., Heumann, D., Männel, D., Bucala, R., and Glauser, M. (2000) Protection from septic shock by neutralization of macrophage migration inhibitory factor (MIF). *Nat Med* **6**, pp. 164–169.
10. de Jong, Y.P., Abadia-Molina, A.C., Satoskar, A.R., Clarke, K., Rietdijk, S.T., Faubion, W.A., Mizoguchi, E., Metz, C.N., Al Sahli, M., ten Hove, T., Keates, A.C., Lubetsky, J.B., Farrell, R.J., Michetti, P., van Deventer, S.J., Lolis, E., David, J.R., Bhan, A.K., and Terhorst, C. (2001) Development of chronic colitis is dependent on the cytokine MIF. *Nat Immunol* **2**, pp. 1061–1066.
11. Bernhagen, J., Bacher, M., Calandra, T., Metz, C.N., Doty, S.B., Donnelly, T., and Bucala, R. (1996) An essential role for macrophage migration inhibitory factor in the tuberculin delayed-type hypersensitivity reaction. *J Exp Med* **183**, pp. 277–282.
12. Lan, H.Y., Bacher, M., Yang, N., Mu, W., Nikolic-Paterson, D.J., Metz, C., Meinhardt, A., Bucala, R., and Atkins, R.C. (1997) The pathogenic role

of macrophage migration inhibitory factor in immunologically induced kidney disease in the rat. *J Exp Med* **185**, pp. 1455–1465.

13. Donnelly, S.C., Haslett, C., Reid, P.T., Grant, I.S., Wallace, W.A., Metz, C.N., Bruce, L.J., and Bucala, R. (1997) Regulatory role for macrophage migration inhibitory factor in acute respiratory distress syndrome. *Nat Med* **3**, pp. 320–323.
14. Morand, E.F., Leech, M., and Bernhagen, J. (2006) MIF: A new cytokine link between rheumatoid arthritis and atherosclerosis. *Nat Rev Drug Discov* **5**, pp. 399–410.
15. Bernhagen, J., Krohn, R., Lue, H., Gregory, J.L., Zernecke, A., Koenen, R.R., Dewor, M., Georgiev, I., Schober, A., Leng, L., Kooistra, T., Fingerle-Rowson, G., Ghezzi, P., Kleemann, R., McColl, S.R., Bucala, R., Hickey, M.J., and Weber, C. (2007) MIF is a noncognate ligand of CXC chemokine receptors in inflammatory and atherogenic cell recruitment. *Nat Med* **13**, pp. 587–596.
16. Gregory, J.L., Leech, M.T., David, J.R., Yang, Y.H., Dacumos, A., and Hickey, M.J. (2004) Reduced leukocyte-endothelial cell interactions in the inflamed microcirculation of macrophage migration inhibitory factor-deficient mice. *Arthritis Rheum* **50**, pp. 3023–3034.
17. Gregory, J.L., Morand, E.F., McKeown, S.J., Ralph, J.A., Hall, P., Yang, Y.H., McColl, S.R., and Hickey, M.J. (2006) Macrophage migration inhibitory factor induces macrophage recruitment via CC chemokine ligand 2. *J. Immunol.* **177**, pp. 8072–8079.
18. Zernecke, A., Bernhagen, J., and Weber, C. (2008) Macrophage migration inhibitory factor in cardiovascular disease. *Circulation* **117**, pp. 1594–1602.
19. Calandra, T., Bernhagen, J., Metz, C.N., Spiegel, L.A., Bacher, M., Donnelly, T., Cerami, A., and Bucala, R. (1995) MIF as a glucocorticoid-induced modulator of cytokine production. *Nature* **377**, pp. 68–71.
20. Flaster, H., Bernhagen, J., Calandra, T., and Bucala, R. (2007) The MIF-glucocorticoid dyad: Regulation of inflammation and immunity. *Mol. Endocrinol.* **21**, pp. 1267–1280.
21. Noels, H., Bernhagen, J., and Weber, C. (2009) Macrophage migration inhibitory factor: A noncanonical chemokine important in atherosclerosis. *Trends Cardiovasc Med* **19**, pp. 76–86.
22. Schober, A., Bernhagen, J., and Weber, C. (2008) Chemokine-like functions of MIF in atherosclerosis. *J Mol Med* **86**, pp. 761–770.
23. Muhlhahn, P., Bernhagen, J., Czisch, M., Georgescu, J., Renner, C., Ross, A., Bucala, R., and Holak, T.A. (1996) NMR characterization of structure,

backbone dynamics, and glutathione binding of the human macrophage migration inhibitory factor (MIF). *Protein Sci* **5**, pp. 2095–2103.

24. Sun, H.W., Bernhagen, J., Bucala, R., and Lolis, E. (1996) Crystal structure at 2.6-A resolution of human macrophage migration inhibitory factor. *Proc Natl Acad Sci U S A* **93**, pp. 5191–5196.
25. Weiser, W.Y., Temple, D.M., Witek-Gianotti, J.S., Remold, H.G., Clark, S.C., and David, J.R. (1989) Molecular cloning of cDNA encoding a human macrophage migration inhibtion factor. *Proc Natl Acad Sci U S A* **86**, pp. 7522–7526.
26. Mischke, R., Kleemann, R., Brunner, H., and Bernhagen, J. (1998) Cross-linking and mutational analysis of the oligomerization state of the cytokine macrophage migration inhibitory factor (MIF). *FEBS Lett* **427**, pp. 85–90.
27. Philo, J.S., Yang, T.H., and LaBarre, M. (2004) Re-examining the oligomerization state of macrophage migration inhibitory factor (MIF) in solution. *Biophys Chem* **108**, pp. 77–87.
28. Kleemann, R., Kapurniotu, A., Frank, R.W., Gessner, A., Mischke, R., Flieger, O., Juttner, S., Brunner, H., and Bernhagen, J. (1998) Disulfide analysis reveals a role for macrophage migration inhibitory factor (MIF) as thiol-protein oxidoreductase. *J Mol Biol* **280**, pp. 85–102.
29. Thiele, M., and Bernhagen, J. (2005) Link between macrophage migration inhibitory factor and cellular redox regulation. *Antioxid Redox Signal* **7**, pp. 1234–1248.
30. Kleemann, R., Hausser, A., Geiger, G., Mischke, R., Burger-Kentischer, A., Flieger, O., Johannes, F.J., Roger, T., Calandra, T., Kapurniotu, A., Grell, M., Finkelmeier, D., Brunner, H., and Bernhagen, J. (2000) Intracellular action of the cytokine MIF to modulate AP-1 activity and the cell cycle through Jab1. *Nature* **408**, pp. 211–216.
31. Burger-Kentischer, A., Goebel, H., Seiler, R., Fraedrich, G., Schaefer, H.E., Dimmeler, S., Kleemann, R., Bernhagen, J., and Ihling, C. (2002) Expression of macrophage migration inhibitory factor in different stages of human atherosclerosis. *Circulation* **105**, pp. 1561–1566.
32. Simons, D., Grieb, G., Hristov, M., Pallua, N., Weber, C., Bernhagen, J., and Steffens, G. (2010) Hypoxia-induced endothelial secretion of macrophage migration inhibitory factor and role in endothelial progenitor cell recruitment. *J Cell Mol Med* **Epub ahead of print**.
33. Miller, E.J., Li, J., Leng, L., McDonald, C., Atsumi, T., Bucala, R., and Young, L.H. (2008) Macrophage migration inhibitory factor stimulates AMP-activated protein kinase in the ischaemic heart. *Nature* **451**, pp. 578–582.

34. Flieger, O., Engling, A., Bucala, R., Lue, H., Nickel, W., and Bernhagen, J. (2003) Regulated secretion of macrophage migration inhibitory factor is mediated by a non-classical pathway involving an ABC transporter. *FEBS Lett* **551**, pp. 78–86.

35. Merk, M., Baugh, J., Zierow, S., Leng, L., Pal, U., Lee, S.J., Ebert, A.D., Mizue, Y., Trent, J.O., Mitchell, R., Nickel, W., Kavathas, P.B., Bernhagen, J., and Bucala, R. (2009) The Golgi-associated protein p115 mediates the secretion of macrophage migration inhibitory factor. *J Immunol* **182**, pp. 6896–6906.

36. Lue, H., Thiele, M., Franz, J., Dahl, E., Speckgens, S., Leng, L., Fingerle-Rowson, G., Bucala, R., Luscher, B., and Bernhagen, J. (2007) Macrophage migration inhibitory factor (MIF) promotes cell survival by activation of the Akt pathway and role for CSN5/JAB1 in the control of autocrine MIF activity. *Oncogene* **26**, pp. 5046–5059.

37. Leng, L., Metz, C.N., Fang, Y., Xu, J., Donnelly, S., Baugh, J., Delohery, T., Chen, Y.B., Mitchell, R.A., and Bucala, R. (2003) MIF signal transduction initiated by binding to CD74. *J Exp Med* **197**, pp. 1467–1476.

38. Borghese, F., and Clanchy, F.I. (2011) CD74: An emerging opportunity as a therapeutic target in cancer and autoimmune disease. *Expert Opin Ther Targets*

39. Matza, D., Kerem, A., and Shachar, I. (2003) Invariant chain, a chain of command. *Trends Immunol* **24**, pp. 264–268.

40. Binsky, I., Haran, M., Starlets, D., Gore, Y., Lantner, F., Harpaz, N., Leng, L., Goldenberg, D.M., Shvidel, L., Berrebi, A., Bucala, R., and Shachar, I. (2007) IL-8 secreted in a macrophage migration-inhibitory factor- and CD74-dependent manner regulates B cell chronic lymphocytic leukemia survival. *Proc Natl Acad Sci U S A* **104**, pp. 13408–13413.

41. Gore, Y., Starlets, D., Maharshak, N., Becker-Herman, S., Kaneyuki, U., Leng, L., Bucala, R., and Shachar, I. (2008) Macrophage migration inhibitory factor induces B cell survival by activation of a CD74-CD44 receptor complex. *J Biol Chem* **283**, pp. 2784–2792.

42. Shi, X., Leng, L., Wang, T., Wang, W., Du, X., Li, J., McDonald, C., Chen, Z., Murphy, J.W., Lolis, E., Noble, P., Knudson, W., and Bucala, R. (2006) CD44 Is the Signaling Component of the Macrophage Migration Inhibitory Factor-CD74 Receptor Complex. *Immunity* **25**, pp. 595–606.

43. Thelen, M. (2001) Dancing to the tune of chemokines. *Nat Immunol* **2**, pp. 129–134.

44. Thelen, M., and Baggiolini, M. (2001) Is dimerization of chemokine receptors functionally relevant? *Sci STKE* **2001**, p. PE34.

45. Thelen, M., Munoz, L.M., Rodriguez-Frade, J.M., and Mellado, M. (2010) Chemokine receptor oligomerization: Functional considerations. *Curr Opin Pharmacol* **10**, pp. 38–43.

46. Thelen, M., and Stein, J.V. (2008) How chemokines invite leukocytes to dance. *Nat Immunol* **9**, pp. 953–959.

47. Schwartz, V., Lue, H., Kraemer, S., Korbiel, J., Krohn, R., Ohl, K., Bucala, R., Weber, C., and Bernhagen, J. (2009) A functional heteromeric MIF receptor formed by CD74 and CXCR4. *FEBS Lett* **583**, pp. 2749–2757.

48. Lin, S.G., Yu, X.Y., Chen, Y.X., Huang, X.R., Metz, C., Bucala, R., Lau, C.P., and Lan, H.Y. (2000) De novo expression of macrophage migration inhibitory factor in atherogenesis in rabbits. *Circ Res* **87**, pp. 1202–1208.

49. Calandra, T., Bernhagen, J., Mitchell, R.A., and Bucala, R. (1994) The macrophage is an important and previously unrecognized source of macrophage migration inhibitory factor. *J Exp Med* **179**, pp. 1895–1902.

50. Burger-Kentischer, A., Gobel, H., Kleemann, R., Zernecke, A., Bucala, R., Leng, L., Finkelmeier, D., Geiger, G., Schaefer, H.E., Schober, A., Weber, C., Brunner, H., Rutten, H., Ihling, C., and Bernhagen, J. (2006) Reduction of the aortic inflammatory response in spontaneous atherosclerosis by blockade of macrophage migration inhibitory factor (MIF). *Atherosclerosis* **184**, pp. 28–38.

51. Chen, Z., Sakuma, M., Zago, A.C., Zhang, X., Shi, C., Leng, L., Mizue, Y., Bucala, R., and Simon, D. (2004) Evidence for a role of macrophage migration inhibitory factor in vascular disease. *Arterioscler Thromb Vasc Biol* **24**, pp. 709–714.

52. Schober, A., Bernhagen, J., Thiele, M., Zeiffer, U., Knarren, S., Roller, M., Bucala, R., and Weber, C. (2004) Stabilization of atherosclerotic plaques by blockade of macrophage migration inhibitory factor after vascular injury in apolipoprotein E-deficient mice. *Circulation* **109**, pp. 380–385.

53. Schmeisser, A., Marquetant, R., Illmer, T., Graffy, C., Garlichs, C.D., Bockler, D., Menschikowski, D., Braun-Dullaeus, R., Daniel, W.G., and Strasser, R.H. (2005) The expression of macrophage migration inhibitory factor 1alpha (MIF 1alpha) in human atherosclerotic plaques is induced by different proatherogenic stimuli and associated with plaque instability. *Atherosclerosis* **178**, pp. 83–94.

54. Kong, Y.Z., Huang, X.R., Ouyang, X., Tan, J.J., Fingerle-Rowson, G., Bacher, M., Mu, W., Scher, L.A., Leng, L., Bucala, R., and Lan, H.Y. (2005) Evidence

for vascular macrophage migration inhibitory factor in destabilization of human atherosclerotic plaques. *Cardiovasc Res* **65**, pp. 272–282.

55. Kong, Y.Z., Yu, X., Tang, J.J., Ouyang, X., Huang, X.R., Fingerle-Rowson, G., Bacher, M., Scher, L.A., Bucala, R., and Lan, H.Y. (2005) Macrophage migration inhibitory factor induces MMP-9 expression: Implications for destabilization of human atherosclerotic plaques. *Atherosclerosis* **178**, pp. 207–215.
56. Verschuren, L., Lindeman, J.H., van Bockel, J.H., Abdul-Hussien, H., Kooistra, T., and Kleemann, R. (2005) Up-regulation and coexpression of MIF and matrix metalloproteinases in human abdominal aortic aneurysms. *Antioxid Redox Signal* **7**, pp. 1195–1202.
57. Pan, J.H., Sukhova, G.K., Yang, J.T., Wang, B., Xie, T., Fu, H., Zhang, Y., Satoskar, A.R., David, J.R., Metz, C.N., Bucala, R., Fang, K., Simon, D.I., Chapman, H.A., Libby, P., and Shi, G.P. (2004) Macrophage migration inhibitory factor deficiency impairs atherosclerosis in low-density lipoprotein receptor-deficient mice. *Circulation* **109**, pp. 3149–3153.
58. Verschuren, L., Kooistra, T., Bernhagen, J., Voshol, P.J., Ouwens, D.M., van Erk, M., de Vries-van der Weij, J., Leng, L., van Bockel, J.H., van Dijk, K.W., Fingerle-Rowson, G., Bucala, R., and Kleemann, R. (2009) MIF deficiency reduces chronic inflammation in white adipose tissue and impairs the development of insulin resistance, glucose intolerance, and associated atherosclerotic disease. *Circ Res* **105**, pp. 99–107.
59. Korshunov, V.A., Nikonenko, T.A., Tkachuk, V.A., Brooks, A., and Berk, B.C. (2006) Interleukin-18 and macrophage migration inhibitory factor are associated with increased carotid intima-media thickening. *Arterioscler Thromb Vasc Biol* **26**, pp. 295–300.
60. Herder, C., Illig, T., Baumert, J., Muller, M., Klopp, N., Khuseyinova, N., Meisinger, C., Martin, S., Thorand, B., and Koenig, W. (2008) Macrophage migration inhibitory factor (MIF) and risk for coronary heart disease: Results from the MONICA/KORA Augsburg case-cohort study, 1984–2002. *Atherosclerosis* **200**, pp. 380–388.
61. Donn, R.P., Shelley, E., Ollier, W.E., and Thomson, W. (2001) A novel 5'-flanking region polymorphism of macrophage migration inhibitory factor is associated with systemic-onset juvenile idiopathic arthritis. *Arthritis Rheum* **44**, pp. 1782–1785.
62. Tereshchenko, I.P., Petrkova, J., Mrazek, F., Lukl, J., Maksimov, V.N., Romaschenko, A.G., Voevoda, M.I., and Petrek, M. (2009) The macrophage migration inhibitory factor (MIF) gene polymorphism in Czech and Russian patients with myocardial infarction. *Clin Chim Acta* **402**, pp. 199–202.

63. Palomino-Morales, R., Gonzalez-Juanatey, C., Vazquez-Rodriguez, T.R., Torres, O., Miranda-Filloy, J.A., Llorca, J., Martin, J., and Gonzalez-Gay, M.A. (2010) Lack of association between macrophage migration inhibitory factor-173 gene polymorphism with disease susceptibility and cardiovascular risk in rheumatoid arthritis patients from northwestern Spain. *Clin Exp Rheumatol* **28**, pp. 68–72.

64. Makino, A., Nakamura, T., Hirano, M., Kitta, Y., Sano, K., Kobayashi, T., Fujioka, D., Saito, Y., Watanabe, K., Watanabe, Y., Kawabata, K., Obata, J.E., and Kugiyama, K. (2010) High plasma levels of macrophage migration inhibitory factor are associated with adverse long-term outcome in patients with stable coronary artery disease and impaired glucose tolerance or type 2 diabetes mellitus. *Atherosclerosis* **213**, pp. 573–578.

65. Schweitzer, K., Bozko, P.M., Dubiel, W., and Naumann, M. (2007) CSN controls NF-kappaB by deubiquitinylation of IkappaBalpha. *Embo J* **26**, pp. 1532–1541.

66. Bianchi, E., Denti, S., Granata, A., Bossi, G., Geginat, J., Villa, A., Rogge, L., and Pardi, R. (2000) Integrin LFA-1 interacts with the transcriptional co-activator JAB1 to modulate AP-1 activity. *Nature* **404**, pp. 617–621.

67. Perez, O.D., Mitchell, D., Jager, G.C., South, S., Murriel, C., McBride, J., Herzenberg, L.A., Kinoshita, S., and Nolan, G.P. (2003) Leukocyte functional antigen 1 lowers T cell activation thresholds and signaling through cytohesin-1 and Jun-activating binding protein 1. *Nat Immunol* **4**, pp. 1083–1092.

68. Mitchell, R.A., Liao, H., Chesney, J., Fingerle-Rowson, G., Baugh, J., David, J., and Bucala, R. (2002) Macrophage migration inhibitory factor (MIF) sustains macrophage proinflammatory function by inhibiting p53: Regulatory role in the innate immune response. *Proc Natl Acad Sci U S A* **99**, pp. 345–350.

69. Hudson, J.D., Shoaibi, M.A., Maestro, R., Carnero, A., Hannon, G.J., and Beach, D.H. (1999) A proinflammatory cytokine inhibits p53 tumor suppressor activity. *J Exp Med* **190**, pp. 1375–1382.

70. Mercer, J., Figg, N., Stoneman, V., Braganza, D., and Bennett, M.R. (2005) Endogenous p53 protects vascular smooth muscle cells from apoptosis and reduces atherosclerosis in ApoE knockout mice. *Circ Res* **96**, pp. 667–674.

71. Atsumi, T., Nishihira, J., Makita, Z., and Koike, T. (2000) Enhancement of oxidised low-density lipoprotein uptake by macrophages in response to macrophage migration inhibitory factor. *Cytokine* **12**, pp. 1553–1556.

72. Chen, L., Yang, G., Zhang, X., Wu, J., Gu, Q., Wei, M., Yang, J., Zhu, Y., NanpingWang, and Guan, Y. (2009) Induction of MIF expression by oxidized LDL via activation of NF-κB in vascular smooth muscle cells. *Atherosclerosis* **207**, pp. 428–433.

73. Schrans-Stassen, B.H., Lue, H., Sonnemans, D.G., Bernhagen, J., and Post, M.J. (2005) Stimulation of vascular smooth muscle cell migration by macrophage migration inhibitory factor. *Antioxid Redox Signal* **7**, pp. 1211–1216.

74. Zernecke, A., Bot, I., Talab, Y.D., Shagdarsuren, E., Bidzhekov, K., Meiler, S., Krohn, R., Schober, A., Sperandio, M., Soehnlein, O., Bornemann, J., Tacke, F., Biessen, E.A., and Weber, C. (February 1, 2008) Protective role of CXC receptor 4/CXC ligand 12 unveils the importance of neutrophils in atherosclerosis. Circ Res. 102(2), pp. 209–217. Epub 2007 Nov 8.

75. Roscic-Mrkic, B., Fischer, M., Leemann, C., Manrique, A., Gordon, C.J., Moore, J.P., Proudfoot, A.E., and Trkola, A. (2003) RANTES (CCL5) uses the proteoglycan CD44 as an auxiliary receptor to mediate cellular activation signals and HIV-1 enhancement. *Blood* **102**, pp. 1169–1177.

76. Huo, Y., Weber, C., Forlow, S.B., Sperandio, M., Thatte, J., Mack, M., Jung, S., Littman, D.R., and Ley, K. (2001) The chemokine KC, but not monocyte chemoattractant protein-1, triggers monocyte arrest on early atherosclerotic endothelium. *J Clin Invest* **108**, pp. 1307–1314.

77. Zernecke, A., Bot, I., Djalali-Talab, Y., Shagdarsuren, E., Bidzhekov, K., Meiler, S., Krohn, R., Schober, A., Sperandio, M., Soehnlein, O., Bornemann, J., Tacke, F., Biessen, E.A., and Weber, C. (2008) Protective role of CXC receptor 4/CXC ligand 12 unveils the importance of neutrophils in atherosclerosis. *Circ Res* **102**, pp. 209–217.

78. Murphy, P.M., Baggiolini, M., Charo, I.F., Hebert, C.A., Horuk, R., Matsushima, K., Miller, L.H., Oppenheim, J.J., and Power, C.A. (2000) International union of pharmacology. XXII. Nomenclature for chemokine receptors. *Pharmacol Rev* **52**, pp. 145–176.

79. Hebert, C.A., Vitangcol, R.V., and Baker, J.B. (1991) Scanning mutagenesis of interleukin-8 identifies a cluster of residues required for receptor binding. *J Biol Chem* **266**, pp. 18989–18994.

80. Kraemer, S., Lue, H., Zernecke, A., Kapurniotu, A., Andreetto, E., Frank, R., Lennartz, B., Weber, C., and Bernhagen, J. (2010) MIF-chemokine receptor interactions in atherogenesis are dependent on an N-loop-based 2-site binding mechanism. *FASEB J.*

81. Weber, C., Kraemer, S., Drechsler, M., Lue, H., Koenen, R.R., Kapurniotu, A., Zernecke, A., and Bernhagen, J. (October 21, 2008) Structural

determinants of MIF functions in CXCR2-mediated inflammatory and atherogenic leukocyte recruitment. *Proc Natl Acad Sci U S A* 105(42), pp. 16278–16283. Epub 2008 Oct 13.

82. Wakasugi, K., and Schimmel, P. (1999) Two distinct cytokines released from a human aminoacyl-tRNA synthetase. *Science* **284**, pp. 147–151.
83. Wakasugi, K., Slike, B.M., Hood, J., Ewalt, K.L., Cheresh, D.A., and Schimmel, P. (2002) Induction of angiogenesis by a fragment of human tyrosyl-tRNA synthetase. *J Biol Chem* **277**, pp. 20124–20126.
84. Yang, D., Chertov, O., Bykovskaia, S.N., Chen, Q., Buffo, M.J., Shogan, J., Anderson, M., Schroder, J.M., Wang, J.M., Howard, O.M., and Oppenheim, J.J. (1999) Beta-defensins: Linking innate and adaptive immunity through dendritic and T cell CCR6. *Science* **286**, pp. 525–528.
85. Hoover, D.M., Boulegue, C., Yang, D., Oppenheim, J.J., Tucker, K., Lu, W., and Lubkowski, J. (2002) The structure of human macrophage inflammatory protein-3alpha /CCL20. Linking antimicrobial and CC chemokine receptor-6-binding activities with human beta-defensins. *J Biol Chem* **277**, pp. 37647–37654.
86. Aliberti, J., Valenzuela, J.G., Carruthers, V.B., Hieny, S., Andersen, J., Charest, H., Reis e Sousa, C., Fairlamb, A., Ribeiro, J.M., and Sher, A. (2003) Molecular mimicry of a CCR5 binding-domain in the microbial activation of dendritic cells. *Nat Immunol* **4**, pp. 485–490.
87. Alcami, A. (2003) Viral mimicry of cytokines, chemokines and their receptors. *Nat Rev Immunol* **3**, pp. 36–50.
88. Rubartelli, A., Cozzolino, F., Talio, M., and Sitia, R. (1990) A novel secretory pathway for interleukin-1 beta, a protein lacking a signal sequence. *EMBO J* **9**, pp. 1503–1510.
89. Nickel, W. (2010) Pathways of unconventional protein secretion. *Curr Opin Biotechnol* **21**, pp. 621–626.
90. Nickel, W., and Rabouille, C. (2009) Mechanisms of regulated unconventional protein secretion. *Nat Rev Mol Cell Biol* **10**, pp. 148–155.
91. Nickel, W., and Seedorf, M. (2008) Unconventional mechanisms of protein transport to the cell surface of eukaryotic cells. *Annu Rev Cell Dev Biol* **24**, pp. 287–308.
92. Pagler, T.A., Wang, M., Mondal, M., Murphy, A.J., Westerterp, M., Moore, K.J., Maxfield, F.R., and Tall, A.R. (2011) Deletion of ABCA1 and ABCG1 impairs macrophage migration because of increased Rac1 signaling. *Circ Res* **108**, pp. 194–200.

93. Chen, Z., Sakuma, M., Zago, A.C., Zhang, X., Shi, C., Leng, L., Mizue, Y., Bucala, R., and Simon, D. (2004) Evidence for a role of macrophage migration inhibitory factor in vascular disease. *Arterioscler Thromb Vasc Biol* **24**, pp. 709–714.

94. Leech, M., Metz, C.N., Santos, L., Peng, T., Holdsworth, S.R., Bucala, R., and Morand, E.F. (1998) Involvement of macrophage migration inhibitory factor in the evolution of rat adjuvant arthritis. *Arthritis Rheum* **41**, pp. 910–917.

95. Qi, D., Hu, X., Wu, X., Merk, M., Leng, L., Bucala, R., and Young, L.H. (2009) Cardiac macrophage migration inhibitory factor inhibits JNK pathway activation and injury during ischemia/reperfusion. *J Clin Invest* **119**(12), pp. 3807–3816.

96. Gao, X.M., Liu, Y., White, D., Su, Y., Drew, B.G., Bruce, C.R., Kiriazis, H., Xu, Q., Jennings, N., Bobik, A., Febbraio, M.A., Kingwell, B.A., Dart, A.M., Morand, E.F., and Du, X.J. (2011) Deletion of macrophage migration inhibitory factor protects the heart from severe ischemia-reperfusion injury: A predominant role of anti-inflammation. *J Mol Cell Cardiol* **50**(6), pp. 991–999.

97. Horuk, R., and Proudfoot, A.E. (2009) Drug discovery targeting the chemokine system--where are we? *Front Biosci (Elite Ed)* **1**, pp. 209–219.

98. Liang, X. (2008) CXCR4, inhibitors and mechanisms of action. *Chem Biol Drug Des* **72**, pp. 97–110.

99. Rosengren, E., Bucala, R., Åman, P., Jacobsson, L., Odh, G., Metz, C.N., and Rorsman, H. (1996) The immunoregulatory mediator macrophage migration inhibitory factor (MIF) catalyzes a tautomerization reaction. *Mol Med* **2**, pp. 143–149.

100. Al-Abed, Y., Dabideen, D., Aljabari, B., Valster, A., Messmer, D., Ochani, M., Tanovic, M., Ochani, K., Bacher, M., Nicoletti, F., Metz, C., Pavlov, V.A., Miller, E.J., and Tracey, K.J. (2005) ISO-1 binding to the tautomerase active site of MIF inhibits its pro-inflammatory activity and increases survival in severe sepsis. *J Biol Chem* **280**, pp. 36541–36544.

101. Dios, A., Mitchell, R.A., Aljabari, B., Lubetsky, J., O'Connor, K., Liao, H., Senter, P.D., Manogue, K.R., Lolis, E., Metz, C., Bucala, R., Callaway, D.J., and Al-Abed, Y. (2002) Inhibition of MIF bioactivity by rational design of pharmacological inhibitors of MIF tautomerase activity. *J Med Chem* **45**, pp. 2410–2416.

102. Senter, P.D., Al-Abed, Y., Metz, C.N., Benigni, F., Mitchell, R.A., Chesney, J., Han, J., Gartner, C.G., Nelson, S.D., Todaro, G.J., and Bucala, R. (2002) Inhibition of macrophage migration inhibitory factor (MIF)

tautomerase and biological activities by acetaminophen metabolites. *Proc Natl Acad Sci U S A* **99**, pp. 144–149.

103. Fingerle-Rowson, G., Kaleswarapu, D.R., Schlander, C., Kabgani, N., Brocks, T., Reinart, N., Busch, R., Schutz, A., Lue, H., Du, X., Liu, A., Xiong, H., Chen, Y., Nemajerova, A., Hallek, M., Bernhagen, J., Leng, L., and Bucala, R. (2009) A tautomerase-null macrophage migration-inhibitory factor (MIF) gene knock-in mouse model reveals that protein interactions and not enzymatic activity mediate MIF-dependent growth regulation. *Mol Cell Biol* **29**, pp. 1922–1932.
104. Nissen, S.E., Tardif, J.C., Nicholls, S.J., Revkin, J.H., Shear, C.L., Duggan, W.T., Ruzyllo, W., Bachinsky, W.B., Lasala, G.P., and Tuzcu, E.M. (2007) Effect of torcetrapib on the progression of coronary atherosclerosis. *N Engl J Med* **356**, pp. 1304–1316.
105. Nissen, S.E., Tuzcu, E.M., Brewer, H.B., Sipahi, I., Nicholls, S.J., Ganz, P., Schoenhagen, P., Waters, D.D., Pepine, C.J., Crowe, T.D., Davidson, M.H., Deanfield, J.E., Wisniewski, L.M., Hanyok, J.J., and Kassalow, L.M. (2006) Effect of ACAT inhibition on the progression of coronary atherosclerosis. *N Engl J Med* **354**, pp. 1253–1263.

Chapter 3

Peptide-Based Vaccination Strategies to Promote Treg-Mediated Atheroprotection

Hafid Ait-Oufella,[a,b] Olivier Herbin,[a,b] Alain Tedgui,[a,b] and Ziad Mallat[a,b,c]

[a] *Paris Cardiovascular Research Center, INSERM and Assistance Publique-Hôpitaux de Paris, Hôpital Européen Georges Pompidou, 75015 Paris, France*

[b] *Université Paris Descartes, Paris, France*

[c] *Department of Medicine, Division of Cardiovascular Medicine, University of Cambridge, Addenbrooke's Hospital, Cambridge CB2 2QQ, England, UK*

zm255@medschl.cam.ac.uk

Atherosclerosis is a chronic arterial inflammatory process driven mainly by innate and adaptive immune mechanisms in response to modified lipoproteins. Genetically invalidated mouse models have identified several pathogenic T cell subsets implicated in atherogenesis. Th1 T cells that produce Interferon-γ accelerate atherosclerosis development and induce a "vulnerable" plaque phenotype [1]. Experimental studies examining the involvement of Th2 and Th17 T cells are contradictory, with some showing pro-atherogenic effects and others protective or no significant effect [2,

Atherosclerosis: Treatment and Prevention
Edited by Christian Weber and Oliver Soehnlein

ISBN 978-981-4316-26-2 (Hardcover), ISBN 978-981-4364-26-3 (eBook)
www.panstanford.com

3]. In 2006, we have identified for the first time an atheroprotective T cell subset called regulatory T cells, that inhibits pro-atherogenic T cells [4] through several mechanisms, including the production of anti-atherogenic cytokines, such as IL-10 and TGF-β. Subsequently, several vaccination-like strategies have emerged to promote antigen-specific Treg cell responses with the aim of limiting atherosclerotic plaque development and/or vulnerability to rupture.

3.1 Regulatory T cells Maintain Self-Tolerance

Natural Treg cells, characterized by the expression of CD4, CD25, and the transcriptional factor Foxp3 (forkhead/winged helix transcription factor) develop in the thymus and recognize specific self-antigen (for review [5]). They home to peripheral tissues to maintain self-tolerance and to prevent autoimmunity by inhibiting pathogenic T lymphocytes. Subsets of Treg cells, induced Treg cells (iTreg), are also generated in the periphery during an active immune response. Naïve $CD4^+CD25^-$ in the periphery can be converted, in the presence of TGF-β, IL-10, or low dose of antigenic peptide into $CD4^+CD25^+Foxp3^+$ cells. The iTreg cells can be induced by IL-10 (Tr1 cells), TGF-β (Th3 cells), or after repetitive antigen stimulation [6]. They mediate suppressor functions through the production of IL-10 and/or TGF-β.

Under homeostatic conditions, natural Treg cells are the major cells exhibiting suppressive functions. This population is composed of two Treg subsets that have distinct phenotypes and homeostasis in normal unmanipulated mice. One is composed of quiescent cells with long lifespan and the other is a cycling nTreg subset that divides extensively and expresses multiple activation markers, suggesting that it is composed of autoreactive Tregs that are continuously activated by tissue self-antigens [7]. An extremely close TCR clonal homology has been found between regulatory and memory CD4+ T cells, suggesting that a proportion of this regulatory population is generated from rapidly dividing, highly differentiated memory CD4+ T cells [8]. *In vitro*, these cells are anergic. They do not proliferate upon stimulation and strongly suppress effector T cell proliferation [9]. The transcriptional factor, Foxp3 is necessary to mediate the inhibitory effect of Treg cells on pathogenic T cells, since no suppressive function was observed in $CD4^+CD25^+$ isolated from Foxp3 knock-out mice [10]. Foxp3 is specific for Treg cell lineage. However, functional Foxp3 is not required for Treg cell development [11] but is instrumental, through its interaction with other transcription factors such as NFAT [12] and AML1 [13], in transcriptional repression of genes involved in T cell activation such as IL-2, and at the opposite induces genes required for Treg function such as CD25 (IL-2 receptor-α chain) and CTLA-4 (Cytotoxic T-Lymphocyte Antigen 4) [12, 14–16].

Three general modes of suppression have been proposed to explain the inhibitory actions of Treg cells on activated T cells, although these are not completely elucidated. These include cell contact-dependent suppression, consumption and limitation of growth factors such as IL-2, and the production of inhibitory cytokines. Cell contact-dependent inhibition mediated by Treg cells involves engagement of CTLA-4 expressed on Treg cells with CD80 molecules expressed on effector T cells, or interaction of CTLA-4 with CD80/CD86 on DCs [17]. The interaction between Treg cells and DCs induces indoleamine dioxygenase (IDO) which leads to down-regulation of effector T cell responses through tryptophan catabolism [18]. A passive mechanism of effector T cell inactivation mediated by Treg cells was also proposed. Effector T cells secrete IL-2 upon activation, which binds to CD25 on Treg cells, maintains and activates Treg cell genes such as Foxp3, which in turn down-regulates IL-2 secretion in a feedback loop. Once activated, Treg cells suppress effector T cells but also deprive them from IL-2. One recent finding demonstrated that Treg cells induce apoptosis of activated T cells *in vitro* and *in vivo* by depriving them from IL-2 [19]. In addition, Treg cells could inhibit activated lymphocytes by producing soluble inhibitory cytokines, such as IL-10 and TGF-β (see below), or IL-35 [20]. Production of these cytokines may also induce deactivation of DCs, leading to a loss of ability to activate effector T cells with distinct antigen specificity to Treg cells, a mechanism called *bystander immune suppression*. However, the requirement of these soluble cytokines in suppressive function mediated by nTreg *in vivo* is complicated by the existence of iTreg that uses overlapping inhibition mechanisms.

3.2 Two Major Mediators of Treg Cell Function with Relevance to Atherosclerosis: TGF-β and IL-10

3.2.1 TGF-β

3.2.1.1 TGF-β and Treg cell function

The importance of TGF-β in the immune system was highlighted by the discovery that TGF-β-deficient mice develop multiple inflammatory diseases [21, 22]. These were associated with enhanced T cell proliferation, activation, and a switch of T cell differentiation toward both Th1 and Th2 profiles. The activation of T cells in this setting results from the fact that TGF-β inhibits the proliferation, activation, and differentiation of T cells towards Th1 and Th2 [23, 24]. In addition, TGF-β1 has been shown to maintain Treg cells in the periphery by acting as a costimulatory factor for expression of Foxp3 [25]. This dual effect on effector T cells and Treg cells is likely to contribute to TGF-β regulation of peripheral T cell tolerance.

Studies on the modalities of requirement of TGF-β for Treg suppressive function remain controversial [26, 27]. *In vitro*, TGF-β produced by Treg cells appears to be dispensable for the suppressive function of Treg cells [28], but adoptive transfer of Treg cells with specific deletion of TGF-β failed to inhibit T cell-induced colitis *in vivo*, suggesting the importance of Treg cell-derived TGF-β in maintaining self-tolerance [28]. However, previous studies with Treg cells isolated from TGF-β1-deficient mice have generated contrasting results [29–31]. In particular, transfer of Treg cells from DO11.10. TGF-ß1$^{-/-}$ mice, which recognize ovalbumin epitope, together with CD4^{+}CD45RB^{high} cells into lymphopenic mice prevented colitis similarly to the equivalent cells taken from DO11.10/TGF-ß1$^{+/+}$ mice, showing that Treg cells can develop in the absence of TGF-ß1 and retain suppressor function *in vivo* [30]. Interestingly, the suppressor function of TGF-ß1$^{-/-}$ Treg was abrogated by injection of anti-TGF-β, indicating that TGF-ß1 is important for the suppressive function of Treg cells even though these cells do not produce it [30].

Besides maintenance of nTreg in the periphery, several studies demonstrated that TGF-β induced conversion of Foxp3− cells to Foxp3+ cells, in extrathymic sites. Overexpression of TGF-β in mouse T cells increased the proportion of Th3, which are protective in adoptive transfer model of experimental autoimmune encephalomyelitis [32]. Additional studies have extended these findings *in vivo*, particularly in settings of chronic antigen exposure or antigen-specific tolerance induction. For example, oral exposure to antigen induced antigen-specific Foxp3-positive cells in large part dependent on TGF-β [33]. Furthermore, continuous low-dose administration of specific peptide induced a TGF-β-dependent formation of suppressor cells that can persist for long periods in the absence of antigen [34]. Thus, it appears that the induction of Foxp3 positive cells in the periphery depends on TGF-β. The gut environment represents a preferential site of extra-thymic Treg cell development depending on TGF-β. The intestinal immune system has evolved redundant regulatory strategies to maintain immune homeostasis. In this regard, the gut is home to a large number of Treg cells, which have the capacity to inhibit many pathogenic T cells in antigen independent manner, using bystander suppression mechanism (for review [35]). DCs have the capacity to induce Treg cell formation depending on TGF-β and retinoic acid, which is a vitamin A metabolite highly expressed in the gut-associated lymphoid tissue (GALT) [36, 37]. Recent studies proposed a mechanism that explains how DCs induce Treg cell development in the gut [38, 39]. DCs express the integrin $\alpha v\beta 8$, which has the capacity to activate the inactive form of TGF-β. This factor is secreted in inactive complexes with a latency-associated peptide, a protein derived from the N-terminal region of the TGF-β gene product, and extracellular activation of these complexes is critical for TGF-β function. It was reported that DC lacking integrin $\alpha v\beta 8$ fail to induce Treg cells *in vitro*, an effect that depends on TGF-β activity [39]. Furthermore, these mice have reduced proportions of Treg cells in colonic tissue and, thus, increased T cell activation, leading to colitis [39]. Therefore, integrin $\alpha v\beta 8$-mediated TGF-β activation by DC is essential for preventing immune dysfunction. This mechanism appears to be specific for colon, since the Treg number in the spleen of integrin $\alpha v\beta 8$-knockout mice remains unaffected [39].

TGF-β converts naïve T cells into Treg cells that prevent autoimmunity. However, in the presence of IL-6, TGF-β also promotes the differentiation of naïve T lymphocytes into cytokine-producing Th17 cells, which promote autoimmunity and inflammation [40]. This raises the question of how TGF-β can generate such distinct outcomes. Recently, Mucida *et al.* identified the vitamin A metabolite retinoic acid as a key regulator of TGF-β-dependent immune responses, capable of inhibiting the IL-6-driven induction of proinflammatory Th17 cells and promoting anti-inflammatory Treg cell differentiation [36]. The authors concluded that a common metabolite such as retinoic acid can regulate the balance between pro- and anti-inflammatory pathways. However, these data were complicated by recent results showing that TGF-β in combination with IL-6 not only leads to increased IL-17 but also IL-10, which has anti-inflammatory properties [41]. These cells have regulatory effects and are protective against experimental autoimmune encephalomyelitis. Hence, TGF-β and IL-6 drive Th17 regulatory cells, which are different from pathogenic Th17 lineage induced, for example, by IL-23.

3.2.1.2 Role of T cell-dependent TGF-β in atherosclerosis

Previous studies using either TGF-β neutralizing antibodies [42] soluble TGF-β receptors [43] or genetic deficiency in TGF-β [44] demonstrated an anti-atherosclerotic effect of TGF-β in apoE$^{-/-}$ mice. In these murine models, accelerated atherosclerosis development was observed, with increased infiltration of inflammatory cells within lesions, together with reduced collagen content [42, 43]. Therefore, TGF-β has anti-inflammatory effects in addition to its stabilizing effects within the lesions through the induction of extracellular matrix synthesis.

The availability of mice with specific deletion of TGF-β signaling in T cells facilitated the study of the specific role of TGF-β in T cell-induced atherosclerosis [45, 46]. The transplantation of bone marrow from T cell dominant-negative TGF-β receptor type II mice into irradiated LDLr$^{-/-}$ mice showed accelerated atherogenesis [46] and increased differentiation of T cells toward both pathogenic Th1 and Th2 phenotypes [45, 46]. These studies clearly showed a protective role of T cell-specific TGF-β activity against atherogenesis by inhibiting activation of both Th1 and Th2 pathways.

The cellular source of TGF-β within atherosclerotic lesions is multiple, since all atheroma-associated cells have the capacity to produce this cytokine. Treg cells, which can be both source and target of TGF-β, may contribute to its production and/or protective activity. Strategies using mouse models with genetic deficiency of Treg cells or strategies using CD25 neutralizing antibodies clearly demonstrated a protective role of Treg cells against atherogenesis [4]. Moreover, Treg depletion did not influence lesion size or inflammatory phenotype when the host T cells did not respond to TGF-β (see Fig. 3.1), suggesting that this factor is required for the atheroprotective effect of Treg cells. Furthermore, reduction in atherosclerosis in $ApoE^{-/-}$ mice has also been achieved through adoptive transfer of $CD4^+CD25^+$ regulatory T cells [4, 47]. More recently, « vaccination » against Tregs was performed in LDL receptor deficient mice using dendritic cells which were transfected with Foxp3 encoding mRNA. Dendritic cells injection induced a significant decrease of Foxp3 Treg population in blood, lymph nodes, spleen and an acceleration of atherosclerosis in the aortic sinus [48].

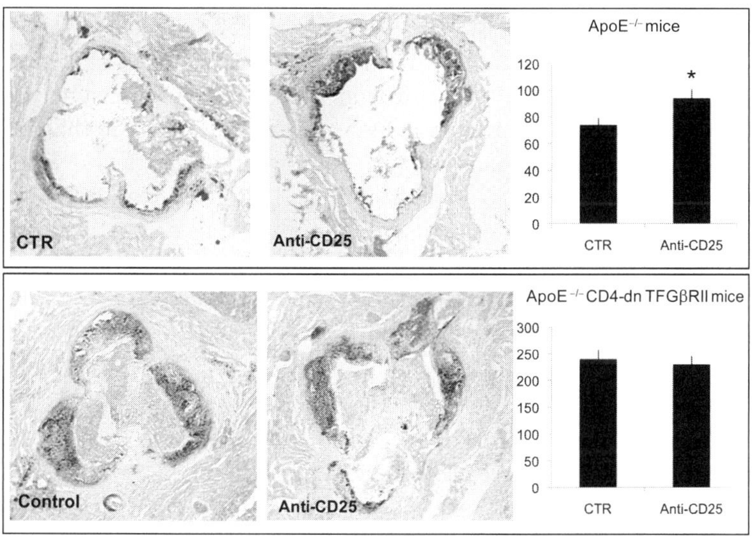

Figure 3.1 Treg depletion induced an increase of lesion size in apoE-/- mice but had no effect in apoE-/- CD4-dn TGFβ RII whose CD4 T cells did not respond to TGFβ (Ait-Oufella *et al.*, *Nat Med* 2006)

3.2.2 IL-10

3.2.2.1 IL-10 and Treg cell function

Experiments using specific deletion of IL-10 in lymphocytes have revealed the importance of this cytokine in the protection against inflammatory processes. Mice with deficiency of IL-10 are susceptible to inflammatory diseases such as colitis [49]. Furthermore, adoptive transfer of IL-10-deficient CD4$^+$ T cells into lymphopenic mice induces severe colitis despite the ability of the recipient's innate immune system to produce IL-10 [50]. In lymphocytes, the production of IL-10 has been associated to Th2 subset and Treg cells. Among the regulatory T cells, both nTreg and induced Tr1 cells have the capacity to produce IL-10. Tr1 cells exhibit their suppressor function by a cell contact-independent, cytokine-dependent mechanism that involves both IL-10 and TGF-β. Several experiments have revealed the requirement of IL-10 to modulate the activation of DCs that prime Tr1 development. Specifically, it has been shown that culture of bone marrow cells in the presence of IL-10 induces the differentiation of tolerogenic DCs expressing CD11c^{low}CD45RB^{high}, which have the capacity to induce Tr1 phenotype *in vitro* and *in vivo* [51]. In addition, repetitive administration of antigens has been shown to induce IL-10 Tregs that originate from Th1 T cells and that suppress immune response [6]. However, more recent study showed that the formation of Tr1 cells expressing IL-10 rather requires the presence of TGF-β and may occur independently of IL-10 [52]. In addition, IL-27 (a member of IL-12 family) was recently involved, together with TGF-β, in promoting the generation of IL-10-producing Tr1 cells [53, 54]. We can, therefore, speculate that TGF-β-induced Treg cells stimulate DC to produce IL-27, which promotes Tr1 formation.

3.2.2.2 Role of IL-10 in atherosclerosis

The role of endogenous IL-10 has been clearly established in mouse models of atherosclerosis. We and others have shown that IL-10 deficiency in C57BL/6 mice fed an atherogenic diet promotes early atherosclerotic lesion formation, characterized by increased infiltration of inflammatory cells, particularly activated T cells, and by increased production of proinflammatory cytokines [55, 56]. Similar results have been reported in IL-10$^{-/-}$/apoE$^{-/-}$ mice fed a chow diet [57]. Using a model of chimeric LDLr$^{-/-}$ mice in which bone marrow cells were deficient in IL-10, we also showed that the absence of IL-10 induced a clear switch toward a Th1 immune response, associated with enhanced accumulation of T cells and macrophages within the lesions [58]. These results provided evidence that leukocyte-derived IL-10 is instrumental in the prevention of atherosclerotic lesion development and in the modulation of cellular and collagen plaque composition, at least in part, through a systemic immune response modulation [58]. The effect of IL-10 disruption in specific cell subtypes (macrophages, DCs, or T cells) on lesion development and progression is still unknown. Consistent with a protective role of IL-10 in atherosclerosis, systemic or local overexpression of IL-10 by adenoviral gene transfer in collar-induced carotid atherosclerosis of LDLr$^{-/-}$ mice was found to be highly efficient in preventing atherosclerosis [59]. It is noteworthy that overexpression of IL-10 by activated T lymphocytes reduced atherosclerosis in LDLr$^{-/-}$ mice [60]. The authors attributed these effects to a switch towards a Th2-like phenotype but failed to report on IL-4 production. In fact, the mouse strain used in that study has been shown to be unable to generate Th2 responses [61], leading us to suggest that the protective effect on atherosclerosis was associated with a Tr1-like phenotype. This is consistent with studies showing that transfer of clones of Tr1 cells reduces lesion development in apoE$^{-/-}$ mice [62] and that promotion of endogenous adaptive Tr1 cell response plays a significant role in limiting disease development during the natural course of atherosclerosis [63] (see below).

3.3 Strategies to Enhance Treg Function in Atherosclerosis

3.3.1 Strategies to Promote CD4$^+$CD25$^+$Foxp3$^+$ Treg Cell Function *in vivo*

Following our initial report on the protective role of CD4$^+$CD25$^+$Foxp3$^+$ Treg cells in atherosclerosis [4], other studies have been published supporting an anti-atherogenic role for this T cell subtype (see Fig. 3.2). Recent studies highlighted the role of inducible costimulatory molecule (ICOS) on regulatory T cell responses in atherosclerosis [64]. LDLr$^{-/-}$ mice transplanted with ICOS-deficient marrow showed accelerated atherosclerosis and enhanced infiltration of CD4$^+$ T cells as well as increased macrophage content. This was associated with decreased numbers of Foxp3$^+$ Treg cells and impaired *in vitro* Treg-suppressive function in ICOS-deficient mice compared with control mice, suggesting that ICOS modulates atherosclerosis through its effect on Treg cell responses [64]. Compound deficient apoE$^{-/-}$/Cxcl10$^{-/-}$ mice fed a Western-style diet demonstrated significant reductions in atherogenesis as compared with *apoE*$^{-/-}$ controls, and this was associated with increased Foxp3 expression, as well as IL-10 and TGF-β1 immunostaining [65].

The identification of a critical role of naturally occurring Treg cells in atherosclerosis has led to the initiation of studies aimed at promoting Treg response *in vivo* (see Table 3.1). Two different strategies have been used. Based on the unique capacity of anti-CD3-specific antibodies to restore self-tolerance in type 1 diabetes [66], Steffens *et al.* applied this strategy in the context of atherosclerosis and showed that anti-CD3 antibody therapy reduced plaque development when administered before a high-cholesterol diet and markedly decreased lesion progression in mice with already established atherosclerosis. This was associated with increased production of TGF-β and enhanced expression of Foxp3 in lymph node and spleen cells, respectively, suggesting a regulatory immune response [67]. Oral administration of anti-CD3 also reduced atherosclerosis in mice through the expansion of a Treg subset called $CD4^+LAP^+$ (LAP for Latent Associated protein) [68]. *In vivo* TGF-β neutralization abolished atheroprotective effects of anti-CD3 treatment, confirming previous studies that reported TGF-β-dependent suppressive functions of $CD4^+LAP^+$ Tregs [69].

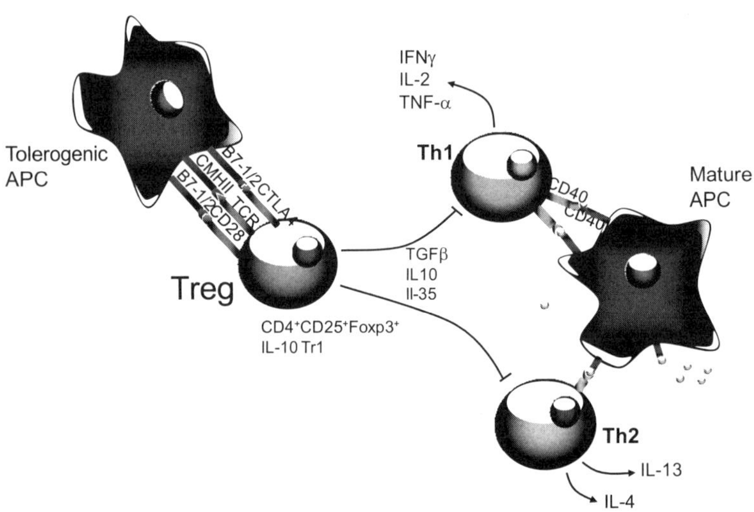

Figure 3.2 Central role of regulatory T cells (Tregs) in the modulation of pathogenic T cell functions in the context of atherosclerosis.

Table 3.1 Examples of strategies to promote Treg expansion in atherosclerotic mouse models

	Delivery	**Regulatory T cell subsets**	**Reference**
Anti-CD3 antibody	Intraperitoneal or intravenous	CD4+CD25+	Steffens *et al.*, *Circulation* 2006
Anti-CD3 antibody	Oral	CD4+LAP+	Sasaki *et al.*, *Circulation* 2009
Viral nucleoprotein	intraperitoneal	Tr-1	Ait-Oufella *et al.*, *Circulation* 2007
Hsp60/65	Nasal or oral	?	Maron *et al.*, *Circulation* 2002 Harats *et al.*, *J Am Coll Cardiol* 2002
OxLDL	Food	Th3	Van Puijvelde *et al.*, *Circulation* 2006
ApoB-derived peptides	Subcutaneous	CD4+CD25+	Herbin *et al.*, Arterioscler Thromb Vasc Biol 2012

The other strategy consisted of the induction of oral tolerance through oral administration of oxLDL or HSP-60 to LDLr$^{-/-}$ mice and resulted in a significant attenuation of the initiation and progression of atherogenesis, associated with increased antigen-specific TGF-β and/or IL-10 production, and increased number of CD4$^+$CD25$^+$Foxp3$^+$ cells in spleen and mesenteric lymph nodes [70, 71]. Even though no direct evidence was presented to relate changes in Treg cell response to disease limitation, these studies suggest novel potential therapeutic avenues in atherosclerosis based on the modulation of Treg response. Von Boehmer's group has also reported that chronic subcutaneous infusion of peptides using osmotic pumps in mice induces expansion of CD4$^+$CD25$^+$ regulatory T cells in lymphoid tissues. Based on this approach, we have recently showed that infusion of apoB-derived peptides subcutaneously in apoE$^{-/-}$ mice induced antigen-specific Treg expansion, inhibited pathogenic T cell responses, and decreased atherosclerosis development and progression [72].

Another strategy may consist of the interference with Treg-inhibitory signals, such as leptin-dependent signaling. Leptin directly affects the immune response, and initial studies reported reversal of starvation-induced immunosuppression *in vivo* following leptin administration, associated with enhanced T cell proliferation and promotion of Th1 proinflammatory response [73]. More recent studies clearly showed that lack or inhibition of leptin/leptin receptor pathway protects against the development of various immuno-inflammatory diseases in experimental models, ranging from colitis [74] to encephalomyelitis [75, 76] or diabetes [77]. Protection was associated, at least in some experiments [76], with a shift of the cytokine profile toward increased Th2/Treg type, and increased number of Treg cells in lymphoid organs of mice with defective leptin signaling. Therefore, leptin signaling may alter Treg cell function and accelerate atherosclerosis. In agreement with this hypothesis, we reported [78] that leptin-deficiency (ob/ob) in $LDLr^{-/-}$ mice induces a marked reduction in atherosclerotic lesion development, compared with $LDLr^{-/-}$ mice having similar total cholesterol levels. $LDLr^{-/-}$/ob/ob mice show reduced Th1 response, enhanced expression of Foxp3, and improved Treg cell function. Leptin receptor-deficient (db/db) mice display marked increase in the number and suppressive function of Treg cells. Supplementation of Treg-deficient lymphocytes with Treg cells from db/db mice in $apoE^{-/-}$ mice induces a significant reduction of lesion size and a marked inhibition of IFN-γ production, compared with supplementation by Treg cells from wild-type mice. Our results are substantiated by those of De Rosa *et al.* [79], showing that leptin inhibits the proliferation of Treg cells *in vitro* and *in vivo*, in part through modulation of cyclin-dependent kinase inhibitor p27 (p27(kip1)) and the phosphorylation of the extracellular-related kinases 1 (ERK1) and ERK2. These results identify a critical role for leptin/leptin receptor pathway in the modulation of the regulatory immune response and point to an important target for therapeutic interventions in immune and autoimmune diseases, such as atherosclerosis.

3.3.2 Strategies to Promote Foxp3-Independent Regulatory T Cell Response

Several studies addressed the role of mucosal tolerance to HSP (expected to induce Treg cells) in the development of experimental atherosclerosis [80, 81]. Both studies showed a reduction in lesion size following oral administration of HSP-65 in $LDLr^{-/-}$ mice immunized with *Mycobacterium tuberculosis* or fed an atherogenic diet [80, 81], suggesting that tolerance induction toward HSP may be protective against atherosclerosis. The mechanisms leading to lesion reduction have not been clearly delineated, but the T cell cytokine profile was switched toward a Th2 phenotype with high production of IL-4 [80] or IL-10 [81]. These results suggest that mucosal administration of antigen reduces plaque development. However, additional mechanistic work is required to understand the potential role of the regulatory immune response in this process.

The hypothesis that an imbalance exists between the effector and the regulatory arms of the immune response suggests that supplementation with Treg cells may lead to the induction of immune suppression and a reduction in pathogenic T cell-mediated responses, ultimately altering plaque development and/or composition. We showed that the administration of a clone of ovalbumin-specific Tr1 cells [82], with its cognate antigen, to apoE$^{-/-}$ mice induced a significant suppression of Th1 (and Th2)-mediated responses and led to an increase in IL-10 production by stimulated peripheral T cells [62]. Tr1 responses were associated with a significant reduction in atherosclerotic plaque development and a marked reduction in the relative accumulation of inflammatory macrophages and T lymphocytes with a preservation of smooth muscle cell and collagen contents of the atherosclerotic plaques. These results showed that modulation of the peripheral immune response is achievable by transfer of Tr1 cells with no specificity to a known plaque antigen and leads to limitation of plaque development in apoE$^{-/-}$ mice, probably through bystander immune suppression. In another study, we showed that treatment of apoE$^{-/-}$ mice with measles virus nucleoprotein, a component of measles virus known to inhibit DC activation [83], induces a DC-dependent Tr1-like phenotype characterized by increased IL-10, but reduced IFN-γ and IL-4 production, and leads to significant inhibition of lesion development and progression [63]. These results suggest that immuno-modulatory properties of measles virus may be harnessed for the treatment of atherosclerosis. More recently, a group has reported that nasal immunization of apoE$^{-/-}$ mice with an ApoB100 peptide fused to the B subunit of cholera toxin (CTB) that binds to mucosal gangliosides reduced atherosclerosis and leads to the induction of ApoB100-specific regulatory Tr1 cells. However, IL-10 and Foxp3 were not significantly increased when the group that received ApoB100-CTB was compared to the group treated with ovalbumine-CTB, suggesting that Tr-1 population was expanded by the toxin itself [84].

3.4 Conclusion

The last decade has witnessed major advances in our understanding of the pathophysiology of atherosclerosis. The discovery of endogenous counter-regulators of the pathogenic immune response in atherosclerosis led to the identification of an important role for Treg cells in the control of lesion development and/or progression. Efforts should be directed toward the delineation of the major determinants of the regulatory response, the critical subtypes of Treg cells responsible for these protective effects, and the molecular mechanisms involved in their survival, migration, homing, and suppressive function. It is also of utmost importance to examine the therapeutic potential of Treg cells specific for plaque-derived antigens or the utility of vaccination-like strategies using such antigens to promote a disease-specific regulatory response and reduce disease development and complications.

References

1. Gupta, S., *et al.*, IFN-gamma potentiates atherosclerosis in apoE knock-out mice. *J Clin Invest*, 1997. **99**(11): 2752–2761.
2. Tedgui, A., and Z. Mallat, Cytokines in atherosclerosis: Pathogenic and regulatory pathways. *Physiol Rev*, 2006. **86**(2): 515–581.
3. Taleb, S., A. Tedgui, and Z. Mallat, Interleukin-17: Friend or foe in atherosclerosis? *Curr Opin Lipidol*, 2010. **21**(5): 404–408.
4. Ait-Oufella, H., *et al.*, Natural regulatory T cells control the development of atherosclerosis in mice. *Nat Med*, 2006. **12**(2): 178–180.
5. Stephens, G.L., and E.M. Shevach, Foxp3+ regulatory T cells: Selfishness under scrutiny. *Immunity*, 2007. **27**(3): 417–419.
6. Gabrysova, L., *et al.*, Negative feedback control of the autoimmune response through antigen-induced differentiation of IL-10-secreting Th1 cells. *J Exp Med*, 2009. **206**(8): 1755–1767.
7. Fisson, S., *et al.*, Continuous activation of autoreactive CD4+ CD25+ regulatory T cells in the steady state. *J Exp Med*, 2003. **198**(5): 737–746.

8. Akbar, A.N., *et al.*, The dynamic co-evolution of memory and regulatory CD4+ T cells in the periphery. *Nat Rev Immunol*, 2007. **7**(3): 231–237.
9. Fontenot, J.D., *et al.*, Regulatory T cell lineage specification by the forkhead transcription factor foxp3. *Immunity*, 2005. **22**(3): 329–341.
10. Fontenot, J.D., M.A. Gavin, and A.Y. Rudensky, Foxp3 programs the development and function of CD4+CD25+ regulatory T cells. *Nat Immunol*, 2003. **4**(4): 330–336.
11. Lin, W., *et al.*, Regulatory T cell development in the absence of functional Foxp3. *Nat Immunol*, 2007. **8**(4): 359–368.
12. Wu, Y., *et al.*, FOXP3 controls regulatory T cell function through cooperation with NFAT. *Cell*, 2006. **126**(2): 375–387.
13. Ono, M., *et al.*, Foxp3 controls regulatory T-cell function by interacting with AML1/Runx1. *Nature*, 2007. **446**(7136): 685–689.
14. Hori, S., T. Nomura, and S. Sakaguchi, Control of regulatory T cell development by the transcription factor Foxp3. *Science*, 2003. **299**(5609): 1057–1061.
15. Williams, L.M., and A.Y. Rudensky, Maintenance of the Foxp3-dependent developmental program in mature regulatory T cells requires continued expression of Foxp3. *Nat Immunol*, 2007. **8**(3): 277-84.
16. Marson, A., *et al.*, Foxp3 occupancy and regulation of key target genes during T-cell stimulation. *Nature*, 2007. **445**(7130): 931–935.
17. Paust, S., *et al.*, Engagement of B7 on effector T cells by regulatory T cells prevents autoimmune disease. *Proc Natl Acad Sci U S A*, 2004. **101**(28): 10398–10403.
18. Fallarino, F., *et al.*, Modulation of tryptophan catabolism by regulatory T cells. *Nat Immunol*, 2003. **4**(12): 1206–1212.
19. Pandiyan, P., *et al.*, CD4(+)CD25(+)Foxp3(+) regulatory T cells induce cytokine deprivation-mediated apoptosis of effector CD4(+) T cells. *Nat Immunol*, 2007. **8**(12): 1353–1362.
20. Collison, L.W., *et al.*, The inhibitory cytokine IL-35 contributes to regulatory T-cell function. *Nature*, 2007. **450**(7169): 566–569.
21. Kulkarni, A.B., and S. Karlsson, Transforming growth factor-beta-1 knockout mice — a mutation in one cytokine gene causes a dramatic inflammatory disease. *Am J Pathol*, 1993. **143**: 3–9.
22. Shull, M.M., *et al.*, Targeted disruption of the mouse transforming growth factor-beta 1 gene results in multifocal inflammatory disease. *Nature*, 1992. **359**(6397): 693–699.
23. Li, M.O., S. Sanjabi, and R.A. Flavell, Transforming growth factor-beta controls development, homeostasis, and tolerance of T cells by

regulatory T cell-dependent and -independent mechanisms. *Immunity*, 2006. **25**(3): 455–471.

24. Marie, J.C., D. Liggitt, and A.Y. Rudensky, Cellular mechanisms of fatal early-onset autoimmunity in mice with the T cell-specific targeting of transforming growth factor-beta receptor. *Immunity*, 2006. **25**(3): 441–454.
25. Cobbold, S.P., *et al.*, Induction of foxP3+ regulatory T cells in the periphery of T cell receptor transgenic mice tolerized to transplants. *J Immunol*, 2004. **172**(10): 6003–6010.
26. Nakamura, K., A. Kitani, and W. Strober, Cell contact-dependent immunosuppression by CD4(+)CD25(+) regulatory T cells is mediated by cell surface-bound transforming growth factor beta. *J Exp Med*, 2001. **194**(5): 629–644.
27. Piccirillo, C.A., *et al.*, CD4(+)CD25(+) regulatory T cells can mediate suppressor function in the absence of transforming growth factor beta1 production and responsiveness. *J Exp Med*, 2002. **196**(2): 237–246.
28. Li, M.O., Y.Y. Wan, and R.A. Flavell, T cell-produced transforming growth factor-beta1 controls T cell tolerance and regulates Th1- and Th17-cell differentiation. Immunity, 2007. 26(5): 579–591.
29. Kullberg, M.C., *et al.*, TGF-beta1 production by CD4+ CD25+ regulatory T cells is not essential for suppression of intestinal inflammation. *Eur J Immunol*, 2005. **35**(10): 2886–2895.
30. Fahlen, L., *et al.*, T cells that cannot respond to TGF-beta escape control by CD4(+)CD25(+) regulatory T cells. *J Exp Med*, 2005. **201**(5): 737–746.
31. Nakamura, K., *et al.*, TGF-beta 1 plays an important role in the mechanism of CD4+CD25+ regulatory T cell activity in both humans and mice. *J Immunol*, 2004. **172**(2): 834–842.
32. Carrier, Y., *et al.*, Th3 cells in peripheral tolerance. I. Induction of Foxp3-positive regulatory T cells by Th3 cells derived from TGF-beta T cell-transgenic mice. *J Immunol*, 2007. **178**(1): 179–185.
33. Mucida, D., *et al.*, Oral tolerance in the absence of naturally occurring Tregs. *J Clin Invest*, 2005. **115**(7): 1923–1933.
34. Apostolou, I., and H. von Boehmer, *In vivo* instruction of suppressor commitment in naive T cells. *J Exp Med*, 2004. **199**(10): 1401–1408.
35. Belkaid, Y., Regulatory T cells and infection: A dangerous necessity. *Nat Rev Immunol*, 2007. **7**(11): 875–888.

36. Mucida, D., *et al.*, Reciprocal TH17 and regulatory T cell differentiation mediated by retinoic acid. *Science*, 2007. **317**(5835): 256–260.

37. Sun, C.M., *et al.*, Small intestine lamina propria dendritic cells promote de novo generation of Foxp3 T reg cells via retinoic acid. *J Exp Med*, 2007. **204**(8): 1775–1785.

38. Lacy-Hulbert, A., *et al.*, Ulcerative colitis and autoimmunity induced by loss of myeloid alphav integrins. *Proc Natl Acad Sci U S A*, 2007. **104**(40): 15823–15828.

39. Travis, M.A., *et al.*, Loss of integrin alpha(v)beta8 on dendritic cells causes autoimmunity and colitis in mice. *Nature*, 2007. **449**(7160): 361–365.

40. Nurieva, R., *et al.*, Essential autocrine regulation by IL-21 in the generation of inflammatory T cells. *Nature*, 2007. **448**(7152): 480–483.

41. McGeachy, M.J., *et al.*, TGF-beta and IL-6 drive the production of IL-17 and IL-10 by T cells and restrain T(H)-17 cell-mediated pathology. *Nat Immunol*, 2007. **8**(12): 1390–1397.

42. Mallat, Z., *et al.*, Inhibition of transforming growth factor-beta signaling accelerates atherosclerosis and induces an unstable plaque phenotype in mice. *Circ Res*, 2001. **89**(10): 930–934.

43. Lutgens, E., *et al.*, Transforming growth factor-beta mediates balance between inflammation and fibrosis during plaque progression. *Arterioscler Thromb Vasc Biol*, 2002. **22**(6): 975–982.

44. Grainger, D.J., *et al.*, Dietary fat and reduced levels of TGFbeta1 act synergistically to promote activation of the vascular endothelium and formation of lipid lesions. *J Cell Sci*, 2000. **113**(Pt 13): 2355–2361.

45. Gojova, A., *et al.*, Specific abrogation of transforming growth factor-{beta} signaling in T cells alters atherosclerotic lesion size and composition in mice. *Blood*, 2003. **102**(12):4052–4058.

46. Robertson, A.K., *et al.*, Disruption of TGF-beta signaling in T cells accelerates atherosclerosis. *J Clin Invest*, 2003. **112**(9): 1342–1350.

47. Mor, A., *et al.*, Role of naturally occurring CD4+ CD25+ regulatory T cells in experimental atherosclerosis. *Arterioscler Thromb Vasc Biol*, 2007. **27**(4): 893–900.

48. van Es, T., *et al.*, Vaccination against Foxp3(+) regulatory T cells aggravates atherosclerosis. *Atherosclerosis*, 2010. **209**(1): 74–80.

49. Davidson, N.J., *et al.*, T helper cell 1-type CD4+ T cells, but not B cells, mediate colitis in interleukin 10-deficient mice. *J Exp Med*, 1996. **184**(1): 241–251.

50. Asseman, C., *et al.*, An essential role for interleukin 10 in the function of regulatory T cells that inhibit intestinal inflammation. *J Exp Med*, 1999. **190**(7): 995–1004.

51. Wakkach, A., *et al.*, Characterization of dendritic cells that induce tolerance and T regulatory 1 cell differentiation *in vivo*. *Immunity*, 2003. **18**(5): 605–617.

52. Maynard, C.L., *et al.*, Regulatory T cells expressing interleukin 10 develop from Foxp3+ and Foxp3- precursor cells in the absence of interleukin 10. *Nat Immunol*, 2007. **8**(9): 931–941.

53. Stumhofer, J.S., *et al.*, Interleukins 27 and 6 induce STAT3-mediated T cell production of interleukin 10. *Nat Immunol*, 2007. **8**(12): 1363–1371.

54. Korn, T., *et al.*, IL-21 initiates an alternative pathway to induce proinflammatory T(H)17 cells. *Nature*, 2007. **448**(7152): 484–487.

55. Mallat, Z., *et al.*, Protective role of interleukin-10 in atherosclerosis. *Circ Res*, 1999. **85**(8): e17–24.

56. Pinderski Oslund, L.J., *et al.*, Interleukin-10 blocks atherosclerotic events In vitro and *In vivo* [In Process Citation]. *Arterioscler Thromb Vasc Biol*, 1999. **19**(12): 2847–2853.

57. Caligiuri, G., *et al.*, Interleukin-10 deficiency increases atherosclerosis, thrombosis, and low-density lipoproteins in apolipoprotein E knockout mice. *Mol Med*, 2003. **9**(1-2): 10–17.

58. Potteaux, S., *et al.*, Leukocyte-derived interleukin 10 is required for protection Against atherosclerosis in low-density lipoprotein receptor knockout mice. *Arterioscler Thromb Vasc Biol*, 2004. **24**(8):1474–1478.

59. Von Der Thusen, J.H., *et al.*, Attenuation of atherogenesis by systemic and local adenovirus-mediated gene transfer of interleukin-10 in LDLr-/- mice *FASEB J*, 2001. **15**(14): 2730–2732.

60. Pinderski, L.J., *et al.*, Overexpression of interleukin-10 by activated T lymphocytes inhibits atherosclerosis in LDL receptor-deficient Mice by altering lymphocyte and macrophage phenotypes. *Circ Res*, 2002. **90**(10): 1064–1071.

61. Hagenbaugh, A., *et al.*, Altered immune responses in interleukin 10 transgenic mice. *J Exp Med*, 1997. **185**(12): 2101–2110.

62. Mallat, Z., *et al.*, Induction of a regulatory T cell type 1 response reduces the development of atherosclerosis in apolipoprotein E-knockout mice. *Circulation*, 2003. **108**(10): 1232–1237.

63. Ait-Oufella, H., *et al.*, Measles virus nucleoprotein induces a regulatory immune response and reduces atherosclerosis in mice. *Circulation*, 2007. **116**(15): 1707–1713.

64. Gotsman, I., *et al.*, Impaired regulatory T-cell response and enhanced atherosclerosis in the absence of inducible costimulatory molecule. *Circulation*, 2006. **114**(19): 2047–2055.

65. Heller, E.A., *et al.*, Chemokine CXCL10 promotes atherogenesis by modulating the local balance of effector and regulatory T cells. *Circulation*, 2006. **113**(19): 2301–2312.

66. Belghith, M., *et al.*, TGF-beta-dependent mechanisms mediate restoration of self-tolerance induced by antibodies to CD3 in overt autoimmune diabetes. *Nat Med*, 2003. **9**(9): 1202–1208.

67. Steffens, S., *et al.*, Short-term treatment with anti-CD3 antibody reduces the development and progression of atherosclerosis in mice. *Circulation*, 2006. **114**(18): 1977–1984.

68. Sasaki, N., *et al.*, Oral anti-CD3 antibody treatment induces regulatory T cells and inhibits the development of atherosclerosis in mice. *Circulation*, 2009. **120**(20): 1996–2005.

69. Zhang, X., *et al.*, Recovery from experimental allergic encephalomyelitis is TGF-beta dependent and associated with increases in CD4+LAP+ and CD4+CD25+ T cells. *Int Immunol*, 2006. **18**(4): 495–503.

70. van Puijvelde, G.H., *et al.*, Induction of oral tolerance to oxidized low-density lipoprotein ameliorates atherosclerosis. *Circulation*, 2006. **114**(18): 1968–1976.

71. van Puijvelde, G.H., *et al.*, Induction of oral tolerance to HSP60 or an HSP60-peptide activates T cell regulation and reduces atherosclerosis. *Arterioscler Thromb Vasc Biol*, 2007. **27**(12): 2677–2683.

72. Herbin O, Ait-Oufella H, Wang Y, Fredrikson GN, Aubier B, MD, Perez N, Barateau V, Nilsson J, Tedgui A, Mallat Z, Taming Atherosclerosis by Promoting a Specific Regulatory T Cell Response to ApoB100-Derived Peptides. 2010: AHA Chicago.

73. Lord, G.M., *et al.*, Leptin modulates the T-cell immune response and reverses starvation-induced immunosuppression. *Nature*, 1998. **394**(6696): 897–901.

74. Siegmund, B., *et al.*, Leptin receptor expression on T lymphocytes modulates chronic intestinal inflammation in mice. *Gut*, 2004. **53**(7): 965–972.

75. Matarese, G., *et al.*, Requirement for leptin in the induction and progression of autoimmune encephalomyelitis. *J Immunol*, 2001. **166**(10): 5909–5916.
76. De Rosa, V., *et al.*, Leptin neutralization interferes with pathogenic T cell autoreactivity in autoimmune encephalomyelitis. *J Clin Invest*, 2006. **116**(2): 447–455.
77. Lee, C.H., *et al.*, Novel leptin receptor mutation in NOD/LtJ mice suppresses type 1 diabetes progression: II. Immunologic analysis. *Diabetes*, 2006. **55**(1): 171–178.
78. Taleb, S., *et al.*, Defective leptin/leptin receptor signaling improves regulatory T cell immune response and protects mice from atherosclerosis. *Arterioscler Thromb Vasc Biol*, 2007. **27**(12):2691–2698.
79. De Rosa, V., *et al.*, A key role of leptin in the control of regulatory T cell proliferation. *Immunity*, 2007. **26**(2): 241–255.
80. Harats, D., *et al.*, Oral tolerance with heat shock protein 65 attenuates Mycobacterium tuberculosis-induced and high-fat-diet-driven atherosclerotic lesions. *J Am Coll Cardiol*, 2002. **40**(7): 1333–1338.
81. Maron, R., *et al.*, Mucosal administration of heat shock protein-65 decreases atherosclerosis and inflammation in aortic arch of low-density lipoprotein receptor-deficient mice. *Circulation*, 2002. **106**(13): 1708–1715.
82. Groux, H., *et al.*, A CD4+ T-cell subset inhibits antigen-specific T-cell responses and prevents colitis. *Nature*, 1997. **389**(6652): 737–742.
83. Lemarie, C.A., *et al.*, Pressure-induced vascular activation of nuclear factor-kappaB: role in cell survival. *Circ Res*, 2003. **93**(3): 207–212.
84. Klingenberg, R., *et al.*, Intranasal immunization with an apolipoprotein B-100 fusion protein induces antigen-specific regulatory T cells and reduces atherosclerosis. *Arterioscler Thromb Vasc Biol*, 2010. **30**(5): 946–952.

Chapter 4

Eicosanoids in Atherosclerosis

Antonio Di Gennaro, Min Wan, M. Dolores Salvado, Jia Sun, and Jesper Z. Haeggström
Department of Medical Biochemistry and Biophysics, Karolinska Institutet, Stockholm, S-171 77, Sweden
jesper.haeggstrom@ki.se

4.1 Introduction

Eicosanoids (from the Greek *eicosa* = twenty; for twenty carbon fatty acid derivatives) are a widespread family of lipid signaling molecules that are derived from polyunsaturated fatty acids (PUFA). In mammalian cells, the major and most abundant precursor of eicosanoid biosynthesis is arachidonic acid (AA; 20:4, ω6). The compounds generated from the reaction of AA with molecular oxygen through the actions of three types of oxygenases, i.e., cyclooxygenase (COX), lipoxygenase (LOX), and cytochrome P450, comprise the major part of a family of structurally related lipid mediators: prostaglandins (PGs), thromboxanes (TXs), leukotrienes (LTs), and lipoxins (LXs) (Fig. 4.1).

Atherosclerosis: Treatment and Prevention
Edited by Christian Weber and Oliver Soehnlein

ISBN 978-981-4316-26-2 (Hardcover), ISBN 978-981-4364-26-3 (eBook)
www.panstanford.com

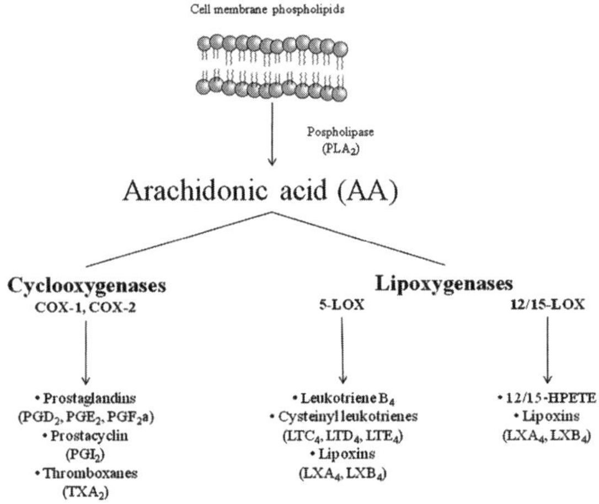

Figure 4.1 Metabolism of arachidonic acid along the cyclooxygenase and lipoxygenase pathways to generate biologically active mediators, i.e., prostanoids, leukotrienes, and lipoxins.

Eicosanoids are hormone-like molecules that exert, in an autocrine and paracrine fashion, complex control over a wide range of physiological processes. Cells of the innate immune system, including tissue macrophages, dendritic cells (DCs), and neutrophils, are the major producers of eicosanoids, which act at nanomolar concentrations, and their effects vary from type to type of cells.

Eicosanoid production is considerably increased during inflammation, and their biosynthetic pathways are of particular clinical relevance because their products are involved in the pathogenesis of various pathologies related to immune functions. During inflammation eicosanoids are present and act as proinflammatory molecules via several mechanisms, e.g., chemoattraction (LTB_4), platelet aggregation (TxA_2), contraction of smooth muscle (cys-LTs, PGs), and modulation of vascular permeability (LTs). On the other hand, LXs appear to play an active role in controlling the resolution of inflammation by stimulating endogenous anti-inflammatory pathways.

In the past decades, research has shown that immune cells (mainly macrophages and some T cells) dominate early atherosclerotic lesions, and their effector molecules accelerate progression of the lesions that finally results in the induction of acute coronary syndromes [64]. That is the reason why the scientific community considers atherosclerosis as an inflammatory disease.

In this scenario, consistent evidences indicate that TxA_2 and PGI_2, and their receptors, play a functional role during atherogenesis as demonstrated by the therapeutic effects of low-dose aspirin (ASA) modulating the vascular inflammatory phenotype typical of the disease and increasing the stability of atherosclerotic plaque [33]. More recently, several studies have brought also the LOX branch of eicosanoid pathways to the attention in the context of atherosclerosis; leukotriene-forming enzymes, and leukotriene receptors are expressed within human atherosclerotic lesions.

In the following sections, the involvement of the different eicosanoid pathways during atherosclerosis will be discussed.

4.2 Prostanoids and Atherosclerosis

Atherosclerosis involves a complex array of factors, including leukocyte adhesion and platelet vasoactive factors. ASA is the most widely used therapeutic agent for the secondary prevention of acute, clinical complications of atherosclerotic cardiovascular diseases (CVD) [33, 122]. Its therapeutic effect is widely attributed to its anti-platelet actions [46, 120, 121], which are mediated by the irreversible inhibition of COX-1, and subsequent suppression of COX-1-derived platelet TxA_2 formation [34, 165]. Prostanoids (PGs and TXs) are bioactive lipids derived from AA by the action of COX isoenzymes and exert important roles in regulation of vascular homeostasis, gastric mucose protection, immune function, and inflammation [119].

Among prostanoids, prostacyclin (PGI_2) and TxA_2 have attracted particular attention for their importance in CVD [23]: the former, generated by COX-2 activity in vascular ECs, is a potent platelet inhibitor and vasodilator, and the latter, released from platelets and their COX-1 activity, is a potent vasoconstrictor and platelet-aggregating agent. Indeed, biosynthesis of TxA_2 and PGI_2 is increased in patients with atherosclerosis [46, 48], reflecting an enhancement of platelet-vessel wall interactions, which has been reported to contribute to the evolution of the atherosclerotic lesion. The effects of TxA_2 and PGI_2 are mediated by specific G-protein-coupled receptors called TP and IP, respectively. Specific deletion of these receptors provided evidence of suppression and significant enhancement of atherosclerosis in apo$E^{-/-}TP^{-/-}$ and apo$E^{-/-}IP^{-/-}$mice, respectively, suggesting strongly proatherogenic and anti-atherogenic actions of TxA_2 and PGI_2. In addition, these results indicate that deletion of the IP enhances the response to thrombogenic stimuli but does not result in spontaneous thrombosis. Hence, the PGI_2-IP signaling axis is important in preventing the initiation of atherosclerosis. However, the opposing biological effects of PGI_2 and TxA_2 on atherogenesis might also be secondary to modulation of the interactions between endothelial cells, platelets and leukocytes, since differential regulation of adhesion molecules such as ICAM-1 and PECAM-1 has been observed in TP and IP deficient mice. In fact, activation of TP receptors on endothelial cells increases the expression of ICAM-1 [78] which promotes monocyte adherence [147]. ICAM-1 is expressed in human atherosclerotic lesions [155], and its circulating levels are associated with atherosclerosis progression [96]. Concordantly, data from Cayatte et al. indicate that inhibition of platelet TxA_2 synthesis with aspirin has no significant effect on atherogenesis or adhesion molecule levels, therefore suggesting that blockade of TP receptors inhibits atherosclerosis by a mechanism independent of platelet-derived TxA_2, perhaps by preventing the expression of adhesion molecules whose expression is stimulated by eicosanoids other than TxA_2 [21]. In fact, TP receptors could be stimulated not only by TxA_2 but also by virtually all eicosanoids; and low doses of ASA do not prevent the formation of other TP-receptor ligands such as hydroxyeicosatetraenoic acids (HETEs) [101] and F_2-isoprostanes (F2-IPs) [110, 129], that are formed by endothelial cells, circulating monocytes and macrophages in the atherosclerotic plaque in response to oxidative stress (Fig. 4.2).

In recent years, atherosclerosis has been redefined as a chronic inflammatory disease [64], where COX-2-derived inflammatory PGs (such as PGE_2 and PGI_2) may directly influence the disease progression by modulating the inflammatory response [33], the expression of metalloproteinases [55], and the growth of cells implicated in the process, such as vascular smooth muscle cells (VSMC) [30].

Controversy has surrounded the role of COX-2 in atherogenesis [97]. Given its importance in inflammation and its colocalization with monocytes and macrophages in atherosclerotic areas, it has been suggested as a rational drug target for reduction of plaque burden and plaque stabilization in humans [26]. In fact, studies have tested the beneficial effect of a combined therapy with TP antagonist and COX-2 selective inhibitor on retarding atherogenesis [41]. Nevertheless, the observation of plaque destabilization ruled out this combined (TP antagonist and COX-2 selective inhibitor) therapeutic option. Surprisingly, COX-2 inhibitors have been reported varyingly not to influence [11, 13, 117], to accelerate

[137], not to accelerate [130], or to retard atherogenesis [15]. This conundrum may reflect differences in timing of the intervention, duration of treatment, or differences among mouse models and drug and dosing regimens.

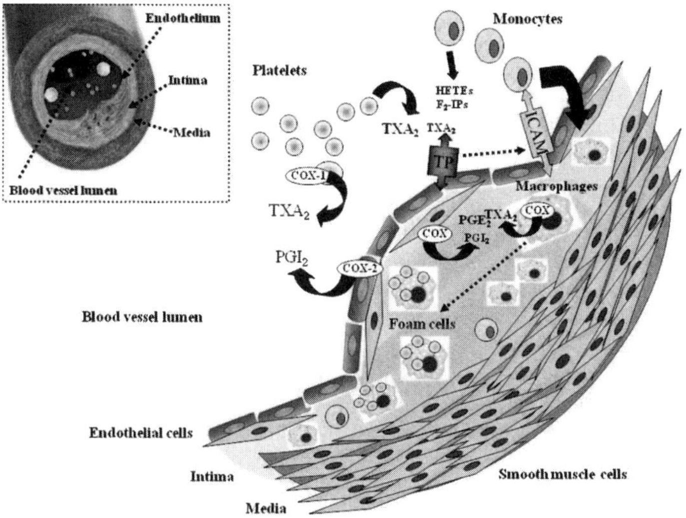

Figure 4.2 Effects of prostanoids on different cell types (i.e., endothelial cells, platelets, smooth muscle cells, monocytes) at the atherosclerotic plaque. Endothelial COX-2-derived PGI_2 counteracts the platelet COX-1-derived TXA_2. TXA_2 produced by platelets, but also by macrophages triggers TX receptor (TP)-dependent ICAM-1 expression, responsible of monocyte recruitment to endothelium, adherence/extravasation and differentiation into macrophages, which will turn into foam cells. Additionally, smooth muscle cells from the media layer may release proinflammatory and proangiogenic PGE_2 and PGI_2, which may cause plaque instability and disruption.

It has been well established that COX-2 is the dominant source of PGI_2 biosynthesis in humans [106], and although PGI_2 (and PGE_2) may mediate inflammation, they also counter the effects of TxA_2 on platelet activation, atherogenesis, vascular proliferation in response to injury, and vascular tone [23, 87]. Indeed, suppression of COX-2-dependent PGI_2 formation, while leaving COX-1-dependent TxA_2 intact, appears likely to explain the augmented risk of myocardial infarction (MI) and stroke observed with structurally distinct selective inhibitors of COX-2.

The severe side effects of NSAIDs and COXIBs [47, 54, 60] have highlighted the need of more specific approaches by targeting effectors downstream of COXs, such as receptors (FP, DP, IP, TP, EPs); or terminal prostanoid synthases (tPGS) [158, 168]. In this regard, PGE_2 effects are transduced by four E prostanoid receptors (EPs), which mediate contrasting biologies. Deletion of EP2, just like the IP, results in salt-sensitive hypertension [49, 86], whereas EP4 mediates anti-inflammatory effects, at least *in vitro* [115, 152]. EP1 and EP3 mediate PGE_2-induced vasoconstriction [79, 115], and PGE_2 can either activate platelets by EP3 or, at higher concentrations, inhibit platelet aggregation by the IP [44, 125]. By contrast, there is one hegemonic inducible PGE_2 terminal synthase, mPGES-1, which is colocalized with COX-2 in activated macrophages in symptomatic atherosclerotic lesions, and its presence in the plaque is reduced by statins [27, 29]. Moreover, data from Wang et al. indicate that mPGES-1 deletion reduces atherogenesis in fat fed hyperlipidemic mice [159]. Interestingly, in addition to the expected depression of PGE_2 production, deletion of mPGES-1 augments systemic biosynthesis of PGI_2, presumably through rediversion of PGH_2 (COX product and substrate of the tPGS) to PGIS observed in VSMC. Additionally, mPGES-1 deletion results in marked depletion of macrophages and macrophage-derived foam cells and limits detrimental angiogenesis in plaque development and instability [65, 111, 159].

Therefore, mPGES-1 pharmacological inhibitors are promising anti-inflammatory drugs with a wide spectrum of applications [139], such as atherosclerosis. Nevertheless, it is currently unclear, whether small molecule inhibitors of mPGES-1 will have the same metabolic and functional effects as gene deletion.

4.3 Leukotrienes and Atherosclerosis: Key Biosynthetic Enzymes

The LTs are biologically active fatty acids, originally isolated from leukocytes and containing a conjugated triene moiety [61, 138]. LT biosynthesis from AA is catalyzed by a series of enzymes, starting with 5-LOX. After cell activation, 5-LOX translocates to the nuclear envelope, where 5-LOX, in concert with 5-lipoxygenase-activating protein (FLAP), oxygenates AA into 5-hydroperoxy-eicosatetraenoic acid (5-HPETE). 5-HPETE is further converted into the unstable epoxide LTA_4, which is transformed by either soluble LTA_4 hydrolase (LTA_4H), producing LTB_4, or conjugated with reduced glutathione by the integral membrane enzyme LTC_4 synthase (LTC_4S), yielding LTC_4. LTC_4 is exported to the extracellular milieu and further metabolized into LTD_4 and LTE_4. LTC_4, LTD_4, and LTE_4 are collectively called cysteinyl leukotrienes (cys-LTs).

More than 20 years ago, it was found that human atherosclerotic plaques have the capacity to produce LTB_4 *ex vivo* [35], and urinary LTE_4 excretion was elevated in patients with either stable coronary artery disease (CAD) [4] or unstable angina (UA) and MI [20]. Moreover, LTC_4 and LTD_4 induced contractions in human atherosclerotic coronary arteries, but not non-atherosclerotic arteries, which indicated that a higher level of CysLT receptors was expressed in human atherosclerotic coronary arteries [3]. Although the cardiovascular actions of LTs have been known for many years, LTs have not been perceived as key players of CVD until recently. Emerging evidence from genetic, biological, and pharmacological studies have indicated that endogenous LTs play an important role in the pathogenesis and clinical progress in CVD, especially in atherosclerosis and its clinical consequences, such as MI and stroke.

4.3.1 5-LOX

Mammalian 5-LOX is a soluble enzyme consisting of 672 or 673 amino acid residues [132]. Very recently, Gilbert and and coworkers reported the crystal structure of a human 5-LOX engineered to improve its stability [56]. The study of the 5-LOX structure revealed that this enzyme contains two domains: the catalytic C-terminal domain, which is mainly helical in structure and contains iron, and the smaller N-terminal C2-like domain. Strikingly, the active site of stable 5-LOX contains a short three-turn helix flanked by extended loops, which is varied from the classic LOX fold in helix α2. The unique orientation of helix α2 in stable-5-LOX greatly limits access to the catalytic iron and yields a distinctive active site cavity.

From mouse genetic studies a locus on chromosome 6 was identified, which confers almost total resistance to atherogenesis [108], and further analysis pointed to 5-LOX as a major gene contributing to atherosclerosis susceptibility in mice [107]. Subsequent studies with genetically modified mice yielded inconsistent results. Thus, Mehrabian et al. reported that LDL receptor-deficient (LDLR$^{-/-}$) mice expressing only one 5-LOX allele (LDLR$^{-/-}$ 5-LOX$^{+/-}$) fed an atherogenic diet for 8 weeks showed around 90% reduction in atherosclerotic lesions [107]. However, this study was based on a small study cohort (*n* = 4), and later, Zhao and coworkers showed that only a modest reduction (24%) in lesion area was observed in ApoE$^{-/-}$5-LOX$^{-/-}$ mice fed an atherogenic diet for 2 months [169]. So far, all other experiments on gene knockout mice have not provided positive results [17, 128, 169]. On the other hand, the LTB_4 signaling cascade may be disrupted in these models, since Qui et al. found segregated expression of 5-LOX and LTA_4H in ApoE–/– mice [131].

For humans it was reported that a 5-LOX promoter variant is associated with increased atherosclerosis [39, 57]. In recent years, upregulated 5-LOX expression at the mRNA and protein levels in human atherosclerotic aorta and coronary and carotid arteries were reported by different groups [3, 131, 140, 148]. Significant 5-LOX expression colocalized mainly with macrophages in atherosclerotic plaques [131, 148] and could also be detected in foam cells, DCs, mast cells, and neutrophils within human atherosclerotic lesions [148]. Moreover, 5-LOX expression was progressively increased with lesion advancement [148], and the leukocytes positive for 5-LOX accumulated at the sites that are most prone to rupture, such as the shoulder regions below the fibrous cap of the atherosclerotic lesion. In addition, 5-LOX expression in human carotid atherosclerotic plaques is associated with symptoms of plaque instability [28, 131].

Pharmacological inhibition of 5-LOX with the compound VIA-2291 in patients with recent acute coronary syndrome demonstrated reduced leukotriene production at 12 weeks after an acute coronary syndrome, which could influence the atherosclerotic process [153]. For pharmacological studies in animals, 5-LOX inhibitor L739010 supplied in an atherogenic diet for 8 weeks did not yield any significant effect in ApoE$^{-/-}$ mice [17]. However, LDLR$^{-/-}$ male mice treated with another 5-LOX inhibitor, ZD4407, for 15 weeks exhibited a reduction of 40% in the intima/media thickness as compared with untreated controls [127]. Moreover, a dual COX/5-LOX inhibitor, licofelone, had similar effects and reduced inflammation in atherosclerotic rabbits [162]. Although the results from animal studies are inconsistent, they revealed that 5-LOX activity could contribute to human atherosclerosis by several processes, including leukocyte recruitment, inflammatory cytokine release, and stimulation of matrix metalloproteinases (MMPs) activity and extracellular matrix breakdown [161]. Effects of inhibiting the LT cascade have been apparent primarily in some short-term studies, whereas the majority of longer studies did not detect any effect of 5-LOX inhibition [127].

4.3.2 FLAP

FLAP was first described in 1990 [38, 135]. It has been shown that FLAP is an AA binding protein [103], and the roles of FLAP could be to present AA to 5-LOX [124], stimulate the utilization of AA by 5-LOX, and increase the efficiency with which 5-LOX converts 5-HPETE into LTA_4 [1].

FLAP is a member of a superfamily of integral membrane proteins designated MAPEG (membrane-associated proteins in eicosanoid and glutathione metabolism) [80]. In 2007, crystal structures of FLAP in complex with FLAP inhibitors were reported, revealing a homotrimeric structure with four transmembrane helices in each monomer [45].

Many studies have implicated FLAP in the pathogenesis of atherosclerosis. Increased expression of FLAP was detected in atherosclerotic lesions from animal models [8, 169] and humans [131, 148]. Furthermore, genetic studies in human cohorts demonstrated that a four-SNP haplotype (HapA) in the FLAP gene confers a nearly two times greater risk of MI and stroke among Icelandic families [69]. Efforts to replicate the data demonstrated variable associations between these FLAP gene variants and risk of developing MI and stroke among different populations. The HapA variant of the FLAP gene was also found to be a risk factor for stroke in a Scottish population [67], while haplotypes different from HapA displayed strong linkage to MI in a British cohort [69] and in a Japanese population [84]. Meanwhile, in one study HapA was significantly associated with stroke in central European population [98], while another study showed opposite results [88]. In a North American population, one study showed a linkage of FLAP gene variants to ischemic stroke among whites, but not among blacks [85]; however, two other studies found no evidence for an association between the FLAP gene variants to risk of ischemic stroke [109, 167]. Interestingly, it was also shown that a stronger association is found in a male population.

Beneficial effects of FLAP inhibitors on both acute and chronic CVD have been demonstrated in animal models and human studies. Inhibition of FLAP by MK-886 significantly reduced the development of atherosclerosis in ApoE/LDL double knockout mice [82] and in transgenic ApoE$^{-/-}$ mice with the dominant-negative transforming growth factor β type II receptor, which displays aggravated atherosclerosis [8]. Another FLAP inhibitor DG-031 (also called BAYx1005) reduced the amount of atherosclerotic lesions in ApoE/LDLR double KO mice [81] and, in a human study, led to significant and dose-dependent suppression of biomarkers that are associated with increased risk of MI events [63]. Although trials were generally suspended, all these studies pointed to inhibition of FLAP as a promising treatment of CVD, and there is still a strong interest in development of FLAP inhibitors for this purpose [161].

4.3.3 LTA_4H

LTA_4H is a monomeric soluble protein containing one zinc atom which is essential for its two catalytic activities. In addition to its epoxide hydrolase activity, i.e., conversion of LTA_4 into LTB_4, LTA_4H also possesses an aminopeptidase activity [62]. The enzyme contains 610 amino acid residues and is highly conserved among various mammalian species. The high resolution crystal structure of LTA_4H in complex with the competitive inhibitor bestatin reveals that this protein is folded into three domains (N-terminal, C-terminal, and catalytic domains) that together create a deep cleft harboring the catalytic Zn^{2+} site [154].

LTA_4H is widely distributed and resides in the cytosol, although nuclear localization has also been reported [14]. The 5-LOX expression is predominantly found in leukocytes, while LTA_4H is present in many cell types that lack significant 5-LOX activity. This uneven distribution of two intimately coupled enzymes has been explained in terms of transcellular biosynthesis. Indeed transfer of LTA_4 from activated leukocytes to a variety of other cell types has been demonstrated *in vitro* [13] and *in vivo* [43, 166], a phenomenon that is promoted by tight cell–cell interactions.

So far, the increased expression of LTA_4H in atherosclerotic lesions from animal models and human samples has been reported [3, 131, 140, 148]. Qiu and coworkers noted that in human plaque, the expression of 5-LOX and LTA_4H correlates with recent or ongoing symptoms of plaque instability. In addition, a selective inhibitor of LTA_4H could block the synthesis of LTB_4 in human carotid plaques [131]. Recently, a haplotype spanning LTA_4H (HapK) was found to confer a moderate relative risk for MI in an Icelandic cohort and European Americans but a much larger risk among African-Americans [68]. All these studies indicated the potential of LTA_4H as a target for pharmacological intervention in treatment of human atherosclerosis.

Since the inhibition of LTA_4H specifically blocks the conversion of LTA_4 to LTB_4, while still allowing LTA_4 to be converted to anti-inflammatory LX, inhibitors of LTA_4H hold promise as potential therapeutic agents against different inflammatory diseases. Several compounds, such as SC-57461A, SA-9499, RP-64966, and DG-051, which inhibit LTA_4H activities, have been developed, and they are potent in whole blood assays and efficacious in preclinical models of inflammation [161]. Among them, DG-051 from deCODE company is currently undergoing human phase II clinical evaluation for the treatment of MI and stroke [141]. Although a potential issue for LTA_4H inhibition could be pathway shunting of LTA_4 to cys-LTs, it was reported that the LTA_4H inhibitor JNJ-26993135 selectively inhibits LTB_4 production, without affecting cys-LTs production, while maintaining or increasing the production of the anti-inflammatory mediator, LXA_4 [133, 134]. Interestingly, the proinflammatory tripeptide Pro-Gly-Pro was recently identified as the endogenous substrate for the aminopeptidase activity of LTA_4H, which suggests that the enzyme is also involved in resolution of inflammation [146]. Inhibitors of LTA_4H that selectively block the epoxide hydrolase activity (generation of LTB_4) while sparing the aminopeptidase activity may therefore be more efficacious anti-inflammatory agents.

4.3.4 LTC_4S

LTC_4S is an 18 kDa integral membrane protein, and the subcellular localization of LTC_4S has been determined to be in the nuclear membrane [24]. Studies on the crystal structure revealed that LTC_4S is a homotrimer, where each monomer is comprised of four transmembrane segments [105]. Similar to FLAP, human LTC_4S belongs to the MAPEG protein family. Moreover, it has been demonstrated that LTC_4S and FLAP interact with each other, and mixed complexes of FLAP and LTC_4S have been detected [104].

Spanbroek and coworkers found an abundant mRNA expression of LTC_4S in human lesions of CVD [148]. However, no significant increase of LTC_4S gene expression was detected in human or mouse atherosclerotic plaques from one study of our group [131]. In contrast, another recent study from our laboratory revealed increased LTC_4S expression and predominant cysteinyl-leukotriene formation in abdominal aortic aneurysms [37]. Thus, increased expression at the mRNA and protein levels of all enzymes involved in cys-LTs pathway (5-LOX, FLAP and LTC_4S) was observed, whereas no increase in LTA_4H expression could be detected. Moreover, these enzymes are present in the media and adventitia layers of aneurysm wall at sites rich in inflammatory cells, and they are able to convert AA primarily into cys-LTs. Interestingly, challenge of the aneurysm wall tissue with exogenous LTD_4 increases the release of MMPs, and selective inhibition of CysLT1 receptor blocks this effect, suggesting a mechanism by which LTs may promote matrix degradation and identifying the components of the cys-LT pathway as potential targets for prevention and treatment of abdominal aortic aneurysm.

Genetic studies in human cohorts have identified several risk polymorphisms in the LTC_4S gene. One study from US showed a strong association between a promoter polymorphism of LTC_4S (-444 A/C) and early predictors of coronary atherosclerosis in young women [77]. Studies in the Danish population showed that another promoter polymorphism of LTC_4S (-1072 G/A) predicts increased risk of ischemic cerebrovascular disease [52]. The same group also found that both of these polymorphisms (-444 A/C and -1072 G/A) are associated with risk of transient ischemic attack and ischemic stroke but not with risk of ischemic heart disease, which indicated that genetically altered LTC_4S activity could play a role in thrombi formation rather than in development of atherosclerosis [50]. Moreover, they also found that four novel mutations that are likely to change the function of LTC_4S were linked to increased risk of venous thrombo-embolism and ischemic stroke [51].

4.4 Leukotrienes and Atherosclerosis: Leukotriene Receptors

The biological effects of LTs are transduced through two subclasses of seven-transmembrane G protein-coupled receptors (GPCRs): BLT receptors, which are activated by LTB_4 and CysLT receptors, which are activated by the cys-LTs [114].

Experimental and genetic studies in mice, rats, rabbits, and humans have revealed a key role for leukotriene-receptor signaling cascades in the pathogenesis/progression of atherosclerosis and its serious consequences such as MI, stroke, and aortic aneurysms [136].

LTB_4 and cys-LTs exert potent proinflammatory actions through interaction with BLT and CysLT-receptor subtypes expressed on inflammatory and structural cells within the vascular wall. LTs may also induce endothelium-dependent and independent vascular responses. Studies have indicated that leukotriene-dependent degradation of the extracellular matrix may associate this pathway to atherosclerotic plaque instability (Fig. 4.3).

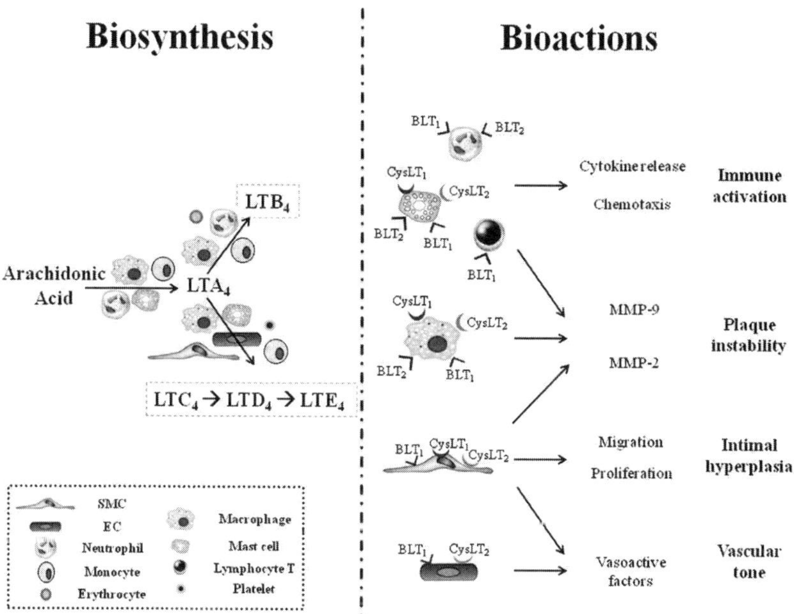

Figure 4.3 Biosynthesis and actions of leukotrienes in the vascular wall. Leukocytes are the main source of LT biosynthesis. In addition, vascular smooth muscle cells, platelets, and endothelial cells are able to convert LTA_4 into cys-LTs (LTC_4, LTD_4, LTE_4). The LT receptors (BLT1, BLT2, CysLT1, CysLT2) are expressed on leukocytes, vascular smooth muscle cells, and endothelial cells. The bioactions downstream of LT receptor signaling in the respective cell types induce alterations associated with atherosclerosis progression and ischemic complications. MMP — matrix metalloproteinase.

Two BLT receptors have been molecularly identified, viz. BLT1 and BLT2. BLT1 is a high-affinity receptor specific for LTB_4, which is expressed primarily in leukocytes and mediates chemotactic responses; BLT2 is a pharmacologically distinct low-affinity receptor for LTB_4, which is ubiquitously expressed and can bind other eicosanoids. Interestingly, 12-hydroxy-heptadecatrienoic acid (12-HHT), which is a side product during TxA_2 synthesis, was shown to be a high-affinity ligand of BLT2, thus connecting this receptor to COX mediated metabolism of AA [116]. The ubiquitous expression and the broader ligand specificity of BLT2 suggest that it may mediate distinct biological and pathophysiological responses from BLT1. In fact, an anti-inflammatory role of BLT2 was recently demonstrated in an animal model of colitis [76].

Receptors activated by cys-LTs were cloned in 1999 and referred to as CysLT1 and CysLT2 [42, 66, 99]. The CysLT1 receptor is activated by all the native ligands, with an order of potency: $LTD_4 > LTC_4 >> LTE_4$, whereas LTD_4 and LTC_4 are equipotent at the CysLT2, and LTE_4 is less potent. In addition to these two classical plasma membrane receptors, alternative activation pathways and evidence for additional CysLT receptor subtypes have been presented. Thus, a purino-like orphan GPCR, GPR17, has been shown to mediate concentration-dependent responses to both LTD_4 and LTC_4 [25]. In later work, GPR17 did not signal with cys-LTs but regulated other CysLT receptors [100]. Two receptors that preferentially signal with LTE_4 have also been identified [5, 118].

In addition, localization of CysLT receptors at the nuclear membrane and cross-talk with other membrane receptors have been observed [19]. Expression of BLT and CysLT receptor subtypes is present on many of the cell types that constitute the atherosclerotic lesions and is highly dependent on transcriptional regulation by pro- and anti-inflammatory mediators. The local production of LTs in atherosclerosis may lead to paracrine and autocrine signaling and exert effects on immunologic and structural cells within the vascular wall.

4.4.1 LTB_4 and BLT Receptor-Induced Immune Responses

Classical immune responses induced by LTB4 include chemotaxis, aggregation and adherence of human leukocytes, in particular neutrophils. LTB_4 formation, catalyzed by the zinc metalloenzyme LTA_4 hydrolase, occurs locally within the vascular wall. Production of LTB_4 is increased in fatty plaques and complicated lesions of atherosclerosis, compared with healthy human vessels and is correlated with the degree of leukocyte infiltration in the tissues [35]. An increase in systemic LTB_4 production has been observed through *ex vivo* stimulation of leukocytes from patients with a history of MI and stroke [69] and in patients with CV risk factors, such as obstructive sleep apnoea [95]. Genetic or pharmacological inhibition of BLT receptors confers beneficial effects in experimental models of atherosclerosis. The effects could potentially be mediated through inhibition of the potent effects induced by LTB_4 both in leukocytes and within the vascular wall [2, 6, 70, 71, 150].

Immune responses participate in every phase of atherosclerosis. In human atherosclerotic lesions, macrophages have been found to stain positive for BLT receptors. Both studies of knockout mice and *in vitro* studies have supported a role for both the high-affinity BLT1 receptor and the low-affinity BLT2 receptor in recruiting macrophages to atherosclerotic lesions [6, 150]. As macrophages are a major source of 5-LOX in the cardiovascular system, LTB_4-induced macrophage recruitment could further exacerbate the inflammatory responses within atherosclerotic lesions. Recently, a novel lipid-peptide signaling circuit involving LTB_4 and the antimicrobial peptide LL-37 was discovered [157]. Since increased expression of LL-37 has been demonstrated in human atherosclerotic plaque [40], these results suggest that LTB_4 may also act in concert with LL-37 to promote vascular inflammation.

In addition to monocytes/macrophages, BLT receptor expression on T-lymphocytes may also play an important role in the immunological responses in the atherosclerotic lesion. In fact, LTB_4 has been identified as a chemotactic factor for T-cells, thus connecting the innate and adaptive immune responses [58, 151]. In addition to macrophages and T-lymphocytes, BLT receptors are also expressed in granulocytes, and although incompletely explored in atherosclerosis, LTB_4 was recently proposed as a mediator of neutrophil chemotaxis and activation in human and animal aortic abdominal aneurysms [16, 73]. Taken together, LTB_4 signaling through BLT receptors provides a link between innate and adaptive immunologic responses, which have been identified as major components in the pathogenesis of atherosclerosis.

The immunologic signaling pathways transducing the atherogenic effects of LTs may also be mediated through enhancement of other proinflammatory mediators. LTB_4 (as well as cys-LTs) upregulates the expression of monocyte chemoattractant protein (MCP)-1, amplifying subsequent MCP-1-induced chemotaxis and other inflammatory responses [160]. LTs also upregulate other proatherogenic genes, including macrophage inflammatory protein 1α, CD36, and interferon-γ [108].

4.4.2 LTB_4 and BLT Receptor-Induced Vascular Responses

LTB_4 can act on the vessel wall via indirect mechanisms involving leukocyte activation. For instance, LTB_4 increases vascular permeability, and it was recently demonstrated that this effect is mediated by a secreted protein azurocidin, also known as heparin binding protein [36]. In addition to leukocyte activation, LTB_4 also has inductive effects on structural components of the vascular wall. Human endothelial cells express BLT1 and BLT2, and the expression and signaling of BLT1 are increased by proinflammatory agents such as LPS and its natural ligand LTB_4 [131]. Human carotid atherosclerotic lesions have been demonstrated to express endothelial BLT1 receptors [6]. Functional studies further show that LTB_4, via BLT1 receptor, induces endothelium-dependent contractile responses *in vitro* [7]. Upregulation of endothelial BLT1 during atherosclerosis may be a mechanism for LTB_4-induced endothelial dysfunction. Additionally, LTB_4 is found to induce contraction of vascular segments lacking a functional endothelium and acts as a chemotactic factor for VSMCs [6, 70]. The importance of LTB_4-induced VSMC migration and proliferation in the development and progression of atherosclerosis is further supported by experimental models targeting the BLT1 receptor [71]. These observations indicate its important role in atherosclerosis-associated intimal hyperplasia and in-stent restenosis. BLT receptor antagonism demonstrates a beneficial effect against intimal hyperplasia induced by balloon angioplasty with stent implantation in hypercholesterolemic rabbits [71]. Use of anti-leukotrienes is, therefore, suggested in the prevention of restenosis subsequent to coronary percutaneous interventions. Finally, targeted disruption of the BLT1 receptor gene in $ApoE^{-/-}$ mice results in decreased SMCs in the aortic lesions [6, 70, 89].

4.4.3 LTB_4 and BLT Receptors in Plaque Instability

In addition to the atherogenic effects, several studies have linked the LTB_4 pathway to plaque instability. A key component in plaque instability and rupture is the degradation of extracellular matrix by specific MMPs. One possible mechanism by which LTB_4 may promote plaque rupture is through activation of MMPs, as suggested by the co-existence of both pathways in atherosclerotic lesions. In addition, LTB_4 release is correlated to MMP-9 both in the saliva and in human aortic abdominal aneurysms, which represent sites of high proteolytic activity. It has been shown that targeting BLT receptor inhibits MMP activities in the context of restenosis and aortic abdominal aneurysms. Targeting 5-LOX or the BLT1 receptor in these contexts confers protective effects against restenosis and aortic abdominal aneurysms by decreasing MMP activities [169].

4.4.4 Cysteinyl-LTs and CysLT Receptors in Atherogenesis

Cysteinyl-LTs are potent inflammatory lipid mediators derived from the 5-LOX pathway of AA metabolism. Several studies have revealed the presence of cys-LTs in atherosclerotic lesions as potential signaling molecules in atherosclerosis, abdominal aneurysm, and intimal hyperplasia. Cysteinyl-LTs, including LTC_4, LTD_4, and LTE_4, can be produced by human coronary arteries [126]. In patients with acute MI and attacks of UA, urinary cys-LTs production is elevated [20]. A similar increase in urinary LTE_4 levels is observed in patients with CAD and after coronary artery bypass surgery [4]. LTC_4 and LTD_4 induce contraction of atherosclerotic coronary arteries, suggesting that atherosclerosis may enhance the vascular reactivity of LTs [3]. In addition to direct activation of VSMCs, cys-LTs also regulate vascular tone through activation of endothelial cells [114]. CysLT receptor subtypes are expressed in diseased human arteries. In endothelial cells, CysLT2 receptors may preferentially transduce the release of contractile factors. CysLT2 receptor activation causes increased endothelial permeability [74], intracellular calcium influx, myosin light-chain kinase activation, stress fiber formation, and endothelial cell contraction through the activity of the pertussis toxin (PTX)-insensitive, Gq protein [136]. In addition to direct action on the vascular tone, LT-induced activation of endothelial cells may also lead to changes in the transcriptional activity. In human umbilical vein endothelial cells (HUVECs), LTD_4 induces upregulation of endothelial P-selectin via a non-CysLT1 receptor [123] and strongly stimulates expression of macrophage inflammatory protein-1α (MIP-1α) in macrophages and MIP-2α in endothelial cells. In HUVEC, this non-CysLT1 receptor has been shown to be CysLT2, which is expressed at much higher levels compared to CysLT1 in these cells [145]. It has also been demonstrated that LTD_4, via CysLT2, and thrombin seem to cooperate in regulating the same genes resulting in a proinflammatory endothelial cell phenotype: *de novo* synthesis of early growth response I protein, IL-8 and tissue factors [156]. CysLT2 receptor and PAR-1 may, therefore, cooperate to augment vascular injury [114]. Although CysLT2 is the dominant CysLT receptor subtype expressed on endothelial cells, CysLT1 receptor expression can also be induced by proinflammatory stimuli [59]. In monocyte/macrophage like U937 cells, which exclusively express the CysLT1 receptor, extracellular nucleotides heterologously desensitize CysLT1 receptor-induced Ca^{2+} transients in a unidirectional way [18]. A number of studies have reported a cross-talk/parallelism between CysLT and purinergic receptor systems [83, 102], which may have profound implications in the regulation of responses at sites of inflammation such as the vascular wall or during brain ischemia. Furthermore, the CysLT1 receptor inhibitor montelukast decreases vascular reactive oxygen species production, significantly improves endothelial function, and ameliorates atherosclerotic plaque generation in a mouse model *in vivo* [112].

In vitro studies of isolated leukocytes have also supported the notion of cys-LTs-induced MMP activity. LTC_4 and LTD_4 but not LTE_4 enhance TNF-α-induced MMP-9 protein concentrations in THP-1 cells, an effect that is inhibited by the CysLT1 receptor antagonist pranlukast [75].

4.4.5 LTs and Atherosclerosis: Summary

Experimental and genetic evidence supports a key role of LTs and leukotriene receptors in the pathogenesis and progression of atherosclerosis and its complications. LT biosynthesis and LT-receptor signaling pathways may, therefore, represent a potential therapeutic target in designing novel anti-inflammatory strategies in the treatment of atherosclerosis and the prevention of its serious consequences such as MI, stroke, aortic aneurysms, and intimal hyperplasia.

Findings in animal models of atherosclerosis and in human genetic studies, based on either genetic association or LT measurement in different patient groups, seem to suggest a beneficial effect on anti-LT treatments in CVD. However, results thus far have been variable, and further studies are needed to conclude what mechanisms and proteins are optimal to target in the LT pathway to achieve therapeutic effects in human diseases. Nevertheless, a number of ongoing clinical studies are exploring the effects of anti-LTs in atherosclerosis and its complications, which will shed further light on the effectiveness and safety of these drugs in CVD.

4.5 12/15-Lipoxygenase and Atherosclerosis

Lipoxygenases are soluble monomeric proteins containing one non-heme iron required for catalysis. These enzymes are named according to their positional specificity for substrate oxygenation. In man, there are four LOXs that can oxygenate AA at C12 and/or C15, i.e., platelet 12(S)-LOX, 12(R)-LOX, 15-LOX type 1, and 15-LOX type 2, which are distinguished not only by their different positional and stereo specificity but also by their unique enzymologic properties and tissue patterns of expression [90]. Early works focused on *in vitro* studies of soybean 15-LOX and human reticulocyte 15-LOX, today known as 15-LOX-1, whereas recent work focuses more on *in vivo* studies taking into account other 12/15-LOX isoforms [94]. Although the 12/15-LOXs generate predominately either 12(S)- or 15(S)-HPETE depending on specific structural elements, those enzymes produce significant amounts of both metabolites [31], and thus will be referred to as the 12/15-LOX in this chapter. Moreover, 12/15-LOX is able to metabolize free fatty acids (e.g., arachidonic and linoleic acids) as well as fatty acids esterified to phospholipids and cholesterol [92]. Here it should be emphasized that there are significant species differences with respect to enzyme properties and expression patterns for 12/15-LOXs and conclusions from animal studies may be difficult to translate into human physiology [53].

In humans, the 12/15-LOX has been implicated in cell development and differentiation. It is constitutively expressed at high levels in immature red blood cells, eosinophils, and airway epithelial cells [113]. Lower expression levels have been reported for polymorphonuclear leukocytes, alveolar macrophages, and vascular cells. 12/15-LOX is absent in unstimulated monocytes, but it is avidly expressed after treatment with IL-4 or IL-13 [22, 32] as well as in atherosclerotic lesional macrophages [164].

A role for 12/15-LOX in mediating pathogenic lipid peroxidation associated with inflammatory vascular disease has been discussed for many years. In the late 1980s, it was demonstrated that soybean 15-LOX incubated with LDL and phospholipase A_2 led to formation of oxidized fatty acids [149]. Subsequent experiments showed direct oxidation of LDL lipid esters by rabbit 15-LOX or recombinant human 12/15-LOX in the absence of phospholipase [10, 91]. Thus, *ex vivo* studies were performed in cholesterol-fed rabbits and in early human atherosclerotic lesions showing evidence for a 12/15-LOX component to oxidize lipids [93, 144]. Moreover, the presence of 12/15-LOX mRNA and protein in macrophages that colocalize with sites of oxidized LDL strongly suggested an association between LOX activity, oxidative modification of LDL, and atherogenesis.

Recently, the advent of 12/15-LOX-deficient mice, transgenic 12/15-LOX over-expressing mice and rabbits, and specific LOX inhibitors have allowed *in vivo* studies. Different groups found that 12/15-LOX/apoE double knockout mice had a pronounced delay and attenuation of lesion development when compared to ApoE-deficient mice at early stages of foamy macrophage-laden fatty streak development. In follow-up studies, atherosclerotic lesion development was significantly reduced at all time points from 10 weeks to 15 months of age [53].

A number of studies have been carried out in rabbits. In one report where 12/15-LOX was overexpressed into iliac arteries by retroviral vectors, rabbits had elevated levels of oxidation-specific lipid protein adducts characteristic of oxidized LDL under diet-induced cholestrolemia [163]. In other independent studies, rabbits fed a diet to induce atherosclerosis were given a specific 12/15-LOX inhibitor, PD146176 [12, 142]. This regimen strikingly attenuated aortic arch lesion coverage and abolished esterified cholesterol content and lipid-laden macrophages in the region, while not affecting plasma total cholesterol and distribution of lipoprotein cholesterol.

Although most of the results obtained in animal atherosclerosis models suggest a pro-atherogenic role of 12/15-LOX, there are also data suggesting an anti-atherogenic activity. When transgenic rabbits, which overexpress 12/15-LOX under the control of the lysozyme promoter, were fed a lipid-rich, Western-style diet, development of atherosclerotic lesions in the aorta was significantly reduced by approximately 50% [143].

Taken together, these results show the controversial role of 12/15-LOX in atherogenesis. Species-specific differences and the complex biologic dynamics of the enzyme may contribute to this controversy. Moreover, the anti-atherogenic activity of 12/15-LOX may be explained by its ability to produce LXs, which have been identified as mediators of the resolution phase of inflammation. Since inflammation is an inherent process of atherogenesis, resolving mediators may counteract, or even reverse, lesion formation [72].

In the recent years, new transgenic animal models are available and new interest in developing specific 12/15-LOX inhibitors is growing. Thus, with those new tools, it should be possible to more clearly define the *in vivo* role of this pathway in atherogenesis.

References

1. Abramovitz, M., Wong, E., Cox, M. E., Richardson, C. D., Li, C., and Vickers, P. J. (1993) 5-lipoxygenase-activating protein stimulates the utilization of arachidonic acid by 5-lipoxygenase. *Eur J Biochem* 215, 105–111.
2. Aiello, R. J., Bourassa, P. A., Lindsey, S., Weng, W., Freeman, A., and Showell, H. J. (2002) Leukotriene B_4 receptor antagonism reduces monocytic foam cells in mice. *Arterioscler Thromb Vasc Biol* 22, 443–449.
3. Allen, S., Dashwood, M., Morrison, K., and Yacoub, M. (1998) Differential leukotriene constrictor responses in human atherosclerotic coronary arteries. *Circulation* 97, 2406–2413.
4. Allen, S. P., Sampson, A. P., Piper, P. J., Chester, A. H., Ohri, S. K., and Yacoub, M. H. (1993) Enhanced excretion of urinary leukotriene E_4 in coronary artery disease and after coronary artery bypass surgery. *Coron Artery Dis* 4, 899–904.
5. Austen, K. F., Maekawa, A., Kanaoka, Y., and Boyce, J. A. (2009) The leukotriene E_4 puzzle: Finding the missing pieces and revealing the pathobiologic implications. *J Allergy Clin Immunol* 124, 406–14; quiz 415–416.

6. Back, M., Bu, D. X., Branstrom, R., Sheikine, Y., Yan, Z. Q., and Hansson, G. K. (2005) Leukotriene B_4 signaling through NF-kappaB-dependent BLT1 receptors on vascular smooth muscle cells in atherosclerosis and intimal hyperplasia. *Proc Natl Acad Sci U S A* 102, 17501–17506.
7. Back, M., Qiu, H., Haeggstrom, J. Z., and Sakata, K. (2004) Leukotriene B_4 is an indirectly acting vasoconstrictor in guinea pig aorta via an inducible type of BLT receptor. *Am J Physiol Heart Circ Physiol* 287, H419–424.
8. Back, M., Sultan, A., Ovchinnikova, O., and Hansson, G. K. (2007) 5-Lipoxygenase-activating protein: A potential link between innate and adaptive immunity in atherosclerosis and adipose tissue inflammation. *Circ Res* 100, 946–949.
9. Bea, F., Blessing, E., Bennett, B. J., Kuo, C. C., Campbell, L. A., Kreuzer, J., and Rosenfeld, M. E. (2003) Chronic inhibition of cyclooxygenase-2 does not alter plaque composition in a mouse model of advanced unstable atherosclerosis. *Cardiovasc Res* 60, 198–204.
10. Belkner, J., Stender, H., and Kuhn, H. (1998) The rabbit 15-lipoxygenase preferentially oxygenates LDL cholesterol esters, and this reaction does not require vitamin E. *J Biol Chem* 273, 23225–23232.
11. Belton, O. A., Duffy, A., Toomey, S., and Fitzgerald, D. J. (2003) Cyclooxygenase isoforms and platelet vessel wall interactions in the apolipoprotein E knockout mouse model of atherosclerosis. *Circulation* 108, 3017–3023.
12. Bocan, T. M., Rosebury, W. S., Mueller, S. B., Kuchera, S., Welch, K., Daugherty, A., and Cornicelli, J. A. (1998) A specific 15-lipoxygenase inhibitor limits the progression and monocyte-macrophage enrichment of hypercholesterolemia-induced atherosclerosis in the rabbit. *Atherosclerosis* 136, 203–216.
13. Brady, H. R., and Serhan, C. N. (1992) Adhesion promotes transcellular leukotriene biosynthesis during neutrophil-glomerular endothelial cell interactions: inhibition by antibodies against CD18 and L-selectin. *Biochem Biophys Res Commun* 186, 1307–1314.
14. Brock, T. G., Maydanski, E., McNish, R. W., and Peters-Golden, M. (2001) Co-localization of leukotriene A_4 hydrolase with 5-lipoxygenase in nuclei of alveolar macrophages and rat basophilic leukemia cells but not neutrophils. *J Biol Chem* 276, 35071–35077.
15. Burleigh, M. E., Babaev, V. R., Oates, J. A., Harris, R. C., Gautam, S., Riendeau, D., Marnett, L. J., Morrow, J. D., Fazio, S., and Linton, M. F. (2002) Cyclooxygenase-2 promotes early atherosclerotic lesion

formation in LDL receptor-deficient mice. *Circulation* 105, 1816–1823.

16. Cao, R. Y., Adams, M. A., Habenicht, A. J., and Funk, C. D. (2007) Angiotensin II-induced abdominal aortic aneurysm occurs independently of the 5-lipoxygenase pathway in apolipoprotein E-deficient mice. *Prostaglandins Other Lipid Mediat* 84, 34–42.
17. Cao, R. Y., St Amand, T., Grabner, R., Habenicht, A. J., and Funk, C. D. (2009) Genetic and pharmacological inhibition of the 5-lipoxygenase/leukotriene pathway in atherosclerotic lesion development in ApoE deficient mice. *Atherosclerosis* 203, 395–400.
18. Capra, V., Ravasi, S., Accomazzo, M. R., Citro, S., Grimoldi, M., Abbracchio, M. P., and Rovati, G. E. (2005) CysLT1 receptor is a target for extracellular nucleotide-induced heterologous desensitization: A possible feedback mechanism in inflammation. *J Cell Sci* 118, 5625–5636.
19. Capra, V., Thompson, M. D., Sala, A., Cole, D. E., Folco, G., and Rovati, G. E. (2007) Cysteinyl-leukotrienes and their receptors in asthma and other inflammatory diseases: Critical update and emerging trends. *Med Res Rev* 27, 469–527.
20. Carry, M., Korley, V., Willerson, J. T., Weigelt, L., Ford-Hutchinson, A. W., and Tagari, P. (1992) Increased urinary leukotriene excretion in patients with cardiac ischemia. *In vivo* evidence for 5-lipoxygenase activation. *Circulation* 85, 230–236.
21. Cayatte, A. J., Du, Y., Oliver-Krasinski, J., Lavielle, G., Verbeuren, T. J., and Cohen, R. A. (2000) The thromboxane receptor antagonist S18886 but not aspirin inhibits atherogenesis in apo E-deficient mice: Evidence that eicosanoids other than thromboxane contribute to atherosclerosis. *Arterioscler Thromb Vasc Biol* 20, 1724–1728.
22. Chaitidis, P., O'Donnell, V., Kuban, R. J., Bermudez-Fajardo, A., Ungethuem, U., and Kuhn, H. (2005) Gene expression alterations of human peripheral blood monocytes induced by medium-term treatment with the TH2-cytokines interleukin-4 and -13. *Cytokine* 30, 366–377.
23. Cheng, Y., Austin, S. C., Rocca, B., Koller, B. H., Coffman, T. M., Grosser, T., Lawson, J. A., and FitzGerald, G. A. (2002) Role of prostacyclin in the cardiovascular response to thromboxane A2. *Science* 296, 539–541.
24. Christmas, P., Weber, B. M., McKee, M., Brown, D., and Soberman, R. J. (2002) Membrane localization and topology of leukotriene C4 synthase. *J Biol Chem* 277, 28902–28908.
25. Ciana, P., Fumagalli, M., Trincavelli, M. L., Verderio, C., Rosa, P., Lecca, D., Ferrario, S., Parravicini, C., Capra, V., Gelosa, P., Guerrini, U., Belcredito,

S., Cimino, M., Sironi, L., Tremoli, E., Rovati, G. E., Martini, C., and Abbracchio, M. P. (2006) The orphan receptor GPR17 identified as a new dual uracil nucleotides/cysteinyl-leukotrienes receptor. *Embo J* 25, 4615–4627.

26. Cipollone, F., Fazia, M., Iezzi, A., Ciabattoni, G., Pini, B., Cuccurullo, C., Ucchino, S., Spigonardo, F., De Luca, M., Prontera, C., Chiarelli, F., Cuccurullo, F., and Mezzetti, A. (2004) Balance between PGD synthase and PGE synthase is a major determinant of atherosclerotic plaque instability in humans. *Arterioscler Thromb Vasc Biol* 24, 1259–1265.

27. Cipollone, F., Fazia, M., Iezzi, A., Zucchelli, M., Pini, B., De Cesare, D., Ucchino, S., Spigonardo, F., Bajocchi, G., Bei, R., Muraro, R., Artese, L., Piattelli, A., Chiarelli, F., Cuccurullo, F., and Mezzetti, A. (2003) Suppression of the functionally coupled cyclooxygenase-2/prostaglandin E synthase as a basis of simvastatin-dependent plaque stabilization in humans. *Circulation* 107, 1479–1485.

28. Cipollone, F., Mezzetti, A., Fazia, M. L., Cuccurullo, C., Iezzi, A., Ucchino, S., Spigonardo, F., Bucci, M., Cuccurullo, F., Prescott, S. M., and Stafforini, D. M. (2005) Association between 5-lipoxygenase expression and plaque instability in humans. *Arterioscler Thromb Vasc Biol* 25, 1665–1670.

29. Cipollone, F., Prontera, C., Pini, B., Marini, M., Fazia, M., De Cesare, D., Iezzi, A., Ucchino, S., Boccoli, G., Saba, V., Chiarelli, F., Cuccurullo, F., and Mezzetti, A. (2001) Overexpression of functionally coupled cyclooxygenase-2 and prostaglandin E synthase in symptomatic atherosclerotic plaques as a basis of prostaglandin E_2-dependent plaque instability. *Circulation* 104, 921–927.

30. Connolly, E., Bouchier-Hayes, D. J., Kaye, E., Leahy, A., Fitzgerald, D., and Belton, O. (2002) Cyclooxygenase isozyme expression and intimal hyperplasia in a rat model of balloon angioplasty. *J Pharmacol Exp Ther* 300, 393–398.

31. Conrad, D. J. (1999) The arachidonate 12/15 lipoxygenases. A review of tissue expression and biologic function. *Clin Rev Allergy Immunol* 17, 71–89.

32. Conrad, D. J., Kuhn, H., Mulkins, M., Highland, E., and Sigal, E. (1992) Specific inflammatory cytokines regulate the expression of human monocyte 15-lipoxygenase. *Proc Natl Acad Sci U S A* 89, 217–221.

33. Cyrus, T., Sung, S., Zhao, L., Funk, C. D., Tang, S., and Pratico, D. (2002) Effect of low-dose aspirin on vascular inflammation, plaque stability, and atherogenesis in low-density lipoprotein receptor-deficient mice. *Circulation* 106, 1282–1287.

34. Davi, G., and Patrono, C. (2007) Platelet activation and atherothrombosis. *N Engl J Med* 357, 2482–2494.

35. De Caterina, R., Mazzone, A., Giannessi, D., Sicari, R., Pelosi, W., Lazzerini, G., Azzara, A., Forder, R., Carey, F., Caruso, D., *et al.* (1988) Leukotriene B_4 production in human atherosclerotic plaques. *Biomed Biochim Acta* 47, S182–S185.

36. Di Gennaro, A., Kenne, E., Wan, M., Soehnlein, O., Lindbom, L., and Haeggstrom, J. Z. (2009) Leukotriene B_4-induced changes in vascular permeability are mediated by neutrophil release of heparin-binding protein (HBP/CAP37/azurocidin). *FASEB J* 23, 1750–1757.

37. Di Gennaro, A., Wagsater, D., Mayranpaa, M. I., Gabrielsen, A., Swedenborg, J., Hamsten, A., Samuelsson, B., Eriksson, P., and Haeggstrom, J. Z. (2010) Increased expression of leukotriene C_4 synthase and predominant formation of cysteinyl-leukotrienes in human abdominal aortic aneurysm. *Proc Natl Acad Sci U S A* 107(49):21093-7

38. Dixon, R. A., Diehl, R. E., Opas, E., Rands, E., Vickers, P. J., Evans, J. F., Gillard, J. W., and Miller, D. K. (1990) Requirement of a 5-lipoxygenase-activating protein for leukotriene synthesis. Nature 343, 282–284.

39. Dwyer, J. H., Allayee, H., Dwyer, K. M., Fan, J., Wu, H., Mar, R., Lusis, A. J., and Mehrabian, M. (2004) Arachidonate 5-lipoxygenase promoter genotype, dietary arachidonic acid, and atherosclerosis. *N Engl J Med* 350, 29–37.

40. Edfeldt, K., Agerberth, B., Rottenberg, M. E., Gudmundsson, G. H., Wang, X. B., Mandal, K., Xu, Q., and Yan, Z. Q. (2006) Involvement of the antimicrobial peptide LL-37 in human atherosclerosis. *Arterioscler Thromb Vasc Biol* 26, 1551–1557.

41. Egan, K. M., Wang, M., Fries, S., Lucitt, M. B., Zukas, A. M., Pure, E., Lawson, J. A., and FitzGerald, G. A. (2005) Cyclooxygenases, thromboxane, and atherosclerosis: Plaque destabilization by cyclooxygenase-2 inhibition combined with thromboxane receptor antagonism. *Circulation* 111, 334–342.

42. Evans, J. F. (2003) The cysteinyl leukotriene receptors. *Prostaglandins Leukot Essent Fatty Acids* 69, 117–122.

43. Fabre, J. E., Goulet, J. L., Riche, E., Nguyen, M., Coggins, K., Offenbacher, S., and Koller, B. H. (2002) Transcellular biosynthesis contributes to the production of leukotrienes during inflammatory responses in vivo. *J Clin Invest* 109, 1373–1380.

44. Fabre, J. E., Nguyen, M., Athirakul, K., Coggins, K., McNeish, J. D., Austin, S., Parise, L. K., FitzGerald, G. A., Coffman, T. M., and Koller, B. H.

(2001) Activation of the murine EP3 receptor for PGE_2 inhibits cAMP production and promotes platelet aggregation. *J Clin Invest* 107, 603–610.

45. Ferguson, A. D., McKeever, B. M., Xu, S., Wisniewski, D., Miller, D. K., Yamin, T. T., Spencer, R. H., Chu, L., Ujjainwalla, F., Cunningham, B. R., Evans, J. F., and Becker, J. W. (2007) Crystal structure of inhibitor-bound human 5-lipoxygenase-activating protein. *Science* 317, 510–512.
46. FitzGerald, G. A. (1991) Mechanisms of platelet activation: Thromboxane A_2 as an amplifying signal for other agonists. *Am J Cardiol* 68, 11B–15B.
47. FitzGerald, G. A., and Patrono, C. (2001) The coxibs, selective inhibitors of cyclooxygenase-2. *N Engl J Med* 345, 433–442.
48. FitzGerald, G. A., Smith, B., Pedersen, A. K., and Brash, A. R. (1984) Increased prostacyclin biosynthesis in patients with severe atherosclerosis and platelet activation. *N Engl J Med* 310, 1065–1068.
49. Francois, H., Athirakul, K., Howell, D., Dash, R., Mao, L., Kim, H. S., Rockman, H. A., Fitzgerald, G. A., Koller, B. H., and Coffman, T. M. (2005) Prostacyclin protects against elevated blood pressure and cardiac fibrosis. *Cell Metab* 2, 201–207.
50. Freiberg, J. J., Dahl, M., Tybjaerg-Hansen, A., Grande, P., and Nordestgaard, B. G. (2009) Leukotriene C_4 synthase and ischemic cardiovascular disease and obstructive pulmonary disease in 13,000 individuals. *J Mol Cell Cardiol* 46, 579–586.
51. Freiberg, J. J., Tybjaerg-Hansen, A., and Nordestgaard, B. G. (2010) Novel mutations in leukotriene C_4 synthase and risk of cardiovascular disease based on genotypes from 50,000 individuals. *J Thromb Haemost* 8, 1694–1701.
52. Freiberg, J. J., Tybjaerg-Hansen, A., Sillesen, H., Jensen, G. B., and Nordestgaard, B. G. (2008) Promotor polymorphisms in leukotriene C_4 synthase and risk of ischemic cerebrovascular disease. *Arterioscler Thromb Vasc Biol* 28, 990–996.
53. Funk, C. D., and Cyrus, T. (2001) 12/15-lipoxygenase, oxidative modification of LDL and atherogenesis. *Trends Cardiovasc Med* 11, 116–124.
54. Funk, C. D., and FitzGerald, G. A. (2007) COX-2 inhibitors and cardiovascular risk. *J Cardiovasc Pharmacol* 50, 470–479.
55. Galis, Z. S., Sukhova, G. K., Lark, M. W., and Libby, P. (1994) Increased expression of matrix metalloproteinases and matrix degrading activity in vulnerable regions of human atherosclerotic plaques. *J Clin Invest* 94, 2493–2503.

56. Gilbert, N. C., Bartlett, S. G., Waight, M. T., Neau, D. B., Boeglin, W. E., Brash, A. R., and Newcomer, M. E. (2011) The structure of human 5-lipoxygenase. *Science* 331, 217–219.

57. Gonzalez, P., Reguero, J. R., Lozano, I., Moris, C., and Coto, E. (2007) A functional Sp1/Egr1-tandem repeat polymorphism in the 5-lipoxygenase gene is not associated with myocardial infarction. *Int J Immunogenet* 34, 127–130.

58. Goodarzi, K., Goodarzi, M., Tager, A. M., Luster, A. D., and von Andrian, U. H. (2003) Leukotriene B_4 and BLT1 control cytotoxic effector T cell recruitment to inflamed tissues. *Nat Immunol* 4, 965–973.

59. Gronert, K., Martinsson-Niskanen, T., Ravasi, S., Chiang, N., and Serhan, C. N. (2001) Selectivity of recombinant human leukotriene D_4, leukotriene B_4, and lipoxin A_4 receptors with aspirin-triggered 15-epi-LXA_4 and regulation of vascular and inflammatory responses. *Am J Pathol* 158, 3–9.

60. Grosser, T., Yu, Y., and Fitzgerald, G. A. (2010) Emotion recollected in tranquility: Lessons learned from the COX-2 saga. *Annu Rev Med* 61, 17–33.

61. Haeggstrom, J. Z., and Funk, C. D. (2011) Lipoxygenase and leukotriene pathways: biochemistry, biology, and roles in disease. Chem Rev 111, 5866–5898.

62. Haeggstrom, J. Z., Wetterholm, A., Vallee, B. L., and Samuelsson, B. (1990) Leukotriene A_4 hydrolase: an epoxide hydrolase with peptidase activity. *Biochem Biophys Res Commun* 173, 431–437.

63. Hakonarson, H., Thorvaldsson, S., Helgadottir, A., Gudbjartsson, D., Zink, F., Andresdottir, M., Manolescu, A., Arnar, D. O., Andersen, K., Sigurdsson, A., Thorgeirsson, G., Jonsson, A., Agnarsson, U., Bjornsdottir, H., Gottskalksson, G., Einarsson, A., Gudmundsdottir, H., Adalsteinsdottir, A. E., Gudmundsson, K., Kristjansson, K., Hardarson, T., Kristinsson, A., Topol, E. J., Gulcher, J., Kong, A., Gurney, M., and Stefansson, K. (2005) Effects of a 5-lipoxygenase-activating protein inhibitor on biomarkers associated with risk of myocardial infarction: A randomized trial. *JAMA* 293, 2245–2256.

64. Hansson, G. K. (2005) Inflammation, atherosclerosis, and coronary artery disease. *N Engl J Med* 352, 1685–1695.

65. Harada, S., Nagy, J. A., Sullivan, K. A., Thomas, K. A., Endo, N., Rodan, G. A., and Rodan, S. B. (1994) Induction of vascular endothelial growth factor expression by prostaglandin E_2 and E_1 in osteoblasts. *J Clin Invest* 93, 2490–2496.

66. Heise, C. E., O'Dowd, B. F., Figueroa, D. J., Sawyer, N., Nguyen, T., Im, D. S., Stocco, R., Bellefeuille, J. N., Abramovitz, M., Cheng, R., Williams, D. L., Jr., Zeng, Z., Liu, Q., Ma, L., Clements, M. K., Coulombe, N., Liu, Y., Austin, C. P., George, S. R., O'Neill, G. P., Metters, K. M., Lynch, K. R., and Evans, J. F. (2000) Characterization of the human cysteinyl leukotriene 2 receptor. *J Biol Chem* 275, 30531–30536.

67. Helgadottir, A., Gretarsdottir, S., St Clair, D., Manolescu, A., Cheung, J., Thorleifsson, G., Pasdar, A., Grant, S. F., Whalley, L. J., Hakonarson, H., Thorsteinsdottir, U., Kong, A., Gulcher, J., Stefansson, K., and MacLeod, M. J. (2005) Association between the gene encoding 5-lipoxygenase-activating protein and stroke replicated in a Scottish population. *Am J Hum Genet* 76, 505–509.

68. Helgadottir, A., Manolescu, A., Helgason, A., Thorleifsson, G., Thorsteinsdottir, U., Gudbjartsson, D. F., Gretarsdottir, S., Magnusson, K. P., Gudmundsson, G., Hicks, A., Jonsson, T., Grant, S. F., Sainz, J., O'Brien, S. J., Sveinbjornsdottir, S., Valdimarsson, E. M., Matthiasson, S. E., Levey, A. I., Abramson, J. L., Reilly, M. P., Vaccarino, V., Wolfe, M. L., Gudnason, V., Quyyumi, A. A., Topol, E. J., Rader, D. J., Thorgeirsson, G., Gulcher, J. R., Hakonarson, H., Kong, A., and Stefansson, K. (2006) A variant of the gene encoding leukotriene A_4 hydrolase confers ethnicity-specific risk of myocardial infarction. *Nat Genet* 38, 68–74.

69. Helgadottir, A., Manolescu, A., Thorleifsson, G., Gretarsdottir, S., Jonsdottir, H., Thorsteinsdottir, U., Samani, N. J., Gudmundsson, G., Grant, S. F., Thorgeirsson, G., Sveinbjornsdottir, S., Valdimarsson, E. M., Matthiasson, S. E., Johannsson, H., Gudmundsdottir, O., Gurney, M. E., Sainz, J., Thorhallsdottir, M., Andresdottir, M., Frigge, M. L., Topol, E. J., Kong, A., Gudnason, V., Hakonarson, H., Gulcher, J. R., and Stefansson, K. (2004) The gene encoding 5-lipoxygenase activating protein confers risk of myocardial infarction and stroke. *Nat Genet* 36, 233–239.

70. Heller, E. A., Liu, E., Tager, A. M., Sinha, S., Roberts, J. D., Koehn, S. L., Libby, P., Aikawa, E. R., Chen, J. Q., Huang, P., Freeman, M. W., Moore, K. J., Luster, A. D., and Gerszten, R. E. (2005) Inhibition of atherogenesis in BLT1-deficient mice reveals a role for LTB_4 and BLT1 in smooth muscle cell recruitment. *Circulation* 112, 578–586.

71. Hlawaty, H., Jacob, M. P., Louedec, L., Letourneur, D., Brink, C., Michel, J. B., Feldman, L., and Back, M. (2009) Leukotriene receptor antagonism and the prevention of extracellular matrix degradation during atherosclerosis and in-stent stenosis. *Arterioscler Thromb Vasc Biol* 29, 518–524.

72. Ho, K. J., Spite, M., Owens, C. D., Lancero, H., Kroemer, A. H., Pande, R., Creager, M. A., Serhan, C. N., and Conte, M. S. (2010) Aspirin-triggered

lipoxin and resolvin E_1 modulate vascular smooth muscle phenotype and correlate with peripheral atherosclerosis. *Am J Pathol* 177, 2116–2123.

73. Houard, X., Ollivier, V., Louedec, L., Michel, J. B., and Back, M. (2009) Differential inflammatory activity across human abdominal aortic aneurysms reveals neutrophil-derived leukotriene B_4 as a major chemotactic factor released from the intraluminal thrombus. *FASEB J* 23, 1376–1383.
74. Hui, Y., Cheng, Y., Smalera, I., Jian, W., Goldhahn, L., Fitzgerald, G. A., and Funk, C. D. (2004) Directed vascular expression of human cysteinyl leukotriene 2 receptor modulates endothelial permeability and systemic blood pressure. *Circulation* 110, 3360–3366.
75. Ichiyama, T., Kajimoto, M., Hasegawa, M., Hashimoto, K., Matsubara, T., and Furukawa, S. (2007) Cysteinyl leukotrienes enhance tumour necrosis factor-alpha-induced matrix metalloproteinase-9 in human monocytes/macrophages. *Clin Exp Allergy* 37, 608–614.
76. Iizuka, Y., Okuno, T., Saeki, K., Uozaki, H., Okada, S., Misaka, T., Sato, T., Toh, H., Fukayama, M., Takeda, N., Kita, Y., Shimizu, T., Nakamura, M., and Yokomizo, T. (2010) Protective role of the leukotriene B4 receptor BLT2 in murine inflammatory colitis. FASEB J 24, 4678–4690.
77. Iovannisci, D. M., Lammer, E. J., Steiner, L., Cheng, S., Mahoney, L. T., Davis, P. H., Lauer, R. M., and Burns, T. L. (2007) Association between a leukotriene C_4 synthase gene promoter polymorphism and coronary artery calcium in young women: The Muscatine Study. *Arterioscler Thromb Vasc Biol* 27, 394–399.
78. Ishizuka, T., Suzuki, K., Kawakami, M., Hidaka, T., Matsuki, Y., and Nakamura, H. (1996) Thromboxane A_2 receptor blockade suppresses intercellular adhesion molecule-1 expression by stimulated vascular endothelial cells. *Eur J Pharmacol* 312, 367–377.
79. Jadhav, V., Jabre, A., Lin, S. Z., and Lee, T. J. (2004) EP1- and EP3-receptors mediate prostaglandin E_2-induced constriction of porcine large cerebral arteries. *J Cereb Blood Flow Metab* 24, 1305–1316.
80. Jakobsson, P. J., Morgenstern, R., Mancini, J., Ford-Hutchinson, A., and Persson, B. (1999) Common structural features of *MAPEG* — A widespread superfamily of membrane associated proteins with highly divergent functions in eicosanoid and glutathione metabolism. *Protein Sci* 8, 689–692.
81. Jawien, J., Gajda, M., Olszanecki, R., and Korbut, R. (2007) BAY x 1005 attenuates atherosclerosis in apoE/LDLR-double knockout mice. *J Physiol Pharmacol* 58, 583-8.

82. Jawien, J., Gajda, M., Rudling, M., Mateuszuk, L., Olszanecki, R., Guzik, T. J., Cichocki, T., Chlopicki, S., and Korbut, R. (2006) Inhibition of five lipoxygenase activating protein (FLAP) by MK-886 decreases atherosclerosis in apoE/LDLR-double knockout mice. *Eur J Clin Invest* 36, 141–146.

83. Jiang, Y., Borrelli, L., Bacskai, B. J., Kanaoka, Y., and Boyce, J. A. (2009) P2Y6 receptors require an intact cysteinyl leukotriene synthetic and signaling system to induce survival and activation of mast cells. *J Immunol* 182, 1129–1137.

84. Kajimoto, K., Shioji, K., Ishida, C., Iwanaga, Y., Kokubo, Y., Tomoike, H., Miyazaki, S., Nonogi, H., Goto, Y., and Iwai, N. (2005) Validation of the association between the gene encoding 5-lipoxygenase-activating protein and myocardial infarction in a Japanese population. *Circ J* 69, 1029–1034.

85. Kaushal, R., Pal, P., Alwell, K., Haverbusch, M., Flaherty, M., Moomaw, C., Sekar, P., Kissela, B., Kleindorfer, D., Chakraborty, R., Broderick, J., Deka, R., and Woo, D. (2007) Association of ALOX5AP with ischemic stroke: A population-based case-control study. *Hum Genet* 121, 601–607.

86. Kennedy, C. R., Zhang, Y., Brandon, S., Guan, Y., Coffee, K., Funk, C. D., Magnuson, M. A., Oates, J. A., Breyer, M. D., and Breyer, R. M. (1999) Salt-sensitive hypertension and reduced fertility in mice lacking the prostaglandin EP2 receptor. *Nat Med* 5, 217–220.

87. Kobayashi, T., Tahara, Y., Matsumoto, M., Iguchi, M., Sano, H., Murayama, T., Arai, H., Oida, H., Yurugi-Kobayashi, T., Yamashita, J. K., Katagiri, H., Majima, M., Yokode, M., Kita, T., and Narumiya, S. (2004) Roles of thromboxane A_2 and prostacyclin in the development of atherosclerosis in apoE-deficient mice. *J Clin Invest* 114, 784–794.

88. Koch, W., Hoppmann, P., Mueller, J. C., Schomig, A., and Kastrati, A. (2007) No association of polymorphisms in the gene encoding 5-lipoxygenase-activating protein and myocardial infarction in a large central European population. *Genet Med* 9, 123–129.

89. Kondo, K., Umemura, K., Ohmura, T., Hashimoto, H., and Nakashima, M. (1998) Suppression of intimal hyperplasia by a 5-lipoxygenase inhibitor, MK-886: studies with a photochemical model of endothelial injury. *Thromb Haemost* 79, 635–639.

90. Kuhn, H. (2005) Biologic relevance of lipoxygenase isoforms in atherogenesis. *Expert Rev Cardiovasc Ther* 3, 1099–1110.

91. Kuhn, H., Barnett, J., Grunberger, D., Baecker, P., Chow, J., Nguyen, B., Bursztyn-Pettegrew, H., Chan, H., and Sigal, E. (1993) Overexpression,

purification and characterization of human recombinant 15-lipoxygenase. *Biochim Biophys Acta* 1169, 80–89.

92. Kuhn, H., Belkner, J., Suzuki, H., and Yamamoto, S. (1994) Oxidative modification of human lipoproteins by lipoxygenases of different positional specificities. *J Lipid Res* 35, 1749–1759.

93. Kuhn, H., Heydeck, D., Hugou, I., and Gniwotta, C. (1997) *In vivo* action of 15-lipoxygenase in early stages of human atherogenesis. *J Clin Invest* 99, 888–893.

94. Kuhn, H., Romisch, I., and Belkner, J. (2005) The role of lipoxygenase-isoforms in atherogenesis. *Mol Nutr Food Res* 49, 1014–1029.

95. Lefebvre, B., Pepin, J. L., Baguet, J. P., Tamisier, R., Roustit, M., Riedweg, K., Bessard, G., Levy, P., and Stanke-Labesque, F. (2008) Leukotriene B_4: Early mediator of atherosclerosis in obstructive sleep apnoea? *Eur Respir J* 32, 113–120.

96. Lind, L. (2003) Circulating markers of inflammation and atherosclerosis. *Atherosclerosis* 169, 203–214.

97. Linton, M. F., and Fazio, S. (2004) Cyclooxygenase-2 and inflammation in atherosclerosis. *Curr Opin Pharmacol* 4, 116–123.

98. Lohmussaar, E., Gschwendtner, A., Mueller, J. C., Org, T., Wichmann, E., Hamann, G., Meitinger, T., and Dichgans, M. (2005) ALOX5AP gene and the PDE4D gene in a central European population of stroke patients. *Stroke* 36, 731–736.

99. Lynch, K. R., O'Neill, G. P., Liu, Q., Im, D. S., Sawyer, N., Metters, K. M., Coulombe, N., Abramovitz, M., Figueroa, D. J., Zeng, Z., Connolly, B. M., Bai, C., Austin, C. P., Chateauneuf, A., Stocco, R., Greig, G. M., Kargman, S., Hooks, S. B., Hosfield, E., Williams, D. L., Jr., Ford-Hutchinson, A. W., Caskey, C. T., and Evans, J. F. (1999) Characterization of the human cysteinyl leukotriene CysLT1 receptor. *Nature* 399, 789–793.

100. Maekawa, A., Balestrieri, B., Austen, K. F., and Kanaoka, Y. (2009) GPR17 is a negative regulator of the cysteinyl leukotriene 1 receptor response to leukotriene D_4. *Proc Natl Acad Sci U S A* 106, 11685–11690.

101. Mallat, Z., Nakamura, T., Ohan, J., Leseche, G., Tedgui, A., Maclouf, J., and Murphy, R. C. (1999) The relationship of hydroxyeicosatetraenoic acids and F_2-isoprostanes to plaque instability in human carotid atherosclerosis. *J Clin Invest* 103, 421–427.

102. Mamedova, L., Capra, V., Accomazzo, M. R., Gao, Z. G., Ferrario, S., Fumagalli, M., Abbracchio, M. P., Rovati, G. E., and Jacobson, K. A. (2005) CysLT1 leukotriene receptor antagonists inhibit the effects of nucleotides acting at P2Y receptors. *Biochem Pharmacol* 71, 115–125.

103. Mancini, J. A., Abramovitz, M., Cox, M. E., Wong, E., Charleson, S., Perrier, H., Wang, Z., Prasit, P., and Vickers, P. J. (1993) 5-lipoxygenase-activating protein is an arachidonate binding protein. *FEBS Lett* 318, 277–281.

104. Mandal, A. K., Skoch, J., Bacskai, B. J., Hyman, B. T., Christmas, P., Miller, D., Yamin, T. T., Xu, S., Wisniewski, D., Evans, J. F., and Soberman, R. J. (2004) The membrane organization of leukotriene synthesis. *Proc Natl Acad Sci U S A* 101, 6587–6592.

105. Martinez Molina, D., Wetterholm, A., Kohl, A., McCarthy, A. A., Niegowski, D., Ohlson, E., Hammarberg, T., Eshaghi, S., Haeggstrom, J. Z., and Nordlund, P. (2007) Structural basis for synthesis of inflammatory mediators by human leukotriene C_4 synthase. *Nature* 448, 613–616.

106. McAdam, B. F., Catella-Lawson, F., Mardini, I. A., Kapoor, S., Lawson, J. A., and FitzGerald, G. A. (1999) Systemic biosynthesis of prostacyclin by cyclooxygenase (COX)-2: The human pharmacology of a selective inhibitor of COX-2. *Proc Natl Acad Sci U S A* 96, 272–277.

107. Mehrabian, M., Allayee, H., Wong, J., Shi, W., Wang, X. P., Shaposhnik, Z., Funk, C. D., and Lusis, A. J. (2002) Identification of 5-lipoxygenase as a major gene contributing to atherosclerosis susceptibility in mice. *Circ Res* 91, 120–126.

108. Mehrabian, M., Wong, J., Wang, X., Jiang, Z., Shi, W., Fogelman, A. M., and Lusis, A. J. (2001) Genetic locus in mice that blocks development of atherosclerosis despite extreme hyperlipidemia. *Circ Res* 89, 125–130.

109. Meschia, J. F., Brott, T. G., Brown, R. D., Jr., Crook, R., Worrall, B. B., Kissela, B., Brown, W. M., Rich, S. S., Case, L. D., Evans, E. W., Hague, S., Singleton, A., and Hardy, J. (2005) Phosphodiesterase 4D and 5-lipoxygenase activating protein in ischemic stroke. *Ann Neurol* 58, 351–361.

110. Montuschi, P., Barnes, P. J., and Roberts, L. J., 2nd. (2004) Isoprostanes: Markers and mediators of oxidative stress. *FASEB J* 18, 1791–1800.

111. Moulton, K. S., Heller, E., Konerding, M. A., Flynn, E., Palinski, W., and Folkman, J. (1999) Angiogenesis inhibitors endostatin or TNP-470 reduce intimal neovascularization and plaque growth in apolipoprotein E-deficient mice. *Circulation* 99, 1726–1732.

112. Mueller, C. F., Wassmann, K., Widder, J. D., Wassmann, S., Chen, C. H., Keuler, B., Kudin, A., Kunz, W. S., and Nickenig, G. (2008) Multidrug resistance protein-1 affects oxidative stress, endothelial dysfunction, and atherogenesis via leukotriene C_4 export. *Circulation* 117, 2912–2918.

113. Nadel, J. A., Conrad, D. J., Ueki, I. F., Schuster, A., and Sigal, E. (1991) Immunocytochemical localization of arachidonate 15-lipoxygenase

in erythrocytes, leukocytes, and airway cells. *J Clin Invest* 87, 1139–1145.

114. Nakamura, M., and Shimizu, T. (2011) Leukotriene receptors. Chem Rev 111, 6231–6298.

115. Norel, X., de Montpreville, V., and Brink, C. (2004) Vasoconstriction induced by activation of EP1 and EP3 receptors in human lung: Effects of ONO-AE-248, ONO-DI-004, ONO-8711 or ONO-8713. *Prostaglandins Other Lipid Mediat* 74, 101–112.

116. Okuno, T., Iizuka, Y., Okazaki, H., Yokomizo, T., Taguchi, R., and Shimizu, T. (2008) 12(S)-Hydroxyheptadeca-5Z, 8E, 10E-trienoic acid is a natural ligand for leukotriene B4 receptor 2. J Exp Med 205, 759–766.

117. Olesen, M., Kwong, E., Meztli, A., Kontny, F., Seljeflot, I., Arnesen, H., Lyngdorf, L., and Falk, E. (2002) No effect of cyclooxygenase inhibition on plaque size in atherosclerosis-prone mice. *Scand Cardiovasc J* 36, 362–367.

118. Paruchuri, S., Tashimo, H., Feng, C., Maekawa, A., Xing, W., Jiang, Y., Kanaoka, Y., Conley, P., and Boyce, J. A. (2009) Leukotriene E_4-induced pulmonary inflammation is mediated by the P2Y12 receptor. *J Exp Med* 206, 2543–2555.

119. Patrono, C., and Baigent, C. (2009) Low-dose aspirin, coxibs, and other NSAIDS: A clinical mosaic emerges. *Mol Interv* 9, 31–39.

120. Patrono, C., and Baigent, C. (2010) Antiplatelet therapy: Aspirin for asymptomatic atherosclerosis? *Nat Rev Cardiol* 7, 306–307.

121. Patrono, C., and Rocca, B. (2010) The future of antiplatelet therapy in cardiovascular disease. *Annu Rev Med* 61, 49–61.

122. Paul, A., Calleja, L., Camps, J., Osada, J., Vilella, E., Ferre, N., Mayayo, E., and Joven, J. (2000) The continuous administration of aspirin attenuates atherosclerosis in apolipoprotein E-deficient mice. *Life Sci* 68, 457–465.

123. Pedersen, K. E., Bochner, B. S., and Undem, B. J. (1997) Cysteinyl leukotrienes induce P-selectin expression in human endothelial cells via a non-CysLT1 receptor-mediated mechanism. *J Pharmacol Exp Ther* 281, 655–662.

124. Peters-Golden, M., and Brock, T. G. (2003) 5-lipoxygenase and FLAP. *Prostaglandins Leukot Essent Fatty Acids* 69, 99–109.

125. Petrucci, G., De Cristofaro, R., Rutella, S., Ranelletti, F. O., Pocaterra, D., Lancellotti, S., Habib, A., Patrono, C., and Rocca, B. (2011) Prostaglandin E_2 differentially modulates human platelet function through the EP2 and EP3 receptors. *J Pharmacol Exp Ther* 336 (2): 391-402.

126. Piomelli, D., Feinmark, S. J., and Cannon, P. J. (1987) Leukotriene biosynthesis by canine and human coronary arteries. *J Pharmacol Exp Ther* 241, 763–770.

127. Poeckel, D., and Funk, C. D. (2010) The 5-lipoxygenase/leukotriene pathway in preclinical models of cardiovascular disease. *Cardiovasc Res* 86, 243–253.

128. Poeckel, D., Zemski Berry, K. A., Murphy, R. C., and Funk, C. D. (2009) Dual 12/15- and 5-lipoxygenase deficiency in macrophages alters arachidonic acid metabolism and attenuates peritonitis and atherosclerosis in ApoE knock-out mice. *J Biol Chem* 284, 21077–21089.

129. Pratico, D., Iuliano, L., Mauriello, A., Spagnoli, L., Lawson, J. A., Rokach, J., Maclouf, J., Violi, F., and FitzGerald, G. A. (1997) Localization of distinct F_2-isoprostanes in human atherosclerotic lesions. *J Clin Invest* 100, 2028–2034.

130. Pratico, D., Tillmann, C., Zhang, Z. B., Li, H., and FitzGerald, G. A. (2001) Acceleration of atherogenesis by COX-1-dependent prostanoid formation in low density lipoprotein receptor knockout mice. *Proc Natl Acad Sci U S A* 98, 3358–3363.

131. Qiu, H., Gabrielsen, A., Agardh, H. E., Wan, M., Wetterholm, A., Wong, C. H., Hedin, U., Swedenborg, J., Hansson, G. K., Samuelsson, B., Paulsson-Berne, G., and Haeggstrom, J. Z. (2006) Expression of 5-lipoxygenase and leukotriene A_4 hydrolase in human atherosclerotic lesions correlates with symptoms of plaque instability. *Proc Natl Acad Sci U S A* 103, 8161–8166.

132. Radmark, O., and Samuelsson, B. (2007) 5-lipoxygenase: regulation and possible involvement in atherosclerosis. *Prostaglandins Other Lipid Mediat* 83, 162–174.

134. Rao, N. L., Dunford, P. J., Xue, X., Jiang, X., Lundeen, K. A., Coles, F., Riley, J. P., Williams, K. N., Grice, C. A., Edwards, J. P., Karlsson, L., and Fourie, A. M. (2007) Anti-inflammatory activity of a potent, selective leukotriene A_4 hydrolase inhibitor in comparison with the 5-lipoxygenase inhibitor zileuton. *J Pharmacol Exp Ther* 321, 1154–1160.

134. Rao, N. L., Riley, J. P., Banie, H., Xue, X., Sun, B., Crawford, S., Lundeen, K. A., Yu, F., Karlsson, L., Fourie, A. M., and Dunford, P. J. (2010) Leukotriene A_4 hydrolase inhibition attenuates allergic airway inflammation and hyperresponsiveness. *Am J Respir Crit Care Med* 181, 899–907.

135. Reid, G. K., Kargman, S., Vickers, P. J., Mancini, J. A., Leveille, C., Ethier, D., Miller, D. K., Gillard, J. W., Dixon, R. A., and Evans, J. F. (1990) Correlation between expression of 5-lipoxygenase-activating protein,

5-lipoxygenase, and cellular leukotriene synthesis. J Biol Chem 265, 19818–19823.

136. Riccioni, G., Back, M., and Capra, V. (2010) Leukotrienes and atherosclerosis. *Curr Drug Targets* 11, 882–887.

137. Rott, D., Zhu, J., Burnett, M. S., Zhou, Y. F., Zalles-Ganley, A., Ogunmakinwa, J., and Epstein, S. E. (2003) Effects of MF-tricyclic, a selective cyclooxygenase-2 inhibitor, on atherosclerosis progression and susceptibility to cytomegalovirus replication in apolipoprotein-E knockout mice. *J Am Coll Cardiol* 41, 1812–1819.

138. Samuelsson, B. (1983) Leukotrienes: Mediators of immediate hypersensitivity reactions and inflammation. *Science* 220, 568–575.

139. Samuelsson, B., Morgenstern, R., and Jakobsson, P. J. (2007) Membrane prostaglandin E synthase-1: A novel therapeutic target. *Pharmacol Rev* 59, 207–224.

140. Sanchez-Galan, E., Gomez-Hernandez, A., Vidal, C., Martin-Ventura, J. L., Blanco-Colio, L. M., Munoz-Garcia, B., Ortega, L., Egido, J., and Tunon, J. (2009) Leukotriene B_4 enhances the activity of nuclear factor-kappaB pathway through BLT1 and BLT2 receptors in atherosclerosis. *Cardiovasc Res* 81, 216–225.

141. Sandanayaka, V., Mamat, B., Mishra, R. K., Winger, J., Krohn, M., Zhou, L. M., Keyvan, M., Enache, L., Sullins, D., Onua, E., Zhang, J., Halldorsdottir, G., Sigthorsdottir, H., Thorlaksdottir, A., Sigthorsson, G., Thorsteinnsdottir, M., Davies, D. R., Stewart, L. J., Zembower, D. E., Andresson, T., Kiselyov, A. S., Singh, J., and Gurney, M. E. (2010) Discovery of 4-[(2S)-2-{[4-(4-chlorophenoxy)phenoxy]methyl}-1-pyrrolidinyl]butanoic acid (DG-051) as a novel leukotriene A_4 hydrolase inhibitor of leukotriene B4 biosynthesis. *J Med Chem* 53, 573–585.

142. Sendobry, S. M., Cornicelli, J. A., Welch, K., Bocan, T., Tait, B., Trivedi, B. K., Colbry, N., Dyer, R. D., Feinmark, S. J., and Daugherty, A. (1997) Attenuation of diet-induced atherosclerosis in rabbits with a highly selective 15-lipoxygenase inhibitor lacking significant antioxidant properties. *Br J Pharmacol* 120, 1199–1206.

143. Shen, J., Kuhn, H., Petho-Schramm, A., and Chan, L. (1995) Transgenic rabbits with the integrated human 15-lipoxygenase gene driven by a lysozyme promoter: Macrophage-specific expression and variable positional specificity of the transgenic enzyme. *FASEB J* 9, 1623–1631.

144. Simon, T. C., Makheja, A. N., and Bailey, J. M. (1990) Relationship of vascular 15-lipoxygenase induction to atherosclerotic plaque formation in rabbits. *Prostaglandins Leukot Essent Fatty Acids* 41, 273–278.

145. Sjostrom, M., Johansson, A. S., Schroder, O., Qiu, H., Palmblad, J., and Haeggstrom, J. Z. (2003) Dominant expression of the CysLT2 receptor accounts for calcium signaling by cysteinyl leukotrienes in human umbilical vein endothelial cells. Arterioscler Thromb Vasc Biol 23, e37–41.

146. Snelgrove, R. J., Jackson, P. L., Hardison, M. T., Noerager, B. D., Kinloch, A., Gaggar, A., Shastry, S., Rowe, S. M., Shim, Y. M., Hussell, T., and Blalock, J. E. (2010) A critical role for LTA_4H in limiting chronic pulmonary neutrophilic inflammation. *Science* 330, 90–94.

147. Spagnuolo, P. J., Ellner, J. J., Hassid, A., and Dunn, M. J. (1988) Mediation of augmented monocyte adhesiveness by thromboxane. *Inflammation* 12, 1–9.

148. Spanbroek, R., Grabner, R., Lotzer, K., Hildner, M., Urbach, A., Ruhling, K., Moos, M. P., Kaiser, B., Cohnert, T. U., Wahlers, T., Zieske, A., Plenz, G., Robenek, H., Salbach, P., Kuhn, H., Radmark, O., Samuelsson, B., and Habenicht, A. J. (2003) Expanding expression of the 5-lipoxygenase pathway within the arterial wall during human atherogenesis. *Proc Natl Acad Sci U S A* 100, 1238–1243.

149. Sparrow, C. P., Parthasarathy, S., and Steinberg, D. (1988) Enzymatic modification of low density lipoprotein by purified lipoxygenase plus phospholipase A_2 mimics cell-mediated oxidative modification. *J Lipid Res* 29, 745–753.

150. Subbarao, K., Jala, V. R., Mathis, S., Suttles, J., Zacharias, W., Ahamed, J., Ali, H., Tseng, M. T., and Haribabu, B. (2004) Role of leukotriene B_4 receptors in the development of atherosclerosis: Potential mechanisms. *Arterioscler Thromb Vasc Biol* 24, 369–375.

151. Tager, A. M., Bromley, S. K., Medoff, B. D., Islam, S. A., Bercury, S. D., Friedrich, E. B., Carafone, A. D., Gerszten, R. E., and Luster, A. D. (2003) Leukotriene B4 receptor BLT1 mediates early effector T cell recruitment. Nat Immunol 4, 982–990.

152. Takayama, K., Garcia-Cardena, G., Sukhova, G. K., Comander, J., Gimbrone, M. A., Jr., and Libby, P. (2002) Prostaglandin E_2 suppresses chemokine production in human macrophages through the EP4 receptor. *J Biol Chem* 277, 44147–44154.

153. Tardif, J. C., L'Allier P, L., Ibrahim, R., Gregoire, J. C., Nozza, A., Cossette, M., Kouz, S., Lavoie, M. A., Paquin, J., Brotz, T. M., Taub, R., and Pressacco, J. (2010) Treatment with 5-lipoxygenase inhibitor VIA-2291 (Atreleuton) in patients with recent acute coronary syndrome. *Circ Cardiovasc Imaging* 3, 298–307.

154. Thunnissen, M. M., Nordlund, P., and Haeggstrom, J. Z. (2001) Crystal structure of human leukotriene A_4 hydrolase, a bifunctional enzyme in inflammation. *Nat Struct Biol* 8, 131–135.

155. Tzoulaki, I., Murray, G. D., Lee, A. J., Rumley, A., Lowe, G. D., and Fowkes, F. G. (2005) C-reactive protein, interleukin-6, and soluble adhesion molecules as predictors of progressive peripheral atherosclerosis in the general population: Edinburgh Artery Study. *Circulation* 112, 976–983.

156. Uzonyi, B., Lotzer, K., Jahn, S., Kramer, C., Hildner, M., Bretschneider, E., Radke, D., Beer, M., Vollandt, R., Evans, J. F., Funk, C. D., and Habenicht, A. J. (2006) Cysteinyl leukotriene 2 receptor and protease-activated receptor 1 activate strongly correlated early genes in human endothelial cells. *Proc Natl Acad Sci U S A* 103, 6326-31.

157. Wan, M., Sabirsh, A., Wetterholm, A., Agerberth, B., and Haeggstrom, J. Z. (2007) Leukotriene B_4 triggers release of the cathelicidin LL-37 from human neutrophils: Novel lipid-peptide interactions in innate immune responses. *FASEB J* 21, 2897–2905.

158. Wang, M., Song, W. L., Cheng, Y., and Fitzgerald, G. A. (2008) Microsomal prostaglandin E synthase-1 inhibition in cardiovascular inflammatory disease. *J Intern Med* 263, 500–505.

159. Wang, M., Zukas, A. M., Hui, Y., Ricciotti, E., Pure, E., and FitzGerald, G. A. (2006) Deletion of microsomal prostaglandin E synthase-1 augments prostacyclin and retards atherogenesis. *Proc Natl Acad Sci U S A* 103, 14507–14512.

160. Welch, C. L., Bretschger, S., Latib, N., Bezouevski, M., Guo, Y., Pleskac, N., Liang, C. P., Barlow, C., Dansky, H., Breslow, J. L., and Tall, A. R. (2001) Localization of atherosclerosis susceptibility loci to chromosomes 4 and 6 using the Ldlr knockout mouse model. *Proc Natl Acad Sci U S A* 98, 7946–7951.

161. Whatling, C., McPheat, W., and Herslof, M. (2007) The potential link between atherosclerosis and the 5-lipoxygenase pathway: Investigational agents with new implications for the cardiovascular field. *Expert Opin Investig Drugs* 16, 1879–1893.

162. Vidal, C., Gomez-Hernandez, A., Sanchez-Galan, E., Gonzalez, A., Ortega, L., Gomez-Gerique, J. A., Tunon, J., and Egido, J. (2007) Licofelone, a balanced inhibitor of cyclooxygenase and 5-lipoxygenase, reduces inflammation in a rabbit model of atherosclerosis. *J Pharmacol Exp Ther* 320, 108–116.

163. Yla-Herttuala, S., Luoma, J., Viita, H., Hiltunen, T., Sisto, T., and Nikkari, T. (1995) Transfer of 15-lipoxygenase gene into rabbit iliac arteries

results in the appearance of oxidation-specific lipid-protein adducts characteristic of oxidized low density lipoprotein. *J Clin Invest* 95, 2692–2698.

164. Yla-Herttuala, S., Rosenfeld, M. E., Parthasarathy, S., Glass, C. K., Sigal, E., Witztum, J. L., and Steinberg, D. (1990) Colocalization of 15-lipoxygenase mRNA and protein with epitopes of oxidized low density lipoprotein in macrophage-rich areas of atherosclerotic lesions. *Proc Natl Acad Sci U S A* 87, 6959–6963.
165. Yu, Y., Ricciotti, E., Grosser, T., and Fitzgerald, G. A. (2009) The translational therapeutics of prostaglandin inhibition in atherothrombosis. *J Thromb Haemost* 7(Suppl 1), 222–226.
166. Zarini, S., Gijon, M. A., Ransome, A. E., Murphy, R. C., and Sala, A. (2009) Transcellular biosynthesis of cysteinyl leukotrienes in vivo during mouse peritoneal inflammation. *Proc Natl Acad Sci U S A* 106, 8296–8301.
167. Zee, R. Y., Cheng, S., Hegener, H. H., Erlich, H. A., and Ridker, P. M. (2006) Genetic variants of arachidonate 5-lipoxygenase-activating protein, and risk of incident myocardial infarction and ischemic stroke: A nested case-control approach. *Stroke* 37, 2007–2011.
168. Zeilhofer, H. U., and Brune, K. (2006) Analgesic strategies beyond the inhibition of cyclooxygenases. *Trends Pharmacol Sci* 27, 467–474.
169. Zhao, L., Moos, M. P., Grabner, R., Pedrono, F., Fan, J., Kaiser, B., John, N., Schmidt, S., Spanbroek, R., Lotzer, K., Huang, L., Cui, J., Rader, D. J., Evans, J. F., Habenicht, A. J. and Funk, C. D. (2004) The 5-lipoxygenase pathway promotes pathogenesis of hyperlipidemia-dependent aortic aneurysm. *Nat Med* 10, 966–973.

Chapter 5

Stabilization of Mast Cells for Taming Vulnerable Plaques

Guo-Ping Shi and Peter Libby
Cardiovascular Medicine, Brigham and Women's Hospital and Harvard Medical School, Boston, MA 02115, USA
gshi@rics.bwh.harvard.edu

5.1 Introduction

Mast cells (MCs) participate in the pathophysiology of allergic diseases, notably in IgE-mediated hypersensitivity reactions in airways, skin, and the gastrointestinal tract — such as asthma, allergic rhinitis, atopic dermatitis, and food allergy. These responses result from allergen-specific IgE binding to and cross-linking of the high-affinity IgE receptor FcεRI on MCs, leading to activation and release of inflammatory mediators. Increased MCs localize in bronchial epithelia and airway smooth muscle, in association with pulmonary inflammation, in mice with experimental allergic airway inflammation (Mathias *et al.*, 2009), and in human asthma (Brightling *et al.*, 2002). MC mediators include histamine, cytokines, chemokines, growth factors, arachidonic acid metabolites, reactive oxygen and nitrogen species, heparin, cathepsins, matrix

Atherosclerosis: Treatment and Prevention
Edited by Christian Weber and Oliver Soehnlein

ISBN 978-981-4316-26-2 (Hardcover), ISBN 978-981-4364-26-3 (eBook)
www.panstanford.com

metalloproteinases (MMPs), carboxypeptide A, and the MC-specific proteases chymases and tryptases. Many cell types other than MCs also produce many of these mediators, and some link directly or indirectly to the pathogenesis of atherosclerosis. Neurons, gastric enterochromaffin-like (ECL) cells, hematopoietic cells, basophils, macrophages, and lymphocytes release histamine (Jutel *et al.*, 2005), one of the many vasoactive components that enhance vascular permeability to macromolecules. By releasing histamine, activated MCs in vessels could disturb endothelial cell (EC) barriers, thereby enhancing lipoprotein permeability (Ma and Kovanen, 1997). Histamine causes smooth-muscle cell (SMC) contraction, which in turn causes local vasoconstriction and can promote coronary arterial spasm (Kounis and Zavras, 1991). MC-derived heparin exhibits many pro-atherogenic properties, including binding to low-density lipoproteins (LDLs) and promoting foam-cell formation, stabilizing MC tryptase active tetramers (Lindstedt *et al.*, 1998), and protecting chymase and cathepsin G from their natural inhibitors (Lindstedt *et al.*, 2001a; Ermolieff *et al.*, 1994), yielding enhanced activities of these MC proteases.

Inflammatory cell migration and accumulation within lesions characterize atherogenesis. Monocytes, macrophages, neutrophils, dendritic cells, and lymphocytes (e.g., B cells, $CD4^+$ T cells, $CD8^+$ T cells, natural killer T (NKT) cells) can migrate to atherosclerotic lesions as terminally differentiated mature cells. In contrast, MCs leave bone marrow as $CD34^+CD117^+CD13^+Fc\varepsilon RI^-$ pluripotent hematopoietic progenitors (Galli *et al.*, 2005a; Okayama and Kawakami, 2006) and reach final maturation in target tissues, such as skin and mucosal surfaces. Currently, the mechanisms by which and the forms in which MCs accumulate in human atheromata remain unknown. *In vitro* studies suggest that the chemokines responsible for MC migration include stem cell factor (SCF) from the stromal fibroblast and endotoxin from the MC chemokine receptors CXCR2, CCR3, CXCR4, and CCR5 (Ochi *et al.*, 1999; Haley *et al.*, 2000; Libby, 2002a). These cells also populate perivascular connective tissue structure and the vascular adventitia, positioning them to participate in processes like wound healing, tissue regeneration and remodeling after injury, fibrosis, and angiogenesis (Gonzalez *et al.*, 1999; Weller *et al.*, 2006; Grimbaldeston *et al.*, 2007). MCs are also located close to neurons, whose products — including neuropeptides such as substance P — can activate them (Foreman, 1987; Williams *et al.*, 1995). Despite much progress in understanding the recruitment of MC progenitors to the small intestine and the inflamed lung, little is known about MC progenitor recruitment and their differentiation in the heart or the vascular wall.

Human MCs are grouped by their expression of cell-type–specific chymases and tryptases: those containing tryptase (MC_T) and those containing both tryptase and chymase (MC_{TC}) (Irani *et al.*, 1986). Rodent MCs are grouped by their tissue locations: mucosal MCs express mouse MC protease (mMCP)-1 and mMCP-2 (tryptases) and localize preferentially in the mucosa of the airways and gastrointestinal tract. In contrast, connective tissue MCs express mMCP-4, mMCP-5, mMCP-6, carboxypeptidase A, and cathepsin G and typically localize in the skin, synovium, peritoneum, and perivascular tissues. But MC phenotype can modulate under certain conditions (Kitamura, 1989); interleukin-4 (IL-4) with SCF, for example, promotes the conversion of MC_T cells into MC_{TC} (Toru *et al.*, 1998). IL-4 further regulates chymase expression in MC_{TC} (Ahn *et al.*, 2000). Human atherosclerotic lesions contain both chymase and tryptase (Jeziorska *et al.*, 1997; Ihara *et al.*, 1999). As discussed further below, inhibition of either chymase or tryptase attenuates experimental atherosclerosis, but whether all MCs are MC_{TC} in human atherosclerotic lesions remains uncertain.

Atherosclerosis is an inflammatory disease in which both innate and adaptive immunity contribute to pathogenesis (Weber *et al.*, 2008; Packard *et al.*, 2009). MCs function in both innate and adaptive immunity. They help defend against parasites and bacteria (Féger *et al.*, 2002; Marshall, 2004) and generally induce inflammation (Bischoff, 2009), thus participating in innate immunity. Because they line various body surfaces, MCs are ideally positioned to be among the first responder cells during microbial attack. MCs are one of the first cell types to react against external threats encountered from the environment (Kitamura, 1989; Galli *et al.*, 1999), and they interact early with invading microorganisms and initiate immune responses (Metz *et al.*, 2008). MCs constitutively express MHC-I and increase MHC-II when stimulated with interferon-gamma (IFN-γ), tumor necrosis factor alpha (TNF-α), or lipopolysaccharide (LPS) (Kambayashi *et al.*, 2009; Galli *et al.*, 2005b; Grabbe *et al.*, 1997). MC-derived TNF-α is important and, together with leukotriene-C4 (LTC4) and leukotriene-B4 (LTB4), contributes to the recruitment of neutrophils and eosinophils and thereby to the clearance of infections (Echtenacher *et al.*, 1996; Malaviya *et al.*, 1996; Malaviya and Abraham, 2000). Thus, MC-null mice clear *Escherichia coli* during experimental acute peritonitis less well than wild-type mice, as well as *Klebsiella pneumoniae* and *Francisella tularensis* in experimental lung infections. In these studies, MC-null mice have decreased survival due to impaired innate immune response to pathogens (Echtenacher *et al.*, 1996; Féger *et al.*, 2002; Ketavarapu *et al.*, 2008; Sutherland *et al.*, 2008). Tryptase mMCP-6 has a critical protective role in bacterial and parasitic infection (Thakurdas *et al.*, 2007; Shin *et al.*, 2008). Patients with acquired immunodeficiency syndrome (AIDS) have fewer MC_T in the interstitial mucosa (Irani *et al.*, 1987). Histamine can induce expression of EC toll-like receptor-2 (TLR2) and toll-like receptor 4 (TLR4), which may have relevance in local innate immune responses in atherosclerotic plaques (Talreja *et al.*, 2004).

When an individual encounters an allergen and a low dose of endotoxin lipopolysaccharide, LPS or peptidoglycan (PGN) in the environment, MC activation through TLR signaling may lead to secretion of TNF-α. Dendritic cells that have taken up the allergen may then be activated by TNF-α to express co-stimulatory molecules and lead to Th2 response and allergen sensitization (Nigo *et al.*, 2006; Eisenbarth *et al.*, 2002; Yamashita and Nakayama, 2008), thereby exacerbating allergic diseases. MCs release TNF-α that acts in dendritic cell migration to lymph nodes through the increase of CCR7 (McLachlan *et al.*, 2003), which allows dendritic cells to respond to the homing chemokines — CCL19 and CCL21 — that are produced by the draining nodes and lymphatics (Förster *et al.*, 2008). Upon activation, MCs release the Th2 polarizing cytokines IL-4, IL-10, and IL-13 to induce a stimulated $CD4^+$ T cell to become a Th2 cell (Stelekati *et al.*, 2007). These Th2 cells induce humoral immune responses to pathogens by producing cytokines that stimulate B-cell antibody production. MCs can also enhance T-cell proliferation through FcεR-dependent and FcεR-independent pathways (Nakae *et al.*, 2005). MC modulation of both innate and adaptive immunity can influence atherosclerosis, its complications, and its clinical manifestations. This chapter focuses on MC identification in atherosclerotic lesions, *in vitro* activities pertinent to atherogenesis, results from animal experiments, MC and MC mediator inhibitor development, and their potential clinical applications.

5.2 Mast Cells in Atherosclerotic Lesions

5.2.1 Mast Cell Location and Recruitment in Atherosclerotic Lesions

MCs were first identified in human and animal atherosclerosis more than half a century ago (Constantinides, 1953; Cairns and Constantinides, 1954). Petri Kovanen, Ken Lindstedt, and their colleagues have contributed most of our current knowledge of the potential roles of these inflammatory cells in atherosclerosis during the last 25 years (Lindstedt and Kovanen, 2004). In human atherosclerotic lesions, fewer MCs locate in the cap and core regions, and more MCs locate in the adventitia and the shoulder regions (Fig. 5.1) — regions prone to erosion or rupture (Kaartinen *et al.*, 1994). Importantly, activated (degranulated) MCs localize preferably to the shoulder regions. These activated MCs represent about 20% of total MCs in the normal coronary intima, 50% of those in fatty streaks, and 85% of those in the shoulder regions (Kovanen, 2007; Kaartinen *et al.*, 1994, 1996b). MCs resided at sites of atherosclerotic erosion or rupture in patients who died of acute myocardial infarction (AMI) (Kovanen *et al.*, 1995). MCs also localize to regions of plaque rupture in experimental atherosclerosis, and activation of perivascular MCs correlates with intraplaque hemorrhage, macrophage and EC apoptosis, vascular leakage, and CXCR2-mediated and very late antigen (VLA)-4–mediated recruitment of leukocytes to plaque (Bot *et al.*, 2007).

Currently, no definitive study illuminates the precise molecules or cells that mediate MC recruitment to atherosclerotic lesions. Human aortic ECs, SMCs, and MCs express SCF (Miyamoto *et al.*, 1997) as a potential player in MC progenitor influx into the aortic and coronary intima. Human atherosclerotic lesions also contain eotaxin, a chemokine implicated in MC trafficking (Haley *et al.*, 2000; Libby, 2002a). MC granules from sonicated human leukemic MCs stimulated human umbilical cord vein EC expression of monocyte chemotactic protein-1 (MCP-1) and IL-8 (but not IL-1β, TNF-α, or granulocyte colony-stimulating factor (G-CSF)). Increased expression of these chemokines might help recruit more MCs to human atherosclerotic lesions, but a tryptase-neutralizing antibody can inhibit this effect. Moreover, human tryptase (but not chymase) had the same effect as

MC lysate (Kinoshita *et al.*, 2005), suggesting a role for MC tryptase in the accumulation of MCs or other inflammatory cells in human atherosclerotic plaques.

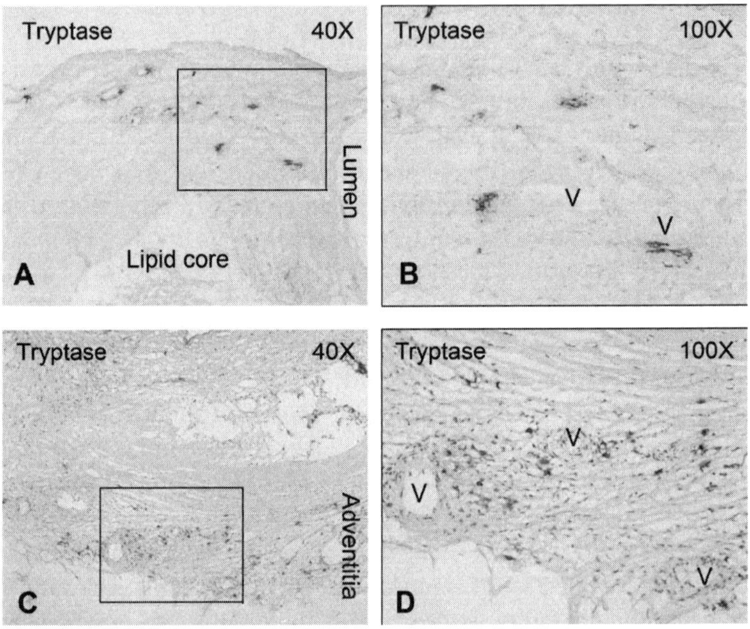

Figure 5.1 Mast cells in human coronary atherosclerotic lesions. Anti-human tryptase antibody immunostaining detected mast cells in the shoulder area (panels A and B) and in the adventitia (panels C and D). Framed areas in panels A and C are shown at higher magnifications in panels B and D, respectively. Lumen, lipid core, and adventitia are indicated. V: microvessel.

5.2.2 Clinical Evidence of Mast Cell Involvement in Atherosclerosis

Recent studies suggest that atherosclerosis associates closely with asthma and allergic diseases, indirectly supporting a role for MCs in atherosclerosis. Allergic disorders, such as asthma and allergic rhinitis, may increase risk for developing atherosclerosis in humans (Knoflach *et al.*, 2005). Epidemiological studies found that increased IgE levels, eosinophilia, positive skin-prick tests, self-reported asthma, and enzymes that regulate leukotriene synthesis (5-lipoxygenase,

5-LO) predict high risk for atherosclerosis, stroke, and MI (Knoflach *et al.*, 2005; Criqui *et al.*, 1987; Langer *et al.*, 1996; Enright *et al.*, 1996; Hospers *et al.*, 1999; Dwyer *et al.*, 2004; Helgadottir *et al.*, 2004). In both the Bruneck Study (826 men and women, 40 to 70 years of age) and the Atherosclerosis Risk Factors in Male Youngsters (ARMY) study (141 men, 17–18 years of age, followed for 5 years) (Knoflach *et al.*, 2005), subjects with allergic disorders had significantly increased risk for high intima-media thickness (OR: 2.5, $P = 0.03$; ARMY study) and for the development and progression of arterial intimal thickening (OR: 3.8, $P = 0.007$; Bruneck Study), even after multivariate adjustment for established and potential vascular risk factors (Knoflach *et al.*, 2005). More directly, patients with coronary artery disease (CAD) have significantly higher serum tryptase levels than those with normal angiography or without CAD (Mito *et al.*, 2002). Most of these studies are relatively small and used various measures of mast cell activity and of disease, highlighting the need for rigorous large studies of biomarkers of MC function and atherosclerotic disease burden and events, appropriately adjusted for potential confounders.

5.3 Mast Cell Functions and Atherosclerosis

5.3.1 Mast Cell Activation

As discussed earlier activated MCs in the shoulder regions of human atherosclerotic lesions may release inflammatory mediators to promote atherosclerotic lesion growth and rupture. MC mediators (e.g., tryptase, chymase, cytokines) can stimulate microvascular tubule formation, fibroblast proliferation, collagen deposition, and MMP activation for plaque formation and destabilization (Fig. 5.2) (Bankl and Valent, 2002; Dvorak, 1986; Marone *et al.*, 1995; Blair *et al.*, 1997; Garbuzenko *et al.*, 2002). Histamine, for example, a classical component of MC granules, derives from L-histidine through histidine decarboxylase (HDC) action (Moya-Garcia *et al.*, 2005) and increases entry of lipoproteins into the arterial wall (Rozenberg *et al.*, 2010). HDC mRNA level increased in atherosclerotic lesions in human aortas, localized to macrophage foam cells and lymphocytes (Higuchi *et al.*, 2001). Histamine may promote SMC proliferation (Miyazawa

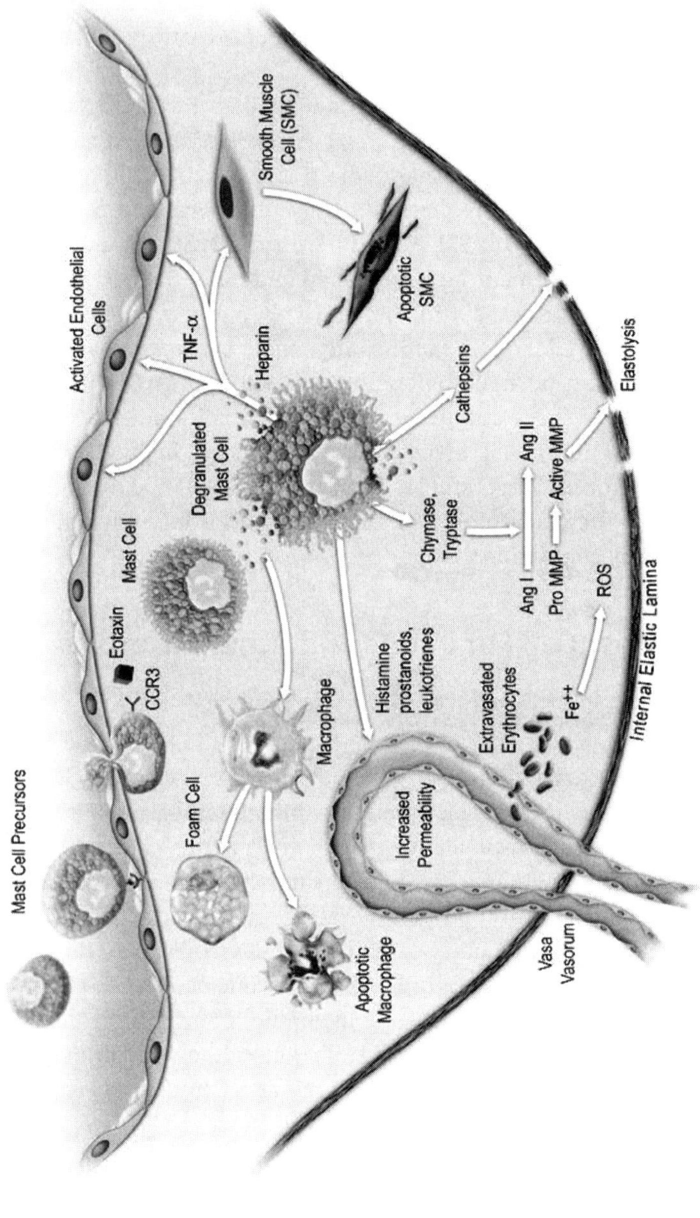

Figure 5.2 Mast cell functions in atherosclerosis. From *Circulation* 2007; 115: 2471–2473.

et al., 1998). After carotid ligation, neointima macrophages and SMCs also expressed HDC (Ohtsu, 2008). HDC gene-deficient mice demonstrated ameliorated atherosclerosis (Tanimoto *et al.*, 2006).

MC activation occurs through multiple mechanisms, most prominently IgE binding to its receptor FcεR1 on MCs (Galli *et al.*, 2005a). Using *Ige*$^{-/-}$ mice, IgE influenced MC number and function, but not MC progenitor recruitment, during *Aspergillus fumigatus* extract-induced pulmonary allergic inflammation (Mathias *et al.*, 2009). The complement-derived anaphylatoxins C3a and C5a (Vlaicu *et al.*, 1985) also activate MCs to release pro-inflammatory cytokines and chemokines (Marshall, 2004; Gilfillan and Tkaczyk, 2006) by binding to their corresponding receptors C3aR and C5aR, thereby enhancing recruitment of eosinophils and more MCs (Daffern *et al.*, 1995; Hartmann *et al.*, 1997). Human atherosclerotic lesions contain both C5a and C5aR (Laine *et al.*, 2002). T cells, ECs, and SMCs also express C5aR and C3aR (Leskinen *et al.*, 2006; Oksjoki *et al.*, 2007), although whether the binding of these anaphylatoxins to T cells and vascular cells participates in atherogenesis remains uncertain. SCF regulates MC development and homeostasis (Broudy, 1997; Tsai *et al.*, 1991); for example, SCF binding to the MC surface receptor CD117 (KIT) can activate MCs (Bischoff and Dahinden, 1992). The TLR signaling pathway also leads to MC activation. MCs express both TLR2 and TLR4; ligands to TLR2 and TLR4 act synergistically on signals mediated by FcεR1, resulting in reinforced cytokine production (e.g., IL-4, IL-6, IL-8, TNF-α) in bone marrow-derived MCs (BMMCs) from mice (Qiao *et al.*, 2006; Masuda *et al.*, 2002; Bachelet and Levi-Schaffer, 2007). BMMC TLR4 stimulation also increases their capacity to produce Th2 cytokines, leading to enhanced eosinophilic airway inflammation (Nigo *et al.*, 2006). Other pathophysiologically relevant MC activators include endogenous peptides (e.g., substance P), lipoproteins, IgG binding to MC surface FcγR (Nieuwenhuizen *et al.*, 2007; Malbec and Daëron, 2007), corticotropin-releasing hormone (Cao *et al.*, 2006), inflammatory cytokines, or even macrophages and T cells in close proximity. Oxidized LDL (oxLDL), for example, induces MC IL-8 expression at both RNA and protein levels *in vitro* (Kelley *et al.*, 2006). IL-1 and TNF-α can induce MC secretion of cytokines in the absence of degranulation (without secretion of histamine and other granule components) (Kandere-Grzybowska *et al.*, 2003; Fischer *et al.*, 2006).

5.3.2 Mast Cells Modulate Vascular Cell Growth and Apoptosis

Binding of IgE to FcεRI or other pathways of MC activation not only regulates MC function, but also directly or indirectly influences cellular survival or resistance to apoptosis (Kawakami and Galli, 2002). MCs can induce SMC death (Leskinen *et al.*, 2003a, 2003b), and EC death (Lätti *et al.*, 2003) or detachment (Mäyränpää *et al.*, 2006), contributing to coronary artery spasm or even superficial erosion — a mechanism that can trigger arterial thrombosis (Kalsner and Richards, 1984; Forman *et al.*, 1985).

Chymases and tryptases may mediate MC-induced modulation of SMC growth and apoptosis. MC-derived chymases activate latent TGF-β1 sequestered by the extracellular matrix (ECM) (Lindstedt *et al.*, 2001b), thereby influencing SMC differentiation, migration, and proliferation, along with ECM synthesis and secretion (Wang *et al.*, 2001). Chymases also induce SMC apoptosis by degrading extracellular fibronectin and thrombin (Tchougounova *et al.*, 2003; Leskinen *et al.*, 2003b), by disrupting focal adhesion complexes and Akt dephosphorylation, and by interrupting NF-κB-mediated survival signalling — processes that promote cell adhesion and survival (Leskinen *et al.*, 2006). Chymase treatment reduces levels of NF-κB and its translocation to the nucleus after LPS or IL-1β stimulation, resulting in decreased Bcl-2 and leading to mitochondrial swelling, cytochrome C release, activation of caspase-8 and caspase-9 (Leskinen *et al.*, 2006), and arterial SMC apoptosis (Leskinen *et al.*, 2003a). MC tryptases also degrade pericellular fibronectin and vitronectin (Vartio *et al.*, 1981), actions that may augment SMC apoptosis. We recently showed that BMMCs from mMCP-4–deficient (*Mcpt4*$^{-/-}$) mice (Fig. 5.3A) (Sun *et al.*, 2009) or mMCP-6–deficient (*Mcpt6*$^{-/-}$) mice (Zhang et al., 2007) had reduced ability to induce apoptosis of vascular SMCs. MCs also weaken the fibrous cap of atherosclerotic plaques by decreasing the production of matrix proteins. Indeed, caps of ruptured coronary arterial plaques contain increased numbers of MCs and reduced numbers of SMCs (Kovanen *et al.*, 1995). Multiple MC mediators can mediate this MC activity; for example, chymase inhibits SMC collagen synthesis by TGF-β–dependent and TGF-β–independent mechanisms (Wang *et al.*, 2001). Heparin sulfate proteoglycans released from rat serosal MCs can inhibit SMC proliferation *in vitro* (Wang and Kovanen, 1999).

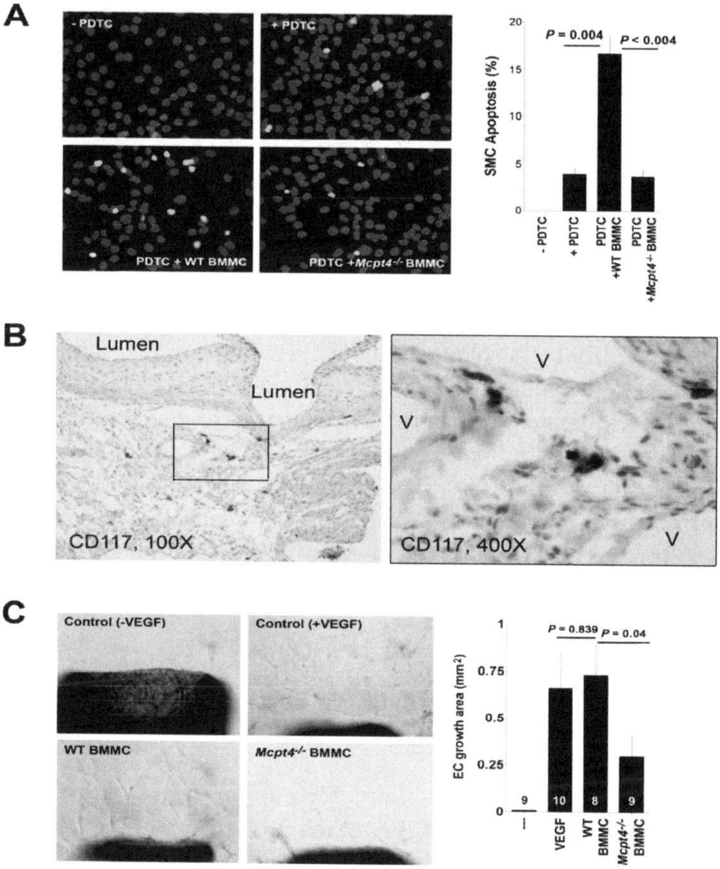

Figure 5.3 Mast cell chymase in smooth-muscle cell (SMC) apoptosis and microvessel growth. A. Fluorescin in situ cell death detection kit (Roche) detected that bone marrow-derived mast cells BMMC from wild-type (WT) mice, but not those from chymase-deficient (Mcpt4$^{-/-}$) mice, enhanced pyrrolidine dithiocarbamate (PDTC)-induced aortic SMC apoptosis. B. Anti-mouse CD117 antibody immunostaining detected MCs in atherosclerotic lesions from aortic roots from Apoe$^{-/-}$ mice that consumed an atherogenic diet for 12 weeks. Lumen areas are indicated. V: microvessel. Framed area in the left panel is shown at higher magnification in the right panel. C. BMMCs from WT mice enhanced microvessel growth from aortic rings, but those from Mcpt4$^{-/-}$ mice showed significantly reduced activity in this aortic ring assay. Representative data in panels A and C are shown to the left. Panels A and C are from *Circulation* 2009; 120: 973–982.

MCs also trigger vascular EC apoptosis. This MC activity depends on TNF-α and chymase, and also involves cytochrome C release from mitochondria to the cytoplasm (Lindstedt and Kovanen, 2004). Crude MC releasate, or a mixture of chymase and TNF-α, causes apoptosis of rat cardiac microvascular ECs or human coronary artery ECs by degrading fibronectin and vitronectin, activating caspase-8 and caspase-9 and inactivating focal adhesion kinase (FAK) and Akt-dependent survival signaling pathway — all partially inhibitable by chymase and TNF-α inhibitors (Heikkilä *et al.*, 2008). MC tryptase and cathepsin G also degrade the subendothelium basement proteins fibronectin, vitronectin, nidogen, and vascular endothelial cadherin (VE-cadherin) and cause EC death (Mäyränpää *et al.*, 2006). Treatment of human coronary arteries *ex vivo* intraluminally with recombinant human tryptase or chymase induced endothelial damage characterized by EC retraction, disruption to cell adhesion, and desquamation, likely because of degradation of VE-cadherin and fibronectin — proteins necessary for cell–cell interactions and EC adhesion — by chymase, tryptase, and possibly cathepsin G (Mäyränpää *et al.*, 2006).

5.3.3 Mast Cell Function in Atherosclerotic Lesion Neovascularization

In early atherosclerotic lesions, MCs often reside superficially just beneath the luminal endothelium, whereas in advanced atherosclerosis, invasion of adventitial microvessels frequently occurs in the deeper regions of plaques (Virmani *et al.*, 2005). These deep parts of human atheroma often lack MCs, unless vascularization has occurred. Indeed, in human atherosclerotic lesions, MCs accompany plaque microvessels (Kaartinen *et al.*, 1996a), particularly in the vasa vasorum (Laine *et al.*, 1999), providing an additional pathway for blood-borne leukocyte recruitment to lesions (Fig. 5.1). In atherosclerotic lesions from apolipoprotein E-deficient (*Apoe*$^{-/-}$) mice, MCs also cluster in microvessel-rich areas (Fig. 5.3B), where there are 10 times as many MCs (Stary, 1990) as in the intima (Atkinson *et al.*, 1994; Budde and Aalberse, 2003). The angiogenic factors acidic fibroblast growth factor and basic fibroblast growth factor (aFGF and bFGF) localize in human plaque MCs in neovascularized areas in both the adventitia and intima (Brogi *et al.*, 1993). The presence of bFGF-positive MCs correlates with the microvascularity of atherosclerotic plaques (Kaartinen *et al.*, 1996a; Lappalainen *et al.*, 2004; Jeziorska and Woolley, 1999).

MCs contribute to angiogenesis through multiple mechanisms. Chymase itself is a pro-angiogenic factor (Muramatsu *et al.*, 2000a, 2000b; Katada *et al.*, 2002), promoting angiogenesis via conversion of angiotensin-I (Ang-I) to angiotensin-II (Ang-II) (Blair *et al.*, 1997; Muramatsu *et al.*, 2000b). BMMCs from *Mcpt4*$^{-/-}$ mice showed impaired activity in promoting microvessel growth in an aortic ring assay (Fig. 5.3C) (Sun *et al.*, 2009). MC tryptases stimulate vessel tubule formation and enhance growth of microvessel ECs. Tryptase cleaves bronchial and interstitial neuropeptides and matrix proteins such as fibronectin and collagen-IV, and may thereby promote proliferation of fibroblasts, ECs, and muscle cells and contribute to angiogenesis and tissue remodeling (Li *et al.*, 2004; Meyer *et al.*, 2005; Tchougounova *et al.*, 2005). Several other MC mediators also are implicated in microvessel growth; MCs produce histamine (Norrby, 2002), leptin (Ribatti *et al.*, 2007), vascular endothelial growth factor (VEGF) (Dvorak, 2005), and Ang-I (Nakayama *et al.*, 2004). Heparin can also stimulate angiogenesis through stimulation of EC migration (Azizkhan *et al.*, 1980).

5.3.4 Mast Cells in Foam-Cell Formation

MCs alter lipid metabolism by interfering with apolipoprotein (Apo) E-dependent and ApoA-II-dependent cholesterol efflux (Lee *et al.*, 2002). When MCs are co-cultured with rat or mouse macrophages and LDL, ApoB-100 of LDL binds to the heparin proteoglycan. The granule-bound complex then undergoes proteolysis by granule-bound chymase, leading to foam-cell formation (Oörni *et al.*, 2000). MCs can promote LDL uptake by macrophages *in vivo*. After intraperitoneal administration of the MC activator compound 48/80 (C48/80) to rats, peritoneal macrophage LDL uptake rose by 7–24-fold (Kokkonen, 1989). In contrast, stabilization of MCs with cromolyn effectively blocked MC-dependent LDL uptake by macrophages *in vitro* (Ma and Kovanen, 2000).

Both chymase and tryptase mediate MC-induced foam-cell formation. Mouse peritoneal MC lysates contain chymase and degrade ApoA-1 in α-high density lipoprotein (HDL) and preβ-HDL particles. Serum or peritoneal fluid from mice with activated

MCs, with intraperitoneal injection of C48/80, showed reduced cholesterol efflux from macrophages (Judström *et al.*, 2010). Chymase and tryptase actively degrade HDL, and, thus generate functionally defective particles that function poorly as acceptors for cholesterol efflux from the arterial wall. HDL_3 particles efficiently remove cholesterol from cultured foam cells, but when MCs are stimulated to degranulate, HDL_3 loses this ability because both tryptase and chymase degrade ApoA-I (Lee-Rueckert and Kovanen, 2006; Kunitake *et al.*, 1990). HDL contributes to cholesterol efflux through two mechanisms (Yokoyama, 2006): Soluble chymases degrade ApoE and ApoA-I and ApoA-IV in mouse or human plasma or peritoneal fluid and reduce macrophage cellular cholesterol efflux (Lee *et al.*, 2002; Lindstedt *et al.*, 1996; Lee *et al.*, 1999; Oksjoki *et al.*, 2007); and MC chymase degrades HDL_3, rendering cholesterol-loaded macrophages (foam cells) unable to mediate cholesterol efflux (Lee *et al.*, 1992). Tryptases also promote macrophage foam-cell formation. In vitro culture of THP-1–derived macrophages in 50 μg/ml oxLDL increases both intracellular lipid levels and total cholesterol after tryptase treatment (1 nmol/L), but the presence of the tryptase inhibitor APC366 inhibits intracellular lipid accumulation or foam-cell formation (Yeong *et al.*, 2010).

5.3.5 MC Products Can Promote the Activation of Protein Mediators by Limited Proteolysis

MC-derived chymases and tryptases function in atherosclerosis and other tissue remodeling-associated diseases through the processing of pro-enzymes, latent cytokines, or other bioactive molecule precursors such as Ang-I. Both human α-chymase and rodent β-chymase can convert Ang-I into Ang-II (Fig. 5.2) (Akasu *et al.*, 1998; Caughey *et al.*, 2000; Miyazaki and Takai, 2001). Ang-II can contribute to many cardiovascular diseases and their complications. Aortic and pulmonary artery SMCs from spontaneously hypertensive rats have elevated chymase mRNA levels. The chymase inhibitor chymostatin can block the associated high Ang-II concentrations (Guo *et al.*, 2001). The angiotensin-converting activity of MC-derived chymase may operate more in rodents than in humans, as in the case of other MC functions. Thus, cross-species extrapolations require care.

Pro-enzyme activation by MC chymases and tryptases can contribute to atherogenesis. Both chymases and tryptases activate pro-MMP-1, -2, -3, and -9 (Fig. 5.2) (Gruber *et al.*, 1989; Saarinen *et al.*, 1994; Tchougounova *et al.*, 2005; Johnson *et al.*, 1998) and further increase ECM degradation and production of matrix protein-bound angiogenic factors (Kanbe *et al.*, 1992). MCs produce urokinase-type plasminogen activator (uPA), which is pro-angiogenic, and may also undergo activation by chymases or tryptases (Carmeliet, 2003). Both MMP and uPA closely associate with atherosclerosis. Chymases, and possibly tryptases, also activate other latent cytokines and bioactive molecules, such as pro-IL-1β (Mizutani *et al.*, 1991) and the peptide endothelin 1-31 (Kido *et al.*, 1998), and promote the expression of MCP-1 and IL-8 expression in human ECs (Kinoshita *et al.*, 2005).

5.4 MC Functions in Experimental Atherosclerosis

MC-deficient mice permit examination of MC functions in pathologic settings — such as experimental asthma, arthritis, allergic encephalitis, bullous pemphigoid, cancer, aortic aneurysm, and bacterial infection. These mice help to probe the causality of MC participation in pathogenesis. For example, angiogenic activities of MC-derived mediators enhance tumor development in early stages and enable metastasis of solid tumors. Evidence of an MC requirement for angiogenesis in skin carcinogenesis (Chen *et al.*, 2001) and pancreatic islet tumors (Soucek *et al.*, 2007) has emerged using MC-deficient $Kit^{W/Wv}$ and $Kit^{W\text{-}sh/W\text{-}sh}$ mice, respectively. In contrast, another study suggested the opposite effect of MCs in cancer progression — a protective role of MCs in intestinal tumorigenesis emerged from observations of experimental gain or loss of MC function (Sinnamon *et al.*, 2008). MCs may, therefore, behave differently in different malignancies. In experimental autoimmune encephalomyelitis and mouse arthritis, MC deficiency protects mice from these chronic inflammatory conditions. In contrast, wild-type mice or MC-deficient mice receiving reconstituted MCs from wild-type mice showed increased induction of these inflammatory conditions and increased severity of symptoms (Lee *et al.*, 2002a). MCs could contribute to these inflammatory conditions by releasing their granular content. Pharmacological stabilization of MCs controls these inflammatory processes (De Filippis *et al.*, 2008). Both *Kit*$^{W/Wv}$ and *Kit*$^{W\text{-}sh/W\text{-}sh}$ mice can serve to test MC functions. *Kit*$^{W/Wv}$ mice are leukopenic and anemic (Galli *et al.*, 2005a), whereas *Kit*$^{W\text{-}sh/W\text{-}sh}$ mice appear normal. We have found that *Kit*$^{W\text{-}sh/W\text{-}sh}$ mice have normal levels of circulating T cells, monocytes, macrophages, and neutrophils. The absence of MCs did not affect many of the tested activities of these inflammatory cells (Sun *et al.*, 2007), although a recent study suggested that *Kit*$^{W\text{-}sh/W\text{-}sh}$ mice develop splenomegaly, neutrophilia, and thrombocytosis (Nigrovic *et al.*, 2008).

5.4.1 Proof of Concept in Experimental Atherosclerosis

Atherosclerotic intimal thickness correlates with MC chymase levels in ovalbumin immunization-induced experimental atherosclerosis in rats (Nishizono *et al.*, 1999), and blood tryptase levels in patients with atherosclerosis correlate with atherosclerotic plaque instability (Deliargyris *et al.*, 2005; Filipiak *et al.*, 2003), but until recently, proof of whether MCs participate directly in atherogenesis was lacking. We recently examined the role of MCs in atherosclerosis by crossbreeding LDL-receptor–deficient (*Ldlr*$^{-/-}$) mice with *Kit*$^{W\text{-}sh/W\text{-}sh}$ mice to generate *Ldlr*$^{-/-}$*Kit*$^{W\text{-}sh/W\text{-}sh}$ double-deficient mice. While *Ldlr*$^{-/-}$ mice developed atherosclerosis after consuming a Western diet for 12 to 26 weeks, *Ldlr*$^{-/-}$*Kit*$^{W\text{-}sh/W\text{-}sh}$ double-deficient mice demonstrated significant protection from Western diet-induced atherosclerosis (Fig. 5.4A, B) (Sun *et al.*, 2007). To prove further the role of MCs and to identify the MC mediators responsible for enhanced experimental atherogenesis, we reconstituted *Ldlr*$^{-/-}$*Kit*$^{W\text{-}sh/W\text{-}sh}$ mice with BMMCs from wild-type mice and those lacking different cytokines, such as IL-6, TNF-α, and IFN-γ. *Ldlr*$^{-/-}$*Kit*$^{W\text{-}sh/W\text{-}sh}$ mice developed levels of atherosclerosis comparable to that in *Ldlr*$^{-/-}$ mice after receiving adoptive transfer of BMMCs from wild-type and *Tnf*$^{-/-}$ mice, but not BMMCs from *Il6*$^{-/-}$ and *Ifng*$^{-/-}$ mice (Fig. 5.4C). This experiment allowed us to conclude that MC-derived IL-6 and IFN-γ, but not TNF-α, contribute to atherogenesis. *In vitro* cell culture studies suggested that MCs use these cytokines to stimulate vascular SMC and EC expression of cysteinyl cathepsins, enzymes previously implicated in atherogenesis (Liu *et al.*, 2004).

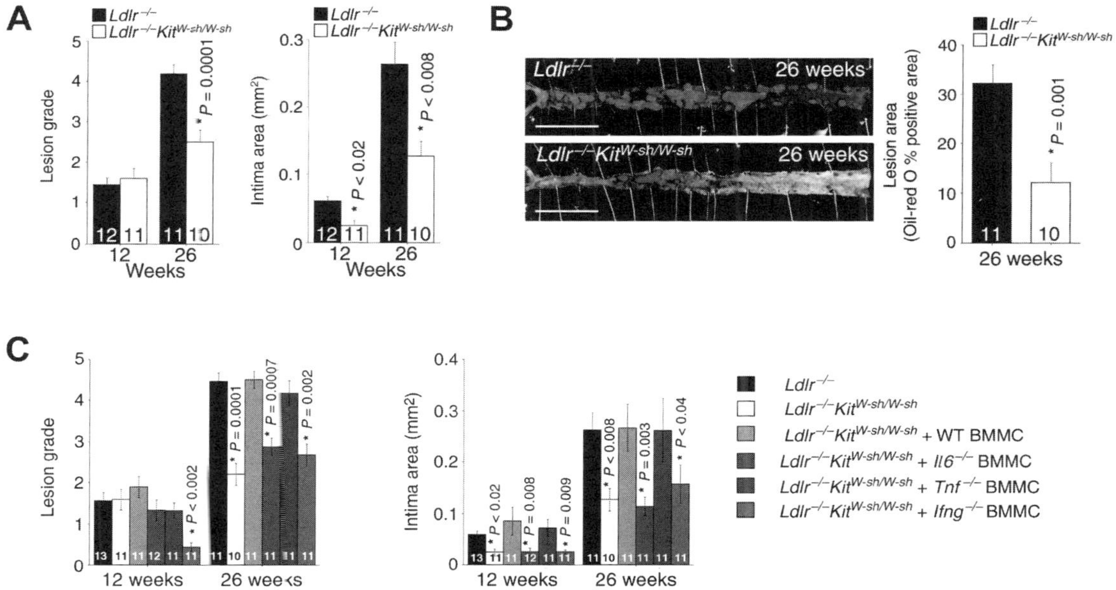

Figure 5.4 Reduced atherosclerosis in mast-cell–deficient mice. A. Atherosclerotic lesion grade and intima area from the aortic arch of Ldlr$^{-/-}$ and Ldlr$^{-/-}$Kit$^{W\text{-}sh/W\text{-}sh}$ mice that consumed an atherogenic diet for 12 weeks and 26-weeks, respectively. B. Oil-red O staining to determine thoracic-abdominal aorta lipid deposition in mice from the 26 week time point. The number of mice is indicated in each bar. Scale bar: 0.5 cm. C. Aortic arch atherosclerotic lesion grade and intima area from Ldlr$^{-/-}$, Ldlr$^{-/-}$Kit$^{W\text{-}sh/W\text{-}sh}$, and Ldlr$^{-/-}Kit^{W\text{-}sh/W\text{-}sh}$ mice receiving adoptive transfer of BMMCs from different mice, indicated in the legend on the right. From *Nat Med* 2007; 13: 719–724.

Heikkilä *et al.* (2010) recently made similar observations. MC-deficient *Ldlr*$^{-/-}$*Kit*$^{W\text{-}sh/W\text{-}sh}$ mice demonstrated a 55% reduction in atherosclerotic lesion sizes in male aortic sinus, and a 33% reduction in aortas and a 45% reduction in female aortic sinus, after consuming a Western diet for 26 weeks. These authors also found a significant correlation between the extent of atherosclerosis and the number of adventitial or perivascular MCs in aortic sinus (r = 0.615, P = 0.015). Serum cholesterol and triglycerides were also lower in *Ldlr*$^{-/-}$*Kit*$^{W\text{-}sh/W\text{-}sh}$ mice, with concomitant decreases in serum intercellular adhesion molecule-1 (ICAM-1) levels, ApoB-containing particles, serum preβ-HDL, and phospholipid transfer protein activity. These observations from two independent studies firmly establish the importance of MCs in atherogenesis in mice.

5.4.2 MC Activation or Stabilization in Experimental Atherosclerosis

Reconstitution of MCs from wild-type mice, but not from IL-6- or IFN-γ-deficient mice, to *Ldlr*$^{-/-}$*Kit*$^{W\text{-}sh/W\text{-}sh}$ mice fully restored atherosclerosis and associated characters in recipient mice (Sun *et al.*, 2007). These observations suggest that MCs contribute to atherogenesis by releasing IL-6 and IFN-γ, and downstream mediators. MC activation or stabilization, therefore, could directly affect atherothrombosis. Several experimental approaches have tested this hypothesis.

In atherosclerosis-prone *Apoe*$^{-/-}$ mice, systemic MC activation by skin sensitization with 0.5% DNFB (dinitrofluorobenzene) followed by intravenous challenge of 1 mg DNP (dinitrophenyl-albumin) increased MC activation threefold and induced bronchiocephalic artery lesion size by more than twofold during 8 weeks of lesion development. Targeted MC activation by perivascular administration of DNP-loaded pluronic F-127 gel with collar-induced carotid artery atherosclerotic plaque nearly doubled lesion MC activation with increased incidence of intraplaque hemorrhage, intima and necrotic core macrophage apoptosis, vascular leakage, and CXCR2/VLA-4–mediated neutrophil and MC recruitment to the carotid artery plaque. Intravital microscopy demonstrated that DNP-induced MC activation also increased leukocyte adhesion to the luminal side of atherosclerotic plaque *in vivo*, an effect reversed by anti-CXCR2 and anti-VLA-4 antibodies *ex vivo*. On the other hand, MC stabilization with cromolyn reduced DNP-induced systemic

MC activation in brachiocephalic artery lesions and reduced total and activated MCs and intraplaque hemorrhage, but did not affect macrophage, neutrophil, or T-cell recruitment (Bot *et al.*, 2007). It was thought that MCs release chymase, tryptase, and histamine after activation to stimulate macrophage apoptosis, leading to plaque rupture and intraplaque hemorrhage formation. *In vitro*, MC supernatants from C48/80-activated MC/9 cell lines, mouse peritoneal MCs, and BMMCs all induced RAW 264.7 macrophage apoptosis. Various proteinase inhibitors inhibited this MC activity — such as soybean trypsin inhibitor (SBTI), which can inhibit chymase and leupeptin, which can inhibit tryptase. Histamine also induced macrophage apoptosis, a process synergized by tryptase. The H_1-receptor antagonist triprolidine can also inhibit this MC activity (Bot *et al.*, 2007). The same group of investigators recently used the neuropeptide substance P to activate MCs in *Apoe*$^{-/-}$ mice, affirming the importance of MC activation in atherogenesis. Substance P associates with stress-related cardiovascular events and inflammation (Black, 2002). Perivascular MC content correlates with the number of nerve fibers in adventitia of human coronary atherosclerotic plaques. These nerve fibers may secrete substance P to activate MCs. Substance P activates MCs via neurokinin-1 receptor (NK1R) or direct interaction with G proteins (Ferry *et al.*, 2002; Lowman *et al.*, 1988). Substance P treatment of *Apoe*$^{-/-}$ mice enhanced the number and activation of adventitial MCs and promoted intraplaque hemorrhage. Co-administration of the NK1R antagonist spantide I prevented these phenotypes (Bot *et al.*, 2010b). After right common carotid collar placement in *Apoe*$^{-/-}$ mice, MC activation by intraperitoneal injection of C48/80 increased plaque size and lumen stenosis, MC degranulation, and densities of SMCs (α-SMC), macrophages (Mac-3), bFGF, and IL-1β (Tang *et al.*, 2009). MC activation, therefore, aggravates the initiation and progression of atherosclerosis.

Several lines of evidence suggest that MC stabilization reduces atherogenesis. As discussed above, Bot *et al.* (2007) used the MC stabilizer cromolyn to prevent atherosclerotic lesion intraplaque hemorrhage, macrophage apoptosis, vascular leakage, and MC recruitment in *Apoe*$^{-/-}$ mice. *N*-(3,4-demethoxycinnamoyl)-anthranilic acid (tranilast), another MC stabilizer, inhibits MC release of mediators and has indications for the treatment of allergic rhinitis, atrophic dermatitis, and asthma (Azuma *et al.*, 1976; Inagaki *et al.*, 2001; Komatsu *et al.*, 1988). In a recent study of Syrian golden hamsters with atherosclerosis induced by consumption of a high-cholesterol diet for 15 weeks, intragastric administration of tranilast for 3 weeks reduced lesion total and activated MC numbers, vascular SMC apoptosis, local chymase activities, Ang-II concentration, and inflammatory markers (e.g., MMP-1, MMP-9, IL-1β, TGF-β1), as well as plaque vulnerability index (Guo *et al.*, 2009). These observations suggest a potential application of anti-allergy drugs for human atherosclerosis prevention and treatment.

5.5 MC Chymase and Tryptase in Atherosclerosis

5.5.1 Chymases and Tryptases in Atherosclerosis

As discussed above, MC chymase and tryptase mediate ECM protein degradation, vascular cell apoptosis, and activation of proenzymes, latent cytokines, and bioactive molecule precursors associated with atherosclerosis (Fig. 5.2). Although direct participation of these MC serine proteases in atherosclerosis remains unconfirmed, indirect evidence suggests their involvement. MC chymase participates in generating Ang-II from Ang-I (Fig. 5.2) (Akasu *et al.*, 1998; Caughey *et al.*, 2000; Miyazaki and Takai, 2001). This pathway may have increased importance in humans treated with angiotensin-converting enzyme inhibitors. Human atherosclerotic lesions have high levels of Ang-II forming activity and chymase expression (Ihara *et al.*, 1999). Using chymase-deficient and tryptase-deficient mice, we proved that both proteases promote aortic SMC apoptosis (Fig. 5.3A) (Sun *et al.*, 2009; Zhang *et al.*, 2011). Activated MCs also induce EC apoptosis by releasing chymases that in turn can inactivate the FAK-mediated cell survival signaling, and TNF-α to trigger apoptosis (Heikkilä *et al.*, 2008). Thus, by inducing EC and SMC apoptosis, MC proteases may contribute to plaque erosion and complications of atherosclerosis. As discussed, chymase-mediated and tryptase-mediated bioactivation of pro-enzyme and latent cytokines also appears important to atherogenesis. Several studies, including ours Xiang *et al.*, 2011 have associated blood tryptase levels with atherosclerotic plaque instability (Deliargyris *et al.*, 2005; Filipiak *et al.*, 2003). Patients with AMI or unstable angina pectoris (UAP) have significantly higher serum tryptase levels than those without significant coronary heart disease (CHD) or with stable angina pectoris (SAP). Serum chymase levels in AMI and UAP patients exceed those in SAP patients or in those without significant CHD (Xiang *et al.*, 2011). *In vitro*, treatment of human coronary arteries intraluminally with recombinant tryptase or chymase induced endothelial damage, characterized by disruption of EC adhesion followed by retraction and desquamation (Mayranpaa *et al.*, 2006). In mice, both chymases and tryptases control the expression of sulfhydryl proteinase cathepsins implicated in atherosclerosis (Sun *et al.*, 2009; Sukhova *et al.*, 2003; Lutgens *et al.*, 2006; Kitamoto *et al.*, 2007).

5.5.2 Chymase and Tryptase Inhibitors in Atherosclerosis

Although evidence supports roles for both chymases and tryptases in MC biology and in the pathogenesis of atherosclerosis and its complications, most current studies focus on the development of chymase inhibitors in experimental cardiovascular disease. Tryptase inhibitors have received relatively less attention, although tryptase may have no less importance than chymase in cardiovascular diseases. In THP-1–derived macrophages, the tryptase inhibitor APC-366 blocked oxLDL-induced foam-cell formation. APC-366 inhibited tryptase activities known to reduce nuclear receptor LXRa (a regulator of lipid homeostasis), ATP-binding cassette transporters A1 and G1 (ABCA1, ABCG1; involved in cellular cholesterol efflux), and sterol regulatory element binding protein-1c (SREBP-1c; a regulator for *de novo* lipogenesis) (Yeong *et al.*, 2010). Chymase expression increases in atherosclerotic lesions (Takai *et al.*, 1997; Uehara *et al.*, 2002). In hamsters that developed atherosclerosis after consuming 12 weeks of a high-cholesterol diet, serum total and LDL cholesterol levels correlated with aortic chymase activity and with lipid deposition in the aorta intima. Administration of the chymase inhibitor SUN-C8257 in drinking water (100 mg/kg/day) for an additional 12 weeks suppressed hamster aortic lesion lipid deposition and adventitial Ang-II immunoreactivity (Arakawa and Urata, 2000; Uehara *et al.*, 2002). In experimental vein graft disease in dogs (Takai *et al.*, 2001), each animal underwent right common carotid artery bypass grafting with the ipsilaterial external jugular vein. Grafting increased vascular cell proliferation, chymase activity, SCF activation, MC accumulation, and intima thickening. Oral administration of the chymase inhibitor NK3201 suppressed these reactions to vein grafting. The same group performed a similar experiment using a balloon catheter-induced carotid artery injury to test the role of NK3201 on intimal hyperplasia (Takai *et al.*, 2003). Both chymase activity and carotid artery intimal thickening decreased significantly in dogs receiving the treatment. In atherosclerotic *Ldlr*$^{-/-}$ mice, periarterial collar placement-induced lesions associated with increased expression of chymase MMCP-1, MMCP-4, and MMCP-5. The newly developed chymase inhibitor RO5066852 (Roche) reduced spontaneous atherosclerosis in the thoracic aorta in *Apoe*$^{-/-}$ mice and prevented accelerated plaque progression in *Apoe*$^{-/-}$ mice that underwent repetitive MC activation. RO5066852 enhanced lesion collagen content, reduced necrotic core size, and normalized the frequency and size of intraplaque hemorrhages in *Apoe*$^{-/-}$ mice after acute perivascular MC activation in advanced atherosclerosis (Bot *et al.*, 2010a).

5.5.3 Chymase Inhibitors in Myocardial Infarction

AMI commonly complicates atherosclerosis. Studies with several chymase inhibitors — including BCEAB, NK3201, TEI-E548, and TY51184 — have examined the role of chymase in experimental MI in hamsters, dogs, and rats. In hamsters, orally active inhibitor BCEAB treatment starting 3 days before coronary ligation suppressed cardiac chymase activity, improved hemodynamics (increased maximal negative and positive rates of pressure development (+dP/dt and –dP/dt) and left ventricular systolic pressure (LVSP)), and reduced mortality (Jin *et al.*, 2002). NK3201 caused similar results in experimental AMI. This compound significantly reduced mortality and improved fractional shortening (Jin *et al.*, 2003). In experimental AMI in hamsters, TEI-E548 completely inhibited chymase-induced microvascular leakage, increased survival rate, and attenuated cardiac hypertrophy and left ventricular end-diastolic pressure. Chymase inhibitor administration also reduced plasma Ang-II levels (Hoshino *et al.*, 2003). In dogs with experimental AMI, the chymase inhibitor TY51184 decreased plasma Ang-II levels and suppressed ventricular arrhythmias by more than 80% (Jin *et al.*, 2004). In rats with AMI, Kanemitsu *et al.*

demonstrated that chymase inhibition with NK3201 decreased TGF-β1 expression, thereby reducing collagen type-I and type-III levels. Rats receiving NK3201 had significantly reduced fibrotic areas, consequently showing significantly reduced left ventricular end-diastolic pressure, increased maximal end-systolic pressure–volume relationship, and decreased time constant of left ventricular relaxation (Kanemitsu *et al.*, 2006, 2008).

5.6 Clinical Implications of MC and MC Mediator Inhibitors

Available knowledge suggests that stabilizing MCs or inactivating MC mediators attenuates or prevents atherogenesis. Although experiments have employed cultured cells or animals, MC stabilizers and MC mediator inhibitors might exhibit similar effects in humans. Patients with allergic disorders commonly use small molecule MC stabilizers. The MC stabilizers cromolyn and ketotifen (Zaditor) have clinical application in pediatric allergic disorders, and tranilast is used broadly in asthma, atopic dermatitis, and allergic conjunctivitis, and has shown anti-angiogenic activity via inhibition of chymase and TGF-β (Patalano and Ruggieri, 1989; Jones *et al.*, 2004). Cromolyn exerts its effect not only on MCs, but also on eosinophils and neutrophils (Moqbel *et al.*, 1986), although its molecular mechanism is poorly understood. One important feature of cromolyn is that it demonstrates less inhibitory effect to intestinal mucosal MCs in rodents (Pearce *et al.*, 1982) and in humans (Befus *et al.*, 1987) — which is particularly important for inhibiting connective tissue MCs while preserving mucosal MC activity and innate immunity to exogenous infections. The oral phosphodiesterase (PDE5) inhibitor zaprinast also stabilizes MCs and exerts a moderate bronchodilator effect (Rudd *et al.*, 1983). Several human oral chymase inhibitors are also currently available (Doggrell and Wanstall, 2004) — including SUN-C8257, BCEAB, NK3201, and TEI-E548. The tryptase inhibitor APC2095 may have use in the therapy of asthma and ulcerative colitis (Tremaine *et al.*, 2002). These MC stabilizers and chymase/tryptase inhibitors could have applicability to treat atherosclerosis or to "stabilize" plaques at risk of rupture and thrombosis in humans, as they have in animal. Other inhibitors of MC functions — such as histamine receptor antagonists, heparin antagonists, FcεR1 antagonists, FcεR1 downstream signaling molecule inhibitors, leukotriene pathway inhibitors, vitamin E, and cannabinomimetic compounds — might also have therapeutic benefit in atherosclerosis.

In Rose Bengal-induced femoral artery injury in mice, histamine from platelets at the site of injury and MCs can stimulate SMC proliferation and migration, thereby causing intimal thickening. Intraperitoneal administration of the histamine H_1-receptor antagonist diphenhydramine (30 mg/kg/day), but not of the H_2-receptor antagonist cimetidine, for 21 days after injury significantly reduced intimal thickening (non-treated vs. treated: 6.2 ± 1.4, 10^{-3} mm^2 vs. 1.1 ± 0.3, 10^{-3} mm^2, $P < 0.01$). The ratio of intima to media fell by 83% in diphenhydramine-treated mice compared to untreated mice. *In vitro*, diphenhydramine also inhibits SMC proliferation (Miyazawa *et al.*, 1998). The heparin antagonists protamine and Polybrene® inhibit tryptase activity by dissociation of active tetrameric tryptase into inactive monomers (Hallgren *et al.*, 2001). Omalizumab is a U.S. Food and Drug Administration (FDA)-approved humanized monoclonal antibody that binds to free IgE for the treatment of allergic diseases (Djukanović *et al.*, 2004). Spleen tyrosine kinase (Syk) plays a central role in IgE receptor FcεRI signaling. Several inhibitors of this kinase are currently in clinical trials (Meltzer *et al.*, 2005; Weinblatt *et al.*, 2010). Leukotriene B4 (LTB4)) is a chemoattractant of MCs, eosinophils, macrophages, and T cells, and it is implicated in atherogenesis (Friedrich *et al.*, 2003; Qiu *et al.*, 2006; Subbarao *et al.*, 2004). Its receptors on MCs, BLT1 and BLT2, mediate chemotaxis to LTB4 (Lundeen *et al.*, 2006). Generation of LTB4 *in vivo* requires LTA4 hydrolase (LTA4H); LTA4H inhibitors (e.g., benzoxazole, benzthiazole, benzinidazole) have anti-inflammatory activity in inflammatory bowel disease in rats (Grice *et al.*, 2008). LTA4H inhibitors might have therapeutic effects on other inflammatory diseases, such as atherosclerosis. Recent observations from a study of the LTB4 antagonist CP105,696 support this hypothesis; in *Apoe*$^{-/-}$ mice, 35 days of treatment with CP105,696 reduced vascular lesions and circulating CD11b$^+$ cells. In *Ldlr*$^{-/-}$ mice fed a Western diet, the same treatment with CP105,696 reduced atherosclerotic lesion area (Aiello *et al.*, 2002). Vitamin E reduces protein kinase C (PKC), protein kinase B (PKB), protein phosphatase 2A, and glycogen synthase kinase 3 (GSKα/β) phosphorylation, leading to modulation of MC proliferation, apoptosis, secretion, and migration (Kempná *et al.*, 2004; Zingg, 2007). Cannabinomimetic compounds modulate endocannabinoid function and control dermatitis, inflammatory gastrointestinal syndrome, and granuloma formation. Palmitoylethanolamide, for example, has been used in human studies to treat severe chronic inflammatory diseases by controlling MC activation (De Filippis *et al.*, 2008).

Although none of these drugs has undergone testing in human atherosclerosis, their application in other diseases through direct or indirect targeting of MCs, MC mediators, or MC pathophysiology could be translated into human atherosclerosis and associated complications. This hypothesis merits future clinical trials and investigations.

5.7 Conclusion

After almost 60 years of speculation and multitudinous *in vitro* observations, recent *in vivo* observations have placed MC functions in experimental atherogenesis on firm ground. While macrophages far outnumber MCs in human atheromata, MC functions not shared by mononuclear phagocytes — such as elaboration of the serine proteinases chymase and tryptase and the small molecule mediators mentioned above — indicate a special place for MCs in inflammatory processes now recognized as fundamental in atherogenesis and its complications. Moreover, the adventitial localization of many MCs positions them strategically for participation in arterial remodeling currently considered capital in the clinical consequences of atherosclerosis. The links between innate and adaptive immunity and MC regulation further fit with current concepts implicating immune functions in this disease. The extension of these recent biological insights to humans and exploration of their clinical therapeutic implications comprise a new translational challenge for atherosclerosis research.

Acknowledgments

We thank Dr. Galina K. Sukhova for her help with the immunohistological analysis of human and mouse atherosclerotic lesions. We also thank Ms. Sara Karwacki for editorial assistance. Some studies cited in this discussion were supported partially by NIH grants HL60942, HL81090, HL88547 (GPS), HL34636, and HL56985 (PL) and American Heart Association EIA award 0840118N (GPS).

References

Ahn, K., Takai, S., Pawankar, R., Kuramasu, A., Ohtsu, H., Kempuraj, D., Tomita, H., Iida, M., Matsumoto, K., Akasawa, A., Miyazaki, M., and Saito, H. (2000). Regulation of chymase production in human mast cell progenitors, *J. Allergy Clin. Immunol.,* **106,** pp. 321–328.

Aiello, R. J., Bourassa, P. A., Lindsey, S., Weng, W., Freeman, A., and Showell, H. J. (2002). Leukotriene B4 receptor antagonism reduces monocytic foam cells in mice, *Arterioscler. Thromb. Vasc. Biol.,* **22,** pp. 443–449.

Akasu, M., Urata, H., Kinoshita, A., Sasaguri, M., Ideishi, M., and Arakawa, K. (1998). Differences in tissue angiotensin II-forming pathways by species and organs in vitro, *Hypertension,* **32,** pp. 514–520.

Arakawa, K., and Urata, H. (2000). Hypothesis regarding the pathophysiological role of alternative pathways of angiotensin II formation in atherosclerosis, *Hypertension,* **36,** pp. 638–641.

Atkinson, J. B., Harlan, C. W., Harlan, G. C., and Virmani, R. (1994). The association of mast cells and atherosclerosis: a morphologic study of early atherosclerotic lesions in young people, *Hum. Pathol.,* **25,** pp. 154-159.

Azizkhan, R. G., Azizkhan, J. C., Zetter, B. R., and Folkman, J. (1980). Mast cell heparin stimulates migration of capillary endothelial cells in vitro, *J. Exp. Med.,* **152,** pp. 931–944.

Azuma, H., Banno, K., and Yoshimura, T. (1976). Pharmacological properties of *N*-(3′,4′-dimethoxycinnamoyl) anthranilic acid (*N*-5′), a new anti-atopic agent, *Br. J. Pharmacol.,* **58,** pp. 483–488.

Bachelet, I., and Levi-Schaffer, F. (2007). Mast cells as effector cells: a co-stimulating question, *Trends Immunol.,* **28,** pp. 360–365.

Bankl, H. C., and Valent, P. (2002). Mast cells, thrombosis, and fibrinolysis: the emerging concept, *Thromb. Res.,* **105,** pp. 359–365.

Befus, A. D., Dyck, N., Goodacre, R., and Bienenstock, J. (1987). Mast cells from the human intestinal lamina propria. Isolation, histochemical subtypes, and functional characterization, *J. Immunol.,* **138,** pp. 2604–2610.

Bischoff, S.C. (2009). Physiological and pathophysiological functions of intestinal mast cells, *Semin. Immunopathol.,* **31,** pp. 185–205.

Bischoff, S. C., and Dahinden, C. A. (1992). c-kit ligand: a unique potentiator of mediator release by human lung mast cells, *J. Exp. Med.,* **175,** pp. 237–244.

Black, P. H. (2002). Stress and the inflammatory response: a review of neurogenic inflammation, *Brain Behav. Immun.*, **16,** pp. 622–653.

Blair, R. J., Meng, H., Marchese, M. J., Ren, S., Schwartz, L. B., Tonnesen, M. G., and Gruber, B. L. (1997). Human mast cells stimulate vascular tube formation. Tryptase is a novel, potent angiogenic factor, *J. Clin. Invest.*, **99,** pp. 2691–2700.

Brightling, C. E., Bradding, P., Symon, F. A., Holgate, S. T., Wardlaw, A. J., and Pavord, I. D. (2002) Mast-cell infiltration of airway smooth muscle in asthma, *N. Engl. J. Med.*, **346,** pp. 1699–1705.

Bot, I., Bot, M., van Heiningen, S. H., van Santbrink, P. J., Lankhuizen, I. M., Hartman, P., Gruener, S., Hilpert, H. , van Berkel, T. J., Fingerle, J., and Biessen, E. A. (2010a) Mast cell chymase inhibition reduces atherosclerotic plaque progression and improves plaque stability in ApoE-/- mice. *Cardiovasc. Res.*, 89, pp. 244–252.

Bot, I., de Jager, S. C., Bot, M., van Heiningen, S. H., de Groot, P., Veldhuizen, R. W., van Berkel, T. J., von der Thüsen, J. H., and Biessen, E. A. (2010b). The neuropeptide substance P mediates adventitial mast cell activation and induces intraplaque hemorrhage in advanced atherosclerosis, *Circ. Res.*, **106,** pp. 89–92.

Bot, I., de Jager, S. C., Zernecke, A., Lindstedt, K. A., van Berkel, T. J., Weber, C., and Biessen, E. A. (2007). Perivascular mast cells promote atherogenesis and induce plaque destabilization in apolipoprotein E-deficient mice, *Circulation,* **115,** pp. 2516–2525.

Brogi, E., Winkles, J. A., Underwood, R., Clinton, S. K., Alberts, G. F., and Libby, P. (1993). Distinct patterns of expression of fibroblast growth factors and their receptors in human atheroma and nonatherosclerotic arteries. Association of acidic FGF with plaque microvessels and macrophages, *J. Clin. Invest.*, **92,** pp. 2408–2418.

Broudy, V. C. (1997). Stem cell factor and hematopoiesis, *Blood.,* **90,** pp. 1345–1364.

Budde, I. K., and Aalberse, R. C. (2003). Histamine-releasing factors, a heterogeneous group of different activities, *Clin. Exp. Allergy,* **33,** pp. 1175–1182.

Cairns, A., and Constantinides, P. (1954). Mast cells in human atherosclerosis, *Science,* **120,** pp. 31–32.

Cao, J., Cetrulo, C. L., and Theoharides, T. C. (2006). Corticotropin-releasing hormone induces vascular endothelial growth factor release from human mast cells via the cAMP/protein kinase A/p38 mitogen-activated protein kinase pathway, *Mol. Pharmacol.,* **69,** pp. 998–1006.

Carmeliet, P. (2003). Angiogenesis in health and disease, *Nat. Med.,* **9,** pp.653–660.

Caughey, G. H., Raymond, W. W., and Wolters, P. J. (2000). Angiotensin II generation by mast cell alpha- and beta-chymases, *Biochim. Biophys. Acta.,* **1480,** pp. 245–257.

Chen, R., Ning, G., Zhao, M. L., Fleming, M. G., Diaz, L. A., Werb, Z., and Liu, Z. (2001). Mast cells play a key role in neutrophil recruitment in experimental bullous pemphigoid, *J. Clin. Invest.,* **108,** pp. 1151–1158.

Constantinides, P. (1953). Mast cells and susceptibility to experimental atherosclerosis, *Science,* **117,** pp. 505–506.

Criqui, M. H., Lee, E. R., Hamburger, R. N., Klauber, M. R., and Coughlin, S. S. (1987). IgE and cardiovascular disease. Results from a population-based study, *Am. J. Med.,* **82,** pp. 964–968.

Daffern, P. J., Pfeifer, P. H., Ember, J. A., and Hugli, T. E. (1995). C3a is a chemotaxin for human eosinophils but not for neutrophils. I. C3a stimulation of neutrophils is secondary to eosinophil activation, *J. Exp. Med.,* **181,** pp. 2119–2127.

De Filippis, D., D'Amico, A., and Iuvone, T. (2008). Cannabinomimetic control of mast cell mediator release: new perspective in chronic inflammation, *J. Neuroendocrinol.,* **20** Suppl 1, pp. 20–25.

Deliargyris, E. N., Upadhya, B., Sane, D. C., Dehmer, G. J., Pye, J., Smith, S. C. Jr., Boucher, W. S., and Theoharides, T. C. (2005). Mast cell tryptase: a new biomarker in patients with stable coronary artery disease, *Atherosclerosis,* **178,** pp. 381–386.

Djukanović, R., Wilson, S. J., Kraft, M., Jarjour, N. N., Steel, M., Chung, K. F., Bao, W., Fowler-Taylor, A., Matthews, J., Busse, W. W., Holgate, S. T., and Fahy, J. V. (2004). Effects of treatment with anti-immunoglobulin E antibody omalizumab on airway inflammation in allergic asthma, *Am. J. Respir. Crit. Care Med.,* **170,** pp. 583–593.

Doggrell, S. A., and Wanstall, J. C. (2004). Vascular chymase: pathophysiological role and therapeutic potential of inhibition, *Cardiovasc. Res.,* **61,** pp. 653–662.

Dvorak, A. M. (1986). Mast-cell degranulation in human hearts, *N. Engl. J. Med.,* **315,** pp. 969–970.

Dvorak, A. M. (2005). Mast cell-derived mediators of enhanced microvascular permeability, vascular permeability factor/vascular endothelial growth factor, histamine, and serotonin, cause leakage of macromolecules through a new endothelial cell permeability organelle, the vesiculo-vacuolar organelle, *Chem. Immunol. Allergy,* **85,** pp. 185–204.

Dwyer, J. H., Allayee, H., Dwyer, K. M., Fan, J., Wu, H., Mar, R., Lusis, A. J., and Mehrabian, M. (2004). Arachidonate 5-lipoxygenase promoter genotype, dietary arachidonic acid, and atherosclerosis, *N. Engl. J. Med.,* **350,** pp. 29–37.

Echtenacher, B., Männel, D. N., and Hültner, L. (1996). Critical protective role of mast cells in a model of acute septic peritonitis, *Nature,* **381,** pp. 75–77.

Eisenbarth, S. C., Piggott, D. A., Huleatt, J. W., Visintin, I., Herrick, C. A., and Bottomly, K. (2002). Lipopolysaccharide-enhanced, toll-like receptor 4-dependent T helper cell type 2 responses to inhaled antigen, *J. Exp. Med.,* **196,** pp.1645–1651.

Enright, P. L., Ward, B. J., Tracy, R. P., and Lasser, E. C. (1996). Asthma and its association with cardiovascular disease in the elderly. The Cardiovascular Health Study Research Group, *J. Asthm.,* **33,** pp. 45–53.

Ermolieff, J., Boudier, C., Laine, A., Meyer, B., and Bieth, J. G. (1994). Heparin protects cathepsin G against inhibition by protein proteinase inhibitors, *J. Biol. Chem.,* **269,** pp. 29502–29508.

Faleiro, L. C., Machado, C. R., Gripp, A., Jr., Resende, R. A., and Rodrigues, P. A. (1981). Cerebral vasospasm: presence of mast cells in human cerebral arteries after aneurysm rupture, *J. Neurosurg.,* **54,** pp. 733–735.

Féger, F., Varadaradjalou, S., Gao, Z., Abraham, S. N., and Arock, M. (2002). The role of mast cells in host defense and their subversion by bacterial pathogens, *Trends Immunol.,* **23,** pp. 151–158.

Ferry, X., Brehin, S., Kamel, R., and Landry, Y. (2002). G protein-dependent activation of mast cell by peptides and basic secretagogues, *Peptides,* **23,** pp. 1507–1515.

Filipiak, K. J., Tarchalska-Krynska, B., Opolski, G., Rdzanek, A., Kochman, J., Kosior, D. A., & Czlonkowski, A. (2003). Tryptase levels in patients after acute coronary syndromes: the potential new marker of an unstable plaque? *Clin. Cardiol.,* **26,** pp. 366–372.

Fischer, M., Harvima, I. T., Carvalho, R. F., Möller, C., Naukkarinen, A., Enblad, G., and Nilsson, G. (2006). Mast cell CD30 ligand is upregulated in cutaneous inflammation and mediates degranulation-independent chemokine secretion, *J. Clin. Invest.,* **116,** pp. 2748–2756.

Foreman, J. C. (1987). Neuropeptides and the pathogenesis of allergy, *Allergy,* **42,** pp. 1–11.

Forman, M. B., Oates, J. A., Robertson, D., Robertson, R. M., Roberts, L. J. 2nd, and Virmani, R. (1985). Increased adventitial mast cells in a patient with coronary spasm, *N. Engl. J. Med.,* **313,** pp. 1138–1141.

Förster, R., Davalos-Misslitz, A. C., and Rot, A. (2008). CCR7 and its ligands: balancing immunity and tolerance, *Nat. Rev. Immunol.,* 2008, **8,** pp. 362–371.

Friedrich, E. B., Tager, A. M., Liu, E., Pettersson, A., Owman, C., Munn, L., Luster, A. D., and Gerszten, R. E. (2003). Mechanisms of leukotriene B4--triggered monocyte adhesion, *Arterioscler. Thromb. Vasc. Biol.,* **23,** pp. 1761–1767.

Galli, S. J., Kalesnikoff, J., Grimbaldeston, M. A., Piliponsky, A. M., Williams, C. M., and Tsai, M. (2005a). Mast cells as "tunable" effector and immunoregulatory cells: recent advances, *Annu. Rev. Immunol.,* **23,** pp. 749–786.

Galli, S. J., Nakae, S., and Tsai, M. (2005b). Mast cells in the development of adaptive immune responses, *Nat. Immunol.,* **6,** pp. 135–142.

Galli, S. J., Maurer, M., and Lantz, C. S. (1999). Mast cells as sentinels of innate immunity, *Curr. Opin. Immunol.,* **11,** pp. 53–59.

Garbuzenko, E., Nagler, A., Pickholtz, D., Gillery, P., Reich, R., Maquart, F. X., and Levi-Schaffer, F. (2002). Human mast cells stimulate fibroblast proliferation, collagen synthesis and lattice contraction: a direct role for mast cells in skin fibrosis, *Clin. Exp. Allergy,* **32,** pp. 237–246.

Gilfillan, A. M., and Tkaczyk, C. (2006). Integrated signalling pathways for mast-cell activation, *Nat. Rev. Immunol.,* **6,** pp. 218–230.

Gonzalez, S., Moran, M., and Kochevar, I. E. (1999). Chronic photodamage in skin of mast cell-deficient mice, *Photochem. Photobiol.,* **70,** pp. 248–253.

Grabbe, J., Karau, L., Welker, P., Ziegler, A., and Henz, B. M. (1997). Induction of MHC class II antigen expression on human HMC-1 mast cells, *J. Dermatol. Sci.,* **16,** pp. 67–73.

Grice, C. A., Tays, K. L., Savall, B. M., Wei, J. , Butler, C. R., Axe, F. U., Bembenek, S. D., Fourie, A. M., Dunford, P. J., Lundeen, K., Coles, F., Xue, X., Riley, J. P., Williams, K. N., Karlsson, L., and Edwards, J. P. (2008). Identification of a potent, selective, and orally active leukotriene a4 hydrolase inhibitor with anti-inflammatory activity, *J. Med. Chem.,* **51,** pp. 4150–4169.

Grimbaldeston, M. A., Nakae, S., Kalesnikoff, J., Tsai, M., and Galli, S. J. (2007). Mast cell-derived interleukin 10 limits skin pathology in contact dermatitis and chronic irradiation with ultraviolet B, *Nat. Immunol.,* **8,** pp.1095–1104.

Gruber, B. L., Marchese, M. J., Suzuki, K., Schwartz, L. B., Okada, Y., Nagase, H., and Ramamurthy, N. S. (1989). Synovial procollagenase activation by human mast cell tryptase dependence upon matrix metalloproteinase 3 activation, *J. Clin. Invest.,* **84,** pp. 1657–1662.

Guo, C., Ju, H., Leung, D., Massaeli, H., Shi, M., and Rabinovitch, M. (2001). A novel vascular smooth muscle chymase is upregulated in hypertensive rats, *J. Clin. Invest.*, **107**, pp. 703–715.

Guo, T., Chen, W. Q., Zhang, C., Zhao, Y. X., and Zhang, Y. (2009). Chymase activity is closely related with plaque vulnerability in a hamster model of atherosclerosis, *Atherosclerosis*, **207**, pp. 59–67.

Haley, K. J., Lilly, C. M., Yang, J. H., Feng, Y., Kennedy, S. P., Turi, T. G., Thompson, J. F., Sukhova, G. K., Libby, P., and Lee, R.T. (2000). Overexpression of eotaxin and the CCR3 receptor in human atherosclerosis: using genomic technology to identify a potential novel pathway of vascular inflammation, *Circulation*, **102**, pp. 2185–2189.

Hallgren, J., Estrada, S., Karlson, U., Alving, K., and Pejler, G. (2001). Heparin antagonists are potent inhibitors of mast cell tryptase, *Biochemistry*, **40**, pp. 7342–7349.

Hartmann, K., Henz, B. M., Krüger-Krasagakes, S., Köhl, J., Burger, R., Guhl, S., Haase, I., Lippert, U., and Zuberbier, T. (1997). C3a and C5a stimulate chemotaxis of human mast cells, *Blood*, **89**, pp. 2863–2870.

Heikkilä, H. M., Lätti, S., Leskinen, M. J., Hakala, J. K., Kovanen, P. T., and Lindstedt, K. A. (2008). Activated mast cells induce endothelial cell apoptosis by a combined action of chymase and tumor necrosis factor-alpha, *Arterioscler. Thromb. Vasc. Biol.*, **28**, pp. 309–314.

Heikkilä, H. M., Trosien, J., Metso, J., Jauhiainen, M., Pentikäinen, M. O., Kovanen, P. T., and Lindstedt, K. A. (2010). Mast cells promote atherosclerosis by inducing both an atherogenic lipid profile and vascular inflammation, *J. Cell. Biochem.*, **109**, pp. 615–623.

Helgadottir, A., Manolescu, A., Thorleifsson, G., Gretarsdottir, S., Jonsdottir, H., Thorsteinsdottir, U., Samani, N. J., Gudmundsson, G., Grant, S. F., Thorgeirsson, G., Sveinbjornsdottir, S., Valdimarsson, E. M., Matthiasson, S. E., Johannsson, H., Gudmundsdottir, O., Gurney, M. E., Sainz, J., Thorhallsdottir, M., Andresdottir, M., Frigge, M. L., Topol, E. J., Kong, A., Gudnason, V., Hakonarson, H., Gulcher. J. R., and Stefansson, K. (2004). The gene encoding 5-lipoxygenase activating protein confers risk of myocardial infarction and stroke, *Nat. Genet.*, **36**, pp. 233–239.

Higuchi, S., Tanimoto, A., Arima, N., Xu, H., Murata, Y., Hamada, T., Makishima, K., and Sasaguri, Y. (2001). Effects of histamine and interleukin-4 synthesized in arterial intima on phagocytosis by monocytes/macrophages in relation to atherosclerosis, *FEBS Lett.*, **505**, pp. 217–222.

Hoshino, F., Urata, H., Inoue, Y., Saito, Y., Yahiro, E., Ideishi, M., Arakawa, K., and Saku, K. (2003). Chymase inhibitor improves survival in hamsters with myocardial infarction, *J. Cardiovasc. Pharmacol.,* **41** Suppl 1, pp. S11–S18.

Hospers, J. J., Rijcken, B., Schouten, J. P., Postma, D. S., and Weiss, S. T. (1999). Eosinophilia and positive skin tests predict cardiovascular mortality in a general population sample followed for 30 years, *Am. J. Epidemiol.,* **150,** pp. 482–491.

Ihara, M., Urata, H., Kinoshita, A., Suzumiya, J., Sasaguri, M., Kikuchi, M., Ideishi, M., and Arakawa, K. (1999). Increased chymase-dependent angiotensin II formation in human atherosclerotic aorta, *Hypertension,* **33,** pp. 1399–1405.

Inagaki, N., Kawasaki, H., and Nagai, H. (2001). High rate of IgE-mediated histamine release from rat mesenteric mast cells, *Exp. Anim.,* **50,** pp. 187–190.

Irani, A. A., Schechter, N. M., Craig, S. S., DeBlois, G., and Schwartz, L. B. (1986). Two types of human mast cells that have distinct neutral protease compositions, *Proc. Natl. Acad. Sci. U S A.,***83,** pp. 4464–4468.

Irani, A. M., Craig, S. S., DeBlois, G., Elson, C. O., Schechter, N. M., and Schwartz, L. B. (1987). Deficiency of the tryptase-positive, chymase-negative mast cell type in gastrointestinal mucosa of patients with defective T lymphocyte function, *J. Immunol.,* **138,** pp. 4381–4386.

Jeziorska, M., McCollum, C., and Woolley, D. E. (1997). Mast cell distribution, activation, and phenotype in atherosclerotic lesions of human carotid arteries, *J. Pathol.,* **182,** pp. 115–122.

Jeziorska, M., and Woolley, D. E. (1999). Local neovascularization and cellular composition within vulnerable regions of atherosclerotic plaques of human carotid arteries, *J. Pathol.,* **188,** pp. 189–196.

Jin, D., Takai, S., Yamada, M., Sakaguchi, M., and Miyazaki, M. (2002). Beneficial effects of cardiac chymase inhibition during the acute phase of myocardial infarction, *Life Sci.,* **71,** pp. 437–446.

Jin, D., Takai, S., Yamada, M., Sakaguchi, M., Kamoshita, K., Ishida, K., Sukenaga, Y., and Miyazaki, M. (2003). Impact of chymase inhibitor on cardiac function and survival after myocardial infarction, *Cardiovasc. Res.,* **60,** pp. 413–420.

Jin, D., Takai, S., Sakaguchi, M., Okamoto, Y., Muramatsu, M., and Miyazaki, M. (2004). An antiarrhythmic effect of a chymase inhibitor after myocardial infarction, *J. Pharmacol. Exp. Ther.,* **309,** pp. 490–497.

Johnson, J. L., Jackson, C. L., Angelini, G. D., and George, S. J. (1998). Activation of matrix-degrading metalloproteinases by mast cell proteases in atherosclerotic plaques, *Arterioscler. Thromb. Vasc. Biol.,* **18,** pp. 1707–1715.

Jones, S. E., Gilbert, R. E., and Kelly, D. J. (2004). Tranilast reduces mesenteric vascular collagen deposition and chymase-positive mast cells in experimental diabetes, *J. Diabetes Complications,* **18,** pp. 309–315.

Judström, I., Jukkola, H., Metso, J., Jauhiainen, M., Kovanen, P. T., and Lee-Rueckert, M. (2010). Mast cell-dependent proteolytic modification of HDL particles during anaphylactic shock in the mouse reduces their ability to induce cholesterol efflux from macrophage foam cells ex vivo, *Atherosclerosis,* **208,** pp. 148–154.

Jutel, M., Blaser, K., and Akdis, C. A. (2005). Histamine in allergic inflammation and immune modulation, *Int. Arch .Allergy. Immunol.,* **137,** pp. 82–92.

Kaartinen, M., Penttilä, A.,and Kovanen, P. T. (1994). Accumulation of activated mast cells in the shoulder region of human coronary atheroma, the predilection site of atheromatous rupture, *Circulation,* **90,** pp. 1669–1678.

Kaartinen, M., Penttilä, A., and Kovanen, P. T. (1996a). Mast cells accompany microvessels in human coronary atheromas: implications for intimal neovascularization and hemorrhage, *Atherosclerosis,* **123,** pp. 123–131.

Kaartinen, M., Penttilä, A., and Kovanen, P. T. (1996b). Mast cells in rupture-prone areas of human coronary atheromas produce and store TNF-alpha, *Circulation,* **94,** pp. 2787–2792.

Kalsner, S., and Richards, R. (1984). Coronary arteries of cardiac patients are hyperreactive and contain stores of amines: a mechanism for coronary spasm, *Science,* **223,** pp. 1435–1437.

Kambayashi, T., Allenspach, E. J., Chang, J. T., Zou, T., Shoag, J. E., Reiner, S. L., Caton, A. J., and Koretzky, G. A. (2009). Inducible MHC class II expression by mast cells supports effector and regulatory T cell activation, *J. Immunol.,* **182,** pp. 4686–4695.

Kanbe, N., Tanaka, A., Kanbe, M., Itakura, A., Kurosawa, M., and Matsuda, H. (1992). Human mast cells produce matrix metalloproteinase 9, *Eur. J. Immunol.,* **29,** pp. 2645–2649.

Kandere-Grzybowska, K., Letourneau, R., Kempuraj, D., Donelan, J., Poplawski, S., Boucher, W., Athanassiou, A., and Theoharides, T. C. (2003). IL-1 induces vesicular secretion of IL-6 without degranulation from human mast cells, *J. Immunol.,* **171,** pp. 4830–4836.

Kanemitsu, H., Takai, S., Tsuneyoshi, H., Nishina, T., Yoshikawa, K., Miyazaki, M., Ikeda, T., and Komeda, M. (2006). Chymase inhibition prevents cardiac fibrosis and dysfunction after myocardial infarction in rats, *Hypertens. Res.,* **29,** pp. 57–64.

Kanemitsu, H., Takai, S., Tsuneyoshi, H., Yoshikawa, E., Nishina, T., Miyazaki, M., Ikeda, T., and Komeda, M. (2008). Chronic chymase inhibition preserves cardiac function after left ventricular repair in rats, *Eur. J. Cardiothorac. Surg.*, **33,** pp. 25–31.

Katada, J., Muramatsu, M., Hayashi, I., Tsutsumi, M., Konishi, Y., and Majima, M. (2002). Significance of vascular endothelial cell growth factor up-regulation mediated via a chymase-angiotensin-dependent pathway during angiogenesis in hamster sponge granulomas, *J. Pharmacol. Exp. Ther.*, **302,** pp. 949–956.

Kawakami, T., and Galli, S. J. (2002). Regulation of mast-cell and basophil function and survival by IgE, *Nat. Rev. Immunol.*, **2,** pp. 773–786.

Kelley, J., Hemontolor, G., Younis, W., Li, C., Krishnaswamy, G., and Chi, D. S. (2006). Mast cell activation by lipoproteins, *Methods. Mol. Biol.*, **315,** pp. 341–348.

Kempná, P., Reiter, E., Arock, M., Azzi, A., and Zingg, J. M. (2004). Inhibition of HMC-1 mast cell proliferation by vitamin E: involvement of the protein kinase B pathway, *J. Biol. Chem.*, **279,** pp. 50700–50709.

Ketavarapu, J. M., Rodriguez, A. R., Yu, J. J., Cong, Y., Murthy, A. K., Forsthuber, T. G., Guentzel, M. N., Klose, K. E., Berton, M. T., and Arulanandam, B. P. (2008). Mast cells inhibit intramacrophage Francisella tularensis replication via contact and secreted products including IL-4, *Proc. Natl. Acad. Sci. U S A.*, **105,** pp. 9313–9318.

Kido, H., Nakano, A., Okishima, N., Wakabayashi, H., Kishi, F., Nakaya ,Y., Yoshizumi, M., and Tamaki, T. (1998). Human chymase, an enzyme forming novel bioactive 31-amino acid length endothelins, *Biol. Chem.*, **379,** pp. 885–891.

Kinoshita, M., Okada, M., Hara, M., Furukawa, Y., and Matsumori, A. (2005). Mast cell tryptase in mast cell granules enhances MCP-1 and interleukin-8 production in human endothelial cells, *Arterioscler. Thromb. Vasc. Biol.*, **25,** pp. 1858–1863.

Kitamoto, S., Sukhova, G. K., Sun, J., Yang, M., Libby, P., Love, V., Duramad, P., Sun, C., Zhang, Y., Yang, X., Peters, C., and Shi, G.-P. (2007). Cathepsin L deficiency reduces diet-induced atherosclerosis in low-density lipoprotein receptor-knockout mice, Circulation, **115,** pp. 2065–2075.

Kitamura, Y. (1989). Heterogeneity of mast cells and phenotypic change between subpopulations, *Annu. Rev. Immunol.*, **7,** pp. 59–76.

Knoflach, M., Kiechl, S., Mayr, A., Willeit, J., Poewe, W., and Wick, G. (2005). Allergic rhinitis, asthma, and atherosclerosis in the Bruneck and ARMY studies, *Arch. Intern. Med.*, **165,** pp. 2521–2526.

Kokkonen, J. O. (1989). Stimulation of rat peritoneal mast cells enhances uptake of low density lipoproteins by rat peritoneal macrophages in vivo, *Atherosclerosis,* **79,** pp. 213–223.

Komatsu, H., Kojima, M., Tsutsumi, N., Hamano, S., Kusama, H., Ujiie, A., Ikeda, S., and Nakazawa, M. (1988). Mechanism of inhibitory action of tranilast on the release of slow reacting substance of anaphylaxis (SRS-A) in vitro: effect of tranilast on the release of arachidonic acid and its metabolites, *Jpn. J. Pharmacol.,* **46,** pp. 53–60.

Kounis, N. G., and Zavras, G. M. (1991). Histamine-induced coronary artery spasm: the concept of allergic angina, *Br. J. Clin. Pract.,* **45,** pp. 121–128.

Kovanen, P. T. (2007). Mast cells: multipotent local effector cells in atherothrombosis, *Immunol. Rev.,* **217,** pp. 105–222.

Kovanen, P. T., Kaartinen, M., and Paavonen, T. (1995). Infiltrates of activated mast cells at the site of coronary atheromatous erosion or rupture in myocardial infarction, *Circulation,* **92,** pp. 1084–1088.

Kunitake, S. T., Chen, G. C., Kung, S. F., Schilling, J. W., Hardman, D. A., and Kane, J. P. (1990). Pre-beta high density lipoprotein. Unique disposition of apolipoprotein A-I increases susceptibility to proteolysis, *Arteriosclerosis,* **10,** pp. 25–30.

Laine, P., Kaartinen, M., Penttilä, A., Panula, P., Paavonen, T., and Kovanen, P. T. (1999). Association between myocardial infarction and the mast cells in the adventitia of the infarct-related coronary artery, *Circulation,* **99,** pp. 361–369.

Laine, P., Pentikäinen, M. O., Würzner, R., Penttilä, A., Paavonen, T., Meri, S., and Kovanen, P. T. (2002). Evidence for complement activation in ruptured coronary plaques in acute myocardial infarction, *Am. J. Cardiol.,* **90,** pp. 404–408.

Langer, R. D., Criqui, M. H., Feigelson, H. S., McCann, T. J., and Hamburger, R. N. (1996). IgE predicts future nonfatal myocardial infarction in men, *J. Clin. Epidemiol.,* **49,** pp. 203–209.

Lappalainen, H., Laine, P., Pentikäinen, M. O., Sajantila, A., and Kovanen, P. T. (2004). Mast cells in neovascularized human coronary plaques store and secrete basic fibroblast growth factor, a potent angiogenic mediator, *Arterioscler. Thromb. Vasc. Biol.,* **24,** pp. 1880–1885.

Lätti, S., Leskinen, M., Shiota, N., Wang, Y., Kovanen, P. T., and Lindstedt, K. A. (2003). Mast cell-mediated apoptosis of endothelial cells in vitro: a paracrine mechanism involving TNF-alpha-mediated down-regulation of bcl-2 expression, *J. Cell Physiol.,* **195,** pp. 130–138.

Lee, D. M., Friend, D. S., Gurish, M. F., Benoist, C., Mathis, D., and Brenner, M. B. (2002a). Mast cells: a cellular link between autoantibodies and inflammatory arthritis, *Science,* **297,** pp. 1689–1692.

Lee, M., Calabresi, L., Chiesa, G., Franceschini, G., and Kovanen, P. T. (2002). Mast cell chymase degrades apoE and apoA-II in apoA-I-knockout mouse plasma and reduces its ability to promote cellular cholesterol efflux, *Arterioscler. Thromb. Vasc. Biol.,* **22,** pp. 1475–1481.

Lee, M., Lindstedt, L. K., and Kovanen, P. T. (1992). Mast cell-mediated inhibition of reverse cholesterol transport, *Arterioscler. Thromb.,* **12,** pp. 1329–1335.

Lee, M., von Eckardstein, A., Lindstedt, L., Assmann, G., and Kovanen, P. T. (1999). Depletion of pre beta 1LpA1 and LpA4 particles by mast cell chymase reduces cholesterol efflux from macrophage foam cells induced by plasma, *Arterioscler. Thromb. Vasc. Biol.,* **19,** pp. 1066–1074.

Lee-Rueckert, M., and Kovanen, P. T. (2006). Mast cell proteases: physiological tools to study functional significance of high density lipoproteins in the initiation of reverse cholesterol transport, *Atherosclerosis,* **189,** pp. 8–18.

Leskinen, M. J., Heikkilä, H. M., Speer, M. Y., Hakala, J. K., Laine, M., Kovanen, P. T., and Lindstedt, K. A. (2006). Mast cell chymase induces smooth muscle cell apoptosis by disrupting NF-kappaB-mediated survival signaling, *Exp. Cell. Res.,* **312,** pp. 1289–1298.

Leskinen, M. J., Lindstedt, K. A., Wang, Y., and Kovanen, P. T. (2003a). Mast cell chymase induces smooth muscle cell apoptosis by a mechanism involving fibronectin degradation and disruption of focal adhesions, *Arterioscler. Thromb. Vasc. Biol.,* **23,** pp. 238–243.

Leskinen, M., Wang, Y., Leszczynski, D., Lindstedt, K. A., and Kovanen, P. T. (2003b). Regulation of smooth muscle cell growth, function and death in vitro by activated mast cells--a potential mechanism for the weakening and rupture of atherosclerotic plaques, *Biochem .Pharmacol.,* **66,** pp. 1493–1498.

Li, M., Liu, K., Michalicek, J., Angus, J. A., Hunt, J. E., Dell'Italia, L. J., Feneley, M. P., Graham, R. M., and Husain, A. (2004). Involvement of chymase-mediated angiotensin II generation in blood pressure regulation, *J. Clin. Invest.,* **114,** pp. 112–120.

Libby, P. (2002a). Inflammation in atherosclerosis, *Nature,* **420,** pp. 868–74.

Libby, P. (2002b). Atherosclerosis: the new view, *Sci. Am.,* **286,** pp. 46–55.

Lindstedt, K. A., Kokkonen, J. O., and Kovanen, P. T. (1998). Regulation of the activity of secreted human lung mast cell tryptase by mast cell proteoglycans, *Biochim. Biophys. Acta.,* **1425,** pp. 617–627.

Lindstedt, K. A.,and Kovanen, P. T. (2004). Mast cells in vulnerable coronary plaques: potential mechanisms linking mast cell activation to plaque erosion and rupture, *Curr. Opin. Lipidol.,* **15,** pp. 567–573.

Lindstedt, L., Lee, M., Castro, G. R., Fruchart, J. C., and Kovanen, P. T. (1996). Chymase in exocytosed rat mast cell granules effectively proteolyzes apolipoprotein AI-containing lipoproteins, so reducing the cholesterol efflux-inducing ability of serum and aortic intimal fluid, *J. Clin. Invest.,* **97,** pp. 2174–2182.

Lindstedt, L., Lee, M., and Kovanen, P. T. (2001a). Chymase bound to heparin is resistant to its natural inhibitors and capable of proteolyzing high density lipoproteins in aortic intimal fluid, *Atherosclerosis,* **155,** pp. 87–97.

Lindstedt, K. A., Wang, Y., Shiota, N., Saarinen, J., Hyytiäinen, M., Kokkonen, J. O., Keski-Oja, J., and Kovanen, P. T. (2001b). Activation of paracrine TGF-beta1 signaling upon stimulation and degranulation of rat serosal mast cells: a novel function for chymase, *FASEB J.,* **15,** pp. 1377–1388.

Liu, J., Sukhova, G. K., Sun, J. S., Xu, W. H., Libby, P., and Shi, G. P. (2004). Lysosomal cysteine proteases in atherosclerosis, *Arterioscler. Thromb. Vasc. Biol.,* **24,** pp.1359–1366.

Lowman, M. A., Benyon, R. C., and Church, M. K. (1988). Characterization of neuropeptide-induced histamine release from human dispersed skin mast cells, *Br. J. Pharmacol.,* **95,** pp. 121–130.

Lundeen, K. A., Sun, B., Karlsson, L., and Fourie, A. M. (2006). Leukotriene B4 receptors BLT1 and BLT2: expression and function in human and murine mast cells, *J. Immunol.,* **177,** pp. 3439–3447.

Lutgens, E., Lutgens, S. P., Faber, B. C., Heeneman, S., Gijbels, M. M., de Winther, M. P., Frederik, P., van der Made, I., Daugherty, A., Sijbers, A. M., Fisher, A., Long, C. J., Saftig, P., Black, D., Daemen, M. J., and Cleutjens, K. B. (2006). Disruption of the cathepsin K gene reduces atherosclerosis progression and induces plaque fibrosis but accelerates macrophage foam cell formation, *Circulation,* **113,** pp. 98–107.

Ma, H., and Kovanen, P. T. (1997). Degranulation of cutaneous mast cells induces transendothelial transport and local accumulation of plasma LDL in rat skin in vivo, *J. Lipid Res.,* **38,** pp. 1877–1887.

Ma, H., and Kovanen, P. T. (2000). Inhibition of mast cell-dependent conversion of cultured macrophages into foam cells with antiallergic drugs, *Arterioscler. Thromb. Vasc. Biol.,* **20,** pp. E134–E142.

Malaviya, R., Ikeda, T., Ross, E., and Abraham, S. N. (1996). Mast cell modulation of neutrophil influx and bacterial clearance at sites of infection through TNF-alpha, *Nature,* **381,** pp. 77–80.

Malaviya, R., and Abraham, S. N. (2000). Role of mast cell leukotrienes in neutrophil recruitment and bacterial clearance in infectious peritonitis, *J. Leukoc. Biol.,* **67,** pp. 841–846.

Malbec, O., and Daëron, M. (2007). The mast cell IgG receptors and their roles in tissue inflammation, *Immunol. Rev.,* **217,** pp. 206–221.

Marone, G., de Crescenzo, G., Adt, M., Patella, V., Arbustini, E., and Genovese, A. (1995). Immunological characterization and functional importance of human heart mast cells, *Immunopharmacology,* **31,** pp. 1–18.

Marshall, J. S. (2004). Mast-cell responses to pathogens, *Nat. Rev. Immunol.,* **4,** pp. 787–799.

Masuda, A., Yoshikai, Y., Aiba, K., and Matsuguchi, T. (2002). Th2 cytokine production from mast cells is directly induced by lipopolysaccharide and distinctly regulated by c-Jun N-terminal kinase and p38 pathways, *J. Immunol.,* **169,** pp. 3801–3810.

Mathias, C. B., Freyschmidt, E. J., Caplan, B., Jones, T., Poddighe, D., Xing, W., Harrison, K. L., Gurish, M. F., and Oettgen, H. C. (2009). IgE influences the number and function of mature mast cells, but not progenitor recruitment in allergic pulmonary inflammation, *J. Immunol.,* **182,** pp. 2416–2424.

Mäyränpää, M. I., Heikkilä, H. M., Lindstedt, K. A., Walls, A. F., and Kovanen, P. T. (2006). Desquamation of human coronary artery endothelium by human mast cell proteases: implications for plaque erosion, *Coron. Artery Dis.,* **17,** pp. 611–621.

McLachlan, J. B., Hart, J. P., Pizzo, S. V., Shelburne, C. P., Staats, H. F., Gunn, M. D., and Abraham, S. N. (2003). Mast cell-derived tumor necrosis factor induces hypertrophy of draining lymph nodes during infection, *Nat. Immunol.,* **4,** pp. 1199–1205.

Metz, M., Siebenhaar, F., and Maurer, M. (2008). Mast cell functions in the innate skin immune system, *Immunobiology,* **213,** pp. 251–260.

Meltzer, E. O., Berkowitz, R. B., and Grossbard, E. B. (2005). An intranasal Syk-kinase inhibitor (R112) improves the symptoms of seasonal allergic rhinitis in a park environment, *J. Allergy Clin. Immunol.,* **115,** pp. 791–796.

Meyer, M. C., Creer, M. H., and McHowat, J. (2005). Potential role for mast cell tryptase in recruitment of inflammatory cells to endothelium, *Am. J. Physiol. Cell Physiol.,* **289,** pp. C1485–C1491.

Mito, N., Kitada, C., Hosoda, T., and Sato, K. (2002). Effect of diet-induced obesity on ovalbumin-specific immune response in a murine asthma model, *Metabolism,* **51,** pp. 1241–1246.

Miyamoto, T., Sasaguri, Y., Sasaguri, T., Azakami, S., Yasukawa, H., Kato, S., Arima, N., Sugama, K., and Morimatsu, M. (1997). Expression of stem cell factor in human aortic endothelial and smooth muscle cells, *Atherosclerosis,* **129,** pp. 207–213.

Miyazaki, M., and Takai, S. (2001) Local angiotensin II-generating system in vascular tissues: the roles of chymase, *Hypertens. Res.,* **24,** pp. 189–193.

Miyazawa, N., Watanabe, S., Matsuda, A., Kondo, K., Hashimoto, H., Umemura, K., and Nakashima, M. (1998). Role of histamine H1 and H2 receptor antagonists in the prevention of intimal thickening, *Eur. J. Pharmacol.,* **362,** pp. 53–59.

Mizutani, H., Schechter, N., Lazarus, G., Black, R. A., and Kupper, T. S. (1991). Rapid and specific conversion of precursor interleukin 1 beta (IL-1 beta) to an active IL-1 species by human mast cell chymase, *J .Exp. Med.,* **174**, pp. 821–825.

Moqbel, R., Walsh, G. M., Macdonald, A. J., and Kay, B. (1986). Effect of disodium cromoglycate on activation of human eosinophils and neutrophils following reversed (anti-IgE) anaphylaxis, *Clin. Allergy,* **16,** pp. 73–83.

Moya-Garcia, A. A., Medina, M. A., and Sánchez-Jiménez, F. (2005). Mammalian histidine decarboxylase: from structure to function, *Bioessays,* **27,** pp. 57–63.

Muramatsu, M., Katada, J., Hattori, M., Hayashi, I., and Majima, M. (2000a). Chymase mediates mast cell-induced angiogenesis in hamster sponge granulomas, *Eur. J. Pharmacol.,* **402,** pp. 181–191.

Muramatsu, M., Katada, J., Hayashi, I., and Majima, M. (2000b). Chymase as a proangiogenic factor. A possible involvement of chymase-angiotensin-dependent pathway in the hamster sponge angiogenesis model, *J. Biol. Chem.,* **275,** pp. 5545–5552.

Nakae, S., Suto, H., Kakurai, M., Sedgwick, J. D., Tsai, M., and Galli, S. J. (2005). Mast cells enhance T cell activation: importance of mast cell-derived TNF, *Proc. Natl. Acad. Sci. U S A.,* **102,** pp. 6467–6472.

Nakayama, T., Yao, L., and Tosato, G. (2004). Mast cell-derived angiopoietin-1 plays a critical role in the growth of plasma cell tumors, *J. Clin. Invest,.* **114,** pp. 1317–1325.

Nieuwenhuizen, N., Herbert, D. R., Lopata, A. L., and Brombacher, F. (2007). CD4+ T cell-specific deletion of IL-4 receptor alpha prevents ovalbumin-induced anaphylaxis by an IFN-gamma-dependent mechanism, *J. Immunol.,* **179,** pp. 2758–2765.

Nigo, Y. I., Yamashita, M., Hirahara, K., Shinnakasu, R., Inami, M., Kimura, M., Hasegawa, A., Kohno, Y., and Nakayama, T. (2006). Regulation of allergic airway inflammation through Toll-like receptor 4-mediated modification of mast cell function, *Proc. Natl. Acad. Sci. U S A.,* **103,** pp. 2286–2291.

Nigrovic, P. A., Gray, D. H., Jones, T., Hallgren, J., Kuo, F. C., Chaletzky, B., Gurish, M., Mathis, D., Benoist, C., and Lee, D. M. (2008). Genetic inversion in mast cell-deficient (W(sh)) mice interrupts corin and manifests as hematopoietic and cardiac aberrancy, *Am. J. Pathol.,* **173,** pp. 1693–1701.

Nishizono, S., Kusaba, M., Adan, Y., and Imaizumi, K. (1999). Induction of atherosclerosis in Brown Norway rats by immunization with ovalbumin, *Biosci. Biotechnol. Biochem,.* **63,** pp. 379–383.

Norrby, K. (2002). Mast cells and angiogenesis. *APMIS,* **110,** pp. 355–371.

Ochi, H., Hirani, W. M., Yuan, Q., Friend, D. S., Austen, K. F., and Boyce, J. A. (1999). T helper cell type 2 cytokine-mediated comitogenic responses and CCR3 expression during differentiation of human mast cells in vitro, *J. Exp. Med.,* **190,** pp. 267–280.

Ohtsu, H. (2008). Progress in allergy signal research on mast cells: the role of histamine in immunological and cardiovascular disease and the transporting system of histamine in the cell, *J. Pharmacol. Sci.,* **106,** pp. 347–353.

Okayama, Y., and Kawakami, T. (2006). Development, migration, and survival of mast cells, *Immunol. Res.,* **34,** pp. 97–115.

Oksjoki, R., Laine, P., Helske, S., Vehmaan-Kreula, P., Mäyränpää, M. I., Gasque, P., Kovanen, P. T., and Pentikäinen, M. O. (2007). Receptors for the anaphylatoxins C3a and C5a are expressed in human atherosclerotic coronary plaques, *Atherosclerosis,* **195,** pp. 90–99.

Oörni, K., Pentikäinen, M. O., Ala-Korpela, M., and Kovanen, P. T. (2000). Aggregation, fusion, and vesicle formation of modified low density lipoprotein particles: molecular mechanisms and effects on matrix interactions, *J. Lipid Res.,* **41,** pp. 1703–1714.

Packard, R. R., Lichtman, A. H., and Libby, P. (2009). Innate and adaptive immunity in atherosclerosis, *Semin. Immunopathol.,* **31,** pp. 5–22.

Patalano, F., and Ruggieri, F. (1989). Sodium cromoglycate: a review, *Eur. Respir. J. Suppl.,* **6,** pp. 556s–560s.

Pearce, F. L., Befus, A. D., Gauldie, J., and Bienenstock, J. (1982). Mucosal mast cells. II. Effects of anti-allergic compounds on histamine secretion by isolated intestinal mast cells, *J. Immunol.,* **128,** pp. 2481–2486.

Qiao, H., Andrade, M. V., Lisboa, F. A., Morgan, K., and Beaven, M. A. (2006). FcepsilonR1 and toll-like receptors mediate synergistic signals to markedly augment production of inflammatory cytokines in murine mast cells, *Blood,* **107,** pp. 610–618.

Qiu, H., Gabrielsen, A., Agardh, H. E., Wan, M., Wetterholm, A., Wong, C. H., Hedin, U., Swedenborg, J., Hansson, G. K., Samuelsson, B., Paulsson-Berne, G., and Haeggström, J. Z. (2006). Expression of 5-lipoxygenase and leukotriene A4 hydrolase in human atherosclerotic lesions correlates with symptoms of plaque instability, *Proc. Natl. Acad. Sci. U S A.,* **103,** pp. 8161–8166.

Ribatti, D., Belloni, A. S., Nico, B., Salà, G., Longo, V., Mangieri, D., Crivellato, E., and Nussdorfer, G. G. (2007). Tryptase- and leptin-positive mast cells correlate with vascular density in uterine leiomyomas, *Am. J. Obstet. Gynecol.,* **196,** pp. 470.e1–e7.

Rozenberg, I., Sluka, S. H., Rohrer, L., Hofmann, J., Becher, B., Akhmedov, A., Soliz, J., Mocharla, P., Borén, J., Johansen, P., Steffel, J., Watanabe, T., Lüscher, T. F., and Tanner, F. C. (2010). Histamine H1 receptor promotes atherosclerotic lesion formation by increasing vascular permeability for low-density lipoproteins, *Arterioscler. Thromb. Vasc. Biol.,* **30,** pp. 923–930.

Rudd, R. M., Gellert, A. R., Studdy, P. R., and Geddes, D. M. (1983). Inhibition of exercise-induced asthma by an orally absorbed mast cell stabilizer (M and B 22,948), *Br. J. Dis. Chest,* **77,** pp. 78–86.

Saarinen, J., Kalkkinen, N., Welgus, H. G., and Kovanen, P. T. (1994). Activation of human interstitial procollagenase through direct cleavage of the Leu83-Thr84 bond by mast cell chymase, *J. Biol. Chem.,* **269,** pp. 18134–18140.

Shamamian, P., Schwartz, J. D., Pocock, B. J., Monea, S., Whiting, D., Marcus, S. G., and Mignatti, P. (2001). Activation of progelatinase A (MMP-2) by neutrophil elastase, cathepsin G, and proteinase-3: a role for inflammatory cells in tumor invasion and angiogenesis, *J. Cell Physiol.,* **189,** pp. 197–206.

Shin, K., Watts, G. F., Oettgen, H. C., Friend, D. S., Pemberton, A. D., Gurish, M. F., and Lee, D. M. (2008). Mouse mast cell tryptase mMCP-6 is a critical link between adaptive and innate immunity in the chronic phase of Trichinella spiralis infection, *J. Immunol.,* **180,** pp. 4885–4891.

Sinnamon, M. J., Carter, K. J., Sims, L. P., Lafleur, B., Fingleton, B., and Matrisian, L. M. (2008). A protective role of mast cells in intestinal tumorigenesis, *Carcinogenesis,* **29,** pp. 880–886.

Soucek, L., Lawlor, E. R., Soto, D., Shchors, K., Swigart, L. B., and Evan, G. I. (2007). Mast cells are required for angiogenesis and macroscopic expansion of Myc-induced pancreatic islet tumors, *Nat. Med.,* **13,** pp. 1211–1218.

Stary, H. C. (1990). The sequence of cell and matrix changes in atherosclerotic lesions of coronary arteries in the first forty years of life, *Eur. Heart J.,* **11 Suppl E,** pp. 3–19.

Stelekati, E., Orinska, Z., and Bulfone-Paus, S. (2007). Mast cells in allergy: innate instructors of adaptive responses, *Immunobiology,* **212,** pp. 505–519.

Subbarao, K., Jala, V. R., Mathis, S., Suttles, J., Zacharias, W., Ahamed, J., Ali, H., Tseng, M. T., and Haribabu, B. (2004). Role of leukotriene B4 receptors in the development of atherosclerosis: potential mechanisms, *Arterioscler. Thromb. Vasc. Biol.,* **24,** pp. 369–375.

Sukhova, G. K., Zhang, Y., Pan, J. H., Wada, Y., Yamamoto, T., Naito, M., Kodama, T., Tsimikas, S., Witztum, J. L., Lu, M. L., Sakara, Y., Chin, M. T., Libby, P., and Shi, G.-P. (2003). Deficiency of cathepsin S reduces atherosclerosis in LDL receptor-deficient mice, *J. Clin. Invest.,* **111,** pp. 897–906.

Sun, J., Sukhova, G. K., Wolters, P. J., Yang, M., Kitamoto, S., Libby, P., MacFarlane, L. A., Mallen-St Clair, J., and Shi, G. P. (2007). Mast cells promote atherosclerosis by releasing proinflammatory cytokines, *Nat. Med.,* **13,** pp. 719–724.

Sun, J., Zhang, J., Lindholt, J. S., Sukhova, G. K., Liu, J., He, A., Abrink, M., Pejler, G., Stevens, R. L., Thompson, R. W., Ennis, T. L., Gurish, M. F., Libby, P., and Shi, G. P. (2009). Critical role of mast cell chymase in mouse abdominal aortic aneurysm formation, *Circulation,* **120,** pp. 973–982.

Sutherland, R. E., Olsen, J. S., McKinstry, A., Villalta, S. A., and Wolters, P. J. (2008). Mast cell IL-6 improves survival from Klebsiella pneumonia and sepsis by enhancing neutrophil killing, *J. Immunol.,* **181**, pp. 5598–5605.

Takai, S., Jin, D., Nishimoto, M., Yuda, A., Sakaguchi, M., Kamoshita, K., Ishida, K., Sukenaga, Y., Sasaki, S., and Miyazaki, M. (2001). Oral administration of a specific chymase inhibitor, NK3201, inhibits vascular proliferation in grafted vein, *Life Sci.,* **69,** pp. 1725–1732.

Takai, S., Sakonjo, H., Fukuda, K., Jin, D., Sakaguchi, M., Kamoshita, K., Ishida, K., Sukenaga, Y., and Miyazaki, M. (2003). A novel chymase inhibitor, 2-(5-formylamino-6-oxo-2-phenyl-1,6-dihydropyrimidine-1-yl)-*N*-

[[,4-dioxo-1 -phenyl-7-(2-pyridyloxy)]2-heptyl]acetamide (NK3201), suppressed intimal hyperplasia after balloon injury, *J. Pharmacol. Exp. Ther.,* **304,** pp. 841–844.

Takai, S., Shiota, N., Kobayashi, S., Matsumura, E., and Miyazaki, M. (1997). Induction of chymase that forms angiotensin II in the monkey atherosclerotic aorta, *FEBS Lett.*, **412,** pp. 86–90.

Talreja, J., Kabir, M. H., B. Filla, M., Stechschulte, D. J., and Dileepan, K. N. (2004). Histamine induces Toll-like receptor 2 and 4 expression in endothelial cells and enhances sensitivity to Gram-positive and Gram-negative bacterial cell wall components, *Immunology,* **113,** pp. 224–233.

Tang, Y. L., Yang, Y. Z., Wang, S., Huang, T., Tang, C. K., Xu, Z. X., and Sun, Y. H. (2009). Mast cell degranulator compound 48–80 promotes atherosclerotic plaque in apolipoprotein E knockout mice with perivascular common carotid collar placement, *Chin. Med. J. (Engl.),* **122,** pp. 319–325.

Tanimoto, A., Sasaguri, Y., and Ohtsu, H. (2006). Histamine network in atherosclerosis, *Trends Cardiovasc. Med.*, **16,** pp. 280–284.

Tchougounova, E., Lundequist, A., Fajardo, I., Winberg, J. O., Abrink, M., and Pejler, G. (2005). A key role for mast cell chymase in the activation of pro-matrix metalloprotease-9 and pro-matrix metalloprotease-2, *J. Biol. Chem.,* **280,** pp. 9291–9296.

Tchougounova, E., Pejler, G., and Abrink, M. (2003). The chymase, mouse mast cell protease 4, constitutes the major chymotrypsin-like activity in peritoneum and ear tissue. A role for mouse mast cell protease 4 in thrombin regulation and fibronectin turnover, *J. Exp. Med.,* **198,** pp. 423–431.

Thakurdas, S. M., Melicoff, E., Sansores-Garcia, L., Moreira, D. C., Petrova, Y., Stevens, R. L., and Adachi, R. (2007). The mast cell-restricted tryptase mMCP-6 has a critical immunoprotective role in bacterial infections, *J. Biol. Chem.,* **282,** pp. 20809–20815.

Toru, H., Eguchi, M., Matsumoto, R., Yanagida, M., Yata, J., and Nakahata, T. (1998). Interleukin-4 promotes the development of tryptase and chymase double-positive human mast cells accompanied by cell maturation, *Blood,* **91,** pp. 187–195.

Tremaine, W. J., Brzezinski, A., Katz, J. A., Wolf, D. C., Fleming, T. J., Mordenti, J., Strenkoski-Nix, L. C., and Kurth, M. C. (2002). AXYS Ulcerative Colitis Study Group. Treatment of mildly to moderately active ulcerative colitis with a tryptase inhibitor (APC 2059): an open-label pilot study, *Aliment Pharmacol. Ther.,* **16,** pp. 407–413.

Tsai, M., Takeishi, T., Thompson, H., Langley, K. E., Zsebo, K. M., Metcalfe, D. D., Geissler, E. N., and Galli, S. J. (1991). Induction of mast cell proliferation, maturation, and heparin synthesis by the rat c-kit ligand, stem cell factor, *Proc. Natl. Acad. Sci. U S A.*, **88,** pp. 6382–6386.

Uehara, Y., Urata, H., Ideishi, M., Arakawa, K., and Saku, K. (2002). Chymase inhibition suppresses high-cholesterol diet-induced lipid accumulation in the hamster aorta, *Cardiovasc. Res.*, **55,** pp. 870–876.

Vartio, T., Seppä, H., and Vaheri, A. (1981). Susceptibility of soluble and matrix fibronectins to degradation by tissue proteinases, mast cell chymase and cathepsin G, *J. Biol. Chem.*, **256,** pp. 471–477.

Virmani, R., Kolodgie, F. D., Burke, A. P., Finn, A. V., Gold, H. K., Tulenko, T. N., Wrenn, S. P., and Narula, J. (2005). Atherosclerotic plaque progression and vulnerability to rupture: angiogenesis as a source of intraplaque hemorrhage, *Arterioscler. Thromb. Vasc. Biol.*, **25,** pp. 2054–2061.

Vlaicu, R., Niculescu, F., Rus, H. G., and Cristea, A. (1985). Immunohistochemical localization of the terminal C5b-9 complement complex in human aortic fibrous plaque, *Atherosclerosis*, **57,** pp. 163–177.

Wang, Y., and Kovanen, P. T. (1999). Heparin proteoglycans released from rat serosal mast cells inhibit proliferation of rat aortic smooth muscle cells in culture, *Circ. Res.*, **84,** pp. 74–83.

Wang, Y., Shiota, N., Leskinen, M. J., Lindstedt, K. A., and Kovanen, P. T. (2001). Mast cell chymase inhibits smooth muscle cell growth and collagen expression in vitro: transforming growth factor-beta1-dependent and -independent effects, *Arterioscler. Thromb. Vasc. Biol.*, **21,** pp. 1928–1933.

Weber, C., Zernecke, A., Libby, P. (2008). The multifaceted contributions of leukocyte subsets to atherosclerosis: lessons from mouse models. The multifaceted contributions of leukocyte subsets to atherosclerosis: lessons from mouse models, *Nat. Rev. Immunol.*, **8,** pp. 802–815.

Weller, K., Foitzik, K., Paus, R., Syska, W., and Maurer, M. (2006). Mast cells are required for normal healing of skin wounds in mice, *FASEB J.*, **20,** pp. 2366–2368.

Williams, R. M., Bienenstock, J., and Stead, R. H. (1995). Mast cells: the neuroimmune connection, *Chem. Immunol.*, **61,** pp. 208–235.

Xiang, M., Sun, J., Lin, Y., Zhang, J., Chen, H., Yang, D., Wang, J., Shi, G. P. (2011) Usefulness of serum tryptase level as an independent biomarker for coronary plaque instability in a Chinese population. *Atherosclerosis.*, **215**, pp. 492–499.

Yamashita, M., and Nakayama, T. (2008). Progress in allergy signal research on mast cells: regulation of allergic airway inflammation through toll-like receptor 4-mediated modification of mast cell function, *J. Pharmacol. Sci.*, **106,** pp. 332–335.

Yeong, P., Ning, Y., Xu, Y., Li, X., and Yin, L. (2010). Tryptase promotes human monocyte-derived macrophage foam cell formation by suppressing LXRalpha activation, *Biochim. Biophys. Acta.,* **1801,** pp. 567–576.

Yokoyama, S. (2006). Assembly of high-density lipoprotein, *Arterioscler. Thromb. Vasc Biol.,* **26,** pp. 20–27.

Zhang, J., Sun, J., Linkholt, J. S., Sukhova, G. K., Sinnamon, M., Stevens, R. L., Adachi, R., Libby, P., Thompson, R. W., Shi, G. P. (2011) Mast cell tryptase deficiency attenuates mouse abdominal aortic aneurysm formation. *Circ. Res.*, **108**, pp. 1316–1327.

Zingg, J. M. (2007). Vitamin E and mast cells, *Vitam. Horm.,* **76,** pp. 393–418.

Chapter 6

HDL, ABC Transporters, and Cholesterol Efflux as Therapeutic Targets in Atherosclerosis

Kazuhiro Nakaya,[a,b] Katsunori Ikewaki,[b] and Daniel J. Rader[a]

[a] *Institute for Translational Medicine and Therapeutics and Cardiovascular Institute, University of Pennsylvania, Philadelphia, PA 19104, USA*

[b] *Division of Anti-aging, Department of Internal Medicine, National Defense Medical College, 3-2 Namiki, Tokorozawa, Saitama 359-8513, Japan*

rader@mail.med.upenn.edu

Reverse cholesterol transport (RCT) is a term used to describe the return of excess cholesterol from peripheral tissues to the liver for excretion in the bile and ultimately the feces. RCT from arterial macrophages (macrophage RCT) is believed to be a critical mechanism by which high-density lipoproteins (HDL) exert a protective effect on the development of atherosclerosis. In this paradigm, cholesterol is effluxed from arterial macrophages to extracellular HDL-based acceptors through the action of transporters such as ATP-binding cassette transporter A1 (ABCA1) and ATP-binding cassette transporter G1 (ABCG1). Macrophage cholesterol efflux is the first

Atherosclerosis: Treatment and Prevention
Edited by Christian Weber and Oliver Soehnlein

ISBN 978-981-4316-26-2 (Hardcover), ISBN 978-981-4364-26-3 (eBook)
www.panstanford.com

and one of the most crucial mechanisms underlying macrophage RCT. Recent research has provided important insights into the molecular mechanisms of RCT, and both the private sector and academia are attempting to develop novel therapies based on pharmacologic enhancement of RCT. This chapter discusses therapeutic strategies for augmenting macrophage RCT via improved macrophage cholesterol efflux and cholesterol efflux acceptor functionality of circulating HDL.

6.1 Introduction

While statins have revolutionized the treatment of atherosclerotic cardiovascular disease, they reduce cardiovascular events by about 20–40% in association with the degree of low-density lipoprotein (LDL) reduction [1], leaving a large burden of residual risk. HDL-C levels have been recognized as a strong inverse predictor of cardiovascular risk based on various epidemiological studies conducted since 1970s [2]. A recent study also showed that even in patients treated with statins to reduce LDL-C levels, HDL-C levels remained an independent predictor of the likelihood of suffering cardiovascular events [3]. However, despite intense efforts to develop new pharmacological strategies to increase HDL-C levels, its robust associations with improved clinical outcomes remain sparse [4, 5].

Reverse cholesterol transport is thought to be a major anti-atherogenic function of HDL. First proposed in 1968 by Glomset [6], RCT involves the return of excess cholesterol from peripheral tissues to the liver, then ultimate biliary excretion into the intestinal lumen and fecal excretion. Although macrophage-specific RCT represents only a small fraction of total flux through the pathway, it may warrant particular focus given the critical importance of cholesterol-laden macrophage foam cells in the development of atheromatous lesions [7, 8]. Indeed, a murine assay that quantifies macrophage RCT has proven a better predictor of atherosclerosis in mice than HDL cholesterol concentration [9]. Furthermore, a robust measure of the "efflux capacity" of HDL in human serum was recently reported to be a better predictor of atherosclerotic cardiovascular disease than HDL-C concentrations themselves [10]. Thus, factors that influence the rate of egress of cholesterol from the macrophage may be critical in influencing the risk of cardiovascular disease.

Table 6.1 Summary of therapeutic strategies to promote macrophage cholesterol efflux and reverse cholesterol transport

Therapeutic strategy	**Effect on HDL-C levels**	**Effect on macrophage RCT *in vivo***	**Effect on atherosclerosis**	**Limitations**
Strategy for increasing macrophage cholesterol efflux				
LXR agonists	Variable	Increase	Decrease	Induction of hepatic steatosis
PPARα agonists	Increase	Increase	Decrease	Specificity and selectivity
Strategy for improving quantity and functionality of HDL-based acceptors				
Small molecule upregulationof apoA-I	Increase	Unknown	Unknown	Limited human efficacy data
ApoA-I/ Reconstituted HDL infusions	None/ increase	Unknown	Decrease	Limited human efficacy data, need for intravenous administration
ApoA-I mimetic peptides	None	Increase	Decrease	Limited human efficacy data, need for intravenous administration
CETP inhibitors	Increase	Variable	Unknown	Failure of one molecule raised doubts about mechanism

The removal of excess cholesterol from macrophage foam cells by HDL-based acceptors, including its principal apolipoprotein, apoA-1, is thought to be one of key mechanisms underlying the macrophage RCT [11]. ATP-binding cassette transporters ABCA1 and ABCG1 play a pivotal role in cholesterol efflux from macrophage foam cells. ABCA1 and ABCG1 also show additive activity in promoting macrophage RCT *in vivo* [12], and combined deficiency of these transporters in bone marrow-derived hematopoietic cells leads to severe defects in cholesterol efflux to HDL, resulting in massive cholesteryl ester accumulation in macrophages and accelerated atherogenesis in susceptible mouse models [13, 14].

Collectively, scrutiny of the subtleties of the RCT pathway and HDL particle heterogeneity might offer a way forward in the development of HDL-centric therapeutics. This article aims to review methodologies of strategies for augmenting macrophage cholesterol efflux, which in turn promotes overall macrophage RCT, by regulating specific cellular transporters and enhancing acceptor functionality of circulating HDL (Table 6.1).

6.2 The Role of ABC Transporters, and the Nature and Quantity of Extracellular HDL-Based Acceptors in Macrophage Cholesterol Efflux

The maintenance of optimal cellular cholesterol concentrations is essential for proper cell function and viability, since excess cholesterol is toxic to cells. Macrophages can protect against cholesterol toxicity by converting free cholesterol to cholesteryl ester or by effluxing cholesterol to extracellular acceptors. The rate of cellular cholesterol efflux is function of cholesterol status in the cell, the level of expression of cholesterol transporters, and the composition and concentration of extracellular cholesterol acceptors, generally HDL or its specific subfractions. The most abundant protein in HDL is apoA-I, which in a lipid-poor form is one type of acceptor; mature HDL particles also serve as acceptors of cellular cholesterol efflux (Fig. 6.1).

A variety of specific pathways of cholesterol efflux have been defined, including: (1) efflux to lipid-poor apolipoproteins, particularly apoA-I, mediated by ABCA1; (2) efflux to mature HDL particles mediated by ABCG1; (3) efflux to mature HDL particles by other pathways, including scavenger receptor-BI (SR-BI); and finally (4) passive diffusion. While it was once assumed that passive diffusion was the primary process, recent research has demonstrated that macrophage cholesterol efflux occurs largely via ABCA1 and ABCG1.

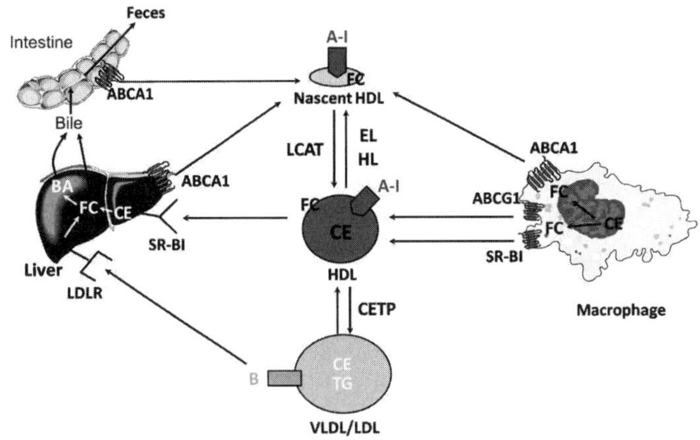

Figure 6.1 Reverse cholesterol transport.

Loss of function mutations in both alleles of ABCA1 in humans, a condition called Tangier disease, is characterized by severe HDL deficiency and cholesterol accumulation in peripheral tissues, including macrophages, characteristics also seen in mice lacking ABCA1. Macrophages deficient in ABCA1 expression have significantly impaired cholesterol efflux to lipid-poor apoA-I *in vitro*. Consistent with this observation, mice that were transplanted with bone marrow from ABCA1 knockout mice have increased the development of atherosclerotic lesion despite maintaining normal plasma HDL-C levels [15], whereas mice that were transplanted with bone marrow from ABCA1-overexpressing mice have reduced atherosclerosis [16]. Further supporting these findings, ABCA1-deficient macrophages also demonstrate significantly reduced RCT *in vivo* [12].

ABCG1 facilitates cholesterol efflux to mature HDL, but not to lipid-poor apoA-I [17, 18]. Mice that are deficient in ABCG1 have lipid accumulation in macrophages within multiple tissues when they are fed a high-fat high-cholesterol diet [18]. Macrophages lacking ABCG1 expression have impaired cholesterol efflux to mature HDL *ex vivo* and demonstrate significantly reduced RCT *in vivo* [12]. However, macrophage deficiency of ABCG1 is paradoxically associated with decreased atherosclerosis [19, 20], possibly due to compensatory upregulation of macrophage ABCA1 and apoE [20] or increased susceptibility of ABCG1-deficient macrophages to induce oxidized LDL-mediated apoptosis [19].

ABCA1 and ABCG1 also act in concert to promote macrophage cellular cholesterol efflux. For example, ABCA1 can lipidate lipid-poor apoA-I to generate nascent HDL particles, which can then serve as substrates for ABCG1-mediated cholesterol efflux [21]. In fact, knockdown of both ABCA1 and ABCG1 in macrophage reduced cholesterol efflux *ex vivo* and macrophage RCT *in vivo* to a greater extent than loss of function of either transporter alone [12]. Moreover, transplantation of ABCA1/G1 double-knockout bone marrow into atherosclerosis-prone mice resulted in substantially greater atherosclerosis than bone marrow from either single knockout [13].

6.3 Therapeutic Strategies for Increasing Macrophage Cholesterol Efflux

Liver X receptors (LXRs), including LXRα and LXRβ, are nuclear receptors that are critical to maintain lipid homeostasis. LXRs serve as the major regulators of macrophage ABCA1 and ABCG1 expression by forming heterodimers with their partner, retinoid X receptor (RXR) [22]. Synthetic LXR agonists have been shown to promote macrophage RCT and decrease atherosclerosis in mouse models [23–25]. However, development of first generation LXR agonists has been hampered by their induction of hepatic steatosis, which might be due to increased fatty acid biosynthesis via increased expression of sterol response element binding protein (SREBP 1-c) [26]. Recent studies have highlighted the primary role of the macrophage to exert anti-atherogenic activity of LXR agonists [27, 28].

A proof-of-concept study was performed in humans using LXR-623 (Wyeth Pharmaceuticals), a nonselective small molecule agonist of LXR [29]. This compound increased expression of ABCA1 and ABCG1 in blood leukocytes from human subjects. However, adverse central nervous system (CNS)-related effects were noted in more than half of the patients, leading to termination of the study. While this may have been related to LXR agonism, it is probably more likely due to off-target effects of this compound.

Because LXRα is the predominant subtype in the liver, selective agonism of LXRβ may help overcome the unfavorable hepatic effects observed in nonselective stimulation. Indeed, LXRβ-selective agonists have been developed to show the ability to promote macrophage cholesterol efflux [30]. Alternatively, restricting LXR activation to the small intestine might also result in an increase in intestinal HDL formation via ABCA1, without developing fatty liver [31]. As such, LXR agonists remain a highly plausible and conceptually attractive therapeutic target, particularly if it can be accomplished with selective targeting of the macrophage or intestine.

Peroxisome proliferator-activate receptor α (PPARα) is a member of nuclear receptor superfamily that regulate gene expression in response to the binding of fatty acids and their metabolites [32]. Although PPARα stimulation has multiple effects on lipid metabolism, including increased apoA-I production [33], we recently found that a specific PPARα agonist GW7647 (GlaxoSmithKline) promoted macrophage RCT *in vivo*, and this promotion was due to the enhanced macrophage cholesterol efflux by increasing ABCA1 and ABCG1 expression through the PPARα-LXR pathway even under condition of increased human apoA-I levels (*Arteriosclerosis, Thrombosis, and Vascular Biology*, in press). However, disappointing results of two recent large clinical trials using the weak PPARα agonist fenofibrate [34, 35] have reduced the enthusiasm for this approach. While fibrates are weak PPARα agonists, several agents with substantially increased potency and selectivity for PPARα have been developed. One of these compounds was shown to upregulate apoA-I production by 30% in humans, though was not assessed for its effects on blood leukocyte ABCA1 upregulation [36]. Combined with the above data suggesting that more potent PPARα agonists have greater potential to activate macrophage RCT, it remains possible that more potent PPARα agonists would have a greater effect on atherosclerotic cardiovascular disease than fibrates have shown.

6.4 Therapeutic Strategies for Improving Quantity and Functionality of HDL-based Acceptors

HDL particles are highly heterogeneous in to size, lipid, and protein composition. Multiple approaches attempt to enhance the plasma concentration or efflux capacity of circulating plasma via oral or infusion therapies.

ApoA-I, which comprises 70% of HDL protein, is well known to have anti-atherogenic properties. Enhancement of apoA-I expression is shown to increase plasma HDL levels and promote RCT, consequently lead to decrease atherosclerosis in several animal models [37, 38]. Small molecules that promote hepatic apoA-I expression in humans may also recapitulate these beneficial effects. One such compound, RVX-208 (Resverlogix Corp), recently entered early phase clinical trials. Serum from human patients or African green monkeys treated with RVX-208 exhibited increased cholesterol efflux capacity despite modest increases in HDL-C levels [39]. It will be of substantial interest to the field to determine whether this approach is anti-atherogenic in humans.

An alternate strategy has been to directly infuse apoA-I or reconstituted HDL (rHDL) into the circulation. These infusions were associated with attenuation, and even regression, of atherosclerosis in rabbit models [40, 41]. Subsequent preclinical studies in humans have noted transient increases in apoA-I levels and lipid poor pre-β HDL concentrations, resulting in increased *ex vivo* cholesterol efflux capacity and fecal sterol excretion [42–44]. A human trial studied the effects of reconstituted HDL-apoA-I disks on coronary atherosclerosis using angiography or intravascular ultrasound (IVUS) and demonstrated the reduction in atheroma volume, consistent with plaque regression, when compared to baseline [45]. While intriguing, the study was underpowered to detect differences from the placebo group and, thus, awaits replication in a larger cohort.

Beyond infusions of wild type apoA-I, several groups have explored the use of apoA-I engineered to be atheroprotective. ApoA-I Milano is a point mutation that is associated with low HDL and apoA-I levels but no dramatic increase in vascular disease, leading to hypothesis that this mutation may have improved atheroprotective properties [46]. This hypothesis, however, remains controversial, since mice expressing wild-type and ApoA-I Milano exhibit no difference in macrophage RCT *in vivo* [47]. In contrast, weekly infusions of ApoA-I Milano — phosphatidylcholine disks were associated with reduction from baseline coronary atheroma volume noted on IVUS within the relatively short term of 5 weeks [48]. While the optimal formulation remains unclear, results in both humans and animal models suggest that infusions of apoA-I/rHDL may increase RCT and reduce atherosclerotic lesions. Larger clinical trials with cardiovascular event outcomes will be important and of major interest to the field.

Recent studies have focused on the development of small apoA-I mimetic peptides, which could mimic the effects of full-length apoA-I but would be cheaper to synthesize and easier to administer [49]. One such peptide, D-4F, was engineered to contain only 18 amino acids but retain its lipid-binding properties. Furthermore, the use of only D-amino acids allows the molecule to escape from gastrointestinal peptidase breakdown. In fact, oral D-4F was associated with improved HDL anti-inflammatory function, enhanced RCT, and decreased atherosclerosis in mouse models [50, 51]. Early-phase clinical investigation of single-dose oral administration of D-4F in humans demonstrated proof of concept with regard to safety, modest oral bioavailability, and a dose-dependent improvement in measures of isolated HDL anti-inflammatory activity [52]. A subsequent study of parenteral administration of L-4F (the same peptide made of L amino acids) indicated relatively little pharmacodynamic effect on HDL function despite good plasma levels of peptide [53] . No other studies of apoA-I mimetic peptides in humans have been reported in the peer-reviewed literature. The future of apoA-I mimetic peptides will likely depend on larger scale evidence of enhanced HDL functionality with acceptable safety.

Cholesteryl ester transfer protein (CETP) has a well-established role in mediating transfer of cholesteryl esters from HDL to apoB-containing lipoproteins (LDL or VLDL) in exchange for triglycerides (Fig. 6.1). A therapeutic approach to pharmacologic CETP inhibition was first suggested by the dramatic high-HDL/low-LDL phenotype of human genetic CETP deficiency [54]. This concept was reinforced when both genetic deficiency and pharmacologic CETP inhibition were associated with increased cholesterol efflux capacity, primarily via the ABCG1 transporter [55, 56]. However, the influence of CETP on RCT remains uncertain [57]. A kinetic study in healthy human subjects involving injection of HDL labeled with a CE tracer suggested that the HDL-derived labeled cholesterol that was ultimately excreted into bile was mostly transferred to apoB-containing lipoproteins (presumably by CETP) [58]. Mice naturally lack CETP and studies in which CETP expression was reconstituted in mice showed that CETP expression facilitated macrophage RCT in wild-type mice but not affected macrophage RCT in LDL-receptor deficient mice [59]. Studies in hamsters (which have CETP) with CETP inhibitors showed variable effects of small molecule CETP inhibitors on macrophage RCT [60]. Additionally, no increase in fecal sterol excretion was noted in a human study of pharmacological CETP inhibition, although the limitations of the methodology preclude definitive conclusions regarding RCT [61]. Collectively, the impact of CETP on RCT, and thus potentially cardiovascular disease, may vary according to hepatic apoB-containing lipoprotein clearance efficiency.

Hope for this new HDL treatment was dealt a major blow when a Phase III clinical trial of one potent CETP inhibitor, torcetrapib (Pfizer), was terminated after an increase in mortality and cardiovascular events was noted in the treatment group. This occurred despite the positive effects on lipid profiles, with a 72% increase in HDL-C and 25% reduction in LDL-C [62]. Unfortunately, torcetrapib was associated with off-target elevations in aldosterone levels and blood pressure, potentially explaining a portion of the adverse effects. Two other CETP inhibitors currently in late-stage clinical development, anacetrapib (Merck and Co.) and dalcetrapib (Roche Pharmaceuticals), show no adverse effects on blood pressure and are likely to provide much-needed insight into the mechanism's utility [63, 64].

6.5 Conclusion

Recent data have highlighted the longstanding hypothesis that macrophage cholesterol efflux and HDL particle heterogeneity play a critical role in the reverse cholesterol transport. Although these molecular mechanisms regulating macrophage RCT have yet to be fully elucidated, the promotion of macrophage RCT by modifying either the macrophage transport pathways or the HDL acceptor particles (or both) remains a promising target for future drug development as a novel anti-atherogenic strategy. Development of a robust assay for RCT, ideally from the macrophage, in humans will also be critical to the development and early assessment of therapeutics that are designed to increase macrophage RCT. In the future, RCT-focused therapy that is safe and efficacious might play a critical role in the treatment of human atherosclerotic diseases.

References

1. Kearney PM, Blackwell L, Collins R, *et al.* 2008; Efficacy of cholesterol-lowering therapy in 18,686 people with diabetes in 14 randomised trials of statins: a meta-analysis. *Lancet* 371:117–125.

2. Miller GJ, Miller NE. 1975; Plasma-high-density-lipoprotein concentration and development of ischaemic heart-disease. *Lancet* 1:16–19.

3. Barter P, Gotto AM, LaRosa JC, *et al.* 2007; HDL cholesterol, very low levels of LDL cholesterol, and cardiovascular events. *N Engl J Med* 357:1301–1310.

4. Singh IM, Shishehbor MH, Ansell BJ. 2007; High-density lipoprotein as a therapeutic target: a systematic review. *JAMA* 298:786–798.

5. Briel M, Ferreira-Gonzalez I, You JJ, *et al.* 2009; Association between change in high density lipoprotein cholesterol and cardiovascular disease morbidity and mortality: systematic review and meta-regression analysis. *BMJ* 338:b92.

6. Glomset JA. 1968; The plasma lecithins:cholesterol acyltransferase reaction. *J Lipid Res* 9:155–167.

7. Tall AR, Wang N, Mucksavage P. 2001; Is it time to modify the reverse cholesterol transport model? *J Clin Invest* 108:1273–1275.

8. Cuchel M, Rader DJ. 2006; Macrophage reverse cholesterol transport: key to the regression of atherosclerosis? *Circulation* 113:2548–2555.

9. Rader DJ, Alexander ET, Weibel GL, *et al.* 2009; The role of reverse cholesterol transport in animals and humans and relationship to atherosclerosis. *J Lipid Res* 50 Suppl:S189–194.

10. Khera AV, Cuchel M, de la Llera-Moya M, *et al.* 2011; Cholesterol efflux capacity, high-density lipoprotein function, and atherosclerosis. *N Engl J Med* 364:127–135.

11. Rader DJ. 2007; Mechanisms of disease: HDL metabolism as a target for novel therapies. *Nat Clin Pract Cardiovasc Med* 4:102–109.

12. Wang X, Collins HL, Ranalletta M, *et al.* 2007; Macrophage ABCA1 and ABCG1, but not SR-BI, promote macrophage reverse cholesterol transport *in vivo*. *J Clin Invest* 117:2216–2224.

13. Yvan-Charvet L, Ranalletta M, Wang N, *et al.* 2007; Combined deficiency of ABCA1 and ABCG1 promotes foam cell accumulation and accelerates atherosclerosis in mice. *J Clin Invest* 117:3900–3908.

14. Out R, Hoekstra M, Habets K, *et al.* 2008; Combined deletion of macrophage ABCA1 and ABCG1 leads to massive lipid accumulation in tissue macrophages and distinct atherosclerosis at relatively low plasma cholesterol levels. *Arterioscler Thromb Vasc Biol* 28:258–264.

15. Van Eck M, Bos IS, Kaminski WE, *et al.* 2002; Leukocyte ABCA1 controls susceptibility to atherosclerosis and macrophage recruitment into tissues. *Proc Natl Acad Sci U S A* 99:6298–6303.

16. Van Eck M, Singaraja RR, Ye D, *et al.* 2006; Macrophage ATP-binding cassette transporter A1 overexpression inhibits atherosclerotic lesion progression in low-density lipoprotein receptor knockout mice. *Arterioscler Thromb Vasc Biol* 26:929–934.

17. Wang N, Lan D, Chen W, *et al.* 2004; ATP-binding cassette transporters G1 and G4 mediate cellular cholesterol efflux to high-density lipoproteins. *Proc Natl Acad Sci U S A* 101:9774–9779.

18. Kennedy MA, Barrera GC, Nakamura K, *et al.* 2005; ABCG1 has a critical role in mediating cholesterol efflux to HDL and preventing cellular lipid accumulation. *Cell Metab* 1:121–131.

19. Baldan A, Pei L, Lee R, *et al.* 2006; Impaired development of atherosclerosis in hyperlipidemic Ldlr-/- and ApoE-/- mice transplanted with Abcg1-/- bone marrow. *Arterioscler Thromb Vasc Biol* 26:2301–2307.

20. Ranalletta M, Wang N, Han S, *et al.* 2006; Decreased atherosclerosis in low-density lipoprotein receptor knockout mice transplanted with Abcg1-/- bone marrow. *Arterioscler Thromb Vasc Biol* 26:2308–2315.

21. Gelissen IC, Harris M, Rye KA, *et al.* 2006; ABCA1 and ABCG1 synergize to mediate cholesterol export to apoA-I. *Arterioscler Thromb Vasc Biol* 26:534–540.

22. Repa JJ, Turley SD, Lobaccaro JA, *et al.* 2000; Regulation of absorption and ABC1-mediated efflux of cholesterol by RXR heterodimers. *Science* 289:1524–1529.

23. Naik SU, Wang X, Da Silva JS, *et al.* 2006; Pharmacological activation of liver X receptors promotes reverse cholesterol transport *in vivo*. *Circulation* 113:90–97.

24. Terasaka N, Hiroshima A, Koieyama T, *et al.* 2003; T-0901317, a synthetic liver X receptor ligand, inhibits development of atherosclerosis in LDL receptor-deficient mice. *FEBS Lett* 536:6–11.

25. Joseph SB, McKilligin E, Pei L, *et al.* 2002; Synthetic LXR ligand inhibits the development of atherosclerosis in mice. *Proc Natl Acad Sci U S A* 99:7604–7609.

26. Li AC, Glass CK. 2004; PPAR- and LXR-dependent pathways controlling lipid metabolism and the development of atherosclerosis. *J Lipid Res* 45:2161–2173.

27. Levin N, Bischoff ED, Daige CL, *et al.* 2005; Macrophage liver X receptor is required for antiatherogenic activity of LXR agonists. *Arterioscler Thromb Vasc Biol* 25:135 142.

28. Teupser D, Kretzschmar D, Tennert C, *et al.* 2008; Effect of macrophage overexpression of murine liver X receptor-alpha (LXR-alpha) on atherosclerosis in LDL-receptor deficient mice. *Arterioscler Thromb Vasc Biol* 28:2009–2015.

29. Katz A, Udata C, Ott E, *et al.* 2009; Safety, pharmacokinetics, and pharmacodynamics of single doses of LXR-623, a novel liver X-receptor agonist, in healthy participants. *J Clin Pharmacol* 49:643–649.

30. Molteni V, Li X, Nabakka J, *et al.* 2007; N-Acylthiadiazolines, a new class of liver X receptor agonists with selectivity for LXRbeta. *J Med Chem* 50:4255–4259.

31. Brunham LR, Kruit JK, Pape TD, *et al.* 2006; Tissue-specific induction of intestinal ABCA1 expression with a liver X receptor agonist raises plasma HDL cholesterol levels. *Circ Res* 99:672–674.

32. Barbier O, Torra IP, Duguay Y, *et al.* 2002; Pleiotropic actions of peroxisome proliferator-activated receptors in lipid metabolism and atherosclerosis. *Arterioscler Thromb Vasc Biol* 22:717–726.

33. Duffy D, Rader DJ. 2009; Update on strategies to increase HDL quantity and function. *Nat Rev Cardiol* 6:455–463.

34. Keech A, Simes RJ, Barter P, *et al.* 2005; Effects of long-term fenofibrate therapy on cardiovascular events in 9795 people with type 2 diabetes mellitus (the FIELD study): randomised controlled trial. *Lancet* 366:1849–1861.

35. Ginsberg HN, Elam MB, Lovato LC, *et al.* 2010; Effects of combination lipid therapy in type 2 diabetes mellitus. *N Engl J Med* 362:1563–1574.

36. Millar JS, Duffy D, Gadi R, *et al.* 2009; Potent and selective PPAR-alpha agonist LY518674 upregulates both ApoA-I production and catabolism in human subjects with the metabolic syndrome. *Arterioscler Thromb Vasc Biol* 29:140–146.

37. Tangirala RK, Tsukamoto K, Chun SH, *et al.* 1999; Regression of atherosclerosis induced by liver-directed gene transfer of apolipoprotein A-I in mice. *Circulation* 100:1816–1822.

38. Zhang Y, Zanotti I, Reilly MP, *et al.* 2003; Overexpression of apolipoprotein A-I promotes reverse transport of cholesterol from macrophages to feces *in vivo*. *Circulation* 108:661–663.

39. Bailey D, Jahagirdar R, Gordon A, *et al.* 2010; RVX-208: a small molecule that increases apolipoprotein A-I and high-density lipoprotein cholesterol *in vitro* and *in vivo*. *J Am Coll Cardiol* 55:2580–2589.

40. Badimon JJ, Badimon L, Fuster V. 1990; Regression of atherosclerotic lesions by high density lipoprotein plasma fraction in the cholesterol-fed rabbit. *J Clin Invest* 85:1234–1241.

41. Miyazaki A, Sakuma S, Morikawa W, *et al.* 1995; Intravenous injection of rabbit apolipoprotein A-I inhibits the progression of atherosclerosis in cholesterol-fed rabbits. *Arterioscler Thromb Vasc Biol* 15:1882–1888.

42. Patel S, Drew BG, Nakhla S, *et al.* 2009; Reconstituted high-density lipoprotein increases plasma high-density lipoprotein anti-inflammatory properties and cholesterol efflux capacity in patients with type 2 diabetes. *J Am Coll Cardiol* 53:962–971.

43. Eriksson M, Carlson LA, Miettinen TA, Angelin B. 1999; Stimulation of fecal steroid excretion after infusion of recombinant proapolipoprotein A-I. Potential reverse cholesterol transport in humans. *Circulation* 100:594–598.

44. Nanjee MN, Cooke CJ, Garvin R, *et al.* 2001; Intravenous apoA-I/lecithin discs increase pre-beta-HDL concentration in tissue fluid and stimulate reverse cholesterol transport in humans. *J Lipid Res* 42:1586–1593.

45. Tardif JC, Gregoire J, L'Allier PL, *et al.* 2007; Effects of reconstituted high-density lipoprotein infusions on coronary atherosclerosis: a randomized controlled trial. *JAMA* 297:1675–1682.

46. Chiesa G, Sirtori CR. 2003; Apolipoprotein A-I(Milano): current perspectives. *Curr Opin Lipidol* 14:159–163.

47. Alexander ET, Weibel GL, Joshi MR, *et al.* 2009; Macrophage reverse cholesterol transport in mice expressing ApoA-I Milano. *Arterioscler Thromb Vasc Biol* 29:1496–1501.

48. Nissen SE, Tsunoda T, Tuzcu EM, *et al.* 2003; Effect of recombinant ApoA-I Milano on coronary atherosclerosis in patients with acute coronary syndromes: a randomized controlled trial. *JAMA* 290:2292–2300.

49. Van Lenten BJ, Wagner AC, Anantharamaiah GM, *et al.* 2009; Apolipoprotein A-I mimetic peptides. *Curr Atheroscler Rep* 11:52–57.

50. Navab M, Anantharamaiah GM, Hama S, *et al.* 2002; Oral administration of an Apo A-I mimetic Peptide synthesized from D-amino acids dramatically reduces atherosclerosis in mice independent of plasma cholesterol. *Circulation* 105:290–292.

51. Navab M, Anantharamaiah GM, Reddy ST, *et al.* 2004; Oral D-4F causes formation of pre-beta high-density lipoprotein and improves high-density lipoprotein-mediated cholesterol efflux and reverse cholesterol

transport from macrophages in apolipoprotein E-null mice. *Circulation* 109:3215–3220.

52. Bloedon LT, Dunbar R, Duffy D, *et al.* 2008; Safety, pharmacokinetics, and pharmacodynamics of oral apoA-I mimetic peptide D-4F in high-risk cardiovascular patients. *J Lipid Res* 49:1344–1352.
53. Watson CE, Weissbach N, Kjems L, *et al.* 2011; Treatment of patients with cardiovascular disease with L-4F, an apo-A1 mimetic, did not improve select biomarkers of HDL function. *J Lipid Res* 52:361–373.
54. Brown ML, Inazu A, Hesler CB, *et al.* 1989; Molecular basis of lipid transfer protein deficiency in a family with increased high-density lipoproteins. *Nature* 342:448–451.
55. Matsuura F, Wang N, Chen W, *et al.* 2006; HDL from CETP-deficient subjects shows enhanced ability to promote cholesterol efflux from macrophages in an apoE- and ABCG1-dependent pathway. *J Clin Invest* 116:1435–1442.
56. Yvan-Charvet L, Matsuura F, Wang N, *et al.* 2007; Inhibition of cholesteryl ester transfer protein by torcetrapib modestly increases macrophage cholesterol efflux to HDL. *Arterioscler Thromb Vasc Biol* 27:1132–1138.
57. Tall AR, Yvan-Charvet L, Wang N. 2007; The failure of torcetrapib: was it the molecule or the mechanism? *Arterioscler Thromb Vasc Biol* 27:257–260.
58. Schwartz CC, VandenBroek JM, Cooper PS. 2004; Lipoprotein cholesteryl ester production, transfer, and output *in vivo* in humans. *J Lipid Res* 45:1594–1607.
59. Tanigawa H, Billheimer JT, Tohyama J, *et al.* 2007; Expression of cholesteryl ester transfer protein in mice promotes macrophage reverse cholesterol transport. *Circulation* 116:1267–1273.
60. Niesor EJ, Magg C, Ogawa N, *et al.* 2010; Modulating cholesteryl ester transfer protein activity maintains efficient pre-beta-HDL formation and increases reverse cholesterol transport. *J Lipid Res* 51:3443–3454.
61. Brousseau ME, Diffenderfer MR, Millar JS, *et al.* 2005; Effects of cholesteryl ester transfer protein inhibition on high-density lipoprotein subspecies, apolipoprotein A-I metabolism, and fecal sterol excretion. *Arterioscler Thromb Vasc Biol* 25:1057–1064.
62. Barter PJ, Caulfield M, Eriksson M, *et al.* 2007; Effects of torcetrapib in patients at high risk for coronary events. *N Engl J Med* 357:2109–2122.

63. Krishna R, Anderson MS, Bergman AJ, *et al.* 2007; Effect of the cholesteryl ester transfer protein inhibitor, anacetrapib, on lipoproteins in patients with dyslipidaemia and on 24-h ambulatory blood pressure in healthy individuals: two double-blind, randomised placebo-controlled phase I studies. *Lancet* 370:1907–1914.
64. Stein EA, Stroes ES, Steiner G, *et al.* 2009; Safety and tolerability of dalcetrapib. *Am J Cardiol* 104:82–91.

Chapter 7

Role of Selective Phospholipase A_2 Inhibition in the Treatment of Atherosclerosis

Colin H. Macphee
2301 Renaissance Boulevard, King of Prussia, PA 19406, 610-787-3851, USA
colin.h.macphee@gsk.com

7.1 Introduction

Atherosclerosis is the main cause of coronary heart disease (CHD), with evidence suggesting that it can begin during childhood. Despite considerable progress in treating CHD (including treatment with statins, anti-platelet therapy, renin–angiotensin–aldosterone system, and/or beta adrenergic blockade and diabetes control), patients at high risk continue to experience major cardiovascular events such as cardiovascular death, myocardial infarction, and stroke (Steg *et al.*, 2007). Thus, there is clear need to identify new complementary approaches, particularly for those patients at high cardiovascular risk.

The etiology of atherogenesis can be best described as a chronic inflammatory disease of the arterial intima, dominated by a leukocyte infiltrate comprising predominately T-lymphocytes and monocyte-

Atherosclerosis: Treatment and Prevention
Edited by Christian Weber and Oliver Soehnlein

ISBN 978-981-4316-26-2 (Hardcover), ISBN 978-981-4364-26-3 (eBook)
www.panstanford.com

derived macrophages (Libby *et al.*, 2009). A critical primary step in the formation of atherosclerotic coronary lesions is the accumulation and oxidation of low-density lipoprotein (LDL) particles (Tabas *et al.*, 2007). Oxidized-LDL favors leukocyte recruitment and activation as well as cell death, and this leads to generation of complex atherosclerotic plaques. These plaques have a high content of necrotic core, a thin inflamed fibrous cap (intense accumulation of macrophages) and scarce presence of smooth muscle cells. These lesions have been identified as vulnerable plaques, inferring to their association with cardiovascular clinical events.

The recognition of atherosclerosis as an inflammatory disease has had two important consequences. First, intensive research efforts have been initiated to identify novel inflammatory markers that may be helpful in assessing cardiovascular risk beyond that, which can be achieved with conventional risk factors such as LDL cholesterol levels. Second, the identification of numerous inflammatory pathways led to a number of novel therapeutic approaches to reduce the inflammatory response and stabilize atherosclerotic plaques. From the many different inflammatory signaling pathways that have been implicated in atherogenesis, two approaches have recently successfully completed Phase II clinical trials, and Phase III outcome trials are now in progress. Although the two drugs in question, **darapladib** (SB-480848, (Blackie *et al.*, 2003)) and **varespladib** (A-001 or previously LY315920 (Snyder *et al.*, 1999; Mihelich and Schevitz, 1999)), target the same enzyme superfamily, the phospholipase A_2s (PLA_2s) (Schaloske and Dennis, 2006), each is inhibitor of different and functionally distinct members of this group of enzymes. For darapladib, the target is a single secreted PLA_2 called lipoprotein-associated PLA_2 (Lp-PLA_2), whereas varespladib is an inhibitor of several members of a different subgroup of structurally related PLA_2s historically referred to as the secretory PLA_2s (sPLA_2s) (Lambeau and Gelb, 2008). The purpose of this article is to review and compare the evidence that has supported these enzymes as novel therapeutic targets for the treatment of atherosclerosis.

7.2 Secreted PLA_2s: Targets for Intervention

Over the past 20 years, there have been a number of significant advances in our knowledge about the superfamily of PLA_2 enzymes. PLA_2 hydrolyzes the fatty acid from the *sn*-2 position of phospholipids. *In vivo*, the *sn-2* position of phospholipids frequently contains polyunsaturated fatty acids such as arachidonic acid, and when released, these can be metabolized to form various eicosanoids and related bioactive lipid mediators (Funk, 2001). The metabolism of arachidonic acid, of course, is a very familiar signaling pathway to cardiologists as it represents the target of the class of drugs known as non-steroidal anti-inflammatory drugs (NSAIDs), such as aspirin, that exert their effects through inhibition of the enzyme cyclooxygenase (Vane and Botting, 2003). The remaining products of PLA_2 action, lysophospholipids, can also have a number of important roles in biological processes (Rivera and Chun, 2008).

The secreted PLA_2s were the first type of PLA_2 enzymes discovered (Lambeau and Gelb, 2008) with the human genome containing nine $sPLA_2$ genes (i.e., groups IB, IIA, IID, IIE, IIF, III, V, X, and XIIA). These proteins are disulphide-rich and have molecular weights of around 16 kDa except for the group III $sPLA_2$, whose cDNA predicts a protein with a molecular weight of ~55 kDa. These enzymes share a common aspartic acid/histidine catalytic dyad that cleaves substrate in a calcium-dependent manner via interfacial kinetics, i.e., when substrate is presented as a large lipid aggregate (Scott *et al.*, 1990). Varespladib is a broad inhibitor of these $sPLA_2$ enzymes with IC_{50} values in the low nanomolar range (e.g., group IIA IC_{50}: 9–14 nM; group V IC_{50}: 77 nM; and group X IC_{50}: 15 nM) (Snyder *et al.*, 1999; Mihelich and Schevitz, 1999). Although varespladib has the ability to inhibit all of the $sPLA_2$ enzymes listed above, this article will focus primarily on groups IIA, V, and X, since there is evidence that these enzymes are implicated in the pathogenesis of atherosclerosis.

Lp-PLA_2, also known as platelet-activating factor acetylhydrolase (PAF-AH) or PLA_2 type VIIA (Schaloske and Dennis, 2006), is also secreted but is a calcium-independent PLA_2. Lp-PLA_2 is different from other secreted PLA_2s in that it utilizes a distinct Ser/His/Asp triad active site (Tjoelker *et al.*, 1995; Burke and Dennis, 2009). Unlike the $sPLA_2s$ described above, which contain a His/Asp dyad active site, Lp-PLA_2 accesses its substrate in the aqueous phase (Min *et al.*, 1999). This property of Lp-PLA_2 enables a broad substrate specificity that is governed primarily by aqueous phase solubility. Since the active site of Lp-PLA_2 is not related to those of the other secreted PLA_2s, it is not surprising that although darapladib is an extremely potent inhibitor of Lp-PLA_2 (IC_{50} 270 pM), it is a relatively poor inhibitor of the $sPLA_2s$ listed above demonstrating $IC_{50}s > 1\ \mu M$

(Wilensky *et al.*, 2008). Darapladib is also a significantly less potent inhibitor of the structurally related but intracellular enzyme, PLA_2 type VIIB (IC_{50} 600 nM, Macphee *et al.*, unpublished data) (Schaloske and Dennis, 2006).

7.3 Substrates Preferences, Lipoprotein Metabolism, and Activity Against Pathogens

7.3.1 Lp-PLA_2

Lp-PLA_2 was first discovered and originally named for its ability to cleave the acetyl group from the *sn*-2 position of PAF *in vitro*, for example, when micromolar concentrations of PAF were added to isolated plasma (Blank *et al.*, 1983). This observation led naturally to the assumption that this enzyme was responsible for the inactivation of PAF *in vivo* and that Lp-PLA_2 inhibition could enhance PAF-mediated biology (Prescott *et al.*, 2000; Stafforini, 2009). However, little to no direct evidence exists implicating a role for Lp-PLA2 in the cleavage and inactivation of physiologically relevant concentrations of PAF *in vivo*. Although the Km of Lp-PLA_2 for PAF is reported to be around 10 μM (Tew *et al.*, 1996), PAF elicits responses at nanomolar concentrations (Snyder, 1995). Furthermore, it has been reported that the half-life for PAF in plasma or whole blood (which contains secreted Lp-PLA_2) from healthy individuals is approximately 5 minutes (Yoshida *et al.*, 1996). These enzyme characteristics tend to question a role for Lp-PLA_2 in hydrolyzing and inactivating physiologically meaningful concentrations of PAF *in vivo*, since this phospholipid mediator is biologically active in the low nM range, having a calculated Kd for its receptor of around 1 nM (Hwang, 1990), a concentration of PAF that is closer to levels found circulating in humans (Vadas *et al.*, 2008). Indeed, the most direct study conducted thus far has suggested a lack of a prominent role of Lp-PLA_2 in modifying PAF-mediated responses. Naoki *et al.* (2004) made use of a natural deficiency in Lp-PLA_2 (Stafforini *et al.*, 1996) amongst the Japanese population to explore PAF responsiveness. This clinical study demonstrated no statistically significant differences in either pulmonary function or transient neutropenia following PAF inhalation in individuals deficient in Lp-PLA_2 when compared with age- and sex-matched controls. These data are entirely consistent with observations made in a very recent article by Liu *et al.* (2011), suggesting that rapid clearance of PAF by endothelial cell-rich organs such as the liver represents the major route of *in vivo* PAF catabolism rather than Lp-PLA_2 activity.

The observation that the catalytic site of Lp-PLA_2 is uniquely exposed to the aqueous phase allows broad substrate recognition. Thus, in addition to hydrolyzing PAF, Lp-PLA_2 notably catalyzes oxidized phospholipids that can be both short (i.e., fragmented) or long chain in nature, including even F_2-isoprostane esterified phospholipids (Stremler *et al.*, 1991; Tew *et al.*, 1996; Min *et al.*, 2001; Stafforini *et al.*, 2006; Kriska *et al.*, 2007; and Davis *et al.*, 2008). It is exactly this unique capability of Lp-PLA_2 to cleave oxidized phospholipids that has implicated it as a potential key player in atherosclerosis (Zalewski and Macphee, 2005). One process, therefore, that Lp-PLA_2 is definitely not involved in is the release of unmodified arachidonic acid for eicosanoid formation.

Unlike $sPLA_2$s, Lp-PLA_2, as its name suggests, associates with lipoproteins in human plasma (Stafforini *et al.*, 1987; Caslake *et al.*, 2000). The vast majority of Lp-PLA_2 is found associated with LDL due primarily to a specific interaction between two domains on human Lp-PLA_2 and the carboxy terminus of apolipoprotein B-100 Stafforini, D. M., Tjoelker, L. W., McCormick, S. P. A., Vaitkus, D., McIntyre, T. M., Gray, P. W., . . . Prescott, S. M. (1999). Molecular basis of the interaction between plasma platelet-activating factor acetylhydrolase and low density lipoprotein. Journal of Biological Chemistry, 274(11), 7018-7024.. Intriguingly, it has been demonstrated that Lp-PLA_2 is enriched on two highly atherogenic apolipoprotein B-100 containing particles, small dense LDL and lipoprotein(a) (Lp(a)) (Tselepsis *et al.*, 1995; Blencowe *et al.*, 1995). Recent findings have shown a more pronounced association of Lp-PLA_2 with allele-specific levels of small size apo(a) (Enkhmaa *et al.*, 2010), which is interesting as several studies have demonstrated an association between small size apo(a) and elevated cardiovascular risk (Clarke *et al.*, 2009). Critically, these apo B-100 containing lipoproteins are viewed to be especially atherogenic once they become oxidized (Tabas et. al., 2007; Libby *et al.*, 2009), thus providing Lp-PLA_2 with a ready supply of substrate, in this instance, oxidized phosphatydylcholine. In short, Lp-PLA_2 remains latent until these lipoproteins undergo oxidative modification, thereafter Lp-PLA_2 rapidly generates biologically meaningful quantities of lysophosphatidylcholine (LPC) and oxidized free fatty acids, both of which have been demonstrated to be causal agents in promoting atherosclerosis (Wilensky and Macphee, 2009) (Wilensky, R. L., & Macphee, C. H. (2009). Lipoprotein-associated phospholipase A2 and atherosclerosis. *Current Opinion in Lipidology*, 20(5), 415–420). Cleavage of oxidized phosphatidylcholines by Lp-PLA_2 has been demonstrated for oxidized LDL, oxidized small dense LDL as well as oxidized Lp(a) (Tselepis *et al.*, 1995; Karabina *et al.*, 1996; Macphee *et al.*, 1999). The situation for Lp(a) is even more interesting as this lipoprotein particle appears to be a preferential carrier of oxidized phospholipids (oxPLs) in human plasma (Tsimikas *et al.*, 2005) and therefore potentially provides a continuous supply of substrate for Lp-PLA_2. Evidence exists for a regulatory role for LPC, in particular, in promoting atherosclerotic plaque development that could ultimately lead to the formation of a necrotic core. These steps include recruitment and activation of leukocytes, induction of apoptosis, and impaired removal of dead cells (Matsumoto *et al.*, 2007; Wilensky and Macphee, 2009; Schmitz and Ruebsaamen, 2010). Thus, through both its lipoprotein association and substrate preferences, Lp-PLA_2 is uniquely placed amongst PLA_2s to directly influence oxidized lipoprotein-mediated inflammatory responses.

Oxidized phospholipids have been proposed by several groups to directly promote inflammatory responses with much of the data originating from *in vitro* studies using exogenously added oxPLs (McIntyre *et al.*, 1999; Berliner and Watson, 2005). Thus, inhibition of Lp-PLA_2 may lead to an accumulation of oxPLs, its substrate, and potentially augment putative processes directly dependent upon intact oxPLs. Accumulation of oxPLs does not appear to be an issue with chronic Lp-PLA_2 inhibition, since long-term darapladib treatment did not influence atherosclerotic lesion oxidized phosphatidylcholine content in a porcine model while reducing significantly the elevated lesion LPC content (Wilensky *et al.*, 2008). This observation suggests that Lp-PLA_2 substrates can be alternatively metabolized or, perhaps, even actively removed through specific transport mechanisms such as Lp(a). It should be noted that more recent studies have demonstrated that oxPLs can induce anti-inflammatory effects through inhibition of Toll-like receptors, an action that could aid resolution of chronic inflammatory states (Bochkov, 2007; Von Schlieffen *et al.*, 2009; Feige *et al.*, 2010).

Another feature worth considering is the role of the various secreted PLA_2s in host defense, in particular in modulating bacterial infection, and how this could impact atherosclerosis. Recent evidence indicates that Lp-PLA_2 can degrade lipoteichoic acid (LTA), a polyphosphate attached to the cell membrane via a diacyl glycolipid that is an abundant component of the envelopes of gram-positive bacteria (Ho and Nahm, 2009). LTA is a ligand for the Toll-like receptor, TLR2, a pattern recognition receptor that is a component of the innate immune system that acts as a defense mechanism against pathogen invasion (O'Neill *et al.*, 2010). Diacylation of LTA is required for TLR2 signaling, thus deacylation by Lp-PLA_2 leads to inactivation of LTA (Ho and Nahm, 2009), which potentially could lead to a reduction in the detection of LTA-containing bacteria. It is interesting in this respect to note that Lp-PLA_2-deficient mice displayed decreased mortality compared to wild-type mice in a model of septic enterocolitis (Lu *et al.*, 2010). Clearly, much more work is needed to elucidate a role for Lp-PLA_2 in bacterial infection, but such a connection could be relevant for atherosclerosis, since compelling data exists indicating that infection contributes to atherogenesis and the acute complications caused by plaque rupture (Epstein *et al.*, 2009). A recent study of human carotid plaques showed a significant association of plaque Lp-PLA_2 with both macrophages and *chlamydia pneumoniae* that prompted the authors to suggest an interactive role of infection and Lp-PLA_2 in accelerating inflammation in atherosclerosis (Atik *et al.*, 2010).

7.3.2 sPLA_2

While group V and X sPLA_2s hydrolyzes both anionic (e.g., phosphatidylglycerol) and zwitterionic (e.g., phosphatidylcholine, PC) phospholipids, group IIA sPLA_2 has extremely low activity on vesicles of high PC content when compared to anionic vesicles (Singer *et al.*, 2002; Gora et al. (2006) Lambeau and Gelb, 2008). These properties have significant physiological consequences particularly when considering hydrolysis of lipoproteins that are PC rich. There is accumulating evidence, however, linking these three sPLA_2s to arachidonic acid release from cellular phospholipids for the biosynthesis of eicosanoids (Lambeau and Gelb, 2008). However, the precise mechanisms remain unclear but appear to require the concomitant participation of cytosolic PLA_2s to fully maximize eicosanoid production (Ghosh *et al.*, 2006; Ni *et al.*, 2006; Henderson *et al.*, 2007). Thus, unlike Lp-PLA_2, these $sPLA_2$s are directly linked with inflammatory pathways resulting from eicosanoid formation.

Of specific interest to atherosclerosis, considerable effort has been invested in evaluating the role of groups IIA, V, and X $sPLA_2$s in the hydrolysis of lipoproteins. It is important to point out that these enzymes, unlike Lp-PLA_2, do not directly associate with human lipoproteins *in vivo* and much of the evidence has been derived from *in vitro* studies where $sPLA_2$s have been added to lipoprotein preparations. Further evidence has been derived from overexpression studies in preclinical animal models that have very different lipoprotein profiles to humans. The relevance of these studies to the human situation could, therefore, be questioned. For instance, the relative ability of groups IIA, V, and X $sPLA_2$s to hydrolyze the major phospholipid within lipoproteins, PC, confirmed previous substrate studies listed above in that only group V and X $sPLA_2$s significantly hydrolyzed LDL and HDL *in vitro* (Gesquiere *et al.*, 2002; Hanasaki *et al.*, 2002; Pruzanski *et al.*, 2005; Jönsson-Rylander *et al.*, 2008). These studies indicated that Groups V and X $sPLA_2$s are potentially physiologically more important than group IIA $sPLA_2$ in lipoprotein metabolism. An important consequence of this lipoprotein remodeling was the finding that LDL modified by either group V and X $sPLA_2$ was demonstrated to induce lipid accumulation in macrophages and activate endothelial cells in culture (Wooten-Kee *et al.*, 2004; Karabina *et al.*, 2006), two proatherogenic activities. It is also speculated that $sPLA_2$-modified LDL could transit the vessel wall more readily than unmodified particles and promote retention of these atherogenic particles in the vessel wall (Rosenson and Gelb, 2009). The finding that lipolysis of LDL by $sPLA_2$ results in a conformational change in apolipoprotein B that enhances LDL binding to intimal proteoglycans certainly supports such a notion (Sartipy *et al.*, 1999; Hakala *et al.*, 2001).

Overexpression studies in mice with group IIA $sPLA_2$ resulted in profound alterations in HDL metabolism, which is somewhat of a surprise given the findings described above (Tietge *et al.*, 2000; Menschikowski *et al.*, 2000). These transgenic mice had significantly lower total cholesterol, which was explained primarily by a reduction in HDL cholesterol due to its enhanced catabolism. Overexpression of group V sPLA2 in mice, in contrast to the above, had no influence on plasma lipoprotein levels (Bostrom *et al.*, 2007). It should be noted that mice have very different lipoprotein profiles to humans, meaning that it is difficult to extrapolate these findings to the human situation. This appears to be borne out by observations made with varespladib in the clinic (section 7.7.2) that consistently demonstrate a reduction in LDL cholesterol levels with no alteration in HDL cholesterol, a result not predicted by the overexpression studies in mice.

The most recognized physiological function of group IIA $sPLA_2$ is its antibacterial activity mediated by its selective and potent ability to attack and degrade the phosphatidylglycerol-rich membranes of bacteria, thereby contributing to the first line of host defense (Koduri *et al.*, 2002; Nevalainen *et al.*, 2008). Importantly, group IIA $sPLA_2$ transgenic mice show decreased mortality following infection by both Gram-positive and Gram-negative bacteria with improved clearance from infected organs. Interestingly, the polyanionic properties of LTA (a possible substrate of Lp-PLA_2 – see above 7.3.1) in the gram-positive bacterial cell wall facilitate the hydrolysis of membrane phospholipids by binding group IIA $sPLA_2$ (Koprivnjak *et al.*, 2002). Several other $sPLA_2$s also exhibit bactericidal activity, with the rank order against Gram-positive bacteria being IIA > X > V > XIIA > IIE > IB (Koduri *et al.*, 2002; Nevalainen *et al.*, 2008). Thus, it appears that $sPLA_2$s and Lp-PLA_2 may have opposite activities against bacteria, which could have implications for varespladib and darapladib in the treatment of coronary artery disease, since infection is thought to contribute to the acute complications caused by atherosclerotic plaque rupture (Epstein *et al.*, 2009).

7.4 Cellular Sources, Expression Within Vulnerable Plaque and Genetically Altered Mouse Studies

7.4.1 Lp-PLA_2

Lp-PLA_2 is expressed and secreted by the following hematopoietic cells, monocytes, macrophages, T-lymphocytes, and mast cells (Zalewski and Macphee, 2005; McIntyre *et al.*, 2009). Lp-PLA_2 is not considered to be an acute phase protein but can be upregulated *in vitro* by lipopolysaccharide, certain inflammatory cytokines (e.g., IL-1β and TNFα), oxLDL but not PAF (Wu *et al.*, 2004; Shi *et al.*, 2007; De Keyzer *et al.*, 2009; Wang *et al.*, 2010). With this leukocyte expression profile, it is not surprising, therefore, to find that Lp-

PLA_2 expression is greatly upregulated in rabbit, pig, and human atherosclerotic lesions (Hakkinen *et al.*, 1999; Kolodgie *et al.*, 2006; Papaspyridonos *et al.*, 2006; Wilensky *et al.*, 2008; De Keyzer *et al.*, 2009). The critical finding that Lp-PLA_2 is highly upregulated in macrophages undergoing apoptosis within the necrotic core and fibrous cap of human coronary vulnerable and ruptured plaques, but not within stable lesions, supports the notion that Lp-PLA_2 products could be crucial in determining plaque instability (Kolodgie *et al.*, 2006). Consistent with this notion is the observation from patients undergoing carotid endarterectomy that Lp-PLA_2 expression along with its product, LPC, was higher in plaques from patients with cardiovascular events than those without suggesting that the enzyme is a key component of a causal pathway for plaque vulnerability (Herrmann *et al.*, 2009).

Pathological studies have shown that thrombotic coronary occlusion after rupture of a lipid-rich atheroma with only a thin fibrous layer of intimal tissue covering the necrotic core (the so-called thin-cap fibroatheroma, TCFA) is the most common cause of myocardial infarction and death from cardiac causes (Virmani *et al.*, 2006). Before discussing preclinical model overexpression studies, it is important to point out that the majority of preclinical animal models, including mice, do not develop complex, human-like, TCFAs. Liver specific overexpression of human Lp-PLA_2 in apolipoprotein E-deficient mice was shown to inhibit injury-induced neointimal formation (Quarck *et al.*, 2001). How such ectopic expression of Lp-PLA_2 by hepatocytes in this mouse model relates to human atherosclerosis is difficult to ascertain but may point to an important interaction between apolipoprotein E and Lp-PLA_2. This study, however, is not consistent with a later study demonstrating a reduction in complex coronary lesion development with darapladib in a porcine model of atherosclerosis with normal apolipoprotein E content (Wilensky *et al.*, 2008; see later section 7.6.1).

7.4.2 sPLA_2

Group IIA sPLA_2 is an acute phase protein whose expression is greatly upregulated by endotoxin, which should come as no surprise given its potent *in vivo* antimicrobial action. Indeed, its expression is markedly induced by proinflammatory stimuli in a wide variety of tissues (Jönsson-Rylander et al., 2008; Murakami *et al.*, 2010). Group V $sPLA_2$ transcripts are also widely expressed, for example high levels have been located in the heart and placenta as well as certain leukocytes, including mouse bone marrow-derived mast cells (Balestrieri and Arm, 2006). Expression of group X $sPLA_2$ has been demonstrated in thymus, spleen, and leukocytes, which suggests an involvement in the immune system (Murakami *et al.*, 2010).

Microarray gene expression studies of human carotid plaques versus non-diseased human vessels failed to show an upregulation of either group IIA or V $sPLA_2$ in disease while clearly demonstrating a large upregulation of Lp-PLA_2 (Zalewski and Macphee, 2005). Indeed, in this study group IIA $sPLA_2$ expression was much lower in the endarterectomy samples when compared with control vessels highlighting the contribution of the smooth muscle-rich media to its expression as this was missing from the tissue sample. These findings were replicated in an analysis of plaque from hypercholesterolemic pigs (De Keyzer *et al.*, 2009). Thus, the only one of the three considered $sPLA_2$ genes that is expressed in atherosclerotic lesions to any great extent is group X $sPLA_2$, which, like Lp-PLA_2, reflects its macrophage expression profile (Karabina *et al.*, 2006; De Keyzer *et al.*, 2009). However, although gene expression studies have been somewhat neutral for Group IIA and V sPLA2s, immunohistochemical analyses have detected their presence within lesions (Hurt-Camejo *et al.*, 1997; Rosengren *et al.*, 2006; Kimura-Matsumoto *et al.*, 2008).

Considerable effort has been invested in genetically altering the expression of $sPLA_2$s in mice to elucidate a role in atherosclerosis (Boyanovsky and Webb, 2009; Murakamo *et al.*, 2010). Interestingly, the common mouse strain used to study atherosclerosis, C57BL/6, is a natural knockout of group IIA $sPLA_2$ due to a frame shift that interferes with gene translation. Thus, group IIA $sPLA_2$ expression is not critical for lesion formation in the mouse. However, overexpession studies in mice, either broadly or ectopically in macrophages, have demonstrated an increased susceptibility to atherosclerosis (Ivandic *et al.*, 1999; Webb *et al.*, 2003; Webb, N. R., Bostrom, M. A., Szilvassy, S. J., Van der Westhuyzen, D. R., Daugherty, A., & De Beer, F. C. (2003). Macrophage-expressed group IIA secretory phospholipase A2 increases atherosclerotic lesion formation in LDL receptor-deficient mice. Arteriosclerosis, Thrombosis, and Vascular Biology, 23(2), 263-268; Tietge *et al.*, 2005). Similarly, as for group IIA, transplantation of bone marrow-derived cells that overexpressed group V $sPLA_2$ in $LDLr^{-/-}$ mice also increased atherosclerotic lesion area. Moreover, group V $sPLA_2$ deficiency in bone-marrow derived cells caused a reduction in atherosclerosis in $LDLr^{-/-}$ (Bostrom *et al.*, 2007) but not in $apoE^{-/-}$ mice (Boyanovsky *et al.*, 2009). Unfortunately, although group X $sPLA_2$ demonstrates perhaps the most convincing profile for a role in atherosclerosis, both in substrate preferences and leukocyte expression, no direct evidence is currently available to support a role in atherosclerotic lesion formation. However, mice deficient in group V $sPLA_2$ are available, with recent data showing that the incidence and severity of angiotensin II-induced abdominal aortic aneurysms were significantly reduced in $apoE^{-/-}$ mice also deficient in group X $sPLA_2$ (Zack *et al.*, 2011). In summary, the accumulated data for $sPLA_2$ involvement in murine atherosclerosis is certainly much stronger than for Lp-PLA_2.

7.5 Human Epidemiology and Genetics

7.5.1 Lp-PLA_2

The first study to highlight the role of Lp-PLA_2 as an independent risk predictor for cardiovascular disease was the West of Scotland Coronary Prevention Study (Packard *et al.*, 2000) Packard, C. J., O'Reilly, D. S. J., Caslake, M. J., McMahon, A. D., Ford, I., Cooney, J., . . . Burczak, J. D. (2000). Lipoprotein-associated phospholipase A2 as an independent predictor of coronary heart disease. New England Journal of Medicine, 343(16), 1148-1155. This study not only showed a positive association between elevated circulating levels of Lp-PLA_2 and risk of coronary events but, critically, demonstrated that the increased risk was not confounded by classical cardiovascular risk factors such as lipids, as well as C-reactive protein (CRP). This observation has now been replicated in many studies covering both primary and secondary prevention and has been summarized in several recent reviews (Caslake and Packard, 2005; Garza *et al.*, 2007; Epps and Wilensky, 2011). In a recent meta-analysis incorporating over 79,000 participants from 32 prospective studies, the risk of developing cardiovascular disease was increased by 11% for each standard deviation unit increase in Lp-PLA_2 activity, after correction for other cardiovascular risk factors (Thompson *et al.*, 2010). The finding that Lp-PLA_2 retains its independence as a predictor of future cardiovascular events following adjustment for classical risk factors is somewhat surprising given that it is consistently found to be significantly associated with LDL (positively), HDL (negatively), and triglycerides (positively).

Although the clinical epidemiology around Lp-PLA$_2$ levels is relatively consistent in demonstrating an independent association between the enzyme and CHD, the same cannot be said for Lp-PLA$_2$ genetics that has provided a somewhat confusing story primarily due to mixed reports on a loss-of-function variant of *PLA2G7* (V279F) first discovered in Japanese individuals (Stafforini *et al.*, 1996). Various reports have since confirmed that homozygous carriers of this variant are lacking Lp-PLA$_2$ in plasma and that heterozygous carriers have around 50% the activity of individuals carrying both copies of the wild-type allele. Moreover, while the 279F null allele is relatively frequent in Japan, with approximately 25% and 2% of the population carrying one or two copies, respectively, its prevalence shows a declining gradient towards the West, with intermediate frequencies in China and Korea and almost complete absence in Europeans (Yamada *et al.*, 2000; Jang *et al.*, 2006). The first studies published reported an association of the loss-of-function variant with an increased risk for myocardial infarction and stroke (Yamada *et al.*, 1998; Yamada *et al.*, 2000), whereas a subsequent study showed only a male- and high cholesterol-specific increased risk (Shimokata *et al.*, 2004). Others reported no association in either Japanese or Chinese subjects (Yamada *et al.*, 2002; Hou *et al.*, 2009). Lastly, a decreased risk of CHD was observed in male carriers of the 279V allele from Korea (Jang *et al.*, 2006), which has very recently been confirmed in a much larger analysis comparing 3,767 male cases with CAD with 4,358 male controls without CAD (Jang *et al.*, 2011). The data from this latest Korean study demonstrated that carriage of one copy of the 279F null allele (approx. 50% reduced plasma activity) conferred a 20% reduction in risk for CHD, which is in line with epidemiological findings on plasma Lp-PLA$_2$ activity. Clearly, further studies are needed to fully understand the association between *PLA2G7* genetic variations and coronary risk.

7.5.2 sPLA$_2$

To date, only a few studies have addressed the utility of plasma sPLA$_2$ as a biomarker of cardiovascular risk. Moreover, when sPLA$_2$ activity is monitored, the contribution of each individual sPLA$_2$ isozyme is unknown. The significant but weak correlation between group IIA

$sPLA_2$ mass and $sPLA_2$ activity ($r = 0.20$) made in one study highlights this issue particularly as a better predictive value was observed for the latter (Mallat *et al.*, 2007). The epidemiology surrounding $sPLA_2$ has been summarized in a recent review by Mallat *et al.* (2010). Two of the larger studies are worth mentioning, EPIC-Norfolk and KAROLA. For EPIC-Norfolk, baseline group IIA $sPLA_2$ mass and $sPLA_2$ activity were shown to be significantly associated with the occurrence of a first coronary event at follow up (Boekholdt *et al.*, 2005; Mallat *et al.*, 2007), with both significantly associated with traditional CV risk factors, including CRP. In KAROLA, which studied stable coronary disease, group IIA $sPLA_2$ mass and $sPLA_2$ activity showed a good correlation ($r = 0.63$) with both demonstrating a significant association with adverse outcomes following multivariate analyses (Koenig *et al.*, 2009). These data support a role for $sPLA_2$ in the prediction of cardiovascular events, although larger studies are needed to further substantiate initial findings.

Several studies have attempted to use a genetic approach to determine whether polymorphisms in the genes for $sPLA_2$s were able to support an etiological role in atherosclerosis. Wootton and colleagues (2006) reported a strong impact of haplotypic variation in the group IIA $sPLA_2$ gene on circulating group IIA $sPLA_2$ levels, although the study was not adequately powered to detect an association between genotype and CHD risk. The same group also found a unique association of group V $sPLA_2$ gene haplotypes with total cholesterol and oxidized LDL, although their association with CHD risk remains to be determined (Wootton *et al.*, 2007). Finally, a polymorphism in the group X $sPLA_2$ gene leading to a R38C substitution demonstrated no detectable impact on cardiovascular risk, even though functional studies found the change resulted in profound reductions in catalytic activity (Gora *et al.*, 2009).

7.6 Pharmacological Intervention: Darapladib

7.6.1 Animal Model

The effect of darapladib on atherosclerotic plaque composition was demonstrated in a diabetic and hypercholesterolemic porcine model of accelerated coronary atherosclerosis (Wilensky *et al.*, 2008). Four weeks after induction of diabetes and hypercholesterolemia, plasma and vascular $Lp\text{-}PLA_2$ activity increased, while 24 weeks of darapladib treatment significantly reduced plasma and vascular Lp-PLA_2 activity to levels nearly equivalent to age-matched non-diabetic, non-hypercholesterolemic controls. Importantly, the administration of darapladib (10 mg/kg/day) not only inhibited coronary artery lesion development but more profoundly reduced progression to advanced coronary lesions. In this model of complex atherosclerosis, macrophage content, plaque area, necrotic core area, and tunica media destruction were all significantly reduced compared to controls. Darapladib has not been studied in mouse models of atherosclerosis primarily, because Lp-PLA_2 associates with different lipoprotein fractions (Wilensky *et al.*, 2008) rendering the species inadequate for studying the effects of Lp-PLA_2 inhibition.

7.6.2 Clinic

Darapladib is currently being studied in two large Phase III trials: STABILITY (Stabilization of Atherosclerotic Plaque by Initiation of Darapladib Therapy Trial, NCT00799903), a fully enrolled trial involving 15,828 patients with CHD (White *et al.*, 2010), and SOLID-TIMI 52 (the Stabilization of Plaques Using Darapladib - Thrombolysis in Myocardial Infarction 52 Trial, NCT01000727), which is estimated to include 11,500 patients with ACS. Both are event-driven trials, using a single daily dose of 160 mg (enteric coated) darapladib, with similar primary end points of cardiovascular death, non-fatal myocardial infarction, and non-fatal stroke.

The 160 mg daily dose of darapladib was selected based upon data obtained from several Phase II clinical trials. Firstly, in a small Phase II trial, treatment with darapladib for two weeks prior to carotid endarterectomy significantly and dose-dependently reduced elevated Lp-PLA_2 activity within the atherosclerotic plaque, demonstrating that the drug could access the critical target site (Johnson *et al.*, 2004). Secondly, a multicenter dose ascending Phase II study was conducted where 959 stable, atorvastatin-treatment CHD patients (with achieved LDL cholesterol concentrations of less than 115 mg/dl) were randomized and treated with darapladib at 40, 80, and 160 mg for 12 weeks. In this study, Lp-PLA_2 activity was reduced by 43, 55, and 66%, respectively at the three dose levels administered (Mohler *et al.*, 2008). Treatment in this trial was not accompanied by changes in lipids, but a reduction in both CRP and Il-6 was noted. Finally, the IBIS-2 (Integrated Biomarker and Imaging Study 2) trial compared the effects of placebo with 12 months of darapladib (160 mg) treatment on plasma CRP levels, coronary atheroma composition, and deformability in 330 patients with angiographically documented CAD (Serruys *et al.*, 2008). Although the primary endpoints of the study were not met, nor did darapladib affect total atheroma volume, treatment did halt the increase in necrotic core volume as assessed by intravascular ultrasound radiofrequency suggesting a stabilization of the overall plaque. These clinical observations of an effect of darapladib on necrotic core formation appear consistent with results obtained in a diabetic pig model of coronary atherosclerosis (Wilensky *et al.*, 2008). Whether these changes translate into differences in clinical outcomes awaits the results of the previously mentioned ongoing Phase III trials, STABILITY and SOLID-TIMI 52.

7.7 Pharmacological Intervention: Varespladib

7.7.1 Animal Model

The effect of $sPLA_2$ inhibition with varespladib on atherosclerosis has been investigated using apo E knockout mice fed a high fat diet (Shaposhnik *et al.*, 2009; Fraser *et al.*, 2009). In these studies, varespladib was shown to significantly reduce atherosclerosis by 40–75% in addition to attenuating the development of angiotensin II-induced aortic aneurysms. In one study (Fraser *et al.*, 2009), plasma total cholesterol that could have contributed to the atheroprotective effect of varespladib was also decreased. Interestingly, a similar reduction in plasma cholesterol in response to varespladib was also observed in the clinic (see below 7.7.2). The fact that varespladib was able to exert an antiatherogenic effect in a mouse strain that does not express group IIA $sPLA_2$ suggests that the benefit is derived through inhibition of one or both of group V and X $sPLA_2$s.

7.7.2 Clinic

Promising preclinical findings were sufficiently encouraging for Eli Lilly to initially explore the potential benefit of LY315920 (varespladib) in a Phase II clinical trial for severe sepsis (Reid, 2005). Although elevated baseline group IIA $sPLA_2$ activity was ablated by LY315920, treatment offered no overall survival benefit to patients and development of this compound for the treatment of sepsis was terminated (Abraham *et al.*, 2003). A later clinical study with LY333013, a more bioavailable methyl ester prodrug of LY315920, was similarly found to be ineffective in rheumatoid arthritis (Bradley *et al.*, 2005). This methyl prodrug of varespladib is now in clinical development for the treatment of atherosclerosis by Anthera Pharmaceuticals (Rosenson *et al.*, 2010 ref 2010b).

Enrollment has already commenced for a pivotal Phase III clinical study named VISTA-16 (Vascular Inflammation Suppression to Treat Acute Coronary Syndrome for 16 Weeks; NCT01130246) designed to evaluate a 16 week therapy with varespladib in combination with statins for the prevention of secondary major adverse coronary events in patients who have recently experienced an acute coronary syndrome. Up to 6500 subjects will be randomized to receive either varespladib 500 mg once daily or placebo in addition to atorvastatin and standard of care. The VISTA-16 study is expected to enroll patients with similar characteristics to those who participated in the Phase IIb FRANCIS (Fewer Recurrent Acute Coronary Events with Near-Term Cardiovascular Inflammatory Suppression; NCT00743925) acute coronary syndrome clinical study.

The first Phase II results for varespladib in cardiovascular patients were from a randomized, double-blind, placebo-controlled parallel arm dose-ranging study that enrolled 393 patients with stable CHD (Rosenson *et al.*, 2009). The primary endpoint was the change in Group IIA $sPLA_2$ mass or activity from baseline to week 8. The authors reported a significant dose-dependent decrease in group IIA $sPLA_2$ mass levels, which reached a 95% reduction in the highest, 500 mg, dose group. However, they could not evaluate the difference in $sPLA_2$ activity, since the enzyme mass was below the limits of detection for the assay. Interestingly, plasma LDL was also significantly lowered by varespladib, attaining a 10% reduction in the highest dose compared with a 1.7% increase in the placebo group. A significant varespladib-mediated reduction in LDL cholesterol beyond standard of care was also observed in the Phase IIb FRANCIS clinical study, which enrolled 624 acute coronary syndrome patients randomized to varespladib 500 mg daily or placebo for a minimum of 6 months (Rosenson *et al.*, 2010 ref 2010a). In addition to the expected large reduction in group IIA $sPLA_2$ mass of 78.5%, trends were also noted for a reduction in CRP with patients treated with varespladib.

7.8 Summary

A significant body of evidence exists demonstrating a role for Lp-PLA_2 and $sPLA_2$s in the development of atherosclerosis (Table 7.1). As such, well-characterized and selective inhibitors of both enzymes have progressed into large Phase III cardiovascular outcome trials. Results from these trials will unequivocally determine whether the supportive observations summarized in this chapter will translate into overall benefit for CHD patients.

Table 7.1 A summary of the evidence for the involvement of Lp-PLA_2 and $sPLA_2$ in atherosclerosis.

	Lp-PLA_2	$sPLA_2$
Inhibited by Darapladib	Yes	No
Inhibited by Varespladib	No	Yes
Resides on LDL	Yes	No
Generates LPC during LDL oxidation	Yes	No
Involved in eicosanoid formation	No	Yes
Expression highly upregulated in complex vulnerable lesions	Yes	No
Protein detected within complex vulnerable lesions	Yes	Yes
Contributes to elevated LPC within lesions	Yes	?
Inhibition reduces atherosclerosis	Yes	Yes
Inhibition results in LDL lowering	No	Yes
Inhibition reduces lesion necrotic core expansion	Yes	?

References

Abraham, E., Naum, C., Bandi, V., Gervich, D., Lowry, S. F., Wunderink, R., *et al.* (2003). Efficacy and safety of LY315920Na/S-5920, a selective inhibitor of 14-kDa group IIA secretory phospholipase A2, in patients with suspected sepsis and organ failure. *Critical Care Medicine,* 31(3), 718–728.

Atik, B., Johnston, S. C., and Dean, D. (2010). Association of carotid plaque lp-PLA(2) with macrophages and chlamydia pneumoniae infection among patients at risk for stroke. *PloS One,* 5(6), e11026.

Balestrieri, B., and Arm, J. P. (2006). Group V sPLA2: Classical and novel functions. *Biochimica Et Biophysica Acta- Molecular and Cell Biology of Lipids,* 1761(11), 1280–1288.

Berliner, J. A., and Watson, A. D. (2005). A role for oxidized phospholipids in atherosclerosis. *New England Journal of Medicine,* 353(1), 9–11.

Bochkov, V. N. (2007). Inflammatory profile of oxidized phospholipids. *Thrombosis and Haemostasis,* 97(3), 348–354.

Blackie, J. A., Bloomer, J. C., Brown, M. J. B., Cheng, H.-, Hammond, B., Hickey, D. M. B., *et al.* (2003). The identification of clinical candidate SB-480848: A potent inhibitor of lipoprotein-associated phospholipase A2. *Bioorganic and Medicinal Chemistry Letters,* 13(6), 1067–1070.

Blank, M. L., Hall, M. N., Cress, E. A., and Snyder, F. (1983). Inactivation of 1-alkyl-2-acetyl-sn-glycero-3-phosphocholine by a plasma acetylhydrolase: Higher activities in hypertensive rats. *Biochemical and Biophysical Research Communications,* 113(2), 666–671.

Blencowe, C., Hermetter, A., Kostner, G. M., and Deigner, H. P. (1995). Enhanced association of platelet-activating factor acetylhydrolase with lipoprotein (a) in comparison with low density lipoprotein. *Journal of Biological Chemistry,* 270(52), 31151–31157.

Bostrom, M. A., Boyanovsky, B. B., Jordan, C. T., Wadsworth, M. P., Taatjes, D. J., De Beer, F. C., *et al.* (2007). Group V secretory phospholipase A2 promotes atherosclerosis: Evidence from genetically altered mice. *Arteriosclerosis, Thrombosis, and Vascular Biology,* 27(3), 600–606.

Boekholdt, S. M., Keller, T. T., Wareham, N. J., Luben, R., Bingham, S. A., Day, N. E., *et al.* (2005). Serum levels of type II secretory phospholipase A2 and the risk of future coronary artery disease in apparently healthy men and women: The EPIC-norfolk prospective population study. *Arteriosclerosis, Thrombosis, and Vascular Biology,* 25(4), 839–846.

Boyanovsky, B., Zack, M., Forrest, K., and Webb, N. R. (2009). The capacity of group V sPLA2 to increase atherogenicity of ApoE-/- and LDLR-/- mouse LDL *in vitro* predicts its atherogenic role *in vivo*. *Arteriosclerosis, Thrombosis, and Vascular Biology,* 29(4), 532–538.

Boyanovsky, B. B., and Webb, N. R. (2009). Biology of secretory phospholipase A2. *Cardiovascular Drugs and Therapy,* 23(1), 61–72.

Bradley, J. D., Dmitrienko, A. A., Kivitz, A. J., Gluck, O. S., Weaver, A. L., Wiesenhutter, C., *et al.* (2005). A randomized, double-blinded, placebo-controlled clinical trial of LY333013, a selective inhibitor of group II secretory phospholipase A 2, in the treatment of rheumatoid arthritis. *Journal of Rheumatology,* 32(3), 417–423.

Burke, J. E., and Dennis, E. A. (2009). Phospholipase A2 structure/function, mechanism, and signaling. *Journal of Lipid Research,* 50 Suppl, S237–S242.

Caslake, M. J., Packard, C. J., Suckling, K. E., Holmes, S. D., Chamberlain, P., and Macphee, C. H. (2000). Lipoprotein-associated phospholipase A2, platelet-activating factor acetylhydrolase: A potential new risk factor for coronary artery disease. *Atherosclerosis,* 150(2), 413–419.

Caslake, M. J., and Packard, C. J. (2005). Lipoprotein-associated phospholipase A2 as a biomarker for coronary disease and stroke. *Nature Clinical Practice Cardiovascular Medicine,* 2(10), 529–535.

Clarke, R., Peden, J. F., Hopewell, J. C., Kyriakou, T., Goel, A., Heath, S. C., *et al.* (2009). Genetic variants associated with lp(a) lipoprotein level and coronary disease. *New England Journal of Medicine,* 361(26), 2518–2528.

Davis, B., Koster, G., Douet, L. J., Scigelova, M., Woffendin, G., Ward, J. M., *et al.* (2008). Electrospray ionization mass spectrometry identifies substrates and products of lipoprotein-associated phospholipase A2 in oxidized human low density lipoprotein. *Journal of Biological Chemistry,* 283(10), 6428–6437.

De Keyzer, D., Karabina, S., Wei, W., Geeraert, B., Stengel, D., Marsillach, J., *et al.* (2009). Increased PAFAH and oxidized lipids are associated with inflammation and atherosclerosis in hypercholesterolemic pigs. *Arteriosclerosis, Thrombosis, and Vascular Biology,* 29(12), 2041–2046.

Enkhmaa, B., Anuurad, E., Zhang, W., Pearson, T. A., and Berglund, L. (2010). Association of lp-PLA2 activity with allele-specific lp(a) levels in a bi-ethnic population. *Atherosclerosis,* 211(2), 526–530.

Epps, K. C., and Wilensky, R. L. (2011). Lp-PLA2- a novel risk factor for high-risk coronary and carotid artery disease. *Journal of Internal Medicine,* 269(1), 94–106.

Epstein, S. E., Zhu, J., Najafi, A. H., and Burnett, M. S. (2009). Insights into the role of infection in atherogenesis and in plaque rupture. *Circulation,* 119(24), 3133–3141.

Feige, E., Mendel, I., George, J., Yacov, N., and Harats, D. (2010). Modified phospholipids as anti-inflammatory compounds. *Current Opinion in Lipidology,* 21(6), 525–529.

Fraser, H., Hislop, C., Christie, R. M., Rick, H. L., Reidy, C. A., Chouinard, M. L., *et al.* (2009). Varespladib (A-002), a secretory phospholipase A2 inhibitor, reduces atherosclerosis and aneurysm formation in ApoE-/- mice. *Journal of Cardiovascular Pharmacology,* 53(1), 60–65.

Funk, C. D. (2001). Prostaglandins and leukotrienes: Advances in eicosanoid biology. *Science,* 294(5548), 1871–1875.

Garza, C. A., Montori, V. M., McConnell, J. P., Somers, V. K., Kullo, I. J., and Lopez-Jimenez, F. (2007). Association between lipoprotein-associated phospholipase A2 and cardiovascular disease: A systematic review. *Mayo Clinic Proceedings,* 82(2), 159–165.

Gesquiere, L., Cho, W., and Subbaiah, P. V. (2002). Role of group IIa and group V secretory phospholipases A2 in the metabolism of lipoproteins. substrate specificities of the enzymes and the regulation of their activities by sphingomyelin. *Biochemistry,* 41(15), 4911–4920.

Ghosh, M., Tucker, D. E., Burchett, S. A., and Leslie, C. C. (2006). Properties of the group IV phospholipase A2 family. *Progress in Lipid Research,* 45(6), 487–510.

Gora, S., Lambeau, G., Bollinger, J. G., Gelb, M., Ninio, E., and Karabina, S. (2006). The proinflammatory mediator platelet activating factor is an effective substrate for human group X secreted phospholipase A2. *Biochimica Et Biophysica Acta- Molecular and Cell Biology of Lipids,* 1761(9), 1093–1099.

Gora, S., Perret, C., Jemel, I., Nicaud, V., Lambeau, G., Cambien, F., *et al.* (2009). Molecular and functional characterization of polymorphisms in the secreted phospholipase A2 group X gene: Relevance to coronary artery disease. *Journal of Molecular Medicine,* 87(7), 723–733.

Hakala, J. K., Öörni, K., Pentikäinen, M. O., Hurt-Camejo, E., and Kovanen, P. T. (2001). Lipolysis of LDL by human secretory phospholipase A2 induces particle fusion and enhances the retention of LDL to human aortic proteoglycans. *Arteriosclerosis, Thrombosis, and Vascular Biology,* 21(6), 1053–1058.

Häkkinen, T., Luoma, J. S., Hiltunen, M. O., Macphee, C. H., Milliner, K. J., Patel, L., *et al.* (1999). Lipoprotein-associated phospholipase A2, platelet-activating factor acetylhydrolase, is expressed by macrophages in human and rabbit atherosclerotic lesions. *Arteriosclerosis, Thrombosis, and Vascular Biology,* 19(12), 2909–2917.

Hanasaki, K., Yamada, K., Yamamoto, S., Ishimoto, Y., Saiga, A., Ono, T., *et al.* (2002). Potent modification of low density lipoprotein by group X secretory phospholipase A2 is linked to macrophage foam cell formation. *Journal of Biological Chemistry,* 277(32), 29116–29124.

Henderson Jr., W. R., Chi, E. Y., Bollinger, J. G., Tien, Y.-, Ye, X., Castelli, L., *et al.* (2007). Importance of group X-secreted phospholipase A2 in allergen-induced airway inflammation and remodeling in a mouse asthma model. *Journal of Experimental Medicine,* 204(4), 865–877.

Herrmann, J., Mannheim, D., Wohlert, C., Versari, D., Meyer, F. B., McConnell, J. P., *et al.* (2009). Expression of lipoprotein-associated phospholipase A2 in carotid artery plaques predicts long-term cardiac outcome. *European Heart Journal,* 30(23), 2930–2938.

Ho, S. S., and Nahm, M. H. (2009). Lipoprotein lipase and hydrofluoric acid deactivate both bacterial lipoproteins and lipoteichoic acids, but platelet-activating factor-acetylhydrolase degrades only lipoteichoic acids. *Clinical and Vaccine Immunology,* 16(8), 1187–1195.

Hou, L., Chen, S., Yu, H., Lu, X., Chen, J., Wang, L., *et al.* (2009). Associations of PLA2G7 gene polymorphisms with plasma lipoprotein-associated phospholipase A2 activity and coronary heart disease in a chinese han population: The beijing atherosclerosis study. *Human Genetics,* 125(1), 11–20.

Hurt-Camejo, E., Andersen, S., Standal, R., Rosengren, B., Sartipy, P., Stadberg, E., *et al.* (1997). Localization of nonpancreatic secretory phospholipase A2 in normal and atherosclerotic arteries: Activity of the isolated enzyme on low-density lipoproteins. *Arteriosclerosis, Thrombosis, and Vascular Biology,* 17(2), 300–309.

Hwang, S. B. (1990). Specific receptors of platelet-activating factor, receptor heterogeneity, and signal transduction mechanisms. *Journal of Lipid Mediators,* 2(3-4), 123–158.

Jönsson-Rylander, A., Lundin, S., Rosengren, B., Pettersson, C., and Hurt-Camejo, E. (2008). Role of secretory phospholipases in atherogenesis. *Current Atherosclerosis Reports,* 10(3), 252–259.

Ivandic, B., Castellani, L. W., Wang, X.- Qiao, J.-, Mehrabian, M., Navab, M., *et al.* (1999). Role of group II secretory phospholipase A2 in atherosclerosis: 1. increased atherogenesis and altered lipoproteins in transgenic mice expressing group IIa phospholipase A2. *Arteriosclerosis, Thrombosis, and Vascular Biology,* 19(5), 1284–1290.

Jang, Y., Oh, Y. K., Soo, J. K., Jey, S. C., Young, G. K., Ji, Y. K., *et al.* (2006). The Val279Phe variant of the lipoprotein-associated phospholipase A2 gene is associated with catalytic activities and cardiovascular disease in korean men. *Journal of Clinical Endocrinology and Metabolism,* 91(9), 3521–3527.

Jang, Y., Waterworth, D., Lee, J., Song, K., Kim, S., Kim, H., Park, K.W., Cho, H., Oh, I., Park, J.E., Lee, B., Ku, H.J., Shin, D., Lee, J.H., Jee, S.H., Han, B., Jang, H., Cho, E., Vallance, P., Whittaker, J., Cardon, L., and Mooser, V. (2011). Carriage of the V279F null allele within the gene encoding Lp-PLA2 is protective from coronary artery disease in South Korean males. *PloS ONE*, 6(4).

Johnson, A., Zalewski, A., Janmohamed, S., *et al.* (2004). Lipoprotein-associated phospholipase A2 (Lp-PLA2) activity, an emerging CV risk marker, can be inhibited in atherosclerotic lesions and plasma by novel pharmacologic intervention: The results of a multicenter clinical study, *Circulation* 110 [17 (Suppl III)] III–590.

Karabina, S. P., Elisaf, M. C., Goudevenos, J., Siamopoulos, K. C., Sideris, D., and Tselepis, A. D. (1996). PAF-acetylhydrolase activity on lp(a) before and during Cu2+-induced oxidative modification *in vitro*. *Atherosclerosis,* 125(1), 121–134.

Karabina, S. A., Brochériou, I., Le Naour, G., Agrapart, M., Durand, H., Gelb, M., *et al.* (2006). Atherogenic properties of LDL particles modified by human group X secreted phospholipase A2 on human endothelial cell function. *The FASEB Journal,* 20(14), 2547–2549.

Kimura-Matsumoto, M., Ishikawa, Y., Komiyama, K., Tsuruta, T., Murakami, M., Masuda, S., *et al.* (2008). Expression of secretory phospholipase A2s in human atherosclerosis development. *Atherosclerosis,* 196(1), 81–91.

Koduri, R. S., Grönroos, J. O., Laine, V. J. O., Calvez, C. L., Lambeau, G., Nevalainen, T. J., *et al.* (2002). Bactericidal properties of human and murine groups I, II, V, X, and XII secreted phospholipases A2. *Journal of Biological Chemistry,* 277(8), 5849–5857.

Koenig, W., Vossen, C. Y., Mallat, Z., Brenner, H., Benessiano, J., and Rothenbacher, D. (2009). Association between type II secretory phospholipase A2 plasma concentrations and activity and cardiovascular events in patients with coronary heart disease. *European Heart Journal,* 30(22), 2742–2748.

Kolodgie, F. D., Burke, A. P., Skorija, K. S., Ladich, E., Kutys, R., Makuria, A. T., *et al.* (2006). Lipoprotein-associated phospholipase A2 protein expression in the natural progression of human coronary atherosclerosis. *Arteriosclerosis, Thrombosis, and Vascular Biology,* 26(11), 2523–2529.

Koprivnjak, T., Peschel, A., Gelb, M. H., Liang, N. S., and Weiss, J. P. (2002). Role of charge properties of bacterial envelope in bactericidal action of human group IIA phospholipase A2 against staphylococcus aureus. *Journal of Biological Chemistry,* 277(49), 47636–47644.

Kriska, T., Marathe, G. K., Schmidt, J. C., McIntyre, T. M., and Girotti, A. W. (2007). Phospholipase action of platelet-activating factor acetylhydrolase, but not paraoxonase-1, on long fatty acyl chain phospholipid hydroperoxides. *Journal of Biological Chemistry,* 282(1), 100–108.

Lambeau, G., and Gelb, M. H. (2008). Biochemistry and physiology of mammalian secreted phospholipases A_2. *Annual Reviews Biochemestry,* 77, 495–520.

Libby, P., Ridker, P. M., and Hansson, G. K. (2009). Inflammation in atherosclerosis. from pathophysiology to practice. *Journal of the American College of Cardiology,* 54(23), 2129–2138.

Liu, J., Chen, R., Marathe, G. K., Febbraio, M., Zou, W., and McIntyre, T. M. (2011). Circulating platelet-activating factor is primarily cleared by transport, not intravascular hydrolysis, by lipoprotein-associated phospholipase A2/PAF acetylhydrolase. *Circulation Research,* 108: 469-477.

Lu, J., Pierce, M., Franklin, A., Jilling, T., Stafforini, D. M., and Caplan, M. (2010). Dual roles of endogenous platelet-activating factor acetylhydrolase in a murine model of necrotizing enterocolitis. *Pediatric Research,* 68(3), 225–230.

Macphee, C. H., Moores, K. E., Boyd, H. F., Dhanak, D., Ife, R. J., Leach, C. A., *et al.* (1999). Lipoprotein-associated phospholipase A2, platelet-activating factor acetylhydrolase, generates two bioactive products during the oxidation of low-density lipoprotein: Use of a novel inhibitor. *Biochemical Journal,* 338(2), 479–487.

Mallat, Z., Benessiano, J., Simon, T., Ederhy, S., Sebella-Arguelles, C., Cohen, A., *et al.* (2007). Circulating secretory phospholipase A2 activity and risk of incident coronary events in healthy men and women: The EPIC-NORFOLK study. *Arteriosclerosis, Thrombosis, and Vascular Biology,* 27(5), 1177–1183.

Mallat, Z., Lambeau, G., and Tedgui, A. (2010). Lipoprotein-associated and secreted phospholipases A2 in cardiovascular disease: Roles as biological effectors and biomarkers. *Circulation,* 122(21), 2183–2200.

Matsumoto, T., Kobayashi, T., and Kamata, K. (2007). Role of lysophosphatidylcholine (LPC) in atherosclerosis. *Current Medicinal Chemistry,* 14(30), 3209–3220.

McIntyre, T. M., Zimmerman, G. A., and Prescott, S. M. (1999). Biologically active oxidized phospholipids. *Journal of Biological Chemistry,* 274(36), 25189–25192.

McIntyre, T. M., Prescott, S. M., and Stafforini, D. M. (2009). The emerging roles of PAF acetylhydrolase. *Journal of Lipid Research,* 50 Suppl, S255–S259.

Menschikowski, M., Eckey, R., Pietzsch, J., Aufenanger, J., Kumpf, R., Nelz, P., *et al.* (2000). Expression of human secretory group IIA phospholipase

A2 is associated with reduced concentrations of plasma cholesterol in transgenic mice. *Inflammation,* 24(3), 227–237.

Min, J. H., Wilder, C., Aoki, J., Arai, H., Inoue, K., Paul, L., *et al.* (2001). Platelet-activating factor acetylhydrolases: Broad substrate specificity and lipoprotein binding does not modulate the catalytic properties of the plasma enzyme. *Biochemistry,* 40(15), 4539–4549.

Min, J. H., Jain, M. K., Wilder, C., Paul, L., Apitz-Castro, R., Aspleaf, D. C., *et al.* (1999). Membrane-bound plasma platelet activating factor acetylhydrolase acts on substrate in the aqueous phase. *Biochemistry,* 38(39), 12935–12942.

Mihelich, E. D., and Schevitz, R. W. (1999). Structure-based design of a new class of anti-inflammatory drugs: Secretory phospholipase A2 inhibitors, SPI. *Biochimica Et Biophysica Acta- Molecular and Cell Biology of Lipids,* 1441(2-3), 223–228.

Mohler III, E. R., Ballantyne, C. M., Davidson, M. H., Hanefeld, M., Ruilope, L. M., Johnson, J. L., *et al.* (2008). The effect of darapladib on plasma lipoprotein-associated phospholipase A2 activity and cardiovascular biomarkers in patients with stable coronary heart disease or coronary heart disease risk equivalent. the results of a multicenter, randomized, double-blind, placebo-controlled study. *Journal of the American College of Cardiology,* 51(17), 1632–1641.

Murakami, M., Taketomi, Y., Girard, C., Yamamoto, K., and Lambeau, G. (2010). Emerging roles of secreted phospholipase A2 enzymes: Lessons from transgenic and knockout mice. *Biochimie,* 92(6), 561–582.

Naoki, K., Asano, K., Satoh, N., Fukunaga, K., Oguma, T., Shiomi, T., *et al.* (2004). PAF responsiveness in japanese subjects with plasma PAF acetylhydrolase deficiency. *Biochemical and Biophysical Research Communications,* 317(1), 205–210.

Nevalainen, T. J., Graham, G. G., and Scott, K. F. (2008). Antibacterial actions of secreted phospholipases A2. review. *Biochimica Et Biophysica Acta - Molecular and Cell Biology of Lipids,* 1781(1–2), 1–9.

Ni, Z., Okeley, N. M., Smart, B. P., and Gelb, M. H. (2006). Intracellular actions of group IIA secreted phospholipase A2 and group IVA cytosolic phospholipase A2 contribute to arachidonic acid release and prostaglandin production in rat gastric mucosal cells and transfected human embryonic kidney cells. *Journal of Biological Chemistry,* 281(24), 16245–16255.

O'Neill, L. A. J., Hennessy, E. J., and Parker, A. E. (2010). Targeting toll-like receptors: Emerging therapeutics? *Nature Reviews Drug Discovery,* 9(4), 293–307.

Papaspyridonos, M., Smith, A., Burnand, K. G., Taylor, P., Padayachee, S., Suckling, K. E., *et al.* (2006). Novel candidate genes in unstable areas of human atherosclerotic plaques. *Arteriosclerosis, Thrombosis, and Vascular Biology,* 26(8), 1837–1844.

Prescott, S. M., Zimmerman, G. A., Stafforini, D. M., and McIntyre, T. M. (2000). Platelet-activating factor and related lipid mediators. *Annual Review of Biochemistry,* 69, 419–445.

Pruzanski, W., Lambeau, L., Lazdunsky, M., Cho, W., Kopilov, J., and Kuksis, A. (2005). Differential hydrolysis of molecular species of lipoprotein phosphatidylcholine by groups IIA, V and X secretory phospholipases A 2. *Biochimica Et Biophysica Acta- Molecular and Cell Biology of Lipids,* 1736(1), 38–50.

Quarck, R., De Geest, B., Stengel, D., Mertens, A., Lox, M., Theilmeier, G., *et al.* (2001). Adenovirus-mediated gene transfer of human platelet-activating factor-acetylhydrolase prevents injury-induced neointima formation and reduces spontaneous atherosclerosis in apolipoprotein E-deficient mice. *Circulation,* 103(20), 2495–2500.

Reid, R. C. (2005). Inhibitors of secretory phospholipase A2 group IIA. *Current Medicinal Chemistry,* 12(25), 3011–3026.

Scott, D. L., White, S. P., Otwinowski, Z., Yuan, W., Gelb, M. H., and Sigler, P. B. (1990). Interfacial catalysis: The mechanism of phospholipase A2. *Science,* 250(4987), 1541–1546.

Rivera, R. and Chun, J. (2008). Biological effects of lysophospholipids *Rev Physiol Biochem Pharmacol.* 160, 25–46.

Rosengren, B., Peilot, H., Umaerus, M., Jönsson-Rylander, A. -., Mattsson-Hultén, L., Hallberg, C., *et al.* (2006). Secretory phospholipase A2 group V: Lesion distribution, activation by arterial proteoglycans, and induction in aorta by a western diet. *Arteriosclerosis, Thrombosis, and Vascular Biology,* 26(7), 1579–1585.

Rosenson, R. S., and Gelb, M. H. (2009). Secretory phospholipase A2: A multifaceted family of proatherogenic enzymes. *Current Cardiology Reports,* 11(6), 445–451.

Rosenson, R. S., Hislop, C., McConnell, D., Elliott, M., Stasiv, Y., Wang, N., *et al.* (2009). Effects of 1-H-indole-3-glyoxamide (A-002) on concentration of secretory phospholipase A2 (PLASMA study): A phase II double-blind, randomised, placebo-controlled trial. *The Lancet,* 373(9664), 649–658.

Rosenson, R. S., Hislop, C., Elliott, M., Stasiv, Y., Goulder, M., and Waters, D. (2010a). Effects of varespladib methyl on biomarkers and major cardiovascular events in acute coronary syndrome patients. *Journal of the American College of Cardiology,* 56(14), 1079–1088.

Rosenson, R. S., Fraser, H., Trias, J., and Hislop, C. (2010b). Varespladib methyl in cardiovascular disease. *Expert Opinion on Investigational Drugs,* 19(10), 1245–1255.

Sartipy, P., Camejo, G., Svensson, L., and Hurt-Camejo, E. (1999). Phospholipase A2 modification of low density lipoproteins forms small high density particles with increased affinity for proteoglycans and glycosaminoglycans. *Journal of Biological Chemistry,* 274(36), 25913–25920.

Schaloske, R. H., and Dennis, E. A. (2006). The phospholipase A2 superfamily and its group numbering system. *Biochimica Et Biophysica Acta-Molecular and Cell Biology of Lipids,* 1761(11), 1246–1259.

Schmitz, G., and Ruebsaamen, K. (2010). Metabolism and atherogenic disease association of lysophosphatidylcholine. *Atherosclerosis,* 208(1), 10–18.

Serruys, P. W., García-García, H. M., Buszman, P., Erne, P., Verheye, S., Aschermann, M., *et al.* (2008). Effects of the direct lipoprotein-associated phospholipase A2 inhibitor darapladib on human coronary atherosclerotic plaque. *Circulation,* 118(11), 1172–1182.

Shaposhnik, Z., Wang, X., Trias, J., Fraser, H., and Lusis, A. J. (2009). The synergistic inhibition of atherogenesis in apoE-/- mice between pravastatin and the sPLA2 inhibitor varespladib (A-002). *Journal of Lipid Research,* 50(4), 623-629.

Shi, Y., Zhang, P., Zhang, L., Osman, H., Mohler III, E. R., Macphee, C., *et al.* (2007). Role of lipoprotein-associated phospholipase A2 in leukocyte activation and inflammatory responses. *Atherosclerosis,* 191(1), 54–62.

Shimokata, K., Yamada, Y., Kondo, T., Ichihara, S., Izawa, H., Nagata, K., *et al.* (2004). Association of gene polymorphisms with coronary artery disease in individuals with or without nonfamilial hypercholesterolemia. *Atherosclerosis,* 172(1), 167–173.

Singer, A. G., Ghomashchi, F., Le Calvez, C., Bollinger, J., Bezzine, S., Rouault, M., *et al.* (2002). Interfacial kinetic and binding properties of the complete set of human and mouse groups I, II, V, X, and XII secreted phospholipases A2. *Journal of Biological Chemistry,* 277(50), 48535–48549.

Snyder, F. (1995). Platelet-activating fator and its analogs: Metabolic pathways and related intracellular processes. *Biochimica Et Biophysica Acta- Lipids and Lipid Metabolism,* 1254(3), 231-249.

Snyder, D. W., Bach, N. J., Dillard, R. D., Draheim, S. E., Carlson, D. G., Fox, N., *et al.* (1999). Pharmacology of LY315920/S-5920, [[3-(aminooxoacetyl)-2-ethyl-1- (phenylmethyl)-1H-indol-4-yl]oxy]acetate, a potent and selective secretory phospholipase A2 inhibitor: A new class of anti-inflammatory drugs, SPI. *Journal of Pharmacology and Experimental Therapeutics,* 288(3), 1117–1124.

Stafforini, D. M., Prescott, S. M., and McIntyre, T. M. (1987). Human plasma platelet-activating factor acetylhydrolase. purification and properties. *Journal of Biological Chemistry,* 262(9), 4223–4230.

Stafforini, D. M., Satoh, K., Atkinson, D. L., Tjoelker, L. W., Eberhardt, C., Yoshida, H., *et al.* (1996). Platelet-activating factor acetylhydrolase deficiency: A missense mutation near the active site of an anti-inflammatory phospholipase. *Journal of Clinical Investigation,* 97(12), 2784–2791.

Stafforini, D. M., Sheller, J. R., Blackwell, T. S., Sapirstein, A., Yull, F. E., McIntyre, T. M., *et al.* (2006). Release of free F2-isoprostanes from esterified phospholipids is catalyzed by intracellular and plasma platelet-activating factor acetylhydrolases. *Journal of Biological Chemistry,* 281(8), 4616–4623.

Stafforini, D. M. (2009). Biology of platelet-activating factor acetylhydrolase (PAF-AH, lipoprotein associated phospholipase A2). *Cardiovascular Drugs and Therapy,* 23(1), 73–83.

Steg, G., Bhatt, D. L., Wilson, P. W. F., D'Agostino Sr., R., Ohman, E. M., Röther, J., *et al.* (2007). One-year cardiovascular event rates in outpatients with atherothrombosis. *Journal of the American Medical Association,* 297(11), 1197–1206.

Stremler, K. E., Stafforini, D. M., Prescott, S. M., and McIntyre, T. M. (1991). Human plasma platelet-activating factor acetylhydrolase: Oxidatively fragmented phospholipids as substrates. *Journal of Biological Chemistry,* 266(17), 11095–11103.

Tabas, I., Williams, K. J., and Borén, J. (2007). Subendothelial lipoprotein retention as the initiating process in atherosclerosis: Update and therapeutic implications. *Circulation,* 116(16), 1832–1844.

Tew, D. G., Southan, C., Rice, S. Q. J., Lawrence, G. M. P., Li, H., Boyd, H. F., *et al.* (1996). Purification, properties, sequencing, and cloning of a lipoprotein-associated, serine-dependent phospholipase involved in the oxidative modification of low-density lipoproteins. *Arteriosclerosis, Thrombosis, and Vascular Biology,* 16(4), 591–599.

Thompson, A., Gao, P., Orfei, L., Watson, S., Di Angelantonio, E., Kaptoge, S., *et al.* (2010). Lipoprotein-associated phospholipase A2 and risk of coronary disease, stroke, and mortality: Collaborative analysis of 32 prospective studies. *The Lancet,* 375(9725), 1536-1544.

Tietge, U. J. F., Maugeais, C., Cain, W., Grass, D., Glick, J. M., De Beer, F. C., *et al.* (2000). Overexpression of secretory phospholipase A2 causes rapid catabolism and altered tissue uptake of high density lipoprotein cholesteryl ester and apolipoprotein A-I. *Journal of Biological Chemistry,* 275(14), 10077–10084.

Tietge, U. J. F., Pratico, D., Ding, T., Funk, C. D., Hildebrand, R. B., Van Berkel, T. J., *et al.* (2005). Macrophage-specific expression of group IIA sPLA2 results in accelerated atherogenesis by increasing oxidative stress. *Journal of Lipid Research,* 46(8), 1604–1614.

Tjoelker, L. W., Eberhardt, C., Unger, J., Hai Le Trong, Zimmerman, G. A., McIntyre, T. M., *et al.* (1995). Plasma platelet-activating factor acetylhydrolase is a secreted phospholipase A2 with a catalytic triad. *Journal of Biological Chemistry,* 270(43), 25481–25487.

Tselepis, A. D., Dentan, C., Karabina, S.-. P., Chapman, M. J., and Ninio, E. (1995). PAF-degrading acetylhydrolase is preferentially associated with dense LDL and VHDL-1 in human plasma: Catalytic characteristics and relation to the monocyte-derived enzyme. *Arteriosclerosis, Thrombosis, and Vascular Biology,* 15(10), 1764–1773.

Tsimikas, S., Brilakis, E. S., Miller, E. R., McConnell, J. P., Lennon, R. J., Kornman, K. S., *et al.* (2005). Oxidized phospholipids, lp(a) lipoprotein, and coronary artery disease. *New England Journal of Medicine,* 353(1), 46–57.

Vane, J. R., and Botting, R. M. (2003). The mechanism of action of aspirin. *Thrombosis Research,* 110(5-6), 255–258.

Vadas, P., Gold, M., Perelman, B., Liss, G. M., Lack, G., Blyth, T., *et al.* (2008). Platelet-activating factor, PAF acetylhydrolase, and severe anaphylaxis. *New England Journal of Medicine,* 358(1), 28–35.

Virmani, R., Burke, A. P., Farb, A., and Kolodgie, F. D. (2006). Pathology of the vulnerable plaque. *Journal of the American College of Cardiology,* 47(8 SUPPL.), C13–C18.

Von Schlieffen, E., Oskolkova, O. V., Schabbauer, G., Gruber, F., Blüml, S., Genest, M., *et al.* (2009). Multi-hit inhibition of circulating and cell-associated components of the toll-like receptor 4 pathway by oxidized phospholipids. *Arteriosclerosis, Thrombosis, and Vascular Biology,* 29(3), 356–362.

Wang, W-Y., Li, J., Yang, D., Xu, W., Zha, R.-, and Wang, Y.- (2010). OxLDL stimulates lipoprotein-associated phospholipase A2 expression in THP-1 monocytes via PI3K and p38 MAPK pathways. *Cardiovascular Research,* 85(4), 845–852.

White, H., Held, C., Stewart, R., Watson, D., Harrington, R., Budaj, A., *et al.* (2010). Study design and rationale for the clinical outcomes of the stability trial (STabilization of atherosclerotic plaque by initiation of darapLadIb TherapY) comparing darapladib versus placebo in patients with coronary heart disease. *American Heart Journal,* 160(4), 655–661.

Wilensky, R. L., Shi, Y., Mohler III, E. R., Hamamdzic, D., Burgert, M. E., Li, J., *et al.* (2008). Inhibition of lipoprotein-associated phospholipase A2 reduces complex coronary atherosclerotic plaque development. *Nature Medicine,* 14(10), 1059–1066.

Wooton-Kee, C. R., Boyanovsky, B. B., Nasser, M. S., De Villiers, W. J. S., and Webb, N. R. (2004). Group V sPLA2 hydrolysis of low-density lipoprotein results in spontaneous particle aggregation and promotes macrophage foam cell formation. *Arteriosclerosis, Thrombosis, and Vascular Biology,* 24(4), 762–767.

Wootton, P. T. E., Drenos, F., Cooper, J. A., Thompson, S. R., Stephens, J. W., Hurt-Camejo, E., *et al.* (2006). Tagging-SNP haplotype analysis of the secretory PLA2IIa gene PLA2G2A shows strong association with serum levels of sPLA2IIa: Results from the UDACS study. *Human Molecular Genetics,* 15(2), 355–361.

Wootton, P. T. E., Arora, N. L., Drenos, F., Thompson, S. R., Cooper, J. A., Stephens, J. W., *et al.* (2007). Tagging SNP haplotype analysis of the secretory PLA2-V gene, PLA2G5, shows strong association with LDL and oxLDL levels, suggesting functional distinction from sPLA2-IIA: Results from the UDACS study. *Human Molecular Genetics,* 16(12), 1437–1444.

Wu, X., Zimmerman, G. A., Prescott, S. M., and Stafforini, D. M. (2004). The p38 MAPK pathway mediates transcriptional activation of the plasma platelet-activating factor acetylhydrolase gene in macrophages stimulated with lipopolysaccharide. *Journal of Biological Chemistry,* 279(34), 36158–36165.

Yamada, Y., Ichihara, S., Fujimura, T., and Yokota, M. (1998). Identification of the G994□ T missense mutation in exon 9 of the plasma platelet-activating factor acetylhydrolase gene as an independent risk factor for coronary artery disease in japanese men. *Metabolism,* 47(2), 177–181.

Yamada, Y., Yoshida, H., Ichihara, S., Imaizumi, T., Satoh, K., and Yokota, M. (2000). Correlations between plasma platelet-activating factor acetylhydrolase (PAF-AH) activity and PAF-AH genotype, age, and atherosclerosis in a japanese population. *Atherosclerosis,* 150(1), 209–216.

Yamada, Y., Izawa, H., Ichihara, S., Takatsu, F., Ishihara, H., Hirayama, H., *et al.* (2002). Prediction of the risk of myocardial infarction from polymorphisms in candidate genes. *New England Journal of Medicine,* 347(24), 1916–1923.

Yoshida, H., Satoh, K., Koyama, M., Hiramoto, M., and Takamatsu, S. (1996). Deficiency of plasma platelet-activating factor acetylhydrolase: Roles of blood cells. *American Journal of Hematology,* 53(3), 158–164.

Zack, M., Boyanovsky, B. B., Shridas, P., Bailey, W., Forrest, K., Howatt, D. A., *et al.* (2011). Group X secretory phospholipase A2 augments angiotensin II-induced inflammatory responses and abdominal aortic aneurysm formation in apoE-deficient mice. *Atherosclerosis,* 214(1), 58–64.

Zalewski, A., and Macphee, C. (2005). Role of lipoprotein-associated phospholipase A2 in atherosclerosis: Biology, epidemiology, and possible therapeutic target. *Arteriosclerosis, Thrombosis, and Vascular Biology,* 25(5), 923–931.

Chapter 8

The Renin Angiotensin System in Atherosclerosis

Hong Lu,[a,b] Lisa A. Cassis,[c] and Alan Daugherty[a,c]
[a]*Saha Cardiovascular Research Center, University of Kentucky, Lexington, KY 40536-40200, USA*
[b]*Department of Cell Biology and Anatomy, University of South Carolina School of Medicine, Columbia, SC 29208, USA*
[c]*Graduate Center for Nutritional Sciences, University of Kentucky, Lexington, KY 40536-40200, USA*
Alan.Daugherty@uky.edu

8.1 Introduction

The renin angiotensin system (RAS) is crucial in the regulation of blood pressure and sodium/water homeostasis. All RAS peptides are derived from a single unique substrate, angiotensinogen, which is cleaved by renin to generate an inactive decapeptide, angiotensin (Ang)I. Subsequently, AngI is cleaved by angiotensin-converting enzyme (ACE) to generate the octapeptide, AngII. AngII is the major bioactive peptide in the RAS, which exerts its effects predominantly through binding AngII type 1 (AT1) receptors. It is now recognized that there are other bioactive peptides in the RAS beyond AngII. Some

Atherosclerosis: Treatment and Prevention
Edited by Christian Weber and Oliver Soehnlein

ISBN 978-981-4316-26-2 (Hardcover), ISBN 978-981-4364-26-3 (eBook)
www.panstanford.com

of the most recently discovered peptides, such as Ang(1-7), have actions that are antagonistic of AngII.[1–5] Therefore, an expanded appreciation for the role of the RAS in atherosclerosis is needed because of the increased complexity of this system with multiple bioactive peptides acting on multiple receptors.

Overactivation of the RAS favoring an increase of AngII has been recognized to promote atherosclerosis.[6] There is also strong evidence that RAS inhibition reduces experimental atherosclerosis[7–17] and reduces atherosclerosis-related cardiovascular events in clinical studies.[18–21] Many cell types present in atherosclerotic tissue express receptors for angiotensin peptides. There have been many studies on cultured cells that demonstrate potential mechanisms for the RAS to influence the development of atherosclerotic lesions, which may be attributable to the events that provoke the acute clinical symptoms of the disease. A current focus of investigation is defining the relevance and contribution of the mechanisms that have been demonstrated in cultured cells to the disease process *in vivo*.

This chapter will present a contemporary update of the RAS that links modulation of this system to development of atherosclerosis through the evidence from both animal and *in vitro* studies as well as the insights from human studies.

8.2 The Renin Angiotensin System

The classically defined RAS contains a major bioactive peptide, AngII, derived from one substrate, angiotensinogen, and two critical enzymes, renin and ACE. The most abundant sources of these components of the RAS are liver for angiotensinogen, kidneys for renin, and lungs for ACE.[22] AngII exerts its bioactive effects through binding to AngII receptors, AT1 and AT2 receptors, that are expressed by many cell types. Many of the AngII actions are via stimulation of AT1 receptors, a seven transmembrane type G-protein-coupled receptor that is encoded by one gene (AGTR1) in humans. Rodents have undergone a chromosomal duplication that leads to expression of two highly homologous isotypes of AT1 receptors, termed Agtr1a and Agtr1b. Numerous intracellular signaling pathways can be activated by AngII stimulation of AT1 receptors.[23] AT2 receptors are transcribed from an X-linked gene.[24] It is also a seven transmembrane type G-protein coupled receptor that has low (34%) homology to AT1 receptors.[25] Several signaling pathways that are stimulated by

AngII interaction with AT2 receptors are inhibitory of AT1 receptor stimulation.[26] This has contributed to the concept that AT2 receptor stimulation opposes the effects of AT1 receptor stimulation, although it has not been uniformly accepted.[27]

More recent studies have led to an expansion of the RAS that has additional bioactive peptides, cellular sources of proteins and enzymes, and other receptors. The complexity of this system includes several aspects. First, there is an identification of a full complement of the RAS components in many organs and specific cell types.[28] In regard to atherosclerosis, cells endowed with the ability to synthesize the RAS components include macrophages,[13] mast cells,[29,30] adipocytes,[31] and smooth muscle cells.[32] Second, there is a recognition of a spectrum of bioactive angiotensin peptides and their corresponding receptors. This includes Ang(1-7) that is synthesized from AngII by ACE2 and exerts its effect via mas receptors.[4,33,34] Also, AngIV, an aminopeptidase product from AngII, interacts with AT4 receptors.[35] Third, some components of the RAS exert effects independent of angiotensin peptides. This includes the direct effect of renin on the renin receptor and the diverse nature of substrates for ACE and ACE2.[36–38] Fourth, the complexity of the RAS is also exhibited by the discovery of alternative enzymes, other than renin and ACE, to generate AngII. This includes chymase, an enzyme produced mainly in mast cells that has been proposed as a major contributor to the conversion of AngI into AngII in atherosclerotic tissues.[30] Overall, while the RAS is a potent regulator of atherosclerosis, its complexity has hindered the determination of the mechanisms of this regulation.

8.3 Regulation of Experimental Atherosclerosis by the RAS

There is considerable evidence that the RAS promotes and augments atherosclerosis. This originates from studies in animal models using pharmacological and genetic approaches that predominantly target the bioactive molecule, AngII. Earlier theories regarding this complex system placed emphasis mostly on indirect effects of AngII, in particular its promotion of lesion formation through increasing blood pressure. However, the more contemporary thought is that AngII has a direct effect on the arterial wall to promote atherosclerosis.[39]

8.3.1 AngII Infusions

A direct approach to defining the role of AngII in atherosclerosis has been to infuse the octapeptide into hypercholesterolemic mice. It has been consistently demonstrated that AngII infusion into either low-density lipoprotein (LDL) receptor −/− or apolipoprotein (apo) E −/− mice augments formation of atherosclerotic lesions.[6,12,40–43] Another line of evidence is that in transgenic mice coexpressing human renin and angiotensinogen genes, extensive aortic root lesions developed after the mice were fed a high fat diet.[44] It has been noticed frequently that AngII-induced augmentation of atherosclerotic lesions is accompanied by increased systolic blood pressure.[41,44] Although it has long been demonstrated that AngII is a potent pressure molecule, the atherogenic effect of AngII does not appear to be related to changes in blood pressure. This assertion is based on studies in which norepinephrine was infused into apoE −/− mice to increase blood pressure equivalently to AngII.[41,45] While norepinephrine infusion promoted small increases in lesion size, its magnitude was dwarfed compared to the profound increase in mice infused with AngII. Similarly, lower doses of AngII that did not raise blood pressure in LDL receptor −/− mice increased atherosclerosis, and reductions in AngII-induced hypertension using a vasodilator had no effect on augmentation of AngII-induced atherosclerosis.[45]

8.3.2 Pharmacological RAS Inhibition

Pharmacological inhibition of the RAS has long been a standard of care for treating hypertension. The first inhibitor of ACE that was discovered was captopril. Subsequently, compounds were developed to antagonize the effects of AngII on AT1 receptors with losartan being the initially approved AT1 receptor antagonist in this class. More recently, aliskiren, a drug that inhibits renin, has been approved. Therefore, there is a large pharmacological armamentarium available to specifically target several different components in the RAS.

8.3.2.1 Angiotensin-converting enzyme inhibition

A large number of studies have demonstrated that ACE inhibitors reduce lesion size in many different animal models. These models include mice, rabbits, hamsters, pigs, and monkeys.[44,46–52] This nearly uniform finding is unusual in the atherosclerotic field for its consistency among different models and species using different classes of ACE inhibitors.

Angiotensin-converting enzyme inhibitors exhibit differences in the chemical structure of their active moieties and many other properties, but despite these differences, all compounds tested in this drug class consistently reduce atherosclerosis. For example, captopril contains a sulfhydryl group with potential antioxidant properties, which have been inferred to be anti-atherosclerotic.[53] Unlike captopril, fosinopril contains a phosphinyl group at its reactive moiety, and enalapril contains a carboxyl moiety. Although no report has compared the efficacy of various ACE inhibitors in reducing atherosclerosis, the benefit to reduce atherosclerosis has been demonstrated for many drugs of these three classes of ACE inhibitors in animal models.[12,16,54] These findings strongly infer a class effect (e.g., ACE inhibition) rather than an ancillary property on this structurally diverse class of drugs to inhibit atherosclerosis.

While ACE inhibition infers a role of AngII in atherosclerosis, this interpretation can be confounded by the numerous other effects of ACE inhibition, since this dicarboxypeptidase has a diverse range of substrates. AngI, the inactive product of renin cleavage of angiotensinogen, is a classic physiological substrate of ACE. ACE converts AngI into the bioactive AngII by removing the C-terminal dipeptides (His-Leu). Another well-known ACE substrate is the vasodilator, bradykinin. ACE inactivates bradykinin by removing the C-terminal dipeptides (His-Leu or Phe-Arg).[55] N-acetyl-Ser-Asp-Lys-Pro (AcSDKP), a putative stem cell suppressor,[56] is also an important substrate of ACE. The importance of ACE cleavage of this substrate has been demonstrated by the finding that ACE deficient mice exhibit anemia.[57] High plasma concentrations of AcSDKP has also been considered a marker for chronic ACE inhibition in patients.[58] The role of ACE-mediated regulation of these non-angiotensin peptides in atherosclerosis has not been clearly defined. The most extensively studied is bradykinin, which is an endogenous vasodilator peptide acting primarily through B2 receptor-dependent pathway.[55,59] A B2 receptor antagonist HOE-140 did not change the effectiveness of perindopril in reducing atherosclerosis in cholesterol-fed rabbits.[60] Furthermore, HOE-140 did not change the effectiveness of ramipril in reducing atherosclerosis in apoE−/− mice.[61] While these two studies do not support bradykinin-dependent anti-atherosclerotic effects of ACE inhibitors, one study has reported that ACE inhibition (lisinopril) exerts its cardioprotective effect in a myocardial infarction model through both B1 and B2 receptor-dependent mechanism.[62] In fact, a recent study has shown that kinin B1 receptor deficiency aggravates atherosclerosis in apoE−/− mice.[63]

8.3.2.2 AngII receptor antagonists

Despite ACE being the direct and predominant enzyme to synthesize AngII and the consistent findings for ACE inhibitors to reduce atherosclerosis, a more direct approach to defining the role of AngII in atherosclerosis is the use of angiotensin receptor blockers, of which currently published studies have predominantly focused on AngII receptor blockers (ARBs). The first reported study using an ARB, SC-51316, failed to define any reduction of lesion size in hypercholesterolemic rabbits.[51] However, later studies have consistently demonstrated a benefit in the reduction of atherosclerosis in experimental animal models treated with ARBs, including mice, rabbits, and monkeys.[8,9,64–70] The study reported by Schuh et al.[51] demonstrating lack of effect of AT1 blockade on atherosclerosis may be attributable to an inability to reach or maintain effective drug concentrations that are needed to sufficiently block the receptor and inhibit atherosclerosis. However, results from the positive studies have the potential for being ambiguous due to the extensive listing of known ancillary properties previously defined for this class of drugs. For example, telmisartan is also well known as a selective modulator of peroxisome proliferator-activated receptor gamma (PPARγ).[71] PPARγ is a central regulator of insulin and glucose metabolism, and it has also been found to change the development of atherosclerosis in animal models.[72]

The mechanistic interpretation of the effects of the AngII receptor antagonists are confounded by blood pressure reductions. Lowering blood pressure has the potential to reduce atherosclerosis rather than any direct effect of AngII on the atherosclerotic tissue. While few studies have directly determined the contribution of blood pressure reductions with ARBs to the regulation of atherosclerosis, two studies have demonstrated that ARBs profoundly reduced atherosclerosis in hypercholesterolemic mice, but equivalent reductions in blood pressure by a calcium channel blocker had no effect on atherosclerosis.[9,73]

As noted above, there is some evidence that AT2 receptor stimulation attenuates the effects of AT1 receptor activation. There is a single pharmacological inhibitor of this receptor, PD123319. Unfortunately, the administration of PD123319 has generated conflicting results in atherosclerosis studies with effects ranging from augmenting atherosclerosis,[74] no change,[75] to reducing atherosclerosis[76] in hypercholesterolemic mice.

8.3.2.3 Renin inhibition

Renin is the rate-limiting enzyme in the process of AngII synthesis by an action on its only known substrate, angiotensinogen. Therefore, renin has long been believed to be an ideal target to efficiently and specifically inhibit the production of AngII. However, the development of renin inhibitors has been hampered primarily by large species-specific variations in inhibitor efficacy and difficulties in achieving sufficient bioavailability of this class of drugs. Recently, the first renin inhibitor, aliskiren, was approved for treatment of hypertension. Renin inhibition using aliskiren has also been shown to profoundly reduce atherosclerosis in animal models, including mice and rabbits.[13–16,77]

8.4 Genetic Manipulation of the RAS

In addition to the pharmacological inhibition of the RAS in atherosclerotic studies, another insightful tool to determine the contribution of the RAS to atherosclerosis is the use of genetically manipulated mouse models. One apparent benefit of using specific mouse models is that pharmacological inhibition may target more than the specific component of the RAS as described above. For example, in mice, since there are two subtypes of AT1 receptors (AT1a and AT1b) that are both inhibited with currently available ARBs, it is impossible to distinguish the effects of AT1a receptors from AT1b receptors by using this pharmacological approach. Hence, the use of mouse models to study AT1 receptor subtypes is particularly important. A potential constraint of this approach is that deficiency of angiotensinogen,[78] renin,[79] ACE,[80] or combined deficiency of AT1a and AT1b receptors[81] causes abnormal renal development and low neonatal survival rate. Therefore, only a few studies reported deficiency of any of these RAS components in the development of atherosclerosis.

8.4.1 Angiotensin Receptors

Mice deficiency of each of the major AngII receptors (AT1a, AT1b, or AT2) has been developed. Many of the physiological and pathological effects of AngII are thought to be mediated through the AT1a receptor subtype in mice. All the studies that have studied deficiency of AT1a receptors in both apoE−/− and LDL receptor −/− mice have demonstrated a profound decrease in the size of lesions.[7,8,82] There is a relatively modest phenotype of the AT1a receptor −/− mice compared to mice with compound deficiency of AT1a and AT1b receptors.[81] Also, AT1b receptors are the only subtype involved in contractile responses of the aorta, the region in which atherosclerosis is typically determined.[83] Although it has been frequently reported that AngII-AT1a receptor activation plays a critical role in the development of atherosclerosis, no studies have reported a role of AT1b receptors in the development of atherosclerosis.

AT2 receptors are highly abundant in many tissues and organs during fetal development, but abundance decreases after birth. Like the pharmacological studies, the application of AT2 receptor −/− mice to atherosclerosis has generated a conflicting literature. This includes AT2 receptor deficiency on atherosclerosis having reductions,[76,84] no effect,[7] no effect on lesion size but compositional changes,[85] and increases.[86] A single study has demonstrated that recombinant adeno-associated virus driven AT2 receptor overexpression reduced atherosclerosis in LDL receptor −/− mice.[84] The basis for these contradictions in the role of AT2 receptors in atherosclerosis is not clear.

8.4.2 Angiotensin-Converting Enzyme

In contrast to the large number of studies using pharmacological inhibitors of ACE, there have been relatively few studies looking at genetic manipulations. This is possibly due to the detrimental developmental effects of mice lacking this enzyme.[87] An initial study of genetic manipulations of ACE used heterozygous deficiency in apoE +/− mice that had no effect on the development of atherosclerosis.[88] Another form of genetic manipulation of ACE generates the truncated protein in mice termed ACE2. Introduction of this truncated ACE protein in both the heterozygous and homozygous forms resulted in decreased atherosclerosis in apoE−/− mice.[89,90]

8.4.3 ACE2

ACE2 is a recently identified monocarboxypeptidase that catalyzes the synthesis of Ang(1-7), primarily from AngII. Therefore, the effects of ACE2 activity may be attributable to either or both of the effects of increasing the availability of Ang(1-7) and decreasing AngII, respectively. ACE2 protein expression has been detected in rabbit atherosclerotic plaques and from early to advanced stages of atherosclerotic plaques in humans.[91,92] Recent studies have also demonstrated that ACE2 deficiency accentuates atherosclerosis in hypercholesterolemic rabbits and mice.[93,94] Conversely, adenoviral overexpression of ACE2 attenuates atherosclerosis in these two animal models.[95,96] In the rabbit model, however, ACE2 overexpression did not reduce the plaque size at an advanced stage (atherogenic diet for 12 to 16 weeks) but reduced lipid deposition and increased collagen contents in the lesions.[96] These studies inferred that the effect of ACE2 deficiency was due to increased AngII. There is no defined evidence whether overexpression of ACE2 reduces atherosclerosis through increased degradation of AngII, increases of Ang(1-7) production, or the synergistic effects of both. The finding that renin inhibition ablates the synthesis of all angiotensin peptides and reduces atherosclerosis[13] is consistent with the hypothesis that ACE2 overexpression attenuates atherosclerosis through the degradation of AngII. However, there is evidence from recent literature that mas receptor antagonism[97] or chronic infusion of Ang(1-7)[98] reduces atherosclerosis in hypercholesterolemic mice. The anti-atherogenic effects of Ang(1-7) is diminished by blocking either mas receptors or AT2 receptors.[98]

8.4.4 Angiotensinogen and Renin

No atherosclerosis studies have been reported using angiotensinogen or renin whole body deficient mice that is likely due to the difficulty in breeding these mice. Conversely, transgenic mouse model with human angiotensinogen and human renin transgenes was developed.[99] Increased atherosclerosis was observed in these mice when fed a high-fat diet.[44]

8.5 Potential Mechanisms of RAS Modulating Atherosclerosis

8.5.1 Hypercholesterolemia Activates the RAS

Epidemiologic evidence and animal studies demonstrate that AngII contributes to the development of atherosclerosis.[6,40] Studies in experimental animal models also indicate that hypercholesterolemia is essential to initiate and accelerate AngII-induced atherosclerosis.[6,17,100] Accumulating evidence exhibits a mechanistic inter-relationship between hypercholesterolemia and the activation of the RAS in the development of atherosclerosis.[17,101]

Hypercholesterolemia has been demonstrated to increase plasma AngII concentrations in mice.[7,13] Modified LDL, such as oxidized LDL, upregulates ACE and AT1 receptors in human umbilical vein endothelial cells.[102] As a consequence, increased AngII-AT1 receptor interaction induces inflammatory gene expression through multiple intracellular signaling pathways to promote the progression of atherosclerosis.[103] In addition to hypercholesterolemia activating the RAS, there are also a few studies focusing on the converse, in which AngII regulates cholesterol metabolism. For example, AngII regulates macrophage cholesterol synthesis,[104] the lipid transporter ABCA1,[105] and lectin-like oxidized LDL receptor-1 (LOX-1) that transports oxidized LDL into cells.[106,107] AngII incubation with macrophages leads to increased LDL oxidation through activating the AT1 receptors,[54,108–113] which may subsequently activate the lipoxygenase-dependent pathway.

In addition to acting on macrophages, AngII also upregulates LOX-1 and lipoxygenase expression in human vascular smooth muscle cells, which may increase susceptibility of this cell type to transform into foam cells.[114] Together hypercholesterolemia and activation of the RAS appear to act as an integral component to induce the initiation and progression of atherosclerosis, although the downstream molecular mechanism by which this integral component promotes atherosclerosis has not been unequivocally defined.

The most common approach to reducing atherosclerosis in humans is to lower plasma cholesterol concentrations using statins, a class of 3-hydroxy-3-methylglutaryl coenzyme A reductase inhibitors.[17] In addition to lowering cholesterol, this class of drugs also downregulate AT1 receptors on neutrophils, platelets, and smooth muscle cells.[115,116] On the other hand, studies have consistently shown that inhibition or genetic disruption of the RAS markedly reduces atherosclerosis in hypercholesterolemic animals, even though plasma cholesterol concentrations remain high.[7,8,13,17] The reciprocal relationship between hypercholesterolemia and the activation of the RAS provide a strong rationale for recommending a combined therapy in order to more effectively inhibit atherosclerosis.[117]

8.5.2 Systemic versus Local Synthesis of Angiotensin Peptides

Traditionally, the RAS has been considered a circulation-driven system, deriving angiotensinogen from the liver, renin from the kidneys, and ACE in the capillary endothelium of the lungs to regulate circulating AngII concentrations. In the development of atherosclerosis, this bioactive peptide from the circulating blood targets blood-born cells or the resident cells in vessel wall. This traditional conception has been challenged by (1) the discovery of all components to form angiotensin peptides in atherosclerotic lesions;[7,13,118–120] (2) Macrophages[13] and arterial vascular smooth muscle cells have the ability to synthesize their own angiotensin peptides[32]; and (3) ACE, the pivotal enzyme in AngII production, has higher affinity as a membrane-bound form (tissue ACE) on cells than as a soluble form in plasma (systemic ACE).[121]

Macrophages are the predominant cell type in atherosclerotic lesions. This cell type contains all the components necessary to synthesize angiotensin peptides. Cultured macrophages secrete angiotensin peptides[13,122] and all the components of the RAS are present in atherosclerotic lesions that are predominantly associated with macrophages.[7,85,91,118,123] Deficiency of renin in bone marrow-derived cells reduces atherosclerosis in hypercholesterolemic mice.[13] The effect of macrophage renin deficiency on reduction of atherosclerosis is comparable to that of the systemic renin inhibitor, aliskiren.[13] This is consistent with macrophages being responsible for local formation of AngII to promote atherosclerosis. No studies have reported the effects of angiotensinogen or ACE deficiency in macrophages in the development of atherosclerosis. AngII exerts its atherogenic role through binding to AT1a receptors. Although whole body deficiency of AT1a receptors has been consistently shown to reduce atherosclerosis in mouse models by many groups,[7,8,124] bone marrow transplantation studies have demonstrated either no effects [13,82,124] or a modest effect[125,126] of AT1a receptor expression on macrophages in the development of atherosclerosis. AT1a receptors are ubiquitously present on many cell types. The findings from these studies imply a potentially important role of AT1a receptors on resident cells of the arterial wall such as endothelial and smooth muscle cells. Therefore, mouse models of cell specific deficiency of the RAS components will be great assets in determining the effects of this receptor on resident cells of the vessel wall. The findings from the bone marrow studies also indicate the complex origin of the RAS components in the development of atherosclerosis.

8.5.3 Angiotensin Peptide Effects on Cells in Atherosclerosis

AngII activation of AT1 receptors may directly or indirectly induce many signaling pathways, such as mitogen-activated protein kinases (MAPK), phosphatidylinositol 3-kinases, and the Janus kinase (JAK)/signal transducer and activator of transcription (STAT) pathways. The induction of these pathways converges on nuclear factor kappa B, a transcription factor that regulates a variety of genes. As a consequence, a cascade of cellular responses are produced, including activation of protein kinase C, mobilization of intracellular calcium, and oxidant signaling through the actions of NADPH complexes. AngII-induced NADPH oxidase activity, in which reactive oxygen species produced serve as intracellular second messengers, promotes endothelial dysfunction, leukocyte infiltration, and vascular smooth muscle cell proliferation, consequently initiating and augmenting atherosclerosis.[103] In addition, AngII has been reported to activate the blood coagulation cascade, contributing to thrombotic formation in atherosclerotic plaques.

8.5.3.1. Endothelial dysfunction and monocyte adhesion

A primary effect of AngII on endothelial cells in the atherogenic process is to promote endothelial dysfunction and monocyte adhesion. It has been consistently demonstrated that AngII increases monocyte adhesion in cultured endothelium.[13,127,128] Conversely, inhibition of ACE or AT1 receptors reduces or reverses endothelial dysfunction and inhibits monocyte adhesion.[129,130] Despite the defined effects on monocyte adhesion, the identification of adhesion molecules responsible for the AngII-induced monocyte adhesion has not been consistent. Vascular cell adhesion molecule-1 (VCAM-1) has been proposed as a pivotal adhesion molecule in endothelial cells. While one study has reported that AngII increases VCAM-1 mRNA and protein in cultured rat aortic endothelial cells,[131] others failed to define increased VCAM-1 expression in endothelial cells isolated from human aortas, coronary arteries, umbilical veins, or rabbit aortas.[13,127,128] ICAM-1 and E-selectin have also been proposed to mediate AngII-induced monocyte adhesion, but the literature has contradictory reports.[12,127,128,132]

8.5.3.2 Macrophage recruitment and vascular inflammation

A pivotal event to the development and progression of atherosclerosis is the recruitment of monocyte/macrophages to the endothelium overlying the evolving lesions. There are several direct cellular effects of AngII that could influence this inflammatory response of the atherogenic process. One of the mechanistic focuses of AngII is its ability to promote macrophage infiltration and vascular inflammation by stimulating monocyte chemoattractant protein-1 (MCP-1). MCP-1 is a potent chemoattractant of monocytes and macrophages.[133] In cultured cells, MCP-1 is detected in all the major cell types present in atherosclerotic lesions, including endothelial cells, smooth muscle cells, and macrophages. MCP-1 has also been directly detected in macrophage rich regions of atherosclerotic lesions.[134,135] As a member of the C-C chemokine family that acts on a chemokine receptor, C-C chemokine receptor-2 (CCR2), there is direct evidence that the MCP-1-CCR2 interaction plays a critical role in experimental atherosclerosis. Genetic deficiency of MCP-1 or CCR2 profoundly reduces atherosclerosis.[136,137] Further evidence indicates that AngII increases MCP-1 expression in aorta[82] and deficiency of CCR2 diminishes aortic macrophage recruitment and reduces atherosclerosis in AngII-infused mice.[138,139] In addition to the crucial role of the MCP-1-CCR2 axis in macrophage recruitment and atherosclerotic lesion formation, several cytokines such as interleukin-6, interleukin-8, and interleukin-18 secreted from blood-borne leukocytes or the cells in the vessel wall have also been reported to play a role in vascular inflammation in the process of atherosclerosis.[126,140–143]

8.5.3.3 Smooth muscle cell proliferation

A major effect in experimental atherosclerosis relates to AngII stimulating smooth muscle cell proliferation. The molecular mechanisms by which AngII promotes smooth muscle cell proliferation have also been extensively studied. AngII-AT1 receptor activation induces activation of MAPK. Among the members of MAPK, extracellular signal regulated kinase (ERK1/2) has been demonstrated to be a critical regulatory factor for AngII-mediated growth in vascular smooth muscle cells.[144–146] While AngII has been consistently shown to induce proliferation of vascular smooth muscle cells,[146–148] divergent effects have been reported for Ang(1-7).[146,149] It has been shown that Ang(1-7) directly inhibits proliferation of rat vascular smooth muscle cells or inhibits AngII-induced mouse smooth muscle cell proliferation.[146,149] Interestingly, Ang(1-7) alone has no effect on mouse smooth muscle cell proliferation.[146] The reason for this discrepancy has not been extensively elucidated.

8.5.3.4 Thrombosis

Thrombus formation adjacent to atheromatous plaques, particularly where ruptured or eroded, contributes to the pathophysiology of acute myocardial infarction. The extrinsic coagulation pathway plays a crucial role in the initiation of blood coagulation in atherosclerotic disease, of which tissue factor has been extensively studied. Tissue factor, an integral membrane protein, is a potent initiator of the extrinsic coagulation cascade situated within the vessel wall. AngII increases tissue factor mRNA abundance and protein activity in macrophages and endothelial cells.[150] Conversely, renin inhibition, ACE inhibition, or AT1 receptor antagonism diminish tissue factor in plasma as well as in monocytes.[151,152] Histological studies have shown that tissue factor is present in all stages of atherosclerotic lesions.[153–155] Abundant tissue factor protein is also found in the extracellular matrix of the necrotic core of the plaques, which may be largely derived from the macrophages present in the plaque.[154,156] Mechanistic studies indicate that locally synthesized AngII in macrophages within the atherosclerotic plaque may activate a series of intracellular signals eventually converging upon nuclear factor kappa B by binding to its specific membrane receptors. This cascade then enhances tissue factor expression. Thus, pharmacological inhibition of the RAS may have the potential to protect against acute ischemic events in patients with atherosclerotic disease through inhibiting tissue factor.[157]

8.6 Clinical Indication of RAS in Atherosclerosis

8.6.1 RAS Components Are Present in Human Atherosclerotic Lesions

One important evidence for the contribution of the RAS to human atherosclerosis is the detection of AngII, AT1 receptors, ACE and ACE2 in lesions. These were predominantly associated with macrophages.[92,118,158] AT2 receptors are also expressed in human atherosclerotic plaque, but no functionally important role of AT2 receptor expression in lesions is defined.[159] There are no reports of the presence of angiotensinogen or renin in human lesions.

8.6.2 RAS Inhibition Reduces Atherosclerosis-Related Cardiovascular Events

Several studies have investigated the inhibition of the RAS in the development of atherosclerosis. To evaluate atherosclerosis, a more direct method of quantitative coronary angiography has been used in the QUIET trial.[160] The QUIET trial investigated whether the ACE inhibitor quinapril influenced progression of atherosclerotic lesions. No net inhibitory effect was found. However, the investigators addressed the concerns of whether the dose was high enough (20 mg/day), that more patients (not statistically significant) treated with quinapril refused a follow-up angiography, and the flow-dependent remodeling after angioplasty may be misinterpreted as progression of the disease by quantitative coronary angiography.[160]

Subsequently, there were reports of clinical outcomes in clinical trials using large populations that extensively investigated ACE inhibition on atherosclerosis associated cardiovascular diseases. The ALLHAT study compared the effectiveness of an ACE inhibitor (lisinopril), a calcium channel antagonist (amlodipine), and a diuretic (chlorthalidone) against the more affordable diuretics on 33,357 high-risk hypertensive patients that were 55 years or older.[161] The ALLHAT study found that thiazide-type diuretics were superior in preventing one or more major forms of cardiovascular diseases. One concern raised regarding the findings in this study is that more than 30% of the patients in each group were African-American, who are considered to be more responsive to diuretics. Hence, this study needs to give respective consideration in the data interpretation and comparison with other clinical trials. HOPE is another large trial of 9,297 patients (older than 55 years) who were at high risk for cardiovascular events. This trial examined the use of ramipril in the prevention of myocardial infarction, stroke, or cardiovascular death.[18] The HOPE study was terminated prematurely because ramipril greatly reduced the rates of death from cardiovascular causes or from any cause. Subsequently, the EUROPA study demonstrated that another ACE inhibitor, perindopril, reduced cardiovascular risks in patients with stable coronary artery disease.[19] However, the treatment with ACE inhibitors did not show additional benefits in terms of the death caused by cardiovascular events in PEACE and IMAGINE studies.[162,163] The PEACE trial used trandolapril to treat patients with stable coronary artery disease who had preserved left ventricular ejection fractions, while quinapril was given to patients after coronary artery bypass graft surgery who also had preserved left ventricular ejection fractions. The results from these studies indicate that ACE inhibition may reduce cardiovascular risk more efficiently in patients with impaired cardiac function.

In addition to clinical trials extensively investigating the benefits of using different ACE inhibitors in patients with high risk to develop cardiovascular events, clinical trials were also performed to compare ACE inhibitors, ARBs, or the combination of these two classes of drugs. Two clinical trials (VALIANT and ONTARGET) compared ACE inhibition, AT1 receptor antagonism, and their combination in patients with cardiovascular diseases and impaired heart or other end organ failure.[21,164] Both studies have demonstrated that ACE inhibition and AT1 receptor antagonism are equivalently effective in preventing death from cardiovascular related causes. However, the combination of these two modes of the RAS inhibition did not provide additional benefits but increased adverse effects.

Taken together, although a few trials have failed to detect a beneficial effect, the majority of the clinical trials provide strong evidence that inhibition of the RAS is a promising therapy in patients with atherosclerotic diseases. However, the mechanistic relationship between the complexity of the RAS and the complex complications of the human atherosclerotic disease are still poorly understood. Further human studies are necessary to help dissect this complex relationship, thus improving treatment of the disease.

8.6.3 Genetic Studies of RAS Components in Human Atherosclerotic Disease

To understand the relationship between a single component of the RAS with atherosclerosis in humans, a number of genetic studies characterized associations between single nucleotide polymorphisms (SNPs) and coronary artery disease. Among the classical components of the RAS, angiotensinogen, ACE and AngII receptor genes have been investigated extensively to link genetic variants of the RAS to atherosclerotic diseases in humans.

M235T is the most studied SNP in the angiotensinogen gene. This polymorphism is caused by a nucleotide substitution in exon 2 that leads to an amino acid replacement from methionine to threonine at position 235. However, the findings from the association studies are not consistent, with some studies showing that this polymorphism is associated with atherosclerotic diseases in humans,[165,166] while some failed to identify any correlation.[167,168]

The most frequently studied polymorphism of the ACE gene is the insertion/deletion (I/D) that represents the presence (I) or absence (D) of a 250 base pair element located within intron 16.[169] The I/I genotype was associated with a markedly reduced serum ACE activity compared to the D/D genotye. Although some studies exhibited a potential link between the I/D polymorphism and atherosclerotic diseases,[170,171] many studies did not find a strong association.[172–174] Sayed-Tabatabaei et al. summarized the studies of the correlation between the I/D polymorphism of ACE and atherosclerosis.[174] The authors suggest that these erratic findings should be considered with regards to genotypic and phenotypic misclassifications, insufficient power in some studies, and the presence of interaction with other genes or environmental factors.

A1166C polymorphism, located in the 3′ untranslated region of the human AT1 receptors, has been exclusively studied in human atherosclerotic diseases. This polymorphism was associated with serum concentrations of C-reactive protein,[175] PPARγ changes and plasma renin activity.[176] While this SNP has been reported to be associated with myocardial infarction and carotid atherosclerosis in various ethnic populations,[177,178] several studies failed to demonstrate an association of this polymorphism with atherosclerotic diseases.[179–181] Polymorphisms of the human AT2 receptor gene have also been investigated in a limited number of studies. One variant in the AT2 receptor gene is G-1332A, located in the promoter. Two studies from the same group reported that this polymorphism is associated with premature coronary artery disease[182] and stenotic atherosclerosis requiring revascularization.[183] Another identified polymorphism is A1675G, located in the intron 1 of the AT2 receptor gene. The G allele of this polymorphism was associated with reduced risk of atherosclerosis in hypertensive patients.[184,185]

Overall, genetic studies of the RAS genes in humans have not been consistent.[186] Many impacting factors should be considered. These include those potential factors recommended by Sayed-Tabatabaei et al.,[174] such as small sample size providing insufficient power, environmental and/or other genetic interactions, and ethnic variations and heterogeneity. Also for consideration is whether the identified SNPs are within the linkage disequilibrium region of an unidentified functional SNP, which may directly influence the expression of the gene through transcriptional and/or translational regulation. While single SNP association analyses are straightforward to carry out, they do not make efficient use of the complex genomic structure, thereby not providing consistently insightful data to understand the association of the RAS gene variants with atherosclerosis. More recent studies have provided evidence that a combination of genotype variants of the RAS genes, M235T of the angiotensinogen gene, I/D of the ACE gene, and A1166C or C573T of the AT1 receptor gene, is a more powerful determinant of coronary artery diseases.[187–190] In addition to these studies, a recent publication recommended to use an exploratory method, logic regression analysis, to study interactions among multiple SNPs of different genes or between SNPs and environmental factors.[191] The authors illustrated this method using data from a US case-control study of myocardial infarction and stroke (1995–1999) carried out among 1,614 hypertensive patients in Washington State who were genotyped for 32 SNPs on five genes in the RAS. This method may provide insights on the pharmacogenetic research of the complex relationship between the RAS and human atherosclerotic disease.

8.7 Conclusions

There is compelling evidence that the RAS is an important component of the atherogenic process. Although studies in animal models have demonstrated that inhibition of the RAS profoundly reduces atherosclerosis, inhibition of the RAS has provided variable efficacy in reducing atherosclerosis-related diseases in humans. One major challenge is how to fully understand the complex nature of the RAS pathway and signaling as well as the complex properties of atherosclerotic disease. Few studies have taken a holistic approach to simultaneously quantify the activity of the entire repertoire of the RAS components during the initiation and progression of atherosclerotic lesions. Studies to identify specific molecular targets in the crucial signaling network that are co-regulated with the RAS in atherosclerosis are also essential in order to rationally predict disease development and guide future therapies.

Acknowledgments

The authors are supported by grants from the National Institutes of Health (HL062846 and HL80100 for AD and HL73085 for LAC). We are grateful to Anju Balakrishnan, Jessica Moorleghen, Aruna Poduri, and Debra Rateri for their constructive comments.

References

1. Cesari M, Rossi GP, Pessina AC. Biological properties of the angiotensin peptides other than angiotensin II: implications for hypertension and cardiovascular diseases. *J Hypertens* 2002; 20: 793–799.
2. Ferrario CM. Angiotensin I, angiotensin II and their biologically active peptides. *J Hypertens* 2002; 20: 805–807.
3. Carey RM, Siragy HM. Newly recognized components of the renin-angiotensin system: potential roles in cardiovascular and renal regulation. *Endocrin Rev* 2003; 24: 261–271.
4. Santos RA, Simoes e Silva AC, Maric C, Silva DM, Machado RP, de Buhr I, Heringer-Walther S, Pinheiro SV, Lopes MT, Bader M, Mendes EP, Lemos VS, Campagnole-Santos MJ, Schultheiss HP, Speth R, Walther T. Angiotensin-(1-7) is an endogenous ligand for the G protein-coupled receptor Mas. *Proc Natl Acad Sci U S A* 2003; 100: 8258–8263.

5. Belova LA. Angiotensin II-generating enzymes. *Biochemistry (Mosc)* 2000; 65: 1337–1345.
6. Daugherty A, Manning MW, Cassis LA. Angiotensin II promotes atherosclerotic lesions and aneurysms in apolipoprotein E-deficient mice. *J Clin Invest* 2000; 105: 1605–1612.
7. Daugherty A, Rateri DL, Lu H, Inagami T, Cassis LA. Hypercholesterolemia stimulates angiotensin peptide synthesis and contributes to atherosclerosis through the AT1A receptor. *Circulation* 2004; 110: 3849–3857.
8. Wassmann S, Czech T, Van Eickels M, Fleming I, Bohm M, Nickenig G. Inhibition of diet-induced atherosclerosis and endothelial dysfunction in apolipoprotein E/Angiotensin II type 1A receptor double-knockout mice. *Circulation* 2004; 110: 3062–3067.
9. Candido R, Allen TJ, Lassila M, Cao Z, Thallas V, Cooper ME, Jandeleit-Dahm KA. Irbesartan but not amlodipine suppresses diabetes-associated atherosclerosis. *Circulation* 2004; 109: 1536–1542.
10. Grothusen C, Bley S, Selle T, Luchtefeld M, Grote K, Tietge UJ, Drexler H, Schieffer B. Combined effects of HMG-CoA-reductase inhibition and renin-angiotensin system blockade on experimental atherosclerosis. *Atherosclerosis* 2005; 182: 57–69.
11. Candido R, Jandeleit-Dahm KA, Cao ZM, Nesteroff SP, Burns WC, Twigg SM, Dilley RJ, Cooper ME, Allen TJ. Prevention of accelerated atherosclerosis by angiotensin-converting enzyme inhibition in diabetic apolipoprotein E-deficient mice. *Circulation* 2002; 106: 246-253.
12. da Cunha V, Tham DM, Martin-McNulty B, Deng G, Ho JJ, Wilson DW, Rutledge JC, Vergona R, Sullivan ME, Wang YX. Enalapril attenuates angiotensin II-induced atherosclerosis and vascular inflammation. *Atherosclerosis* 2005; 178: 9–17.
13. Lu H, Rateri DL, Feldman DL, Jr RJ, Fukamizu A, Ishida J, Oesterling EG, Cassis LA, Daugherty A. Renin inhibition reduces hypercholesterolemia-induced atherosclerosis in mice. *J Clin Invest* 2008; 118: 984–993.
14. Imanishi T, Tsujioka H, Ikejima H, Kuroi A, Takarada S, Kitabata H, Tanimoto T, Muragaki Y, Mochizuki S, Goto M, Yoshida K, Akasaka T. Renin inhibitor aliskiren improves impaired nitric oxide bioavailability and protects against atherosclerotic changes. *Hypertension* 2008; 52: 563–572.
15. Nussberger J, Aubert JF, Bouzourene K, Pellegrin M, Hayoz D, Mazzolai L. Renin inhibition by aliskiren prevents atherosclerosis progression:

comparison with irbesartan, atenolol, and amlodipine. *Hypertension* 2008; 51: 1306–1311.

16. Weiss D, Taylor WR. Deoxycorticosterone acetate salt hypertension in apolipoprotein E-/- mice results in accelerated atherosclerosis: the role of angiotensin II. *Hypertension* 2008; 51: 218–224.
17. Rader DJ, Daugherty A. Translating molecular discoveries into new therapies for atherosclerosis. *Nature* 2008; 451: 904–913.
18. Yusuf S, Sleight P, Pogue J, Bosch J, Davies R, Dagenais G. Effects of an angiotensin-converting-enzyme inhibitor, ramipril, on cardiovascular events in high-risk patients. The heart outcomes prevention evaluation study investigators. *N Engl J Med* 2000; 342: 145–153.
19. Fox KM. Efficacy of perindopril in reduction of cardiovascular events among patients with stable coronary artery disease: randomised, double-blind, placebo-controlled, multicentre trial (the EUROPA study). *Lancet* 2003; 362: 782–788.
20. Pfeffer MA, McMurray J, Leizorovicz A, Maggioni AP, Rouleau JL, Van De Werf F, Henis M, Neuhart E, Gallo P, Edwards S, Sellers MA, Velazquez E, Califf R. Valsartan in acute myocardial infarction trial (VALIANT): rationale and design. *Am Heart J* 2000; 140: 727–750.
21. ONTARGET Investigators, Yusuf S, Teo KK, Pogue J, Dyal L, Copland I, Schumacher H, Dagenais G, Sleight P, Anderson C. Telmisartan, ramipril, or both in patients at high risk for vascular events. *N Engl J Med* 2008; 358: 1547–1559.
22. Dzau VJ. Implications of local angiotensin production in cardiovascular physiology and pharmacology. *Am J Cardiol* 1987; 59: 59A–65A.
23. Mehta PK, Griendling KK. Angiotensin II cell signaling: physiological and pathological effects in the cardiovascular system. *Am J Physiol Cell Physiol* 2007; 292: C82–C97.
24. De Gasparo M, Catt KJ, Inagami T, Wright JW, Unger T. International union of pharmacology. XXIII. The angiotensin II receptors. *Pharmacol Rev* 2000; 52: 415–472.
25. Mukoyama M, Nakajima M, Horiuchi M, Sasamura H, Pratt RE, Dzau VJ. Expression cloning of type 2 angiotensin II receptor reveals a unique class of seven-transmembrane receptors. *J Biol Chem* 1993; 268: 24539–24542.
26. Stegbauer J, Coffman TM. New insights into angiotensin receptor actions: from blood pressure to aging. *Curr Opin Nephrol Hypertens* 2011; 20: 84–88.

27. Siragy HM. The potential role of the angiotensin subtype 2 receptor in cardiovascular protection. *Curr Hypertens Rep* 2009; 11: 260–262.

28. Bader M, Ganten D. Update on tissue renin-angiotensin systems. *J Mol Med* 2008; 86: 615–621.

29. Reid AC, Silver RB, Levi R. Renin: at the heart of the mast cell. *Immunol Rev* 2007; 217: 123–140.

30. Miyazaki M, Takai S, Jin D, Muramatsu M. Pathological roles of angiotensin II produced by mast cell chymase and the effects of chymase inhibition in animal models. *Pharmacol Ther* 2006; 112: 668–676.

31. Cassis LA, Police SB, Yiannikouris F, Thatcher SE. Local adipose tissue renin-angiotensin system. *Curr Hypertens Rep* 2008; 10: 93–98.

32. Fukuda N, Satoh C, Hu WY, Soma M, Kubo A, Kishioka H, Watanabe Y, Izumi Y, Kanmatsuse K. Production of angiotensin II by homogeneous cultures of vascular smooth muscle cells from spontaneously hypertensive rats. *Arterioscler Thromb Vasc Biol* 1999; 19: 1210-1217.

33. Donoghue M, Hsieh F, Baronas E, Godbout K, Gosselin M, Stagliano N, Donovan M, Woolf B, Robison K, Jeyaseelan R, Breitbart RE, Acton S. A novel angiotensin-converting enzyme-related carboxypeptidase (ACE2) converts angiotensin I to angiotensin 1–9. *Circ Res* 2000; 87: E1–9.

34. Tipnis SR, Hooper NM, Hyde R, Karran E, Christie G, Turner AJ. A human homolog of angiotensin-converting enzyme. Cloning and functional expression as a captopril-insensitive carboxypeptidase. *J Biol Chem* 2000; 275: 33238–33243.

35. Albiston AL, McDowall SG, Matsacos D, Sim P, Clune E, Mustafa T, Lee J, Mendelsohn FA, Simpson RJ, Connolly LM, Chai SY. Evidence that the angiotensin IV (AT(4)) receptor is the enzyme insulin- regulated aminopeptidase. *J Biol Chem* 2001; 276: 48623–48626.

36. Nguyen G, Contrepas A. The (pro)renin receptors. *J Mol Med* 2008; 86: 643–646.

37. Tom B, Dendorfer A, Danser AH. Bradykinin, angiotensin-(1-7), and ACE inhibitors: how do they interact? *Int J Biochem Cell Biol* 2003; 35: 792–801.

38. Kalea AZ, Batlle D. Apelin and ACE2 in cardiovascular disease. *Curr Opin Investig Drugs* 2010; 11: 273–282.

39. Dzau VJ. Tissue angiotensin and pathobiology of vascular disease- A unifying hypothesis. *Hypertension* 2001; 37: 1047–1052.

40. Daugherty A, Cassis L. Chronic angiotensin II infusion promotes atherogenesis in low density lipoprotein receptor-/- mice. *Ann NY Acad Sci* 1999; 892: 108–118.

41. Weiss D, Kools JJ, Taylor WR. Angiotensin II-induced hypertension accelerates the development of atherosclerosis in apoE-deficient mice. *Circulation* 2001; 103: 448–454.

42. Ni W, Kitamoto S, Ishibashi M, Usui M, Inoue S, Hiasa KI, Zhao Q, Nishida KI, Takeshita A, Egashira K. Monocyte chemoattractant protein-1 Is an essential inflammatory mediator in angiotensin II-induced progression of established atherosclerosis in hypercholesterolemic mice. *Arterioscler Thromb Vasc Biol* 2004; 24: 534–539.

43. Nobuhiko A, Suganuma E, Babaev VR, Fogo A, Swift LL, Linton MF, Fazio S, Ichikawa I, Kon V. Angiotensin II amplifies macrophage-driven atherosclerosis. *Arterioscler Thromb Vasc Biol* 2004; 24: 2143–2148.

44. Sugiyama F, Haraoka S, Watanabe T, Shiota N, Taniguchi K, Ueno Y, Tanimoto K, Murakami K, Fukamizu A, Yagami K. Acceleration of atherosclerotic lesions in transgenic mice with hypertension by the activated renin-angiotensin system. *Lab Invest* 1997; 76: 835–842.

45. Cassis LA, Gupte M, Thayer S, Zhang X, Charnigo R, Howatt DA, Rateri DL, Daugherty A. Angiotensin II infusion promotes abdominal aortic aneurysms independent of increased blood pressure in hypercholesterolemic mice. *Am J Physiol Heart Circ Physiol* 2009; 296: H1660–H1665.

46. Aberg G, Ferrer P. Effects of captopril on atherosclerosis in cynomolgus monkeys. *J Cardiovasc Pharmacol* 1990; 15: S65–S72.

47. Miyazaki M, Sakonjo H, Takai S. Anti-atherosclerotic effects of an angiotensin converting enzyme inhibitor and an angiotensin II antagonist in Cynomolgus monkeys fed a high-cholesterol diet. *Br J Pharmacol* 1999; 128: 523–529.

48. Hernandez-Presa M, Bustos C, Ortego M, Tunon J, Renedo G, Ruiz-Ortega M, Egido J. Angiotensin-converting enzyme inhibition prevents arterial nuclear factor-kappa B activation, monocyte chemoattractant protein-1 expression, and macrophage infiltration in a rabbit model of early accelerated atherosclerosis. *Circulation* 1997; 95: 1532–1541.

49. Chobanian AV, Haudenschild CC, Nickerson C, Drago R. Antiatherogenic effect of captopril in the Watanabe heritable hyperlipidemic rabbit. *Hypertension* 1990; 15: 327–331.

50. Hoshida S, Nishida M, Yamashita N, Igarashi J, Aoki K, Hori M, Kuzuya T, Tada M. Vascular angiotensin-converting enzyme activity in

cholesterol-fed rabbits: effects of enalapril. *Atherosclerosis* 1997; 130: 53–59.

51. Schuh JR, Blehm DJ, Frierdich GE, Mcmahon EG, Blaine EH. Differential effects of renin-angiotensin system blockade on atherogenesis in cholesterol-fed rabbits. *J Clin Invest* 1993; 91: 1453–1458.
52. Charpiot P, Rolland PH, Friggi A, Piquet P, Scalbert E, Bodard H, Barlatier A, Latrille V, Tranier P, Mercier C, Luccioni R, Calaf R, Garcon D. ACE inhibition with prindopril and atherogenesis-induced structural and functional changes in minipig arteries. *Arterio Thromb* 1993; 13: 1125–1138.
53. Mashima R, Witting PK, Stocker R. Oxidants and antioxidants in atherosclerosis. *Curr Opin Lipidol* 2001; 12: 411–418.
54. Hayek T, Attias J, Coleman R, Brodsky S, Smith J, Breslow JL, Keidar S. The angiotensin-converting enzyme inhibitor, fosinopril, and the angiotensin II receptor antagonist, losartan, inhibit LDL oxidation and attenuate atherosclerosis independent of lowering blood pressure in apolipoprotein E deficient mice. *Cardiovasc Res* 1999; 44: 579–587.
55. Yang HY, Erdos EG, Levin Y. Characterization of a dipeptide hydrolase (kininase II: angiotensin I converting enzyme). *J Pharmacol Exp Ther* 1971; 177: 291–300.
56. Rousseau A, Michaud A, Chauvet MT, Lenfant M, Corvol P. The hemoregulatory peptide N-acetyl-Ser-Asp-Lys-Pro is a natural and specific substrate of the N-terminal active site of human angiotensin-converting enzyme. *J Biol Chem* 1995; 270: 3656–3661.
57. Cole J, Ertoy D, Lin H , Sutliff RL, Ezan E, Guyene TT, Capecchi M, Corvol P, Bernstein KE. Lack of angiotensin II-facilitated erythropoiesis causes anemia in angiotensin-converting enzyme-deficient mice. *J Clin Invest* 2000; 106: 1391–1398.
58. Azizi M, Ezan E, Nicolet L, Grognet JM, Menard J. High plasma level of N-acetyl-seryl-aspartyl-lysyl-proline: a new marker of chronic angiotensin-converting enzyme inhibition. *Hypertension* 1997; 30: 1015–1019.
59. Remme WJ. Bradykinin-mediated cardiovascular protective actions of ACE inhibitors. A new dimension in anti-ischaemic therapy? *Drugs* 1997; 54 Suppl 5: 59–70.
60. Fennessy PA, Campbell JH, Mendelsohn FA, Campbell GR. Angiotensin-converting enzyme inhibitors and atherosclerosis: relevance of animal models to human disease. *Clin Exp Pharmacol Physiol* 1996; 23: S30–S32.

61. Keidar S, Attias J, Coleman R, Wirth J, Scholkens B, Hayek T. Attenuation of atherosclerosis in apolipoprotein E-deficient mice by ramipril is dissociated from its antihypertensive effect and from potentiation of bradykinin. *J Cardiovasc Pharmacol* 2000; 35: 64–72.

62. Duka A, Kintsurashvili E, Duka I, Ona D, Hopkins TA, Bader M, Gavras I, Gavras H. Angiotensin-converting enzyme inhibition after experimental myocardial infarct: role of the kinin B1 and B2 receptors. *Hypertension* 2008; 51: 1352–1357.

63. Merino VF, Todiras M, Mori MA, Sales VM, Fonseca RG, Saul V, Tenner K, Bader M, Pesquero JB. Predisposition to atherosclerosis and aortic aneurysms in mice deficient in kinin B1 receptor and apolipoprotein E *J Mol Med* 2009; 87: 953–963.

64. Warnholtz A, Nickenig G, Schulz E, Macharzina R, Brasen JH, Skatchkov M , Heitzer T, Stasch JP, Griendling KK, Harrison DG, Bohm M, Meinertz T, Munzel T. Increased NADH-oxidase-mediated superoxide production in the early stages of atherosclerosis- Evidence for involvement of the renin-angiotensin system. *Circulation* 1999; 99: 2027–2033.

65. De las Heras N, Aragoncillo P, Maeso R, Vazquez-Perez S, Navarro-Cid J, DeGasparo M, Mann J, Ruilope LM, Cachofeiro V, Lahera V. AT(1) receptor antagonism reduces endothelial dysfunction and intimal thickening in atherosclerotic rabbits. *Hypertension* 1999; 34: 969–975.

66. Strawn WB, Chappell MC, Dean RH, Kivlighn S, Ferrario CM. Inhibition of early atherogenesis by losartan in monkeys with diet-induced hypercholesterolemia. *Circulation* 2000; 101: 1586–1593.

67. Dol F, Martin G, Staels B, Mares AM, Cazaubon C, Nisato D, Bidouard JP, Janiak P, Schaeffer P, Herbert JM. Angiotensin AT(1) receptor antagonist irbesartan decreases lesion size, chemokine expression, and macrophage accumulation in apolipoprotein E-deficient mice. *J Cardiovasc Pharmacol* 2001; 38: 395–405.

68. Johnstone MT, Perez AS, Nasser I, Stewart R, Vaidya A, Al Ammary F, Schmidt B, Horowitz G, Dolgoff J, Hamilton J, Quist WC. Angiotensin receptor blockade with candesartan attenuates atherosclerosis, plaque disruption, and macrophage accumulation within the plaque in a rabbit model. *Circulation* 2004; 110: 2060–2065.

69. Takai S, Jin D, Sakaguchi M, Muramatsu M, Ishii K, Kirimura K, Sakonjo H, Miyazaki M. Comparative effects of candesartan and amlodipine in a monkey atherosclerotic model. *Hypertens Res* 2004; 27: 517–522.

70. Ruan LM, Cai W, Chen JZ , Duan JF. Effects of Losartan on expression of connexins at the early stage of atherosclerosis in rabbits. *Int J Med Sci* 2010; 7: 82–89.

71. Schupp M, Janke J, Clasen R, Unger T, Kintscher U. Angiotensin type 1 receptor blockers induce peroxisome proliferator-activated receptor-gamma activity. *Circulation* 2004; 109: 2054–2057.

72. Li AC, Binder CJ, Gutierrez A, Brown KK, Plotkin CR, Pattison JW, Valledor AF, Davis RA, Willson TM, Witztum JL, Palinski W, Glass CK. Differential inhibition of macrophage foam-cell formation and atherosclerosis in mice by PPARalpha, beta/delta, and gamma. *J Clin Invest* 2004; 114: 1564–1576.

73. Doran DE, Weiss D, Zhang Y, Griendling KK, Taylor WR. Differential effects of AT(1) receptor and Ca(2+) channel blockade on atherosclerosis, inflammatory gene expression, and production of reactive oxygen species. *Atherosclerosis* 2007; 195: 39–47.

74. Daugherty A, Manning MW, Cassis LA. Antagonism of AT2 receptors augments angiotensin II-induced abdominal aortic aneurysms and atherosclerosis. *Br J Pharmacol* 2001; 134: 865–870.

75. Johansson ME, Wickman A, Fitzgerald SM, Gan LM, Bergstrom G. Angiotensin II, type 2 receptor is not involved in the angiotensin II-mediated pro-atherogenic process in ApoE-/- mice. *J Hypertens* 2005; 23: 1541–1549.

76. Koitka A, Cao Z, Koh P, Watson AM, Sourris KC, Loufrani L, Soro-Paavonen A, Walther T, Woollard KJ, Jandeleit-Dahm KA, Cooper ME, Allen TJ. Angiotensin II subtype 2 receptor blockade and deficiency attenuate the development of atherosclerosis in an apolipoprotein E-deficient mouse model of diabetes. *Diabetologia* 2010; 53: 584–592.

77. Poss J, Werner C, Lorenz D, Gensch C, Bohm M, Laufs U. The renin inhibitor aliskiren upregulates pro-angiogenic cells and reduces atherogenesis in mice. *Basic Res Cardiol* 2010; 105: 725-735.

78. Nagata M, Tanimoto K, Fukamizu A, Kon Y, Sugiyama F, Yagami K, Murakami K, Watanabe T. Nephrogenesis and renovascular development in angiotensinogen-deficient mice. *Lab Invest* 1996; 75: 745–753.

79. Yanai K, Saito T, Kakinuma Y, Kon Y, Hirota K, Taniguchi-Yanai K, Nishijo N, Shigematsu Y, Horiguchi H, Kasuya Y, Sugiyama F, Yagami K, Murakami K, Fukamizu A. Renin-dependent cardiovascular functions and renin-independent blood- brain barrier functions revealed by renin-deficient mice. *J Biol Chem* 2000; 275: 5–8.

80. Esther CR Jr, Howard TE, Marino EM, Goddard JM, Capecchi MR, Bernstein KE. Mice lacking angiotensin-converting enzyme have low blood pressure, renal pathology, and reduced male fertility. *Lab Invest* 1996; 74: 953–965.

81. Oliverio MI, Kim HS, Ito M, Le T, Audoly L, Best CF, Hiller S, Kluckman K, Maeda N, Smithies O, Coffman TM. Reduced growth, abnormal kidney structure, and type 2 (AT2) angiotensin receptor-mediated blood pressure regulation in mice lacking both AT1A and AT1B receptors for angiotensin II. *Proc Natl Acad Sci U S A* 1998; 95: 15496–15151.

82. Koga J, Egashira K, Matoba T, Kubo M, Ihara Y, Iwai M, Horiuchi M, Sunagawa K. Essential role of angiotensin II type 1a receptors in the host vascular wall, but not the bone marrow, in the pathogenesis of angiotensin II-induced atherosclerosis. *Hypertens Res* 2008; 31: 1791–1800.

83. Zhou Y, Chen Y, Dirksen WP, Morris M, Periasamy M. AT1b receptor predominantly mediates contractions in major mouse blood vessels. *Circ Res* 2003; 93: 1089–1094.

84. Hu C, Dandapat A, Chen J, Liu Y, Hermonat PL, Carey RM, Mehta JL. Over-expression of angiotensin II type 2 receptor (agtr2) reduces atherogenesis and modulates LOX-1, endothelial nitric oxide synthase and heme-oxygenase-1 expression. *Atherosclerosis* 2008; 199: 288–294.

85. Sales VL, Sukhova GK, Lopez-Ilasaca MA, Libby P, Dzau VJ, Pratt RE. Angiotensin type 2 receptor is expressed in murine atherosclerotic lesions and modulates lesion evolution. *Circulation* 2005; 112: 3328–3336.

86. Iwai M, Chen R, Li Z, Shiuchi T, Suzuki J, Ide A, Tsuda M, Okumura M, Min LJ, Mogi M, Horiuchi M. Deletion of angiotensin II type 2 receptor exaggerated atherosclerosis in apolipoprotein E-null mice. *Circulation* 2005; 112: 1636–1643.

87. Krege JH, John SW, Langenbach LL, Hodgin JB, Hagaman JR, Bachman ES, Jennette JC, O'Brien DA, Smithies O. Male-female differences in fertility and blood pressure in ACE-deficient mice. *Nature* 1995; 375: 146-148.

88. Krege JH, Moyer JS, Langenbach LL, Peng L, Zhang SH, Maeda N, Reddick RL, Smithies O. Angiotensin-converting enzyme gene and atherosclerosis. *Arterioscler Thromb Vasc Biol* 1997; 17: 1245–1250.

89. Hayek T, Pavlotzky E, Hamoud S, Coleman R, Keidar S, Aviram M, Kaplan M. Tissue angiotensin-converting-enzyme (ACE) deficiency leads to a reduction in oxidative stress and in atherosclerosis. Studies in ACE-knockout mice type 2. *Arterioscler Thromb Vasc Biol* 2003; 23: 2090–2096.

90. Weiss D, Bernstein KE, Fuchs S, Adams J, Synetos A, Taylor WR. Vascular wall ACE is not required for atherogenesis in ApoE(-/-) mice. *Atherosclerosis* 2009; 209: 352–358.

91. Zulli A, Burrell LM, Widdop RE, Black MJ, Buxton BF, Hare DL. Immunolocalization of ACE2 and AT2 receptors in rabbit atherosclerotic plaques. *J Histochem Cytochem* 2006; 54: 147–150.

92. Sluimer JC, Gasc JM, Hamming I, van Goor H, Michaud A, van den Akker LH, Jutten B, Cleutjens J, Bijnens AP, Corvol P, Daemen MJ, Heeneman S. Angiotensin-converting enzyme 2 (ACE2) expression and activity in human carotid atherosclerotic lesions. *J Pathol* 2008; 215: 273–279.

93. Zhang C, Zhao YX, Zhang YH, Zhu L, Deng BP, Zhou ZL, Li SY, Lu XT, Song LL, Lei XM, Tang WB, Wang N, Pan CM, Song HD, Liu CX, Dong B, Zhang Y, Cao Y. Angiotensin-converting enzyme 2 attenuates atherosclerotic lesions by targeting vascular cells. *Proc Natl Acad Sci USA* 2010; 107: 15886–15891.

94. Thomas MC, Pickering RJ, Tsorotes D, Koitka A, Sheehy K, Bernardi S, Toffoli B, Nguyen-Huu TP, Head G, Fu Y, Chin-Dusting J, Cooper ME, Tikellis C. Genetic Ace2 deficiency accentuates vascular inflammation and atherosclerosis in the apoE knockout mouse. *Circ Res* 2010; 107: 888–897.

95. Lovren F, Pan Y, Quan A, Teoh H, Wang G, Shukla PC, Levitt KS, Oudit GY, Al-Omran M, Stewart DJ, Slutsky AS, Peterson MD, Backx PH, Penninger JM, Verma S. Angiotensin converting enzyme-2 confers endothelial protection and attenuates atherosclerosis. *Am J Physiol Heart Circ Physiol* 2008 ; 295: H1377–H1384.

96. Dong B, Zhang C, Feng JB, Zhao YX, Li SY, Yang YP, Dong QL, Deng BP, Zhu L, Yu QT, Liu CX, Liu B, Pan CM, Song HD, Zhang MX, Zhang Y. Overexpression of ACE2 enhances plaque stability in a rabbit model of atherosclerosis. *Arterioscler Thromb Vasc Biol* 2008; 28: 1270–1276.

97. Toton-Zuranska J, Gajda M, Pyka-Fosciak G, Kus K, Pawlowska M, Niepsuj A, Wolkow P, Olszanecki R, Jawien J, Korbut R. AVE 0991-angiotensin-(1-7) receptor agonist, inhibits atherogenesis in apoE-knockout mice. *J Physiol Pharmacol* 2010; 61: 181–183.

98. Tesanovic S, Vinh A, Gaspari TA, Casley D, Widdop RE. Vasoprotective and atheroprotective effects of angiotensin (1-7) in apolipoprotein E-deficient mice. *Arterioscler Thromb Vasc Biol* 2010; 30: 1606–1613.

99. Fukamizu A, Sugimura K, Takimoto E, Sugiyama F, Seo MS, Takahashi S, Hatae T, Kajiwara N, Yagami K, Murakami K. Chimeric renin-angiotensin system demonstrates sustained increase in blood pressure of transgenic mice carrying both human renin and human angiotensinogen genes. *J Biol Chem* 1993; 268: 11617–11621.

100. Strehlow K, Wassmann S, Bohm M, Nickenig G. Angiotensin AT1 receptor over-expression in hypercholesterolaemia. *Ann Med* 2000; 32: 386–389.

101. Daugherty A, Lu H, Rateri DL, Cassis LA. Augmentation of the renin-angiotensin system by hypercholesterolemia promotes vascular diseases. *Future Lipidol* 2008; 3: 625–636.

102. Catar RA, Muller G, Heidler J, Schmitz G, Bornstein SR, Morawietz H. Low-density lipoproteins induce the renin-angiotensin system and their receptors in human endothelial cells. *Horm Metab Res* 2007; 39: 801–805.

103. Brasier AR, Recinos A, Eledrisi MS. Vascular inflammation and the renin-angiotensin system. *Arterioscler Thromb Vasc Biol* 2002; 22: 1257–1266.

104. Keidar S, Attias J, Heinrich R, Coleman R, Aviram M. Angiotensin II atherogenicity in apolipoprotein E deficient mice is associated with increased cellular cholesterol biosynthesis. *Atherosclerosis* 1999; 146: 249–257.

105. Takata Y, Chu V, Collins AR, Lyon CJ, Wang W, Blaschke F, Bruemmer D, Caglayan E, Daley W, Higaki J, Fishbein MC, Tangirala RK, Law RE, Hsueh WA. Transcriptional repression of ATP-binding cassette transporter A1 gene in macrophages: a novel atherosclerotic effect of angiotensin II. *Circ Res* 2005; 97: e88–e96.

106. Li DY, Zhang YC, Philips MI, Sawamura T, Mehta JL. Upregulation of endothelial receptor for oxidized low-density lipoprotein (LOX-1) in cultured human coronary artery endothelial cells by angiotensin II type 1 receptor activation. *Circ Res* 1999; 84: 1043–1049.

107. Morawietz H, Rueckschloss U, Niemann B, Duerrschmidt N, Galle J, Hakim K, Zerkowski HR, Sawamura T, Holtz J. Angiotensin II induces LOX-1, the human endothelial receptor for oxidized low-density lipoprotein. *Circulation* 1999; 100: 899–902.

108. Keidar S, Attias J. Angiotensin II injection into mice increases the uptake of oxidized LDL by their macrophages via a proteoglycan-mediated pathway. *Biochem Biophys Res Comm* 1997; 239: 63–67.

109. Keidar S, Attias J, Smith J, Breslow JL, Hayek T. The angiotensin-II receptor antagonist, losartan, inhibits LDL lipid peroxidation and atherosclerosis in apolipoprotein E-deficient mice. *Biochem Biophys Res Comm* 1997; 236: 622–625.

110. Scheidegger KJ, Butler S, Witztum JL. Angiotensin II increases macrophage-mediated modification of low density lipoprotein via a lipoxygenase-dependent pathway. *J Biol Chem* 1997; 272: 21609–21615.

111. Keidar S, Heinrich R, Kaplan M, Hayek T, Aviram M. Angiotensin II administration to atherosclerotic mice increases macrophage uptake

of oxidized LDL- A possible role for interleukin-6. *Arterioscler Thromb Vasc Biol* 2001; 21: 1464–1469.

112. Hayek T, Kaplan M, Raz A, Keidar S, Coleman R, Aviram M. Ramipril administration to atherosclerotic mice reduces oxidized low-density lipoprotein uptake by their macrophages and blocks the progression of atherosclerosis. *Atherosclerosis* 2002; 161: 65–74.

113. Keidar S, Heinrich R, Kaplan M, Aviram M. Oxidative stress increases the expression of the angiotensin-II receptor type 1 in mouse peritoneal macrophages. *J Renin Angiotensin Aldosterone Syst* 2002; 3: 24–30.

114. Limor R, Kaplan M, Sawamura T, Sharon O, Keidar S, Weisinger G, Knoll E, Naidich M, Stern N. Angiotensin II increases the expression of lectin-like oxidized low-density lipoprotein receptor-1 in human vascular smooth muscle cells via a lipoxygenase-dependent pathway. *Am J Hypertens* 2005; 18: 299–307.

115. Guasti L, Marino F, Cosentino M, Maio RC, Rasini E, Ferrari M, Castiglioni L, Klersy C, Gaudio G, Grandi AM, Lecchini S, Venco A. Prolonged statin-associated reduction in neutrophil reactive oxygen species and angiotensin II type 1 receptor expression: 1-year follow-up. *Eur Heart J* 2008; 29: 1118–1126.

116. Nickenig G, Baumer AT, Temur Y, Kebben D, Jockenhovel F, Bohm M. Statin-sensitive dysregulated AT1 receptor function and density in hypercholesterolemic men. *Circulation* 1999; 100: 2131–2134.

117. Koh KK, Han SH, Oh PC, Shin EK, Quon MJ. Combination therapy for treatment or prevention of atherosclerosis: focus on the lipid-RAAS interaction. *Atherosclerosis* 2010; 209: 307–313.

118. Diet F, Pratt RE, Berry GJ, Momose N, Gibbons GH, Dzau VJ. Increased accumulation of tissue ACE in human atherosclerotic coronary artery disease. *Circulation* 1996; 94: 2756–2767.

119. Fukuhara M, Geary RL, Diz DI, Gallagher PE, Wilson JA, Glazier SS, Dean RH, Ferrario CM. Angiotensin-converting enzyme expression in human carotid artery atherosclerosis. *Hypertension* 2000; 35: 353–359.

120. Ohishi M, Ueda M, Rakugi H, Naruko T, Kojima A, Okamura A, Higaki J, Ogihara T. Relative localization of angiotensin-converting enzyme, chymase and angiotensin II in human coronary atherosclerotic lesions. *J Hypertens* 1999; 17: 547–553.

121. Hooper NM. Angiotensin converting enzyme: implications from molecular biology for its physiological functions. *Int J Biochem* 1991; 23: 641–647.

122. Okamura A, Rakugi H, Ohishi M, Yanagitani Y, Takiuchi S, Moriguchi K, Fennessy PA, Higaki J, Ogihara T. Upregulation of renin-angiotensin

system during differentiation of monocytes to macrophages. *J Hyperten* 1999; 17: 537–545.

123. Potter DD, Sobey CG, Tompkins PK, Rossen JD, Heistad DD. Evidence that macrophages in atherosclerotic lesions contain angiotensin II. *Circulation* 1998; 98: 800–807.

124. Cassis LA, Rateri DL, Lu H, Daugherty A. Bone marrow transplantation reveals that recipient AT1a receptors are required to initiate angiotensin II-induced atherosclerosis and aneurysms. *Arterioscler Thromb Vasc Biol* 2007; 27: 380–386.

125. Fukuda D, Sata M, Ishizaka N, Nagai R. Critical role of bone marrow angiotensin II type 1 receptor in the pathogenesis of atherosclerosis in apolipoprotein E deficient mice. *Arterioscler Thromb Vasc Biol* 2007; 28: 72–77.

126. Tsubakimoto Y, Yamada H, Yokoi H, Kishida S, Takata H, Kawahito H, Matsui A, Urao N, Nozawa Y, Hirai H, Imanishi J, Ashihara E, Maekawa T, Takahashi T, Okigaki M, Matsubara H. Bone marrow angiotensin AT1 receptor regulates differentiation of monocyte lineage progenitors from hematopoietic stem cells. *Arterioscler Thromb Vasc Biol* 2009; 29: 1529–1536.

127. Kim JA, Berliner JA, Nadler JL. Angiotensin II increases monocyte binding to endothelial cells. *Biochem Biophys Res Comm* 1996; 226: 862–868.

128. Grafe M, Auch-Schwelk W, Zakrzewicz A, Regitz-Zagrosek V, Bartsch P, Graf K, Loebe M, Gaehtgens P, Fleck E. Angiotensin II-induced leukocyte adhesion on human coronary endothelial cells is mediated by E-selectin. *Circ Res* 1997; 81: 804–811.

129. Kojima C, Kawakami A, Takei T, Nitta K, Yoshida M. Angiotensin-converting enzyme inhibitor attenuates monocyte adhesion to vascular endothelium through modulation of intracellular zinc. *J Pharmacol Exp Ther* 2007; 323: 855–860.

130. Prasad A, TupasHabib T, Schenke WH, Mincemoyer R, Panza JA, Waclawin MA, Ellahham S, Quyyumi AA. Acute and chronic angiotensin-1 receptor antagonism reverses endothelial dysfunction in atherosclerosis. *Circulation* 2000; 101: 2349–2354.

131. Pueyo ME, Gonzalez W, Nicoletti A, Savoie F, Arnal JF, Michel JB. Angiotensin II stimulates endothelial vascular cell adhesion molecule-1 via nuclear factor-kappa B activation induced by intracellular oxidative stress. *Arterioscler Thromb Vasc Biol* 2000; 20: 645–651.

132. Pastore L, Tessitore A, Martinotti S, Toniato E, Alesse E, Bravi MC, Ferri C, Desideri G, Gulino A, Santucci A. Angiotensin II stimulates

intercellular adhesion molecule-1 (ICAM-1) expression by human vascular endothelial cells and increases soluble ICAM-1 release *in vivo*. *Circulation* 1999; 100: 1646–1652.

133. Charo IF, Ransohoff RM. The many roles of chemokines and chemokine receptors in inflammation. *N Engl J Med* 2006; 354: 610–621.

134. Kowala MC, Recce R, Beyer S, Gu C, Valentine M. Characterization of atherosclerosis in LDL receptor knockout mice: macrophage accumulation correlates with rapid and sustained expression of aortic MCP-1/JE. *Atherosclerosis* 2000; 149: 323–330.

135. Ylä-Herttuala S, Lipton BA, Rosenfeld ME, Sarkioja T, Yoshimura T, Leonard EJ, Witztum JL, Steinberg D. Expression of monocyte chemoattractant protein-1 in macrophage-rich areas of human and rabbit atherosclerotic lesions. *Proc Natl Acad Sci U S A* 1991; 88: 5252–5256.

136. Gu L, Okada Y, Clinton SK, Gerard C, Sukhova GK, Libby P, Rollins BJ. Absence of monocyte chemoattractant protein-1 reduces atherosclerosis in low density lipoprotein receptor-deficient mice. *Mol Cell* 1998; 2: 275–281.

137. Boring L, Gosling J, Cleary M, Charo IF. Decreased lesion formation in CCR2(-/-) mice reveals a role for chemokines in the initiation of atherosclerosis. *Nature.* 1998; 394: 894–897.

138. Bush E, Maeda N, Kuziel WA, Dawson TC, Wilcox JN, DeLeon H, Taylor WR. CC chemokine receptor 2 is required for macrophage infiltration and vascular hypertrophy in angiotensin II-induced hypertension. *Hypertension* 2000; 36: 360–363.

139. Ishibashi M, Egashira K, Zhao Q, Hiasa K, Ohtani K, Ihara Y, Charo IF, Kura S, Tsuzuki T, Takeshita A, Sunagawa K. Bone marrow-derived monocyte chemoattractant protein-1 receptor CCR2 is critical in angiotensin II-induced acceleration of atherosclerosis and aneurysm formation in hypercholesterolemic mice. *Arterioscler Thromb Vasc Biol* 2004; 24: e174–e178.

140. Recinos A 3rd, Lejeune WS, Sun H, Lee CY, Tieu BC, Lu M, Hou T, Boldogh I, Tilton RG, Brasier AR. Angiotensin II induces IL-6 expression and the Jak-STAT3 pathway in aortic adventitia of LDL receptor-deficient mice. *Atherosclerosis* 2007; 194: 125–133.

141. Cui R, Tieu B, Recinos A, Tilton RG, Brasier AR. RhoA mediates angiotensin II-induced phospho-Ser536 nuclear factor kappaB/RelA subunit exchange on the interleukin-6 promoter in VSMCs. *Circ Res* 2006; 99: 723–730.

142. Sahar S, Dwarakanath RS, Reddy MA, Lanting L, Todorov I, Natarajan R. Angiotensin II enhances interleukin-18 mediated inflammatory gene expression in vascular smooth muscle cells: a novel cross-talk in the pathogenesis of atherosclerosis. *Circ Res* 2005; 96: 1064–1010.

143. Ito T, Ikeda U. Inflammatory cytokines and cardiovascular disease. *Curr Drug Targets Inflamm Allergy* 2003; 2: 257–265.

144. Xi XP, Graf K, Goetze S, Fleck E, Hsueh WA, Law RE. Central role of the MAPK pathway in ang II-mediated DNA synthesis and migration in rat vascular smooth muscle cells. *Arterioscler Thromb Vasc Biol* 1999; 19: 73–82.

145. Touyz RM, He G, Deng LY, Schiffrin EL. Role of extracellular signal-regulated kinases in angiotensin II-stimulated contraction of smooth muscle cells from human resistance arteries. *Circulation* 1999; 99: 392–399.

146. Zhang F, Hu Y, Xu Q, Ye S. Different effects of angiotensin II and angiotensin-(1–7) on vascular smooth muscle cell proliferation and migration. *PLoS One* 2010; 5: e12323.

147. Daemen MJ, Lombardi DM, Bosman FT, Schwartz SM. Angiotensin II induces smooth muscle cell proliferation in the normal and injured rat arterial wall. *Circ Res* 1991; 68: 450–456.

148. Schiffrin EL, Park JB, Intengan HD, Touyz RM. Correction of arterial structure and endothelial dysfunction in human essential hypertension by the angiotensin receptor antagonist losartan. *Circulation* 2000; 101: 1653–1659.

149. Freeman EJ, Chisolm GM, Ferrario CM, Tallant EA. Angiotensin-(1-7) inhibits vascular smooth muscle cell growth. *Hypertension* 1996; 28: 104–148.

150. Nishimura H, Tsuji H, Masuda H, Nakagawa K, Nakahara Y, Kitamura H, Kasahara T, Sugano T, Yoshizumi M, Sawada S, Nakagawa M. Angiotensin II increases plasminogen activator inhibitor-1 and tissue factor mRNA expression without changing that of tissue type plasminogen activator or tissue factor pathway inhibitor in cultured rat aortic endothelial cells. *Thromb Haemost* 1997; 77: 1189–1195.

151. Zaman AK, Fujii S, Sawa H, Goto D, Ishimori N, Watano K, Kaneko T, Furumoto T, Sugawara T, Sakuma I, Kitabatake A, Sobel BE. Angiotensin-converting enzyme inhibition attenuates hypofibrinolysis and reduces cardiac perivascular fibrosis in genetically obese diabetic mice. *Circulation* 2001; 103: 3123–3128.

152. Napoleone E, Di Santo A, Camera M, Tremoli E, Lorenzet R. Angiotensin-converting enzyme inhibitors downregulate tissue factor synthesis in monocytes. *Circ Res* 2000; 86: 139–143.

153. Wilcox JN, Smith KM, Schwartz SM, Gordon D. Localization of tissue factor in the normal vessel wall and in the atherosclerotic plaque. *Proc Natl Acad Sci U S A* 1989; 86: 2839–2843.

154. Landers SC, Gupta M, Lewis JC. Ultrastructural localization of tissue factor on monocyte-derived macrophages and macrophage loam cells associated with atherosclerotic lesions. *Virchows Archiv- an Internat. J. Pathol* 1994; 425: 49–54.

155. Marmur JD, Thiruvikraman SV, Fyfe BS, Guha A, Sharma SK, Ambrose JA, Fallon JT, Nemerson Y, Taubman MB. Identification of active tissue factor in human coronary atheroma. *Circulation* 1996; 94: 1226–1232.

156. Toschi V, Gallo R, Lettino M, Fallon JT, Gertz SD, FernandezOrtiz A, Chesebro JH, Badimon L, Nemerson Y, Fuster V, Badimon JJ. Tissue factor modulates the thrombogenicity of human atherosclerotic plaques. *Circulation* 1997; 95: 594–599.

157. Celi A, Cianchetti S, Dell'Omo G, Pedrinelli R. Angiotensin II, tissue factor and the thrombotic paradox of hypertension. *Expert Rev Cardiovasc Ther* 2010; 8: 1723–1729.

158. Schieffer B, Schieffer E, HilfikerKleiner D, Hilfiker A, Kovanen PT, Kaartinen M, Nussberger J, Harringer W, Drexler H. Expression of angiotensin II and interleukin 6 in human coronary atherosclerotic plaques- Potential implications for inflammation and plaque instability. *Circulation* 2000; 101: 1372–1378.

159. Johansson ME, Fagerberg B, Bergstrom G. Angiotensin type 2 receptor is expressed in human atherosclerotic lesions. *J Renin Angiotensin Aldosterone Syst* 2008; 9: 17–21.

160. Pitt B, O'Neill B, Feldman R, Ferrari R, Schwartz L, Mudra H, Bass T, Pepine C, Texter M, Haber H, Uprichard A, Cashin-Hemphill L, Lees RS. The QUinapril Ischemic Event Trial (QUIET): evaluation of chronic ACE inhibitor therapy in patients with ischemic heart disease and preserved left ventricular function. *Am J Cardiol* 2001; 87: 1058–1063.

161. ALLHAT Officers. Major outcomes in high-risk hypertensive patients randomized to angiotensin-converting enzyme inhibitor or calcium channel blocker vs diuretic: The Antihypertensive and Lipid-Lowering Treatment to Prevent Heart Attack Trial (ALLHAT). *JAMA* 2002; 288: 2981–2997.

162. Pitt B. ACE inhibitors for patients with vascular disease without left ventricular dysfunction — may they rest in peace? *N Engl J Med* 2004; 351: 2115–2117.

163. Rouleau JL, Warnica WJ, Baillot R, Block PJ, Chocron S, Johnstone D, Myers MG, Calciu CD, Dalle-Ave S, Martineau P, Mormont C, van Gilst WH. Effects of angiotensin-converting enzyme inhibition in low-risk patients early after coronary artery bypass surgery. *Circulation* 2008; 117: 24–31.

164. Aguilar D, Solomon SD, Kober L, Rouleau JL, Skali H, McMurray JJ, Francis GS, Henis M, O'Connor CM, Diaz R, Belenkov YN, Varshavsky S, Leimberger JD, Velazquez EJ, Califf RM, Pfeffer MA. Newly diagnosed and previously known diabetes mellitus and 1-year outcomes of acute myocardial infarction: the VALsartan In Acute myocardial iNfarcTion (VALIANT) trial. *Circulation* 2004; 110: 1572–1578.

165. Katsuya T, Koike G, Yee TW, Sharpe N, Jackson R, Norton R, Horiuchi M, Pratt RE, Dzau VJ, MacMahon S. Association of angiotensinogen gene T235 variant with increased risk of coronary heart disease. *Lancet* 1995; 345: 1600–1603.

166. Rodriguez-Perez JC, Rodriguez-Esparragon F, Hernandez-Perera O, Anabitarte A, Losada A, Medina A, Hernandez E, Fiuza D, Avalos O, Yunis C, Ferrario CM. Association of angiotensinogen M235T and A(-6) G gene polymorphisms with coronary heart disease with independence of essential hypertension: the PROCAGENE study. Prospective Cardiac Gene. *J Am Coll Cardiol* 2001; 37: 1536–1542.

167. Sethi AA, Nordestgaard BG, Gronholdt ML, Steffensen R, Jensen G, Tybjaerg-Hansen A. Angiotensinogen single nucleotide polymorphisms, elevated blood pressure, and risk of cardiovascular disease. *Hypertension* 2003; 41: 1202–1211.

168. Zafarmand MH, van der Schouw YT, Grobbee DE, de Leeuw PW, Bots ML. The M235T polymorphism in the AGT gene and CHD risk: evidence of a Hardy–Weinberg equilibrium violation and publication bias in a meta-analysis. *PLoS One* 2008; 3: e2533.

169. Rigat B, Hubert C, Alhenc-Gelas F, Cambien F, Corvol P, Soubrier F. An insertion/deletion polymorphism in the angiotensin I-converting enzyme gene accounting for half the variance of serum enzyme levels. *J Clin Invest* 1990; 86: 1343–1346.

170. Cambien F, Poirier O, Lecerf L, Evans A, Cambou JP, Arveiler D, Luc G, Bard JM, Bara L, Ricard S, et al. Deletion polymorphism in the gene for angiotensin-converting enzyme is a potent risk factor for myocardial infarction. *Nature* 1992; 359: 641–644.

171. Petrovic D, Peterlin B. Pharmacogenomic considerations of the insertion/deletion gene polymorphism of the angiotensin I-converting enzyme and coronary artery disease. *Curr Vasc Pharmacol* 2004; 2: 271–279.

172. Lindpaintner K, Pfeffer MA, Kreutz R, Stampfer MJ, Grodstein F, LaMotte F, Buring J, Hennekens CH. A prospective evaluation of an angiotensin-converting-enzyme gene polymorphism and the risk of ischemic heart disease. *N Engl J Med* 1995; 332: 706–711.

173. Kitsios G, Zintzaras E. ACE (I/D) polymorphism and response to treatment in coronary artery disease: a comprehensive database and meta-analysis involving study quality evaluation. *BMC Med Genet* 2009; 10: 50.

174. Sayed-Tabatabaei FA, Oostra BA, Isaacs A, van Duijn CM, Witteman JC. ACE polymorphisms. *Circ Res* 2006; 98: 1123–1133.

175. Suchankova P, Henningsson S, Olsson M, Baghaei F, Rosmond R, Holm G, Eriksson E, Ekman A. Association between the AGTR1 polymorphism +1166A>C and serum levels of high-sensitivity C-reactive protein. *Regul Pept* 2009; 152: 28–32.

176. Underwood PC, Sun B, Williams JS, Pojoga LH, Chamarthi B, Lasky-Su J, Raby BA, Hopkins PN, Jeunemaitre X, Brown NJ, Adler GK, Williams GH. The relationship between peroxisome proliferator-activated receptor-gamma and renin: a human genetics study. *J Clin Endocrinol Metab* 2010; 95: E75–E79.

177. Zhu S, Meng QH. Association of angiotensin II type 1 receptor gene polymorphism with carotid atherosclerosis. *Clin Chem Lab Med* 2006; 44: 282–284.

178. Fernandez-Arcas N, Dieguez-Lucena JL, Munoz-Moran E, Ruiz-Galdon M, Espinosa-Caliani S, Aranda-Lara P, Martinez-Espigares S, Banderas-Donaire MJ, De Teresa-Galvan E, Reyes-Engel A. The genotype interactions of methylenetetrahydrofolate reductase and renin-angiotensin system genes are associated with myocardial infarction. *Atherosclerosis* 1999; 145: 293–300.

179. Jeunemaitre X, Ledru F, Battaglia S, Guillanneuf MT, Courbon D, Dumont C, Darmon O, Guize L, Guermonprez JL, Diebold B, Ducimetiere P. Genetic polymorphisms of the renin-angiotensin system and angiographic extent and severity of coronary artery disease: the CORGENE study. *Hum Genet* 1997; 99: 66–73.

180. Gruchala M, Ciecwierz D, Ochman K, Wasag B, Koprowski A, Wojtowicz A, Dubaniewicz W, Targonski R, Sobiczewski W, Grzybowski A, Romanowski P, Limon J, Rynkiewicz A. Left ventricular size, mass

and function in relation to angiotensin-converting enzyme gene and angiotensin-II type 1 receptor gene polymorphisms in patients with coronary artery disease. *Clin Chem Lab Med* 2003; 41: 522–528.

181. Burdon KP, Langefeld CD, Beck SR, Wagenknecht LE, Carr JJ, Freedman BI, Herrington D, Bowden DW. Association of genes of lipid metabolism with measures of subclinical cardiovascular disease in the Diabetes Heart Study. *J Med Genet* 2005; 42: 720–724.

182. Alfakih K, Lawrance RA, Maqbool A, Walters K, Ball SG, Balmforth AJ, Hall AS. The clinical significance of a common, functional, X-linked angiotensin II type 2-receptor gene polymorphism (-1332 G/A) in a cohort of 509 families with premature coronary artery disease. *Eur Heart J* 2005; 26: 584–589.

183. Alfakih K, Brown B, Lawrance RA, Warburton P, Maqbool A, Walters K, Samani NJ, Ball SG, Balmforth AJ, Hall AS. Effect of a common X-linked angiotensin II type 2-receptor gene polymorphism (-1332 G/A) on the occurrence of premature myocardial infarction and stenotic atherosclerosis requiring revascularization. *Atherosclerosis* 2007; 195: e32–38.

184. Jones A, Dhamrait SS, Payne JR, Hawe E, Li P, Toor IS, Luong L, Wootton PT, Miller GJ, Humphries SE, Montgomery HE. Genetic variants of angiotensin II receptors and cardiovascular risk in hypertension. *Hypertension* 2003; 42: 500–506.

185. Tousoulis D, Koumallos N, Antoniades C, Antonopoulos AS, Bakogiannis C, Milliou A, Marinou K, Kallikazarou E, Stefanadi E, Mentzikof D, Stefanadis C. Genetic polymorphism on type 2 receptor of angiotensin II, modifies cardiovascular risk and systemic inflammation in hypertensive males. *Am J Hypertens* 2010; 23: 237–242.

186. Xu M, Sham P, Ye Z, Lindpaintner K, He L. A1166C genetic variation of the angiotensin II type I receptor gene and susceptibility to coronary heart disease: collaborative of 53 studies with 20,435 cases and 23,674 controls. *Atherosclerosis* 2010; 213: 191–199.

187. Kretowski A, McFann K, Hokanson JE, Maahs D, Kinney G, Snell-Bergeon JK, Wadwa RP, Eckel RH, Ogden L, Garg S, Li J, Cheng S, Erlich HA, Rewers M. Polymorphisms of the renin-angiotensin system genes predict progression of subclinical coronary atherosclerosis. *Diabetes* 2007; 56: 863–871.

188. Tsai CT, Hwang JJ, Ritchie MD, Moore JH, Chiang FT, Lai LP, Hsu KL, Tseng CD, Lin JL, Tseng YZ. Renin-angiotensin system gene polymorphisms and coronary artery disease in a large angiographic cohort: detection of high order gene-gene interaction. *Atherosclerosis* 2007; 195: 172–180.

189. Lin J, Hu FB, Qi L, Curhan GC. Genetic polymorphisms of angiotensin-2 type 1 receptor and angiotensinogen and risk of renal dysfunction and coronary heart disease in type 2 diabetes mellitus. *BMC Nephrol* 2009; 10: 9.

190. Franco E, Palumbo L, Crobu F, Anselmino M, Frea S, Matullo G, Piazza A, Trevi GP, Bergerone S. Renin-angiotensin-aldosterone system polymorphisms: a role or a hole in occurrence and long-term prognosis of acute myocardial infarction at young age. *BMC Med Genet* 2007; 8: 27.

191. Kooperberg C, Bis JC, Marciante KD, Heckbert SR, Lumley T, Psaty BM. Logic regression for analysis of the association between genetic variation in the renin-angiotensin system and myocardial infarction or stroke. *Am J Epidemiol* 2007; 165: 334–343.

Chapter 9

Role of Matrix Metalloproteinases as Targets for the Prevention of Atherosclerosis

Andrew C. Newby
Bristol Heart Institute, University of Bristol, Bristol Royal Infirmary, Bristol BS28HW, UK
a.newby@bris.ac.uk

9.1 Key Role of Extracellular Proteolysis at all Stages of Atherosclerosis

Atherosclerosis is defined as the accumulation of excess lipid, foam cells, and connective tissue in the arterial intima [1]. One of the earliest steps is the ingress of inflammatory cells through the junctional complexes of activated endothelial cells (ECs), which may require tightly regulated proteolysis [2]. Subsequent movement of inflammatory cells into the deeper layers of the intima and media also requires proteolysis of extracellular matrix (ECM) [3] to remove physical barriers and release latent factors, such as chemo-attractants [4]. Proteolysis of LDL can promote uptake into macrophages and, therefore, aid foam-cell formation [5]. The ability of foam cells not

Atherosclerosis: Treatment and Prevention
Edited by Christian Weber and Oliver Soehnlein

ISBN 978-981-4316-26-2 (Hardcover), ISBN 978-981-4364-26-3 (eBook)
www.panstanford.com

only to migrate but also to proliferate or undergo apoptosis is also regulated in part by proteolysis [6]. Migration of foam cells to the base of lesions and their subsequent apoptosis and necrosis are key events in generating the lipid pool of atherosclerotic plaques [7]. Proteolysis of the ECM plays a major role in liberating vascular smooth muscle cells (VSMC) from their normal quiescent, contractile state and promoting modulation to a more synthetic phenotype [8]. These modified VSMCs are capable of moving, proliferating, and synthesizing ECM components to build up a fibrous cap over the lipid cores of advanced atherosclerotic plaques. However, VSMCs also have an increased propensity to secrete extracellular proteinases and to undergo apoptosis, which promotes thinning of plaque caps and generation of acellular connective tissue [9]. Proteolysis of such acellular ECM, which has little chance of resynthesis, may be an important trigger for plaque rupture, which precipitates the majority of myocardial infarctions [10]. Detachment of ECs from the ECM, most likely the results of proteolysis, may lead to "endothelial erosion," the cause of most of the remaining myocardial infarctions [10]. Hence extracellular proteolysis appears to be a proximal cause of acute coronary syndromes and an attractive target for therapeutic intervention. However, designing therapies demands clear identification of the proteinase involved and development of clinically useful inhibitors. Progress towards these aims is discussed below for one family of extracellular proteinases, the matrix degrading metalloproteinases (MMPs) also known as matrixins [4].

9.2 Characteristics of the MMP Family

MMPs comprise 23 structurally related Zn^{2+}-dependent endopeptidases [4] that are either secreted into the extracellular space or attached to the external face of the plasma membrane. What makes the MMPs particularly interesting as therapeutic targets is their combined substrate repertoire, which encompasses collagens, elastins, proteoglycan core proteins, and matrix glycoproteins [4]. Hence, the combined action of MMPs should be sufficient to extensively degrade a fully mature ECM. There is also an increasingly long list of cell surface and matrix-associated protein substrates [4]. Shedding of cell surface proteins or activation of latent mediators by MMPs can modulate many cellular functions [4], such as migration, proliferation and apoptosis of connective tissue and other cells [8]. The different MMPs are made up by combinations of eight structural motifs, namely, signal sequence, pro-peptide, catalytic subunit, with or without fibronectin-like inserts, hinge region, haemopexin-like (Pex) domain, and either a membrane spanning domain or Glycosylphosphatidylinositol (GPI) anchor in membrane-type MMPs (MT-MMPs) (Fig. 9.1).

The catalytic domain of the MMPs is the most highly conserved, although it is interrupted in MMP-2 and -9 by fibronectin repeats that confer avidity for gelatin. Several histidines in the catalytic site, which usually make up a motif HEXXHXXGXXH, hold the Zn^{2+} ion. This activates a water molecule, which serves as the nucleophile in the cleavage of peptide bonds. This catalytic domain is found also in the adamalysins, which comprise a membrane attached disintgrin and metalloproteinase group (ADAMs) and a group of secreted proteins that have additional thrombospondin domains (ADAMTSs). Some but not all of the adamlysins have catalytic domains that retain proteolytic activity [11]; they are often inhibited by small molecular weight inhibitors directed at the catalytic site of the MMPs, which complicates their pharmacology. Blockade of the catalytic site by intramolecular and intermolecular protein-protein interaction is important for the normal regulation of MMP activity. Most MMPs are secreted as inactive proforms in which a cysteine residue in the propeptide wraps around and occupies the catalytic site, complexing the Zn^{2+} ion (Fig. 9.1, 9.2A). Multi-step proteolysis of the propeptide releases the so-called "cysteine switch" in all but MMP-23 and allows the MMP to become active [4] (Fig. 9.2A). By cleaving the propeptide at the "bait" region (Fig. 9.2), other MMPs or other classes of proteinase (e.g., trypsin, plasmin, and thrombin) can activate MMPs in proteolytic cascades. Non-proteolytic (e.g., oxidation, nitrosylation) mechanisms are also feasible (Fig. 9.2A). In the case of the MT-MMPs, MMP-11, and MMP-23, pro-peptide processing occurs within the endosome by the action of furin before the MMP appears at the cell surface (Fig. 9.2A). Active MMPs can be inhibited by binding to endogenous tissue inhibitors of metalloproteinases (TIMPs) of which there are four family members (Fig. 9.1). The N-terminal region of TIMPs complexes with the active site Zn^{2+} ion and blocks the active site cleft. In general TIMPs inhibit most MMPs, except that TIMP-1 is a poor inhibitor of MMPs-14, -16, -19, and -24. TIMP-2 has a

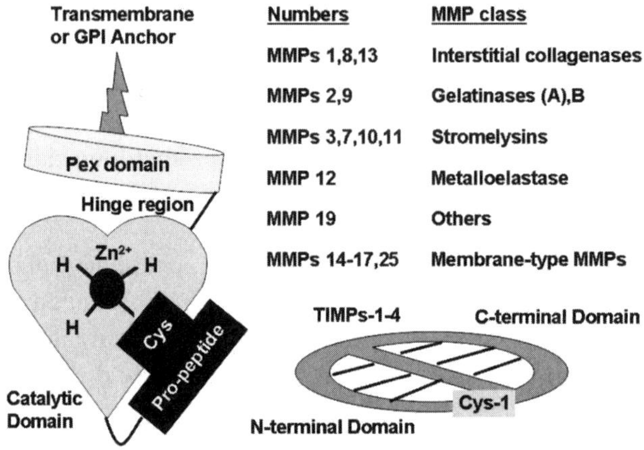

Figure 9.1 Structure and function of metalloproteinases expressed in vascular cells. In the active form of all matrix metalloproteinases (MMPs) the catalytic Zn^{2+} ion is coordinated by three histidines and the fourth co-ordination site activates a water molecule (not shown) that acts as the nucleophile. The fourth co-ordination site may be occupied in an inactive complex with the N-terminal residue of a tissue inhibitor of metalloproteinases (TIMP). Most MMPs have a C-terminal Pex domain linked to the catalytic domain by a hinge region. The Pex domain is absent in the matrilysins, MMP-7 and -26, and is replaced by a cysteine rich domain in MMP-23. The MT-MMPs have an addition membrane spanning domain or a site of attachment for a glycophosphatidylinositol (GPI) anchor. MMPs fall into functional groups based on substrate specificity. Interstitial collagenase can cleave fibrillar collagens, gelatinases denatured collagens, and stromelysins most ECM proteins except fibrillar collagens. MMP-12 is active against elastin. MT-MMPs cleave matrix components but are also active as sheddases. For a fuller description of the ECM and non-ECM substrates of MMPs, see the review by Nagase and colleagues [4]. Each of the four TIMPs has an N-terminal and C-terminal domain with three disulphide bridges each. The N-terminal cysteine (Cys) interacts with the catalytic Zn^{2+} ion of MMPs to inhibit activity.

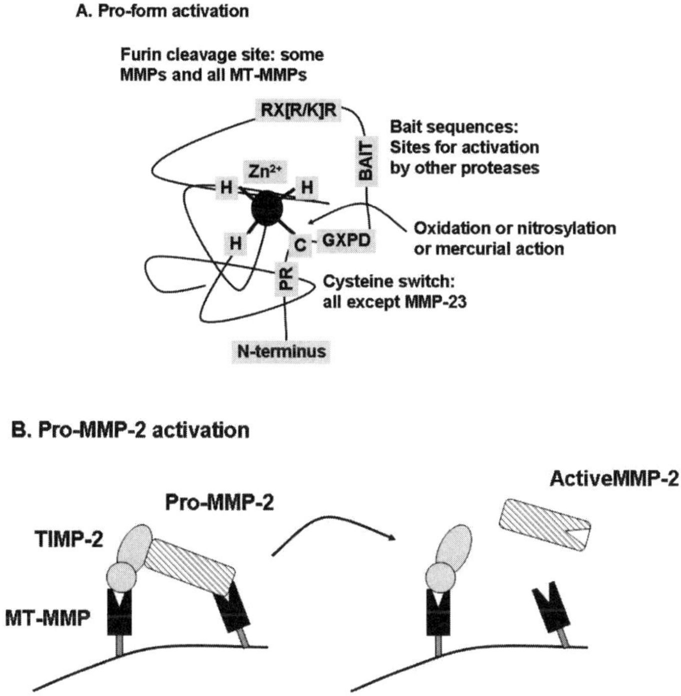

Figure 9.2 Metalloproteinase activation. (A) Pro-form activation can take place by a variety of mechanisms that destabilise the interaction of a crucial cysteine (C) residue that coordinates the catalytic Zn^{2+} ion (in all but MMP-23). This can be brought about by chemical means, such as oxidation, nitrosylation, or *in vitro* with mercurial compounds. The commonest mechanisms are, however, proteolytic, either in the endosome for MMPs that have furin recognition sequences, or extracellularly for MMPs that have susceptible "bait" residues for other proteases. (B) MMP-2 activation occurs at the cell surface by unique mechanism brought about by all MT-MMPs (except MT4-MMP). Only TIMP-2 can act as a cofactor in this mechanism. The N-terminal domain of TIMP-2 sits in the catalytic site and inactivates one molecule of MT-MMP. The C-terminus of the same molecule of TIMP-2 acts as a receptor for a molecule of pro-MMP-2 and presents it to a second un-complexed molecule of MT-MMP. The concentration of TIMP-2 is critical; if there is none, not MMP-2, and MT-MMPs do not come into close contact; if there is too much all the MT-MMP is present as inactive complexes.

unique ability to act as a co-factor in activation of MMP-2 by MMP-14 thanks to its ability to bind also to the haemopexin domain of pro-MMP-2 through its C-terminal domain (Fig. 9.2B). As a result low concentrations of TIMP-2 promote activation of MMP-2 by bringing its pro-peptide into proximity with active MT1-MMP. However, high concentrations inhibit the activity of MT1-MMP and block processing of MMP-2. TIMP-1 and, especially, TIMP-3 inhibit several ADAMs as well as MMPs. TIMP-3 is also unusual in that it binds strongly to the ECM, which appears to stabilise TIMP-3 and confine it to the peri-cellular environment. TIMP-4 is less abundant in vascular cells and is, therefore, less studied. The structurally unrelated membrane attached metalloproteinase inhibitor reversion-inducing cysteine-rich protein with Kazal motifs (RECK) is, however, well described, especially in the context of angiogenesis [12, 13].

All the C-terminal domains of MMPs are lacking in the matrilysins, MMP-7 and -26, and in MMP-25 (MT6-MMP); these domains are, therefore, dispensable for activity, although they confer additional functions. For example, membrane spanning domains or GPI anchor sequences direct attachment of MT-MMPs to the cell membrane. The hemopexin domain helps to confer specificity in the collagenase, MMP-1, and is responsible for binding TIMP-2 to MMP-2 during its activation by MT-MMPs (Fig. 9.2B). Pex domains also mediate binding of proMMP-9 with TIMP-1 and TIMP-3 through their C-terminal domains. ProMMP-9 also binds to CD44 on the cell surface, which may be important to localise its activity during polarised cell movement. Pro-MMP-9 is disulphide bonded to neutrophil gelatinase associated lipocalin-like molecule (NGAL) in neutrophil granules and in the soluble form secreted from many vascular cells, although the functional significance of complex formation is not clear. The Pex domain is replaced by a cysteine rich domain in MMP-23 [4].

9.3 Regulation of MMP Activity in Vascular Cells

Transcriptional control is undoubtedly the most important determinant of the activity of MMPs [14]. Transcriptional control operates at many levels, including, species, cell type, developmental stage as well as in response to activators. For example, MMP-13 appears to substitute in all tissues of mice and rats for the functions of MMP-1 in humans [4]. More subtle differences are also apparent. For example, MMP-2 is a more abundant gelatinase than MMP-9 in mouse macrophages, but the opposite is true in humans and rabbits. MMP-23 is abundantly expressed in mouse but not human macrophages, and MMP-25 in human but not mice. These differences are more than academic when considering the weight placed on mice as models for atherosclerosis research and drug development.

Similarities and differences exist in regulation of the same MMP genes in different vascular cells. However, few studies have quantified expression of a comprehensive range of MMPs, even at the mRNA level, and so findings are frustratingly fragmentary and incomplete. Recent reviews have dealt separately with what is known of the regulation of MMPs in VSMCs [15], ECs [16], and monocyte/macrophages [17], which have been extensively studied. Much less is known about other leukocytes found in plaques but this has been reviewed also [15]. The discussion here will emphasize broad principles and comparisons.

Table 9.1 illustrates the pattern of constitutive expression of MMPs and TIMPs in human vascular cells. Notable is the high constitutive expression of mRNAs for MMP-1, -2, -10 and MT1-MMP in ECs, MMP-2 and MT1/3-MMP in VSMCs, and MMPs -7, -9, -19 and MT1-MMP in mature macrophages. Messenger RNAs TIMPs-1, -2 are highly expressed constitutively in ECs, VSMCs, and monocytes, but TIMP-3 is induced by PDGF and TGF-β in VSMCs and by unknown mechanisms during the maturation of monocytes to macrophages. The mechanisms responsible for these tissue and developmental stage differences remain largely unknown, which raises the intriguing possibility that such mechanisms could be drug targets to reduce MMP activity.

One of the most interesting developments in recent years has been the realisation that many MMPs are induced by inflammatory mediators, although this should not be extrapolated uncritically to all MMPs in all tissues (see Table 9.1). MMPs-1, -3, -7, -9, -10, -12, -14, and -16 are all induced by Toll-like receptor ligands such as bacterial lipopolysaccharide (LPS) and high-mobility group box 1 [18], cytokines such as interleukin-1β (IL-1β) and tumor necrosis factor-α (TNF-α), CD40 ligand (CD40L) acting through its receptor CD40 and cyclophilin A acting through its receptor EMMPRIN [19].

Table 9.1 Expression patterns of some MMPs in primary human vascular cells

Agonist	None	LPS	IL-1β, TNFα, CD40L	Growth Factor	Forskolin (cAMP)	IFNγ	IL-4	Cell type
MMP-1	++	+++	+++	++	S			EC
	–	++	+*	+*				VSMC
	–	++	++	N	++			Monocyte
	–	++	++	N		I	+/–	Macrophage
MMP-3	–		+	+	S			EC
	–		+*	+*				VSMC
	–	+	+	N				Monocyte
	–	+	+	N		I	–	Macrophage
MMP-7	–			+				EC
	–							VSMC
	–	+	+	++	+			Monocyte
	++	++	++	++		I	+/–	Macrophage
MMP-9	–		+	+	S			EC
	–	+	+*	+*				VSMC
	–	+	+	++	+			Monocyte
	++	++	++	++		I	+/–	Macrophage
MMP-10	+		++	+				EC
	–							VSMC
	–		++	++	++			Monocyte
	–		++	++		I	+/–	Macrophage
MMP-12	–		+					EC
	–							VSMC
	–		+	+	+			Monocyte
	+		++	++		I	+++	Macrophage
MMP-14	+		++	++				EC
(MT1-	++							VSMC
MMP)	+	++	++	+	++			Monocyte
	++	+++	+++	++		+++	+	Macrophage
TIMP-1	+		++	+	S			EC
	++		++	++				VSMC
	++	+++	+++	++				Monocyte
	++	+++	+++	++		I	+/–	Macrophage
TIMP-2	+	+	+	+				EC
	++	++	++	++				VSMC
	++	++	++	++	++	++		Monocyte
	++	++	++	++		++	++	Macrophage

Agonist	None	LPS	IL-1β, TNFα, CD40L	Growth Factor	Forskolin (cAMP)	IFNγ	IL-4	Cell type
TIMP-3	–							EC
	–							VSMC
	–	–	–	++		+	+++	Monocyte
	++	++	++	++		+	+++	Macrophage

Note: The table shows constitutive expression levels or levels in the presence of individual agonists. For details, see the text and previous reviews [15, 17]. * = synergy between growth factors and cytokines. S = stimulatory with other agonists, I = inhibitory against other agonists.

There are some interesting cell-type differences. For example, MMP-7 and MMP-9 are inducible in ECs and VSMCs and some monocytic cell lines but constitutive in mature human macrophages and rabbit foam cells [20, 21].

The binding site for activator protein-1 (AP-1) in the proximal promoter of several MMP genes undoubtedly plays an important role in regulation of many MMP genes, and SP-1 sites are important in others [14]. As a result, pharmacological inhibition of activators of these transcription factors, e.g., mitogen activated protein kinases (MAPKs), including extracellular related kinases (ERKs1/2) and c-Jun N-terminal kinase (JNK) selectively block induction of MMPs by inflammatory mediators, while leaving constitutive expression unaffected [21]. Other pathways responsible for stimulated but not constitutive MMP production include protein kinase C (PKC) (including isoforms that respond to phorbol esters and those that do not [22]) and phosphoinositide-3-kinase (PI3K) [14]. MAPKs, PKC, and PI3K are important in a plethora of cellular functions, reducing their attractiveness as therapeutic targets. Induction of several MMPs, but by no means all, depends on nuclear transcription factor-κB (NF-κB) [20, 23], which is a signature transcription factor for inflammatory genes. Futhermore, AP-1 and NF-κB pathways synergise to induce several MMPs in VSMCs [23] and other cells. Surprisingly though, only the MMP-1 and -9 (and possibly the MMP-19) promoters have a clearly definable NF-κB binding sites in their proximal promoters [14]. The basis for the apparent synergy between AP-1 and NF-κB for induction several other MMPs remains an enigma.

The effect of interferon-γ (IFN-γ) on MMP induction is paradoxical. IFN-γ is clearly a pro-inflammatory mediator that gives rise to classical macrophage activation, but it inhibits production of many MMPs in VSMCs [15] and monocyte/macrophages [17].

The underlying mechanism needs further study because it could be a route to anti-MMP therapy. IL-4, a mediator of alternative macrophage activation, also inhibits production of most MMPs but the matrix metalloelastase, MMP-12, is an exception being strongly up-regulated by IL-4 [17]. This pathway of MMP-12 activation is believed to be important in aneurysm formation [24] and is, therefore, deserving of further study.

Consistent with their natures as inflammatory genes, many MMPs are inhibited by anti-inflammatory nuclear hormone receptor ligands, including glucocorticoids, estrogens, and peroxisome proliferator activator receptors (PPARs) [15, 17]. Anti-inflammatory cytokines, including transforming growth factor-β and IL-10, also inhibit transcription of many MMPs [15, 17]. It seems likely that inhibition of MMPs contributes to the beneficial effects of these mediators on atherosclerosis development, although this has only rarely been tested directly. One mouse study highlighted MMP-13 in this context [25] but this gene appears much less important than MMP-1 in humans.

Important roles for other mediators in inducing or repressing MMP genes have also been described. Not surprisingly, MMPs that are inducible by inflammatory mediators can also be up-regulated by reactive oxygen species either by activating ERKs or NFκB. This might also account for the induction of several MMPs by hypoxia. However, strong up-regulation of MMP-7 by hypoxia probably occurs indirectly by triggering the Wnt/β-catenin pathway [26], which acts through TCF/LEF-1 promoter elements [14]. Elevating intracellular cAMP induces several MMPs in ECs [27] and monocytes [17] through poorly defined downstream pathways. Pro-inflammatory prostaglandins are clearly important mediators for cAMP-dependent MMP production in monocytes [17], although prostaglandin independent-pathways run in parallel [21, 28]. The cAMP pathway can antagonise NF-κB under some circumstances, and this might give rise to conflicting results.

Biomechanical factors are also important, in particular stretch and shear force. For example, cyclical stretch was reported to increase

MMP-2 expression from VSMCs [29]. Shear stress is especially relevant for ECs, since high average laminar stress is associated with protection from inflammation, oxidant stress, and atherosclerosis [30]. High shear is associated with reduction in production of inflammatory genes [31] and so one might expect this to extend to MMPs. On the other hand, shear-stress induced enlargement of the mouse carotid artery was mediated by up-regulation and activation of MMP-9 as an indirect consequence of peroxynitrite formation [32].

Other levels of regulation than transcription are undoubtedly important for MMP activity in vascular cells. Up-regulation of most MMPs proteins closely follows the mRNAs, except perhaps for MMP-14. Nevertheless, translational control of the MMP mRNAs is under-researched, and the field may hide some secrets. Secretion of MMP-8 and MMP-9 from preformed, stored pools occurs in neutrophils and to some extent in macrophages. Pro-form activation is clearly of key functional importance for all MMPs. One clear example is the experiment of Gough and colleagues [33], who showed that transgenic ApoE null mice over-expressing wild-type pro-MMP-9 had unaltered plaque development. On the other hand, transgenic mice with an auto-activated form of pro-MMP-9 suffered extensive plaque disruption. The implication is that MMP-9 activation is tightly controlled even in ApoE null mouse plaques, and this limits the possible deleterious effects of the MMP. While it is easy to draw theoretical activation cascades based on *in vitro* work, relatively few studies have examined their operation *in vivo*. Early work showed that plasmin plays a major part in MMP activation in injured myocardium *in vivo* [34], although similar studies have not been reported in atherosclerosis models. Chymase and tryptase from mast cells have also been implicated, at least in vascular injury models [35]. Oxidant stress and nitric oxide can open the cysteine switch and activate MMPs *in vitro* [36], and there is evidence for this mechanism operating *in vivo* [32]. Binding to TIMPs is also an important step in regulating MMP activity. Indeed, constitutively produced TIMPs are probably at higher levels than MMPs in normal vessels [37]. There is obvious redundancy between the TIMPs, and there is also back-up from lower affinity, general protease inhibitors, such as α2macroglogulin [4]. This probably accounts for the mild phenotypes for individual TIMP knockouts. TIMP-3 may be an exception because of its unique localisation through tight binding to the ECM [4]. TIMP-3 null mice have a temporal defect in bone elongation as a result of altered chondroplasia and invasion of the growth plate by macrophages [38].

9.4 Functional Effects of MMPs and TIMPs

9.4.1 Endothelial Cells

The participation of MMPs and their natural inhibitors in angiogenesis have been exhaustively reviewed [12, 13, 39]. The strongest evidence is for involvement of MMP-2 and -9 and MT1-MMP, which probably act together and with other classes of protease, including adamalysins and cathepsins [13, 39]. MMP-2 and -9 and MT1-MMP are all able to degrade basement membrane components, which is necessary for ECs to establish new sprouts and then effect tube formation [40] (Fig. 9.3). ECs can form podosomes or podosome type adhesions (PTAs), which are ring-like, actin-rich adhesive structures that can localise MT1-MMP with its binding partner MMP-2 and MMP-9 with its transmembrane receptor CD44 [41], thereby focusing MMP degradation on the underlying matrix [42]. Other MMPs, including recently MMP-10 [43], have been ascribed roles in ECM remodelling to promote angiogenesis [13, 39]. Other ways for MMPs to promote angiogenesis have also been discussed. For example, cyclical MT1-MMP activation and deactivation may help locomotion of ECs (and indeed other vascular cells) through the ECM [13] (see Fig. 9.3). Several MMPs have the ability to free latent angiogenic growth factors from attachment to the ECM [13, 39] (Fig. 9.3). On the contrary, however, fragmentation of ECM and other proteins by MMPs can generate angiostatic factors and this may account for the paradoxical activity of MMP-12 and -19 to inhibit angiogenesis [39].

9.4.2 Vascular Smooth Muscle Cells

The role of MMPs in the migration, proliferation, and death of VSMCs has been previously reviewed in depth [8]. Under baseline conditions, VSMCs express pro-MMP-2, MT-1 and MT3-MMPs, and TIMPs-1 and -2 [44]. Resting VSMCs have no detectable active MMP-2, and there

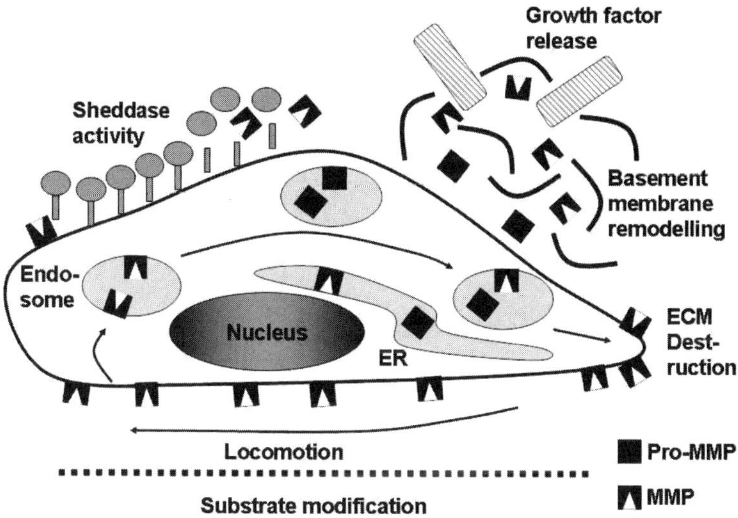

Figure 9.3. Proposed functions for MMPs in vascular cells. MMPs are formed in the endoplasmic reticulum (ER) and passed into endosomes. Soluble MMPs are mostly secreted as pro-forms but become activated in the extracellular matrix . MT-MMPs are presented on the cell surface as active enzymes. Active MMPs can modify the cell surface and surrounding ECM. This may result in the removal of physical barriers to motion or may disturb existing cell-ECM and cell-cell contacts. It may also release factors sequestered in the ECM and promote new cell-ECM interactions. MT-MMPs can act as adhesion sites for directed migration.

is, therefore, a very low level or no turnover of their surrounding basement membrane. After injury or during inflammation, however, they turn on MMP-1, -3, -7, and -12 genes (at least), up-regulate MT1 and 3-MMPs, activate MMP-2, and extensively degrade their basement membrane [45] (Fig. 9.3). MMPs also cleave cell surface components (Fig. 9.3), including, importantly, cadherins [46]. Cleavage of cell-basement membrane and cell-cell cadherin contacts liberates VSMCs to move and proliferate so as to repair damaged tissue and form a neointima [8]. MMPs may also liberate latent growth factors bound to the ECM and remodel specific ECM components so as to generate adhesion sites for cells to migrate over [47] (Fig. 9.3). Cell-ECM and cell-cell contacts are also vital to regulate cell cycle entry and apoptosis of VSMCs [8]. Increased proliferation of VSMCs partly reflects the essential role of cell-matrix contacts in cell cycle progression [48] and partly the permissive effect of cadherin cleavage [49]. Increased migration and proliferation associate with increased propensity for apoptosis, which may prevent excessive neointima formation [8]. Paradoxically, however, TIMP-3 over-expression promotes apoptosis [50], which implies that proteolysis needs to be neither too much nor too little for cells to survive.

9.4.3 Monocytes and Macrophages

Circulating human monocytes express high levels of TIMPs-1 and -2 mRNAs but lower levels of MMPs-8, -9, -19 and MT1-MMP [21, 51], which implies that any MMP activity expressed by monocytes is tightly regulated. Monocytes rapidly up-regulate MMP-1, -7, -10, and -12 and further increase expression of MMP-19 and MT1-MMP after adhesion for just 2 hours [21]. All of these MMPs might, therefore, be involved in endothelial transmigration or early penetration of monocytes into the intima. Interestingly, a similar group of MMPs has been implicated in monocyte migration during xenopus embryo development [3]. *In vitro* experiments show that MMP-14 mediates ICAM-dependent monocyte migration across ECs [2]. More explicit *in vivo* data in atherosclerosis models would be very welcome. Recruitment of macrophages into subcutaneous sponges depends on MMP-12 in mice [52, 53]. Given that pro-inflammatory mediators, including cytokines, pathogen associated molecular patterns, and alarmins, further increase expression of MMPs-1, -3, -7, -9, -10, -12, and MT1-MMP [17, 19, 21], these MMPs may well aid penetration of monocytes to sites of acute inflammation, although this needs to be demonstrated.

Differentiation to macrophages down-regulates MMP-1 and -10 and TIMP-1 but up-regulates MMPs-2,-7, -9 -12, and MT1-MMP expression and greatly increases that of TIMP-3 [21]. What effect these changes have on the ability of macrophages to migrate compared to monocytes is unknown [21]. Pro-inflammatory mediators selectively up-regulate MMP-1, -3, -10, -12, and MT1-MMP and down-regulate TIMP-3 expression in macrophages [17] and presumably facilitate macrophage migration, although direct evidence is lacking. Rabbit foam cell macrophages generated *in vivo* selectively over-express MMP-1, -3, -12, and MT1-MMP and down-regulate TIMP-3 compared to non-foamy macrophages [6, 20, 54]. Hence, foam cell formation *in vivo* seems to replicate the selective changes in MMP expression seen with pro-inflammatory mediators. A further interesting and unexpected conclusion emerges from these studies. Rabbit foam cells contain distinct MT1-MMPhighTIMP-3low and MT1-MMPlowTIMP-3high populations, showing that regulation of MMPs might be heterogeneous between different populations of macrophages. MT1-MMPhighTIMP-3low populations of rabbit foam cells are more destructive in an *in situ* zymography assay, invade matrigel, proliferate and undergo apoptosis more readily than MT1-MMPlowTIMP-3high populations [6]. All these differences are abolished by an inhibitory anti-MT1-MMP antibody [6]. TIMP-3high and TIMP-3low foam cells were also observed in human plaques [6]. Being highly destructive, invasive and readily undergoing apoptosis would make MT1-MMPhighTIMP-3low foam cells likely to thin the fibrous caps and generate the lipid core, making plaques more vulnerable to rupture. A similar role for MT1-MMPs emerges from experiments using gene transfer of TIMP-1 and TIMP-2 [55] in mice. Only TIMP-2 reduces plaque size and promotes foam cell apoptosis in mouse plaques, and MT1-MMP is the most highly expressed MMP that fails to be inhibited by TIMP-1.

9.5 Genetic Manipulation of MMPs and TIMPs in Experimental Models of Atherosclerosis

Rabbits and mice have been extensively used to study initiation and progression of atherosclerosis, but, sadly, we currently have no good experimental models for plaque rupture or erosion. Advanced plaques of aged, chow-fed, ApoE null mice have intra-plaque haemorrhages close to lateral xanthomas (accumulations of foam cells) [56]. Several independent studies showed that similar acute disruptions can occur in fat-fed ApoE mice at early time points [57]. The early lesions are "plaque ruptures" semantically, but they do not look anything like the ones in human plaques; the disrupted part of the fibrous cap is extremely thin and rarely contains smooth muscle cells. Hence, most pathologists are understandably reluctant even to use the term plaque rupture for the mouse disruptions. Multiple smooth muscle cells and connective tissue layers are also seen in early mouse plaques; their occurrence is associated with fibrin deposition and so might be evidence of previous ruptures [57]. Placing a restrictive collar around the carotid artery of fat-fed ApoE null mice produces very rapidly developing lesions that can show intra-plaque haemorrhage if other adverse stimuli are superadded [58, 59]. However, these lesions bear little morphological resemblance to human ruptured plaques. There has been even less progress in generating an animal model of endothelial erosion. Even the plaques of fat-fed ApoE null mice have a high degree of endothelial cover.

In the absence of any good models, a large number of MMP transgenic and knockout studies of MMPs and TIMPs have been conducted in mouse and rabbits (see Table 9.2) using presumptive criteria of plaque vulnerability, including increased plaque size, fewer VSMC, more macrophages, and decreased collagen content, features seen in vulnerable human plaques. Additional markers of instability included disruption of elastic fibres in the media at the base of plaques, intraplaque haemorrhage, and the occurrence of buried fibrous caps.

As noted above, mouse MMP-1 is not expressed, but human MMP-1 transgenic mice have smaller plaques with less collagen [60] (Table 9.2). Over-expressing wild-type pro-MMP-9 in macrophages does not affect atherosclerosis in ApoE null mice, but auto-activatable pro- MMP-9 greatly reduces plaque stability [33]. Similarly, adenovirus-mediated over-expression of MMP-9 disrupted advanced plaques caused by collar implantation into ApoE null mice [59]. Hence, enough active MMP-9 can be disruptive as expected.

When MMP knockouts were studied, both protective and adverse effects were noted (Table 9.2). MMP-2 knockout reduced VSMC accumulation in plaques, suggesting less stable cap formation, perhaps related to the loss of effects on migration and proliferation of VSMCs. MMP-3 knockout increased plaque size and buried fibrous in one study [63], implying less stability, but decreased macrophage content and elastin breaks in another [62], implying greater stability. This might be explained by the balance of effects on migration of macrophages and VSMCs. MMP-7 deletion had little effect except to increase VSMC content in one study [63]. MMP-8 knockout decreased lesion formation but, most likely, via a complex systemic mechanism [65]. MMP-8 null mice showed reduced conversion of angiotensin I to angiotensin II and hence lower blood pressure [65], which would

Table 9.2 Effects of MMP interventions in atherosclerotic plaque development and stability

Number	Site	Size	SMC	Macrophages	ECM Integrity	Overall Stability	References
MMP-1 ++	Root/arch	↓	=	=	↓	=	[60]
MMP-2 null	Root/arch	↓	↓	=	=	↓	[61]
MMP-3 null	Ao, BCA	↑ , ↑	? , ↓	↓ , =	↑ , ?	↑ , ↓	[62, 63]
MMP-7 null	BCA	=	↑	=	?	=	[63]
MMP-9 null	Ao, BCA	↓ , ↑	? , ↓	↓ , ↑	↓↑ , =	↑ , ↓	[63, 64]
MMP-8 null	Ao	↓	=	↓	↑	↑	[65]
MMP-9 ++ MMP-9 ++a	Arch, BCA	=, =	=, =	=, =	=, =	=, ↓	[33, 59]
MMP-12 null	Arch, BCA			=	=	↓	[33]
MMP-12 ++a	Ao, BCA	= , ↓	= , ↑	=, ↓	=, ?	↑ , ↑	[63, 64]
MMP-13 null	Ao	↑	↑	↑	?	?	[66]
MMP-14 null	Root	=	=	=	↑	↓	[67]
TIMP-1 null	Root	=	=	=	↑	↓	[68]
TIMP-1 ++	Root, Aorta	= , ↓	= , ?	=, ↑	↓ , ↓	↓ , ↓	[69, 70]
TIMP-2 ++	Root, BCA	↓ , =	? , =	↓ , =	↑ , ↑	↑ , =	[55, 71]
TIMP-3 ++	BCA	↓	↑	↓	↑	↑	[55]

Note: Results of over-expression (++), over-expression of activated enzymes (++a), and knockout (null) included increases (↑), decreases (↓), or no change (=) in the specified parameters. Missing or uncertain data is indicated as (?). Abbreviations: Ao = aorta, arch = aortic arch, BCA = brachiocephalic artery, root = aortic root. Modified from Newby AC, George SJ, Ismail Y, Johnson JL, Sala-Newby GB, Thomas AC, Vulnerable atherosclerotic plaque metalloproteinases and foam cell phenotypes, Thromb Haemost, 2009;101(6):1006-11 with permission.

be expected to reduce atherosclerosis. MMP-9 knockout produced opposite effects on plaque size and macrophage content and elastin breaks in two studies [63, 64], although the diet, timing, and site of plaques chosen for were different. MMP-12 knockout decreased elastin breaks [64] and buried fibrous layers [63], while active MMP-12 over-expression in rabbits increased plaque size and inflammation [66]. Hence, there is a consensus that MMP-12 contributes to plaque instability. Recently, treatment with a specific inhibitor of MMP-12 was also shown to halt plaque progression, to decrease macrophage recruitment into plaques and subcutaneous sponges, and increase apoptosis in plaques foam cells [52, 63]. Similar effects on apoptosis were replicated by manipulating MMP-12 activity *in vitro*, where cleavage of cadherins played a part in promoting apoptosis [52]. Knockout of the collagenases, MMP-13 and MT1-MMP increased collagen in plaques, which implies greater stability, but had little effect on macrophage or VSMC content. Nevertheless, MT1-MMP may have a role in macrophage recruitment and apoptosis based on the differential effects of TIMP-1 and -2 knockouts [55].

Adenovirus-mediated gene transfer of TIMP-1 improved plaque stability in one study [71] but not another [55]. Moreover, prolonged over-expression of TIMP-2, but not TIMP-1, prevented progression of established brachiocephalic artery plaques [55]. As discussed above, this suggests that at least one MT-MMP, most likely MT1-MMP based on its prevalence, promotes plaque instability. The beneficial effects of TIMP-2 were owing to decreased macrophage invasion and apoptosis, implying a similar effect for MT1-MMP knockout. Interestingly, TIMPs appear to be more effective than low molecular weight MMP inhibitors at inhibiting atherosclerosis in mice [72] for reasons that are not currently clear.

TIMP-1 knockout caused disruption of medial elastic layers in two studies [69, 70] (Table 9.2), associated in one study with increased macrophage content [69, 70]. Gene transfer of TIMP-3 should lead to highly localised effects compared to the other TIMPs but may also affect several ADAMs. Knockout of TIMP-3 selectively in bone marrow cells apparently reduces atherosclerosis [73].

Taken together, the results support the role of several MMPs in plaque development and disruption. They are consistent with the multiple impacts of MMPs on ECM degradation and the migration, proliferation and apoptosis of vascular cells.

9.6 MMPs and TIMPs in Human Atherosclerotic Plaques

A wave of publication starting in the early 1990s [74, 75] established the presence of MMPs-1, -2, -3, -7, -8, -11, -13, -14, and -16 (at least) plus TIMPs-1, -2, and -3 in human atherosclerotic plaques [15]. MMPs are localised with all types of vascular cells but many are especially prominent in macrophages. However, it is worth noting that macrophages make up a minority of the cell population even in the most inflamed plaques [1], so that the bulk of many MMPs may be derived from the much more prevalent VSMC population. Two additional types of evidence support the functional importance of MMPs. Firstly, collagenases were shown to co-localise with cleaved collagen and are, therefore, active in plaques [76]. Secondly, the MMP protein levels in large numbers of plaques were compared with histological parameters and patient outcome. On this basis, MMP-2 may be protective against unstable plaque morphology, whereas MMP-8 and -9 show and adverse relationship [77, 78]. The status of several other prominent MMPs and TIMPs remains to be established.

Attempts have also been made to relate circulating MMP levels of MMP genotypes to atherosclerosis burden and its symptoms [79]. Circulating MMPs most likely derive from neutrophils or ECs from all over the body. The implications for plaque are, therefore, rather indirect. Genetics gives an indication of lifelong risk. Although initial data studying MMP-3 looked promising, clear indications have yet to emerge of which MMPs are harmful and, therefore, preferred targets for intervention [80].

9.7 Inhibition of MMPs as Therapy for Atherosclerosis or Plaque Disruption

The previous sections clearly set out an important role for MMPs in atherosclerotic plaque progression and the acute coronary syndromes that result from plaque rupture or erosion. The most obvious way to translate these observations is to apply a global MMP inhibitor, firstly in a suitable animal model and then in patients. The effects of TIMP-1 or TIMP-2 gene transfer in mice provide encouragement for this approach. A plethora of peptide-mimetic and other small molecular with compounds have been developed to target MMPs [81] and several antibiotic tetracylines proved to be potent inhibitors of MMP production and activity as well [81]. Hence, optimism was high that the MMP inhibitor strategy would provide a new therapy for unstable atherosclerosis.

Unfortunately, until very recently, hopes have been dashed. Carefully conducted studies with global MMP inhibitors in mice [72, 82, 83] and primates [84] failed to show any effect on plaque progression. In addition, underpowered phase II clinical studies with tetracyclines showed no obvious benefit [85]. Taken together with the emerging evidence for dose-limiting, musculo-skeletal side effects of MMP inhibitors in cancer therapy trials [81], enthusiasm for the long-term application of MMP inhibitors as prophylaxis for atherosclerosis and its complications waned.

Some pharmacologists have explored new chemistries to develop more selective MMP inhibitors. An example is the development of a highly selective inhibitor of MMP-12 [86]. Given the strong evidence for a detrimental effect of MMP-12 on atherosclerosis in experimental models (see Table 9.2), we evaluated this inhibitor on progression of established plaques in ApoE null mice [87]. Concentrations of MMP-12 inhibitor designed to spare all other MMPs halted plaque progression. Moreover, the plaques had more VSMCs and collagen but fewer macrophages than in placebo treated mice. The plaques were also less complex, with fewer buried fibrous layers and less calcification. All of these histological features would be consistent with greater stability in human plaques. The effects of MMP-12 inhibition were remarkably similar in this study to those of MMP-12 knockout in the same mouse background [63]. Moreover, the mechanisms by which MMP-12 inhibition altered plaque biology, i.e., reduction in macrophage invasion and protection against macrophage apoptosis, were exactly replicated in MMP-12 null mice. These studies provide renewed hope for translating knowledge of MMP regulation in plaques into a workable therapy, although clinical studies are yet to be initiated.

An alternative strategy may be to target the common causes of plaque inflammation and production of the group of MMPs (MMPs-1, -3, -10, -12 and MT1-MMP) that appear to be classical inflammatory genes. One intervention that undoubtedly achieves this is statin therapy [88], but the benefits of this are already available to patients.

Thiazolidinediones most likely also exert beneficial effects through anti-inflammatory mechanisms that include reduced MMP secretion [89]. Aspirin, other cyclooxygase inhibitors and specific inhibitors of prostaglandin E_2 synthesis inhibit MMP production from monocytes [17] and so could affect plaque stability through this mechanism. However, the presence of cyclooxygenase-independent pathways of MMP production in monocyte and mature macrophages reduces the potential impact of this therapy [21]. Further progress will depend on clearly defining the stimuli of MMP production in plaques, which may be a multiplicity of pro-inflammatory cytokines and growth factors (see above). These may act redundantly and, therefore, be difficult to target with drugs. However, one recent study pointed to an unexpectedly prominent and unique role for agonists of Toll-like receptor-2 [90]. Another paradigm for activation of plaque inflammation is auto-immunity, and this leads to the concept of promoting plaque stability by immune modulation [91]. Studying the relationship of MMP production plaques and immune activation is in its infancy [25] but promises to be an interesting avenue.

In summary, a wealth of basic science has established a role for MMPs and defined their up-regulation during the various stages of atherosclerosis. The pharmacology of MMPs has also advanced substantially but initial attempts at translation to the clinic have been met with frustration. Recent insights have provided new hope of devising therapies either through specifically targeting selected MMPs known to have adverse effects or by exploiting the selective up-regulation of groups of MMPs that cooperate to cause plaque instability.

References

1. Falk, E (2006) Pathogenesis of atherosclerosis. *J Am Coll Cardiol* **47**: C7–C12.
2. Sithu, SD, *et al.* (2007) Membrane-type 1-matrix metalloproteinase regulates intracellular adhesion molecule-1 (ICAM-1)-mediated monocyte transmigration. *J Biol Chem* **282**: 25010–25019.
3. Tomlinson, ML, *et al.* (2008) Three matrix metalloproteinases are required *in vivo* for macrophage migration during embryonic development. *Mech Dev* **125**: 1059–1070.
4. Nagase, H, R Visse, and G Murphy (2006) Structure and function of matrix metalloproteinases and TIMPs. *Cardiovasc Res* **69**: 562–573.

5. Plihtari, R, *et al.* (2010) Proteolysis sensitizes LDL particles to phospholipolysis by secretory phospholipase A2 group V and secretory sphingomyelinase. *J Lipid Res* **51**: 1801–1809.
6. Johnson, JL, *et al.* (2008) Low tissue inhibitor of metalloproteinases 3 and high matrix metalloproteinase 14 levels defines a subpopulation of highly invasive foam-cell macrophages. *Arterioscler Thromb Vasc Biol* **28**: 1647–1653.
7. Tabas, I (2005) Consequences and therapeutic implications of macrophage apoptosis in atherosclerosis: The importance of lesion stage and phagocytic efficiency. *Arterioscler Thromb Vasc Biol* **25**: 2255–2264.
8. Newby, AC (2006) Matrix metalloproteinases regulate migration, proliferation, and death of vascular smooth muscle cells by degrading matrix and non-matrix substrates. *Cardiovasc Res* **69**: 614–624.
9. Clarke, MC, *et al.* (2006) Apoptosis of vascular smooth muscle cells induces features of plaque vulnerability in atherosclerosis. *Nat Med* **12**: 1075–1080.
10. Virmani, R, *et al.* (2006) Pathology of the vulnerable plaque. *J Am Coll Cardiol* **47**: C13–C18.
11. Van Goor, H, *et al.* (2009) Adamalysins in biology and disease. *J Pathol* **219**: 277–286.
12. Clark, JC, *et al.* (2007) RECK--a newly discovered inhibitor of metastasis with prognostic significance in multiple forms of cancer. *Cancer Metastasis Rev* **26**: 675–683.
13. Van Hinsbergh, VW, and P Koolwijk (2008) Endothelial sprouting and angiogenesis: Matrix metalloproteinases in the lead. *Cardiovasc Res* **78**: 203–212.
14. Clark, IM, *et al.* (2008) The regulation of matrix metalloproteinases and their inhibitors. *Int J Biochem Cell Biol* **40**: 1362–1378.
15. Newby, AC (2005) Dual role of matrix metalloproteinases (matrixins) in intimal thickening and atherosclerotic plaque rupture. *Physiol Rev* **85**: 1–31.
16. White, S, and A Newby (2010) Metalloproteinases, the endothelium and atherosclerosis, in *Atherosclerosis*, S. George and J.L. Johnson, Editors. Wiley-VCH: Weinheim. p. 157–172.
17. Newby, AC (2008) Metalloproteinase expression in monocytes and macrophages and its relationship to atherosclerotic plaque instability. *Arterioscler Thromb Vasc Biol* **28**: 2108–2114.

18. Qiu, J, *et al.* (2010) High-mobility group box 1 promotes metalloproteinase-9 upregulation through Toll-like receptor 4 after cerebral ischemia. *Stroke* **41**: 2077–2082.

19. Yuan, W, H Ge, and B He (2010) Pro-inflammatory activities induced by CyPA-EMMPRIN interaction in monocytes. *Atherosclerosis* **213**: 415–421.

20. Chase, A, *et al.* (2002) Role of nuclear factor-κB activation in metalloproteinase-1, -3 and -9 secretion by human macrophages *in vitro* and rabbit foam cells produced *in vivo*. *Arterioscler Thromb Vasc Biol* **22**: 765–771.

21. Reel, B, *et al.* (2011). Diverse patterns of cyclooxygenase-independent metalloproteinase gene regulation in human monocytes. *Br J Pharmacol* **163**: 1679–1690.

22. Hussain, S, *et al.* (2002) Activation of protein kinase Czeta is essential for cytokine-induced metalloproteinase-1, -3, and -9 secretion from rabbit smooth muscle cells and inhibits proliferation. *J Biol Chem* **277**: 27345–27352.

23. Bond, M, *et al.* (2001) Inhibition of transcription factor NF-κB reduces matrix metalloproteinase-1,-3and-9production by vascular smooth muscle cells. *Cardiovasc Res* **50**: 556–565.

24. Shimizu, K, *et al.* (2004) Th2-predominant inflammation and blockade of IFN-gamma signaling induce aneurysms in allografted aortas. *J Clin Invest* **114**: 300–308.

25. Ovchinnikova, O, *et al.* (2009) T-cell activation leads to reduced collagen maturation in atherosclerotic plaques of Apoe(-/-) mice. *Am J Pathol* **174**: 693–700.

26. Deguchi, JO, *et al.* (2009) Chronic hypoxia activates the Akt and beta-catenin pathways in human macrophages. *Arterioscler Thromb Vasc Biol* **29**: 1664–1670.

27. Hanemaaijer, R, *et al.* (1993) Regulation of matrix metalloproteinase expression in human vein and microvascular endothelial cells. Effects of tumour necrosis factor α, interleukin 1 and phorbol ester. *Biochem J* **296**: 803–809.

28. Zhang, Y, *et al.* (1998) Differential regulation of monocyte matrix metalloproteinase and TIMP-1 production by TNF-alpha, granulocyte-macrophage CSF, and IL-1 beta through prostaglandin-dependent and-independent mechanisms. *J Immunol* **161**: 3071–3076.

29. Grote, K, *et al.* (2003) Mechanical stretch enhances mRNA expression and proenzyme release of matrix metalloproteinase-2 (MMP-2) via

NAD(P)H oxidase-derived reactive oxygen species. *Circ Res* **92**: 80e–86e.

30. Dai, GH, *et al.* (2004) Distinct endothelial phenotypes evoked by arterial waveforms derived from atherosclerosis-susceptible and -resistant regions of human vasculature. *Proc Natl Acad Sci U S A* **101**: 14871–14876.
31. Atkins, GB, and MK Jain (2007) Role of Kruppel-like transcription factors in endothelial biology. *Circ Res* **100**: 1686–95.
32. Castier, Y, *et al.* (2005) p47phox-dependent NADPH oxidase regulates flow-induced vascular remodeling. *Circ Res* **97**: 533–540.
33. Gough, PJ, *et al.* (2006) Macrophage expression of active MMP-9 induces acute plaque disruption in apoE-deficient mice. *J Clin Invest* **116**: 59–69.
34. Heymans, S, *et al.* (1999) Inhibition of plasminogen activators or matrix metalloproteinases prevents cardiac rupture but impairs therapeutic angiogenesis and causes cardiac failure. *Nat Med* **5**: 1135–1142.
35. Johnson, JL, *et al.* (1998) Activation of matrix-degrading metalloproteinases by mast cell proteases in atherosclerotic plaques. *Arterioscler Thromb Vasc Biol* **18**: 1707–1715.
36. Rajagopalan, S, *et al.* (1996) Reactive oxygen species produced by macrophage-derived foam cells regulate the activity of vascular matrix metalloproteinases *in vitro*. *J Clin Invest* **98**: 2572–2579.
37. Kranzhöfer, A, *et al.* (1999) Expression of tissue inhibitor of metalloproteinases-1, -2 and -3 during neointima formation in organ cultures of human saphenous vein. *Arterioscler Thromb Vasc Biol* **19**: 255–265.
38. Vu, TH, *et al.* (1998) MMP-9/gelatinase B is a key regulator of growth plate angiogenesis and apoptosis of hypertrophic chondrocytes. *Cell* **93**: 411–422.
39. Deryugina, EI, and JP Quigley (2010) Pleiotropic roles of matrix metalloproteinases in tumor angiogenesis: contrasting, overlapping and compensatory functions. *Biochim Biophys Acta* **1803**: 103–120.
40. Wang, J, *et al.* (2009) GIT1 Mediates VEGF-induced podosome formation in endothelial cells: Critical role for PLCγ. *Arterioscler Thromb Vasc Biol* **29**: 202–208.
41. Chabadel, A, *et al.* (2007) CD44 and beta3 integrin organize two functionally distinct actin-based domains in osteoclasts. *Mol Biol Cell* **18**: 4899–4910.

42. Linder, S (2007) The matrix corroded: Podosomes and invadopodia in extracellular matrix degradation. *Trends Cell Biol* **17**: 107–117.

43. Heo, SH, *et al.* (2010) Expression profiling of ETS and MMP factors in VEGF-activated endothelial cells: Role of MMP-10 in VEGF-induced angiogenesis. *J Cell Physiol* **224**: 734–742.

44. Fabunmi, RP, *et al.* (1996) Divergent regulation by growth factors and cytokines of 95 kDa and 72 kDa gelatinases and tissue inhibitors or metalloproteinases-1, -2, and -3 in rabbit aortic smooth muscle cells. *Biochem J* **315 (Pt 1)**: 335–342.

45. Aguilera, CM, *et al.* (2003) Relationship between type IV collagen degradation, metalloproteinase activity and smooth muscle cell migration and proliferation in cultured human saphenous vein. *Cardiovasc Res* **58**: 679–688.

46. Dwivedi, A, SC Slater, and SJ George (2009) MMP-9 and -12 cause N-cadherin shedding and thereby beta-catenin signalling and vascular smooth muscle cell proliferation. *Cardiovasc Res* **81**: 178-186.

47. Stringa, E, *et al.* (2000) Collagen degradation and platelet-derived growth factor stimulate the migration of vascular smooth muscle cells. *J Cell Sci* **113**: 2055–2064.

48. Bond, M, GB Sala-Newby, and AC Newby (2004) Focal adhesion kinase (FAK)-dependent regulation S-phase kinase associated protein-2 (Skp-2) stability: A novel mechanism regulating smooth muscle cell proliferation. *J Biol Chem* **279**: 37304–37310.

49. Quasnichka, H, *et al.* (2006) Regulation of smooth muscle cell proliferation by beta-catenin/T-cell factor signaling involves modulation of cyclin D1 and p21 expression. *Circ Res* **99**: 1329–1337.

50. Baker, AH, *et al.* (1998) Divergent effects of tissue inhibitors of metalloproteinase-1, -2 or -3 on rat vascular smooth muscle cell invasion, proliferation and death *in vitro*: TIMP-3 promotes apoptosis. *J Clin Invest* **101**: 1478–1487.

51. Bar-Or, A, *et al.* (2003) Analyses of all matrix metalloproteinase members in leukocytes emphasize monocytes as major inflammatory mediators in multiple sclerosis. *Brain* **126**: 2738–2749.

52. Johnson, JL, *et al.* (2011) A selective matrix metalloproteinase-12 inhibitor retards atherosclerotic plaque development in apolipoprotein E-knockout mice. *Arterioscler Thromb Vasc Biol* **31**: 528–535.

53. Shapiro, S, D Kobayashi, and T Ley (1993) Cloning and characterization of a unique elastolytic metalloproteinase produced by human alveolar macrophages. *J Biol Chem* **268**: 23824–23829.

54. Thomas, AC, *et al.* (2007) Genomics of foam cells and nonfoamy macrophages from rabbits identifies arginase-I as a differential regulator of nitric oxide production. *Arterioscler Thromb Vasc Biol* **27**: 571–577.
55. Johnson, JL, *et al.* (2006) Suppression of atherosclerotic plaque progression and instability by tissue inhibitor of metalloproteinase-2: Involvement of macrophage migration and apoptosis. *Circulation* **113**: 2435–2444.
56. Rosenfeld, ME, *et al.* (2000) Advanced atherosclerotic lesions in the innominate artery of the ApoE knockout mouse. *Arterioscler Thromb Vasc Biol* **20**: 2587–2592.
57. Johnson, JL, *et al.* (2005) Plaque rupture after short periods of fat-feeding in the apolipoprotein e knockout mouse: Model characterisation, and effects of pravastatin treatment. *Circulation* **111**: 1422–1430.
58. Cheng, C, *et al.* (2006) Atherosclerotic lesion size and vulnerability are determined by patterns of lluid shear stress. *Circulation* **113**: 2744–2753.
59. De Nooijer, R, *et al.* (2006) Lesional overexpression of matrix metalloproteinase-9 promotes intraplaque hemorrhage in advanced lesions but not at earlier stages of atherogenesis. *Arterioscler Thromb Vasc Biol* **26**: 340–346.
60. Lemaitre, V, *et al.* (2001) ApoE knockout mice expressing human matrix metalloproteinase-1 in macrophages have less advanced atherosclerosis. *J Clin Invest* **107**: 1227–1234.
61. Kuzuya, M, *et al.* (2006) Effect of MMP-2 deficiency on atherosclerotic lesion formation in ApoE-deficient mice. *Arterioscler Thromb Vasc Biol* **26**: 1120–1125.
62. Silence, J, *et al.* (2001) Persistence of atherosclerotic plaque but reduced aneurysm formation in mice with stromelysin-1 (MMP-3) gene inactivation. *Arterioscler Thromb Vasc Biol* **21**: 1440–1445.
63. Johnson, JL, *et al.* (2005) Divergent effects of matrix metalloproteinases 3, 7, 9, and 12 on atherosclerotic plaque stability in mouse brachiocephalic arteries. *Proc Natl Acad Sci U S A* **102**: 15575–15580.
64. Luttun, A, *et al.* (2004) Loss of matrix metalloproteinase-9 or matrix metalloproteinase-12 protects apolipoprotein E-deficient mice against atherosclerotic media destruction but differentially affects plaque growth. *Circulation* **109**: 1408–1414.
65. Laxton, RC, *et al.* (2009) A role of matrix metalloproteinase-8 in atherosclerosis. *Circ Res* **105**: 921–929.

66. Liang, J, *et al.* (2006) Macrophage metalloelastase accelerates the progression of atherosclerosis in transgenic rabbits. *Circulation* **113**: 1993–2001.
67. Deguchi, J-O, *et al.* (2005) Matrix metalloproteinase-13/Collagenase-3 deletion promotes collagen accumulation and organization in mouse atherosclerotic plaques. *Circulation* **112**: 2708–2715.
68. Schneider, F, *et al.* (2008) Matrix-metalloproteinase-14 deficiency in bone-marrow-derived cells promotes collagen accumulation in mouse atherosclerotic plaques. *Circulation* **117**: 931–939.
69. Lemaitre, V, PD Soloway, and J D'Armiento (2003) Increased medial degradation with pseudo-aneurysm formation in apolipoprotein E-knockout mice deficient in tissue inhibitor of metalloproteinases-1. *Circulation* **107**: 333–338.
70. Silence, J, D Collen, and HR Lijnen (2002) Reduced atherosclerotic plaque but enhanced aneurysm formation in mice with inactivation of the tissue inhibitor of metalloproteinase-1 (TIMP-1) gene. *Circ Res* **90**: 897–903.
71. Rouis, M, *et al.* (1999) Adenovirus-mediate overexpression of tissue inhibitor of metalloproteinase-1 reduces atherosclerotic lesions in apolipoprotein E deficient mice. *Circulation* **100**: 533–540.
72. Johnson, JL, *et al.* (2006) Effect of broad-spectrum matrix metalloproteinase inhibition on atherosclerotic plaque stability. *Cardiovasc Res* **71**: 586–595.
73. Casagrande, V., *et al.* (2012) Overexpression of Tissue Inhibitor of Metalloproteinase 3 in Macrophages Reduces Atherosclerosis in Low-Density Lipoprotein Receptor Knockout Mice. *Arterioscler Thromb Vasc Biol* **32**: 74–81.
74. Galis, ZS, *et al.* (1994) Increased expression of matrix metalloproteinases and matrix degrading activity in vulnerable regions of human atherosclerotic plaques. *J Clin Invest* **94**: 2493–2503.
75. Henney, AM, *et al.* (1991) Localization of stromelysin gene expression in atherosclerotic plaques by *in situ* hybridization. *Proc Natl Acad Sci U S A* **88**: 8154–8158.
76. Sukhova, GK, *et al.* (1999) Evidence for increased collagenolysis by interstitial collagenases-1 and-3 in vulnerable human atheromatous plaques. *Circulation* **99**: 2503–2509.
77. Peeters, W *et al.* Collagenase matrix metalloproteinase-8 expressed in atherosclerotic carotid plaques is associated with systemic cardiovascular outcome. *Eur Heart J* **32**: 2314–2325.

78. Sluijter, JPG, *et al.* (2006) Matrix metalloproteinase 2 is associated with stable and matrix metalloproteinases 8 and 9 with vulnerable carotid atherosclerotic lesions- A study in human endarterectomy specimen pointing to a role for different extracellular matrix metalloproteinase inducer glycosylation forms. *Stroke* **37**: 235–239.

79. Newby, AC (2006) Do metalloproteinases destabilize vulnerable atherosclerotic plaques? *Curr Opin Lipidol* **17**: 556–561.

80. Ye, S (2006) Influence of matrix metalloproteinase genotype on cardiovascular disease susceptibility and outcome. *Cardiovasc Res* **69**: 636–645.

81. Peterson, JT (2006) The importance of estimating the therapeutic index in the development of matrix metalloproteinase inhibitors. *Cardiovasc Res* **69**: 677–687.

82. Manning, MW, LA Cassis, and A Daugherty (2003) Differential effects of doxycycline, a broad-spectrum matrix metalloproteinase inhibitor, on angiotensin II-induced atherosclerosis and abdominal aortic aneurysms. *Arterioscler Thromb Vasc Biol* **23**: 483–488.

83. Prescott, MF, *et al.* (1999) Effect of matrix metalloproteinase inhibition on progression of atherosclerosis and aneurysm in LDL receptor-deficient mice overexpressing MMP-3, MMP-12, and MMP-13 and on restenosis in rats after balloon injury. *Ann N Y Acad Sci* **878**: 179–190.

84. Cherr, GS, *et al.* (2002) Metalloproteinase inhibition and the response to angioplasty and stenting in atherosclerotic primates. *Arterioscler Thromb Vasc Biol* **22**: 161–166.

85. Brown, DL, *et al.* (2004) Clinical and biochemical results of the metalloproteinase inhibition with subantimicrobial doses of doxycycline to prevent acute coronary syndromes (MIDAS) pilot trial. *Arterioscler Thromb Vasc Biol* **24**: 733–738.

86. Devel, L, *et al.* (2006) Development of selective inhibitors and substrate of matrix metalloproteinase-12. *J Biol Chem* **281**: 11152–11160.

87. Johnson, JL, *et al.* (2011) A selective matrix metalloproteinase-12 inhibitor retards atherosclerotic plaque development in apolipoprotein E-knockout mice. *Arterioscler Thromb Vasc Biol* **31**: 528–535.

88. Luan, Z, AJ Chase, and AC Newby (2003) Statins inhibit secretion of metalloproteinases-1, -2, -3, and -9 from vascular smooth muscle cells and macrophages. *Arterioscler Thromb Vasc Biol* **23**: 769–775.

89. Marx, N, *et al.* (2003) Antidiabetic PPAR{gamma}-activator rosiglitazone reduces MMP-9 serum levels in type 2 diabetic patients with coronary artery disease. *Arterioscler Thromb Vasc Biol* **23**: 283–288.

90. Monaco, C, *et al.* (2009) Toll-like receptor-2 mediates inflammation and matrix degradation in human atherosclerosis. *Circulation* **120**: 2462–2469.

91. Hansson, GK, and J Nilsson (2009) Vaccination against atherosclerosis? Induction of atheroprotective immunity. *Semin Immunopathol* **31**: 95–101.

Chapter 10

Probucol-Derivatives in the Treatment of Atherosclerosis

Robyn G. Midwinter and Roland Stocker
Centre for Vascular Research, The University of Sydney, Sydney, NSW 2006, Australia
roland.stocker@sydney.edu.au

10.1 Introduction

Deaths from atherosclerotic disease are increasing in the modern world and account for a significant economical burden on society. The progression of atherosclerosis is multifaceted and linked to a number of factors rather than a single initiating event, which has made the disease difficult to treat. Several factors, including hypertension, obesity, hypercholesterolemia, smoking, diabetes, and age, increase the risk of atherosclerosis. Changes to life-style are important for decreasing the incidence of atherosclerosis, yet the development of novel compounds that target specific aspects of the progression of atherosclerosis are essential. However, a hallmark of the disease is the presence of inflammation and increased oxidative damage [18].

There is a continued interest in the development of compounds that exhibit both anti-inflammatory and anti-oxidant activity as

Atherosclerosis: Treatment and Prevention
Edited by Christian Weber and Oliver Soehnlein

ISBN 978-981-4316-26-2 (Hardcover), ISBN 978-981-4364-26-3 (eBook)
www.panstanford.com

protective compounds. Probucol and the more recent probucol analogues are such compounds.

10.2 Probucol and Atherosclerosis

Probucol (4,4′-(isopropylidenedithio)*bis*(2,6-*di*-*tert*-butylphenol)) (Fig. 10.1) is a diphenolic compound with anti-inflammatory and anti-oxidant properties that was introduced in the early 1970s as a cholesterol-lowering drug [1]. Besides its ability to decrease cholesterol, probucol showed good promise by inhibiting atherosclerosis in a number of animal models apparently independent of its cholesterol-lowering abilities.

10.2.1 Anti-Atherosclerotic Effects of Probucol

An early study showed that probucol was able to regress Achilles tendon xanthoma in patients with familial hypercholesterolemia (FH) [32, 33]. The resulting PQRST clinical trial investigated if treatment of hypercholesterolemic patients with probucol for 3 years affected femoral atherosclerosis [27]. Disappointingly, no significant benefits over placebo were observed and concerns were raised over probucol's efficacy. In addition, there was a significant undesirable alteration in the lipid profiles of participants receiving probucol, with a decrease in HDL-cholesterol [27]. The negative results of the PQRST trial, together with the probucol-associated tachyarrhythmic events and QT prolongation [15], prompted the withdrawal of probucol from the US market. Despite this, however, probucol was shown later to decrease atherosclerosis in carotid arteries of hypercholesterolemic patients, and this was associated with reduced cardiac events [17]. Indeed, the drug continues to be used, albeit rarely, in some countries. Most recently, a randomized trial with polymer-free dual drug eluting stents reported prolonged patency of sirolimus- and probucol-eluting stents than siroimus only eluting stents in humans [Byrne RA, Kastrati A, Tiroch K, et al. 2-year clinical and angiographic outcomes from a randomized trial of polymer-free dual drug-eluting stents versus polymer-based Cypher and Endeavor [corrected] drug-eluting stents. J Am Coll Cardiol. 2010;55:2536-2543].

A number of animal studies showed that probucol inhibits the progression of athcrosclerosis and intimal hyperplasia in various models [20, 22]. While the exact mechanisms for probucol's protective effects have not been identified, these studies indicated a number of beneficial activities of the drug, including modulation of lipid metabolism, anti-inflammatory and anti-oxidant activities, promotion of endothelial cell growth and re-endothelialization, as well as inhibition of vascular smooth muscle cells (VSMC).

10.2.2 Probucol's Mode of Action

10.2.2.1 Anti-inflammatory activity

Inflammation plays a significant role in all phases of atherosclerosis through impaired endothelial function and the release of compounds that can lead to tissue damage and the promotion of lipoprotein modifications. Probucol has only limited anti-inflammatory activities *in vitro*. It is unable to inhibit tumor necrosis factor-α (TNF-α) induced expression of vascular cell adhesion protein 1 (VCAM-1) [12] nor suppress the lipopolysaccharide-induced production of TNF-α, interleukin-1β, or interleukin-6 from human mononuclear cells [9]. However, probucol exhibits anti-inflammatory actions *in vivo* that can contribute to the inhibition of experimental atherosclerosis. Thus, probucol was shown to inhibit the expression of VCAM-1 [30] to reduce endothelial adhesion of inflammatory cells in hypercholesterolemic rabbits [7]. In addition, probucol treatment decreased the number of macrophages in lesions of LDL receptor-deficient Watanabe heritable hyperlipidemic rabbits [3] and apolipoprotein E gene deficient (*Apoe*$^{-/-}$) mice [30]. The reduced macrophage accumulation was associated with a decrease in both the production and activity of matrix metalloproteinase-2 and -9 [30]. The activation of metalloproteases has been shown to participate in plaque rupture, so that the ability of probucol to decrease the presence of inflammatory cells could conceivably translate into increased stability of plaques. The apparent difference between *in vivo* and *in vitro* efficacy likely relates to probucol's highly lipophillic nature [2], the associated inefficient delivery to cells [9], and its metabolism in vivo.

10.2.2.2 Anti-oxidant activity

Containing two phenol moieties, both with adjacent tertiary butyl groups, probucol was designed originally as a hindered radical-scavenging anti-oxidant. Consistent with this, the ability of probucol to scavenge peroxyl radicals is ~14% of that of the biologically most abundant phenolic anti-oxidant, α-tocopherol [14]. Early studies reported probucol to decrease lipoprotein lipid oxidation in the vessel wall [8]. However, vascular protection by probucol was subsequently dissociated from its ability to affect lipoprotein lipid oxidation. Specifically, probucol inhibited intimal hyperplasia in aortic balloon-injured rabbits and atherosclerosis in *Apoe*$^{-/-}$ mice unrelated to inhibition of arterial lipid oxidation [4, 10]. Instead, the drug improved endothelial function and promoted re-endothelialization. Thus, while probucol undoubtedly has radical scavenging anti-oxidant activity that may translate into attenuation of lipoprotein lipid oxidation, it appears the latter is not how probucol exerts its anti-atherosclerotic activity.

While probucol is less reactive towards peroxyl radicals compared with α-tocopherol, the former is able to scavenge a greater number of radicals than the vitamin [14]. A recent structure-function study suggested that the sulphur atoms of probucol importantly contribute to the *in vivo* protection seen with probucol [29], although it remains unknown whether this relates to oxidant scavenging and, if so, which oxidants are likely involved. Typically, sulphur engages in two-electron redox reactions rather than radical scavenging. Also, these recent studies suggested that the central isopropylidene moiety of probucol (Fig. 10.1) is neither required for inhibition of atherosclerosis and intimal hyperplasia nor for increasing re-endothelialization by this class of drugs [29].

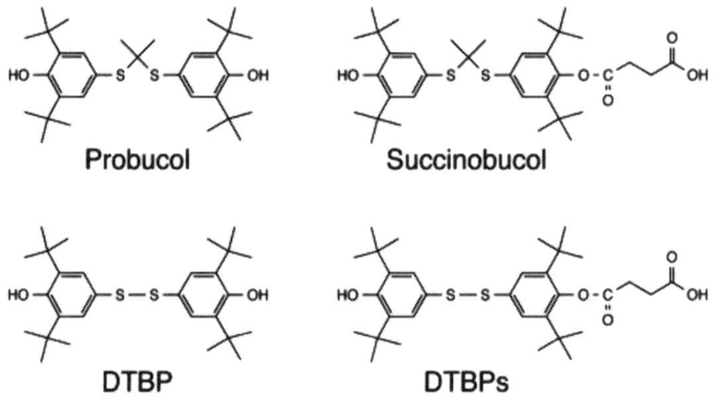

Figure 10.1 Chemical structures of probucol and some of its derivatives.

10.2.2.3 Induction of heme oxygenase-1

There is increasing evidence that the stress protein heme oxygenase-1 (HO-1) plays an important role in atherosclerotic progression [16, 19]. Interestingly, probucol is able to induce heme oxygenase-1 in both VSMC and endothelial cells [6, 29], with the drug inhibiting VSMC proliferation but increasing endothelial cell proliferation [10]. Blockade of HO-1 induction by molecular means prevented probucol from inhibiting VSMC proliferation *in vitro* [6]. Similarly, inhibition of HO-1 activity blocked the ability of probucol to promote re-endothelialization in rabbits following vascular injury [29, 31]. Significantly, probucol was able to increase the number of circulating endothelial progenitor cells in rabbits after vascular injury, and this increase was dependent on HO-1 activity [31].

These findings indicated that the ability of probucol to promote endothelial cell growth and to inhibit VSMC proliferation are mediated via HO-1 induction, suggesting HO-1 induction as novel mechanism by which probucol exerts its biological protection. It is currently not known whether probucol induces HO-1 in humans and, if this occurs, whether it protects against atherosclerosis.

10.3 Analogues of Probucol

The adverse side effects of probucol treatment, poor solubility, lowering of HDL cholesterol and prolongation of QT interval, encouraged the development of probucol analogues.

10.3.1 Succinobucol

As the name suggests, succinobucol (also known as AGI-1067) contains a monosuccinate group esterified to one of the two phenol groups of probucol (Fig. 10.1) [12]. The adjacent tertiary butyl groups render the ester bond resistant to hydrolysis or subsequent metabolism when administered to animals or humans [12]. Compared with probucol, succinobucol has increased hydrophilicity, cellular uptake, and retention [9], and hence overcomes one of the disadvantages of probucol, its poor cellular uptake.

10.3.1.1 Succinobucol as an anti-inflammatory

The addition of the succinyl ester turned succinobucol into a surprisingly potent inhibitor of TNF-α inducible VCAM-1 expression with an IC_{50} of 6 μM (versus > 100 μM for probucol) [9, 12]. *In vitro* succinobucol treatment of TNF-α stimulated endothelial cells attenuated the expression of VCAM-1, monocyte chemotactic protein-1, and E-selectin [9, 12]. Interestingly, succinobucol had no effect on the expression of inter-cellular adhesion molecule 1, suggesting that succinobucol was not a global inhibitor of the inflammatory response and that treatment with this analogue may maintain rather than suppress the immune system. Furthermore, the *in vitro* formation of inflammatory mediators such as TNF-α, interleukin-1β, and interleukin-6 was decreased by low levels of succinobucol (<10 μM) but were unaffected by similar concentrations of probucol [9]. Surprisingly, given its selective and strong anti-inflammatory activities *in vitro*, information of the anti-inflammatory activity of succinobucol was not included in the preclinical atherosclerosis studies (see below), even though those studies did report inhibition of VCAM-1 and monocyte chemotactic protein-1 mRNA levels in lungs of lipopolysaccharide-stimulated mice [21]. Also, the anti-inflammatory activity of succinobucol has not been assessed widely in clinical studies. In humans succinobucol (280 mg per day) decreased plasma concentrations of myeloperoxidase, but not those of C-reactive protein [24], without providing information on endothelial adhesion factors. A recent report showed that in non-injured mice, succinobucol was able to significantly increase the number of progenitor cells in both the bone marrow ($CD34^+$/$Flk1^+$/$CD45^-$) and the circulation ($CD34^+$/$CD45^+lin^-$) [31]. This new and potentially exciting property may contribute to the ability of succinobucol to promote re-endothelialization of damaged vessels.

10.3.1.2 Succinobucol as an anti-oxidant

Although possessing only a single phenol group, succinobucol was reported to have comparable anti-oxidant activity to that of probucol in its ability to prevent the *in vitro* oxidation of *N*-benzoylleukomethylene blue by linoleic acid hydroperoxide [9]. The same study reported ≤ 10 μM succinobucol, but not probucol, to lower basal levels of reactive oxygen species in human artery endothelial cells and the pro-monocytic cell line U937, as assessed by fluorescence due to oxidation of 2′,7′-dichlorofluorescin-diacetate [9]. It has been suggested that succinobucol acts as a lipophilic anti-oxidant based on its association with and protection of plasma lipoproteins from *ex vivo* oxidation by Cu_2SO_4 [21].

10.3.1.3 Heme oxygenase-1 and succinobucol

In a manner similar to probucol, there is increasing evidence that induction of HO-1 plays a key role in succinobucol's ability to protect arteries from disease. *In vitro* succinobucol induced HO-1 in rat VSMC with greater molar efficiency than probucol (Midwinter RG, Maghzal GJ, Dennis JM, et al. Succinobucol induces apoptosis in vascular smooth muscle cells. Free Radic Biol Med. 2012;52:871-879.). Also, succinobucol induced HO-1 in balloon-injured rabbit arteries, and HO-1 induction was required for succinobucol to promote re-endothelialization [31]. That study was the first to report succinobucol to increase circulating progenitor cells in vascular injury. This increase in circulating progenitor cells was blocked when rabbits were treated with a HO-1 inhibitor, indicating a requirement for enzyme activity in inducing progenitor mobilization [31]. Intriguingly, however, the ability of succinobucol to inhibit rat VSMC proliferation was recently observed to be independent of HO-1 activity (Midwinter RG, Maghzal GJ, Dennis JM, et al. Succinobucol induces apoptosis in vascular smooth muscle cells. Free Radic Biol Med. 2012;52:871-879.), unlike the situation with probucol [6, 29]. Indeed, succinobucol (but not probucol) was shown to be pro-apoptotic for VSMC [Midwinter RG, Maghzal GJ, Dennis JM, et al. Succinobucol induces apoptosis in vascular smooth muscle cells. Free Radic Biol Med. 2012;52:871-879.] This recent result further highlights important differences in the multiple biological activities of succinobucol versus probucol.

10.3.1.4 Succinobucol in pre-clinical studies

Pre-clinical studies with succinobucol showed promising results. Cynomolgus monkeys rendered hypercholesterolemic by a high-fat diet before treatment by gavage with succinobucol at 150 mg/kg/day for 1 year lowered LDL cholesterol by 90% and increased HDL cholesterol 107% [21]. At 150 but not 50 mg/kg/day, succinobucol demonstrated a qualitative inhibitory effect on atherosclerosis, although the group size was small and there was variable degree and incidence of atherosclerosis in the control group that precluded statistical analyses of the data [21]. Different to the situation with hypercholesterolemic monkeys, succinobucol at 150 mg/kg/day for 12 weeks did not lower circulating lipids in either $Apoe^{-/-}$ or LDL receptor gene knockout mice, yet the drug decreased atherosclerosis in the arch, thoracic, and abdominal aorta of both models [21].

10.3.1.5 Succinobucol clinical trials

The Canadian Antioxidant Restenosis Trial (CART-1) assessed the effect of succinobucol versus on restenosis after percutaneous coronary intervention (PCI), with or without stent placement. The drugs were given 2 weeks before PCI and continued 4 weeks after

PCI. The primary outcome, minimal lumen area, was measured by intravascular ultrasound and was found to be significantly greater at follow up 5–7 months after PCI in the highest succinobucol group (280 mg/day) and the probucol group (500 mg/twice daily). However, the minimal lumen areas in the 70 and 140 mg/day succinobucol groups were not significantly different to placebo, although there appeared to be a dose related effect [23]. However, the secondary endpoint of restenosis rate did not differ significantly between placebo, probucol, or any of the succinobucol treatment groups [23].

As most patients undergo non-elective PCI without the possibility for drug pre-treatment, CART-2 was designed to assess whether pre-treatment with succinobucol for a short time when combined with extended (12 months) treatment after non-elective PCI reduces restenosis [24]. Although designed originally with restenosis as a primary endpoint, this study was modified subsequently to primarily investigate the effects of succinobucol on coronary atherosclerosis. At the 12 month follow-up, there was a significant decrease in the plaque volume in the succinobucol treated group, but there was no significant difference in plaque volume between the succinobucol and placebo groups [24]. Interestingly, there was a small but significant drop in white blood cell count in the succinobucol treated patients, suggesting that succinobucol was exhibiting anti-inflammatory properties. Furthermore, and as noted earlier, there was a significant decrease in plasma myeloperoxidase levels in the succinobucol-treated group while no difference in the C-reactive protein was observed [24]. As high levels of plasma myeloperoxidase have been associated with long-term mortality after myocardial infarct [13], this decrease in myeloperoxidase could be highly significant.

In ARISE, the effect of succinobucol (300 mg/day) over standard care on cardiovascular death, resuscitated cardiac arrest, myocardial infarction, stroke, the need for coronary revascularization and admission to hospital for unstable angina was examined in 6144 patients with acute coronary syndrome [26]. After a follow up of 24 months, succinobucol was found to be no better than placebo in reducing the primary outcome, indeed the drug appeared to increase the incidence of unstable angina [26]. However, succinobucol did decrease the incidence of the pre-defined secondary endpoint composed of cardiovascular death, cardiac arrest, myocardial infarction, or stroke. These results suggest that an unexpected side effect of succinobucol may be the promotion of plaque instability leading to unstable angina and potentially the need for coronary revascularization. We observed recently that *in vitro* succinobucol at > 20 μM has unexpected pro-apoptotic activity in VSMC [Midwinter RG, Maghzal GJ, Dennis JM, et al. Succinobucol induces apoptosis in vascular smooth muscle cells. Free Radic Biol Med. 2012;52:871-879.]. As VSMC apoptosis alone is sufficient to induce plaque vulnerability [5], our recent results may help explain the disappointing outcome of ARISE. Unfortunately, circulating concentrations of succinobucol were not reported for either CART-1, CART-2, or ARISE, so that it is presently unclear what pharmacologically relevant concentrations of succinobucol are.

10.3.1.6 Safety of succinobucol

Unlike the situation with probucol, administration of succinobucol was not associated with the prolongation of the QT interval [23], nor was there an increase in weight or waist circumference [26]. In ARISE, however, more patients in the succinobucol than the placebo group reported adverse bleeding episodes or anemia as serious adverse effects [26]. Also, and reminiscent to the situation with probucol, succinobucol significantly decreased HDL-cholesterol, although to a level less than that observed for probucol [23, 25, 26]. Furthermore, there was a potentially adverse effect on blood pressure and an increase in new onset atrial fibrillation with succinobucol treatment [26]. The occurrence of new onset atrial fibrillation may be attributed to the slight increase in blood pressure [26] or perhaps C-reactive protein in the succinobucol group [11].

10.4 Other Probucol Derivatives

Structure optimization studies suggest that even small substitutions, such as extending the side chain of probucol by one methylene group, significantly decreased the drug's ability to inhibit VCAM-1 expression [12]. Other probucol analogues that have been synthesized, such as 4,4′-dithiobis(2,6-di-tert-butyl-phenol) (DTBP or probucol dithiobisphenol, Fig. 10.1), protect against oxidant-induced endothelial dysfunction [28] and promote re-endothelialization in rabbits [29]. Like probucol, DTBP also inhibited intimal hyperplasia in rabbits in response to injury, and atherosclerosis in *Apoe*$^{-/-}$ mice [29]. In addition, DTBP showed anti-inflammatory properties in *Apoe*$^{-/-}$ mice as assessed by the reduced macrophage infiltrate in the lesions [29], although other inflammatory makers were not investigated. The monosuccinate ester of DTBP (DTBPs, Fig. 10.1) was tested recently in rabbits against vascular injury-induced hyperplasia. Supplementation of the diet with 0.02% (wt/wt) DTBPs decreased the intima to media ratio: 0.84 ± 0.05 versus 1.07 ± 0.06 for DTBPs ($n = 11$) and control ($n = 12$), respectively ($P < 0.05$) (Stocker et al., unpublished). Furthermore, this decrease in intimal hyperplasia was achieved without lowering plasma cholesterol (Stocker et al., unpublished). Interestingly, DTBPs is a more effective inhibitor of *in vitro* VSMC proliferation when compared with succinobucol (Stocker et al., unpublished).

10.5 Conclusion

Over the past decades, probucol has been shown to be a strong anti-oxidant that can inhibit atherosclerosis in both humans and animals by a variety of potential mechanisms. However, due to its adverse effects, in particular the lowering of HDL cholesterol and prolongation of the QT interval, probucol is no longer used in most countries. Compounds that share the beneficial activities of probucol but lack its undesirable effects would be highly advantageous. In search of such an agent, succinobucol, the monosuccinate ester of probucol was developed and evaluated. While this drug shows anti-inflammatory activity, and preclinical studies have yielded encouraging results, clinical trials have not met the high expectations and side effects, some reminiscent of those of probucol, have (re-)emerged. One potentially unresolved issue pertains to the concentration of the drug used, as plasma concentrations of succinobucol have not been reported and the drug may have pro-apoptotic activity at higher concentrations.

Acknowledgments

We thank past and present members of the Stocker laboratory for their contributions to this area of research. R.G.M. is supported by a Program Grant from the National Health and Medical Research Council of Australia (NHMRC) (to R.S.). R.S. is supported by a NHMRC Senior Principal Research Fellowship and a University of Sydney Professorial Fellowship.

References

1. Barnhart, J. W., Sefranka, J. A., and McIntosh, D. D. (1970). Hypocholesterolemic effect of 4,4′-(isopropylidenedithio)-bis(2,6-di-*t*-butylphenol) (Probucol), *Am. J. Clin. Nutr.*, **23**, pp. 1229–1233.
2. Barnhart, J. W., Wagner, E. R., and Jackson, R. L. (1991). The synthesis, metabolism, and biological activity of probucol and its analogs, In *Antilipidemic Drugs* (eds. Witiak, D. T., Newman, H. A. I., and Feller, D. R.), Elsevier, Amsterdam, pp. 277–298.
3. Bräsen, J. H., Koenig, K., Bach, H., Kontush, A., Heinle, H., Witting, P. K., Ylä-Herttuala, S., Stocker, R., and Beisiegel, U. (2002). Comparison of the effects of alpha-tocopherol, ubiquinone-10 and probucol at therapeutic doses on atherosclerosis in WHHL rabbits, *Atherosclerosis*, **163**, pp. 249–259.
4. Choy, K., Beck, K., Png, F. Y., Wu, B. J., Leichtweis, S. B., Thomas, S. R., Hou, J. Y., Croft, K. D., Mori, T. A., and Stocker, R. (2005). Processes involved in the site-specific effect of probucol on atherosclerosis in apolipoprotein E gene knockout mice, *Arterioscl. Thromb. Vasc. Biol.*, **25**, pp. 1684–1690.
5. Clarke, M. C., Figg, N., Maguire, J. J., Davenport, A. P., Goddard, M., Littlewood, T. D., and Bennett, M. R. (2006). Apoptosis of vascular smooth muscle cells induces features of plaque vulnerability in atherosclerosis, *Nat. Med.*, **12**, pp. 1075–1080.
6. Deng, Y. M., Wu, B. J., Witting, P. K., and Stocker, R. (2004). Probucol protects against smooth muscle cell proliferation by upregulating heme oxygenase-1, *Circulation*, **110**, pp. 1855–1860.
7. Fruebis, J., Gonzalez, V., Silvestre, M., and Palinski, W. (1997). Effect of probucol treatment on gene expression of VCAM-1, MCP-1, and M-CSF in the aortic wall of LDL receptor-deficient rabbits during early atherogenesis, *Arterioscler. Thromb. Vasc. Biol.*, **17**, pp. 1289–1302.
8. Hodis, H. N., Chauhan, A., Hashimoto, S., Crawford, D. W., and Sevanian, A. (1992). Probucol reduces plasma and aortic wall oxysterol levels in cholesterol-fed rabbits independently of its plasma cholesterol lowering effect, *Atherosclerosis*, **96**, pp. 125–134.
9. Kunsch, C., Luchoomun, J., Grey, J. Y., Olliff, L. K., Saint, L. B., Arrendale, R. F., Wasserman, M. A., Saxena, U., and Medford, R. M. (2004). Selective inhibition of endothelial and monocyte redox-sensitive genes by AGI-1067: a novel antioxidant and anti-inflammatory agent, *J. Pharmacol. Exp. Ther.*, **308**, pp. 820–829.

10. Lau, A. K., Leichtweis, S. B., Hume, P., Mashima, R., Hou, J. Y., Chaufour, X., Wilkinson, B., Hunt, N. H., Celermajer, D. S., and Stocker, R. (2003). Probucol promotes functional reendothelialization in balloon-injured rabbit aortas, *Circulation*, **107**, pp. 2031–2036.

11. Liu, T., and Li, G. (2009). Probucol and succinobucol in atrial fibrillation: pros and cons, *Int. J. Cardiol.*, **144**, pp. 295–296.

12. Meng, C. Q., Somers, P. K., Rachita, C. L., Holt, L. A., Hoong, L. K., Zheng, X. S., Simpson, J. E., Hill, R. R., Olliff, L. K., Kunsch, C., Sundell, C. L., Parthasarathy, S., Saxena, U., Sikorski, J. A., and Wasserman, M. A. (2002). Novel phenolic antioxidants as multifunctional inhibitors of inducible VCAM-1 expression for use in atherosclerosis, *Bioorg. Med. Chem. Lett.*, **12**, pp. 2545–2548.

13. Mocatta, T. J., Pilbrow, A. P., Cameron, V. A., Senthilmohan, R., Frampton, C. M., Richards, A. M., and Winterbourn, C. C. (2007). Plasma concentrations of myeloperoxidase predict mortality after myocardial infarction, *J. Am. Coll. Cardiol.*, **49**, pp. 1993–2000.

14. Pryor, W. A., Strickland, T., and Church, D. F. (1988). Comparison of the efficiencies of several natural and synthetic antioxidants in aqueous sodium sulfate micelle solutions, *J. Am. Chem. Soc.*, **110**, pp. 2224–2229.

15. Reinoehl, J., Frankovich, D., Machado, C., Kawasaki, R., Baga, J. J., Pires, L. A., Steinman, R. T., Fromm, B. S., and Lehmann, M. H. (1996). Probucol-associated tachyarrhythmic events and QT prolongation: importance of gender, *Am. Heart J.*, **131**, pp. 1184–1191.

16. Ryter, S. W., Alam, J., and Choi, A. M. (2006). Heme oxygenase-1/carbon monoxide: from basic science to therapeutic applications, *Physiol. Rev.*, **86**, pp. 583–650.

17. Sawayama, Y., Maeda, S., Ohnishi, H., Okada, K., and Hayashi, J. (2006). Effect of probucol on elderly hypercholesterolemic patients in the FAST study, *Fukuoka Igaku Zasshi*, **97**, pp. 15–24.

18. Stocker, R., and Keaney, J. F., Jr. (2004). Role of oxidative modifications in atherosclerosis, *Physiol. Rev.*, **84**, pp. 1381–1478.

19. Stocker, R., and Perrella, M. A. (2006). Heme oxygenase-1. A novel drug target for atherosclerotic diseases?, *Circulation*, **114**, pp. 2178–2189.

20. Stocker, R. (2009). Molecular mechanisms underlying the antiatherosclerotic and antidiabetic effects of probucol, succinobucol, and other probucol analogues, *Curr. Opin. Lipidol.*, **20**, pp. 227–235.

21. Sundell, C. L., Somers, P. K., Meng, C. Q., Hoong, L. K., Suen, K. L., Hill, R. R., Landers, L. K., Chapman, A., Butteiger, D., Jones, M., Edwards, D.,

Daugherty, A., Wasserman, M. A., Alexander, R. W., Medford, R. M., and Saxena, U. (2003). AGI-1067: a multifunctional phenolic antioxidant, lipid modulator, anti-inflammatory and antiatherosclerotic agent, *J. Pharmacol. Exp. Ther.*, **305**, pp. 1116–1123.

22. Tanous, D., Hime, N., and Stocker, R. (2008). Anti-atherosclerotic and anti-diabetic properties of probucol and related compounds, *Redox Rep.*, **13**, pp. 48–59.

23. Tardif, J. C., Grégoire, J., Schwartz, L., Title, L., Laramee, L., Reeves, F., Lesperance, J., Bourassa, M. G., L'Allier, P. L., Glass, M., Lambert, J., and Guertin, M. C. (2003). Effects of AGI-1067 and probucol after percutaneous coronary interventions, *Circulation*, **107**, pp. 552–558.

24. Tardif, J. C., Gregoire, J., L'Allier, P. L., Ibrahim, R., Anderson, T. J., Reeves, F., Title, L. M., Schampaert, E., LeMay, M., Lesperance, J., Scott, R., Guertin, M. C., Brennan, M. L., Hazen, S. L., and Bertrand, O. F. (2008). Effects of the antioxidant succinobucol (AGI-1067) on human atherosclerosis in a randomized clinical trial, *Atherosclerosis*, **197**, pp. 480–486.

25. Tardif, J. C., Grégoire, J., L'Allier, P. L., Ibrahim, R., Anderson, T. J., Reeves, F., Title, L. M., Schampaert, E., LeMay, M., Lespérance, J., Scott, R., Guertin, M. C., Brennan, M. L., Hazen, S. L., and Bertrand, O. F. (2008). Effects of the antioxidant succinobucol (AGI-1067) on human atherosclerosis in a randomized clinical trial, *Atherosclerosis*, **197**, pp. 480–486.

26. Tardif, J. C., McMurray, J. J., Klug, E., Small, R., Schumi, J., Choi, J., Cooper, J., Scott, R., Lewis, E. F., L'Allier, P. L., and Pfeffer, M. A. (2008). Effects of succinobucol (AGI-1067) after an acute coronary syndrome: a randomised, double-blind, placebo-controlled trial, *Lancet*, **371**, pp. 1761–1768.

27. Walldius, G., Erikson, U., Olsson, A. G., Bergstrand, L., Hådell, K., Johansson, J., Kaijser, L., Lassvik, C., Mölgaard, J., Nilsson, S., Schäfer-Elinder, L., Stenport, G., and Holme, I. (1994). The effect of probucol on femoral atherosclerosis: the Probucol Quantitative Regression Swedish Trial (PQRST), *Am. J. Cardiol.*, **74**, pp. 875–883.

28. Witting, P. K., Wu, B. J., Raftery, M., Southwell-Keely, P., and Stocker, R. (2005). Probucol protects against hypochlorite-induced endothelial dysfunction. Identification of a novel pathway of probucol oxidation to a biologically active intermediate, *J. Biol. Chem.*, **280**, pp. 15612–15618.

29. Wu, B. J., Kathir, K., Witting, P. K., Beck, K., Choy, K., Li, C., Croft, K. D., Mori, T. A., Tanous, D., Adams, M. R., Lau, A. K., and Stocker, R. (2006). Antioxidants protect from atherosclerosis by a heme oxygenase-1

pathway that is independent of free radical scavenging, *J. Exp. Med.*, **203**, pp. 1117–1127.

30. Wu, B. J., Di Girolamo, N., Beck, K., Hanratty, C. G., Choy, K., Hou, J. Y., Ward, M. R., and Stocker, R. (2007). Probucol [4,4′-[(1-methylethylidene) bis(thio)]bis-[2,6-bis(1,1-dimethylethyl)phenol]] inhibits compensatory remodeling and promotes lumen loss associated with atherosclerosis in apolipoprotein E-deficient mice, *J. Pharmacol. Exp. Ther.*, **321**, pp. 477–484.
31. Wu, B. J., Midwinter, R. G., Cassano, C., Beck, K., Wang, Y., Changsiri, D., Gamble, J. R., and Stocker, R. (2009). Heme oxygenase-1 increases endothelial progenitor cells, *Arterioscler. Thromb. Vasc. Biol.*, **29**, pp. 1537–1542.
32. Yamamoto, A., Matsuzawa, Y., Yokoyama, S., Funahashi, T., Yamamura, T., and Kishino, B. (1986). Effects of probucol on xanthomata regression in familial hypercholesterolemia, *Am. J. Cardiol.*, **57**, pp. 29H–35H.
33. Yamamoto, A., Hara, H., Takaichi, S., Wakasugi, J., and Tomikawa, M. (1988). Effect of probucol on macrophages, leading to regression of xanthomas and atheromatous vascular lesions, *Am. J. Cardiol.*, **62**, pp. 31B–36B.

Chapter 11

Interference with ER Stress and Restoration of Efferocytosis in the Treatment of Advanced Atherosclerosis

Edward Thorp, Lale Ozcan, and Ira Tabas
Department of Medicine, Division of Molecular Medicine, Columbia University, New York, NY 10032, USA
iat1@columbia.edu

11.1 Overview of ER Stress and Efferocytosis in Atherosclerosis

A number of cellular events in the inflammatory advanced atherosclerotic milieu conspire to form the characteristic vulnerable plaque that is strongly associated with acute myocardial infarction and sudden death. A key component of plaque vulnerability is expansion of the lipid necrotic core, which also contains remnants of dead or dying macrophages (Ball *et al.*, 1995). This focal concentration of inflammation, cell death, and tissue destabilization arises through a combination of advanced lesional macrophage apoptosis and defective clearance of these dead cells, a process called defective efferocytosis (Vandivier *et al.*, 2006). In the case of macrophage

Atherosclerosis: Treatment and Prevention
Edited by Christian Weber and Oliver Soehnlein

ISBN 978-981-4316-26-2 (Hardcover), ISBN 978-981-4364-26-3 (eBook)
www.panstanford.com

apoptosis, chronic activation of ER stress pathways tip the balance from adaptive pro-survival ER stress signaling to networks that promote cell death. The significance of ER stress in other lesional cell types is less well understood, however the current evidence strongly supports roles for regulation of cell survival in smooth muscle cells and endothelial cells (ECs) (Kedi *et al.*, 2009b; Nakano *et al.*, 2006). Importantly, the consequences of ER stress-mediated apoptosis are tightly linked to efferocytosis. That efferocytosis is defective in human advanced plaque suggests that the combination of ER stress-induced apoptosis and defective efferocytosis create the "perfect storm", which enables a continuous cycle of cell death, reduced clearance, and chronic inflammation (Tabas, 2010; Schrijvers *et al.*, 2005). The causes of defective efferocytosis in atherosclerosis are not well understood. To date, genetic causation experiments in pre-clinical animal models implicate a handful of clearance signaling pathways that may malfunction during advanced lesional maturation. In this chapter, we provide an overview of the critical and relevant pathways of ER stress and efferocytosis in advanced atheromata. Furthermore, we discuss new therapeutic strategies designed to target these pathways and promote inflammation resolution and plaque stabilization.

11.2 Part I. ER Stress Therapy

11.2.1 Introduction to ER Stress in Atherosclerosis

Atherosclerosis is a maladaptive inflammatory response to subendothelially-retained apolipoprotein B-containing lipoproteins. Atherosclerotic progression involves complex interactions between lipoproteins and the cells of the arterial wall, namely ECs, macrophages, and vascular smooth muscle cells (VSMCs) (Lusis, 2000). Decades of experimental evidence indicate that subendothelial retention of apolipoprotein B-containing lipoproteins is the key initiating event of atherogenesis (Williams and Tabas, 1995). This is followed by recruitment of inflammatory monocytes to activated ECs and their differentiation into macrophages. Macrophage phagocytes ingest oxidatively-modified lipoproteins, become foam cells, and secrete inflammatory cytokines and chemokines that promote recruitment of VSMCs and other types of immune cells. Through a number of cell biological events that remain incompletely elucidated, a small percentage of stable early atherosclerotic lesions convert into complex and rupture-prone plaques that ultimately are the precursor to acute clinical events such as myocardial infarction and stroke (Tabas, 2010). One particular cellular event that has emerged as a prominent feature of atherosclerotic progression is endoplasmic reticulum (ER) stress and the induction of the ER-derived unfolded protein response (UPR) (Tabas, 2009).

The ER is a membranous network where protein maturation, folding, and transport occur (Rutkowski and Kaufman, 2004). The ER also acts as the major site for the production of cholesterol and other membrane lipid components. In addition to its vital role in protein folding and lipid biosynthesis, the ER also functions as a major calcium storage and signaling organelle. ER-regulated changes in calcium flux occur through ER-resident multimeric ion channels (Wu and Kaufman, 2006). Perturbations that interfere with proper functioning of the ER, such as the accumulation of misfolded proteins or an imbalance of ER calcium, can in turn lead to activation of the UPR ER stress response (Ron and Walter, 2007a). Initially, the UPR is an adaptive reaction that acts to restore cellular homeostasis. For example, the UPR signaling network can restore ER homeostasis through downregulation of ER protein client load concomitant with increased expression of protein-folding chaperones. This manifests through the activation and cross-talk of three upstream ER-localized transmembrane receptors. These include: PKR-like eukaryotic initiation factor 2α kinase (PERK), inositol-requiring enzyme-1 (IRE-1), and activating transcription factor-6 (ATF-6) (Rutkowski and Kaufman, 2004; Rutkowski *et al.*, 2008; Ron and Walter, 2007b; Wu and Kaufman, 2006; Marciniak and Ron, 2006). In cells undergoing ER stress, activated PERK phosphorylates eukaryotic translation initiation factor 2 alpha (eIF2α) at Ser51, and this results in global translational attenuation and reduced ER protein load. Stimulation of IRE-1 leads to its autophosphorylation and activation of an endoribonuclease domain. The endoribonuclease splices mRNA to encode for spliced X-box binding protein-1 (XBP-1s). XBP-1s is a transcriptional factor that upregulates many essential UPR genes in order to increase ER folding capacity and expansion of ER membrane surface area (Glimcher, 2010). Finally, a third UPR pathway is initiated by ATF-6, which is proteolytically-processed and translocates to the nucleus. In the nucleus, ATF-6 also acts to increase the expression of ER chaperones such as Grp78 (Wu and Kaufman, 2006). Collectively, these three arms of the UPR attempt to relieve the stress and promote cell survival. However, if the stress is prolonged or severe, the UPR can trigger programmed cell death. UPR-mediated cell death appears to contribute to the pathogenesis of many diseases, including cancer, diabetes, neurodegeneration, and atherosclerosis (Marciniak and Ron, 2006).

The mechanisms of ER stress-induced apoptosis are complex and involve two principle signaling pathways: the extrinsic or death receptor pathway and the intrinsic or mitochondrial pathway, both of which exhibit crosstalk with each other. The best characterized ER stress-induced pro-apoptotic factor is CHOP/GADD153. CHOP is a transcription factor that is induced via a pathway in which P-eIF2α increases the translation of ATF4, a transcription factor for CHOP (Zinszner *et al.*, 1998). CHOP triggers apoptosis, in part, through downregulation of the anti-apoptotic factor B cell lymphoma-2 (Bcl-2) and upregulation of Bim, a proapoptotic BH3-only member of the Bcl-2 family (Szegezdi *et al.*, 2006). CHOP also upregulates ERO-1, which is involved in disulfide bond formation. This not only is critical for protein folding but also generates reactive oxygen species (ROS) that may contribute to the activation of the apoptotic program (Marciniak *et al.*, 2004). Recently, ERO-1 has been shown to activate inositol 1,4,5-triphosphate receptor (IP3R1) through formation of a disulfide bond in the lumenal loop of IP3R1. This, in turn, increases IP3R1 calcium channel activity and leads to an increase in the cytoplasmic calcium, which is a critical process in apoptosis (Li *et al.*, 2009b). Studies have shown that deletion of CHOP partially protects both cells and mice from ER stress-mediated cell death (Thorp *et al.*, 2009; Oyadomari *et al.*, 2002; Tamaki *et al.*, 2008; Song *et al.*, 2008a; Tsukano *et al.*, 2010). In addition, IRE-1 signaling pathways can also promote apoptosis, specifically by activating the c-Jun N-terminal Kinase (JNK). This pathway involves recruitment of TNF receptor-associated factor (TRAF2) and the apoptosis signal regulating kinase-1 (ASK1) complex (Urano *et al.*, 2000). Besides CHOP and JNK, ER resident cysteine protease caspase 12 has also been linked to ER stress-induced apoptosis. For example, caspase $12^{-/-}$ mice and cultured cells exhibit reduced ER stress-mediated apoptosis relative to controls (Nakagawa *et al.*, 2000).

In the context of the intrinsic/mitochondrial death pathway, the mechanisms that lead to cell death are more complex. For example, increased calcium transfer from ER to mitochondria is implicated in mitochondrial programmed cell death, however the nature of the signaling pathways remains incompletely understood (Giorgi *et al.*, 2009). There are a number of molecules that have been implicated in control of calcium transfer to mitochondria during ER stress (Chami *et al.*, 2008; Hayashi and Su, 2007; Kornmann *et al.*, 2009). For example, a calcium sensing enzyme, calcium/calmodulin-dependent protein kinase II (CaMKII), which is activated by ER stress, has been shown to play a role in mitochondrial calcium accumulation upon ER stress in macrophages (Timmins *et al.*, 2009). As discussed below, given that CaMKII acts as an upstream molecule that regulates multiple apoptosis pathways, targeting CaMKII for inhibition may be a viable target in reducing ER stress-induced cell death during advanced atherosclerosis (Ozcan and Tabas, 2010).

11.2.2 Candidate Targets for ER Stress Therapy in Advanced Lesions

11.2.2.1 Targeting macrophage apoptosis

Macrophages play a key role during atherogenesis by ingesting lipoprotein-derived cholesterol and storing cholesterol ester as lipid-laden foam cells in early lesions. As lesions progress, dead and dying macrophages contribute to the development of a necrotic core, which promotes inflammation and plaque instability (Tabas *et al.*, 2009). Necrotic cores originate through a combination of post-apoptotic macrophage necrosis and defective phagocytic clearance of apoptotic macrophages (Tabas, 2005). Necrotic cores are a reservoir of matrix proteases, inflammatory mediators, and pro-thrombotic molecules. Thus, macrophage apoptosis is a key factor in converting lesions from a benign to an unstable phenotype by promoting necrotic core formation. One cause of macrophage apoptosis in advanced atherosclerosis is the activation of proapoptotic branches of the UPR (Seimon and Tabas, 2009). In addition to macrophages, UPR activation is also found in other vascular cell types during atherosclerotic progression, namely ECs and VSMCs, which will be discussed below (see Figure 11.1).

As lesions advance in age, macrophages accumulate increasing amounts of free cholesterol and, in combination with other ER stressors found in plaque, this likely drives macrophages to die. *In vitro* proof of this concept originated from cell culture models where macrophages loaded with AcLDL-derived cholesterol and Acetyl-Coenzyme A acetyltransferase (ACAT) inhibitors exhibited activation of the UPR followed later by CHOP-dependent apoptosis (Thorp *et al.*, 2009; Feng *et al.*, 2003a). Recent studies have shown that the key initiating event in the apoptosis cascade in ER-stressed macrophages is release of calcium from ER stores into the cytosol (Seimon *et al.*, 2006). Additionally, the UPR itself amplifies this calcium release by activating inositol-3-phosphate receptor via CHOP-induced ERO1α (Li *et al.*, 2009b). The concomitant increase in cytoplasmic calcium activates CaMKII and this in turn activates a number of apoptotic pathways, including pro-apoptotic signal transducer and activator of transcription-1 (STAT1), cell-surface death receptor Fas, pro-apoptotic mitochondrial dysfunction, and accumulation of ROS through activation of NADPH oxidase (Timmins *et al.*, 2009; Lim *et al.*, 2008).

In vitro and *in vivo* genetic evidence have demonstrated a strong, causal relationship between atherosclerosis, particularly the formation of necrotic lesions, and ER stress. For example, a collection of studies have shown that advanced lesional macrophage death and plaque necrosis are decreased in atherosclerotic apolipoprotein E-deficient (Apoe–/–) mice in the setting of ER stress prevention, CHOP deficiency, or Stat-1 deficiency in $LDLR^{-/-}$ mice (Feng *et al.*, 2003b; Thorp *et al.*, 2009; Tsukano *et al.*, 2010; Lim *et al.*, 2008). Moreover, Myoishi *et al.* have documented a close correlation among CHOP expression, apoptosis, and plaque vulnerability in human coronary artery lesions (Myoishi *et al.*, 2007). Cooperatively, these studies provide the evidence that ER stress-induced macrophage apoptosis plays a major role in the etiology of advanced lesion development and that compounds that inhibit therapeutic targets such as CHOP or STAT1 could be considered for atherosclerosis therapy.

As mentioned above, prolonged activation of the IRE-1 pathway also functions as a proapoptotic pathway through recruiting a TRAF2 and ASK1 complex and activating JNK. Recent evidence has also shown that prolonged ER stress can activate JNK through activation of CaMKII (Timmins *et al.*, 2009). Once JNK is activated, it can induce proapoptotic Bim and inhibit Bcl-2 (Lei and Davis, 2003; Putcha *et al.*, 2003). In this context, macrophages deficient in JNK2 were shown to be protected from ER stress-induced cell death (DeVries-

Seimon *et al.*, 2005). Furthermore, ApoE-null mice that were treated with the JNK1/2 pathway inhibitor SP600125 were found to develop significantly less atherosclerosis than ApoE-null mice treated with vehicle. Similarly, irradiated Apoe$^{-/-}$ mice transplanted with Jnk2$^{-/-}$ bone marrow exhibited reduced atherosclerotic lesion formation (Ricci *et al.*, 2004). Thus, pharmacological agents that specifically target proapototic JNK in macrophages could be used in therapeutic applications.

In humans, *in situ* hybridization with riboprobes has shown an association of ER-associated chaperone ORP150 (150-kDa oxygen-regulated protein) with macrophages in atherosclerotic plaques (Tsukamoto *et al.*, 1996). ORP150 may play a role in promoting cellular adaptive responses during ER stress in plaque. Interestingly, auto-antibodies to ORP150 have been identified in the serum of patients with severe atherosclerosis. In addition, a recent study reported that ER stress markers and ORP150 chaperones are co-expressed in lesional areas containing oxLDLs (Sanson *et al.*, 2009). *In vitro*, ORP150 is induced by oxLDLs and oxidized lipids in tissue culture cells. These studies provide an important proof of principle that targeting ER stress at the level of molecular chaperones may have therapeutic potential during athero-progresion.

Chemical or pharmaceutical chaperones are a group of low molecular-weight compounds that can increase ER folding capacity and decrease the accumulation and aggregation of misfolded proteins in the ER lumen (Loo and Clarke, 2007). 4-Phenyl butyrate (4-PBA), trimethylamine N-Oxide (TMAO), glycerol, dimethyl sulfoxide (DMSO), and taurine-conjugated deoxycholic acid (TUDCA) have been reported to have chemical chaperone activities (Vilatoba *et al.*, 2005; Tatzelt *et al.*, 1996; de Almeida *et al.*, 2007). However, the exact mechanism of how these chaperones act is still not understood. It is believed that these agents induce the stabilization of misfolded proteins and reduce protein accumulation by preventing the interactions between hydrophobic patches, a characteristic of unfolded proteins. At the level of the arterial wall, a recent study showed that the chemical chaperone PBA, an FDA approved drug for the treatment of urea cycle disorders, alleviated saturated fatty acid-induced ER stress in cultured macrophages and reduced lesion area, ER stress and apoptosis in Western diet-fed Apoe$^{-/-}$ mice (Erbay *et al.*, 2009a). However, the same compound in diabetes-induced atherosclerosis in hamsters failed to decrease ER stress in aorta and had no effect on atherosclerotic lesion size (Kurokawa *et al.*, 2009). The differences in experimental design, such as differences in genetic background, diets and duration of the treatment, may have contributed to the disparate outcomes in these studies. On the other hand, the other chemical chaperone TUDCA, which is now being used in the treatment of cholestatic liver disease in Europe, has been shown to suppress both the development of aortic lesions and ER stress in Ldlr$^{-/-}$/Ampk-2$^{-/-}$ mice (Dong *et al.*, 2010). However, the mechanism of how these chemicals act to relieve ER stress or whether these chemicals affect the other cell types relevant to atherosclerosis is not known and remains to be investigated.

11.2.2.2 Targeting endothelial cells

ER function in the presence of atherosclerosis-relevant stimuli has been shown to influence other cells of the arterial wall besides macrophages. ECs express all key proteins involved in regulating ER stress (Luo *et al.*, 2008) and are capable of initiating ER stress signaling after exposure to oxidized phospholipids (Gharavi *et al.*, 2007) or homocysteine (Outinen *et al.*, 1999). In human atherosclerotic lesions, makers of ER stress are increased in areas containing oxidized phospholipids. Thus, ER stress might contribute to reduced NO availability and be responsible for EC dysfunction in atherosclerosis (Gargalovic *et al.*, 2006). In addition, atherosclerosis preferentially develops in regions with slow or disturbed blood flow where low shear stress can affect the phenotype of ECs. Glucose regulated protein 78 (GRP78), a chaperone protein and marker of ER stress, can be regulated by hemodynamic shear stress in the endothelium of atherosclerotic-prone regions in C57BL/6 mice (Feaver *et al.*, 2008). Also, in normal swine aorta, ATF-6 and IRE-1/Xbp-1 pathways are activated in the endothelium of the athero-susceptible aortic arch (Civelek *et al.*, 2009). However, when XBP-1 was overexpressed in lesions, ECs exhibited more apoptosis, and atherosclerosis development was accelerated (Zeng *et al.*, 2009). Further studies are needed to evaluate the exact mechanisms responsible for this effect.

Another piece of evidence supporting the relationship between endothelial ER stress and atherosclerosis came from a study where Apoe–/– mice were made hyperglycemic by streptozocin injection. This lead to increased endothelial cell ER stress markers that preceded the development of atherosclerosis (Khan *et al.*, 2009). However, markers of ER stress were also increased in macrophage cells, suggesting that the effect of hyperglycemia on the development of atherosclerosis is not endothelial specific. Finally, hyperhomocystinemia, which is an independent risk factor for cardiovascular disease, has been shown to induce endothelial dysfunction in many studies using animal models and human subjects (Hossain *et al.*, 2003; Woo *et al.*, 1997). *In vitro* work has shown that homocysteine promotes endothelial cell dysfunction through a pathway involving the activation of IRE1-JNK (Zhang *et al.*, 2001a; Zhang *et al.*, 2001b). Thus, chemical inhibitors of the endothelial IRE1-JNK pathway might be a therapeutic option.

11.2.2.3 Targeting vascular smooth muscle cells

In advanced plaque, VSMC death compromises plaque integrity and weakens the fibrous cap (Geng and Libby, 2002). *In vitro* evidence suggests that ER stressors like cholesterol loading, hyperhomocysteinemia or high glucose and glucosamine upregulate ER stress markers such as CHOP, which also has been implicated in the death of SMCs (Kedi *et al.*, 2009a; Werstuck *et al.*, 2006). Also, 7-keto-cholesterol, an oxysterol that is elevated in the plasma of patients with a high cardiovascular risk, has been shown to activate the UPR and induce apoptosis of cultured human SMCs (Pedruzzi *et al.*, 2004). Moreover, fibrous caps of thin-cap human atheroma lesions were found to be positive by immunohistochemistry for 7-KC, a finding consistent with the increase UPR markers (Myoishi *et al.*, 2007). In addition, VSMCs has been shown to display markers of ER stress in hyperhomocystinemic Apoe$^{-/-}$ mice. The mechanism is thought to be mediated through changes in ER calcium release (Dickhout *et al.*, 2007). In this context, pretreatment of SMCs with taurine, an amino-sulphonic acid, has been shown to reduce homocysteine-induced ER stress parameters such as PERK phosphorylation and GRP 78 induction (Nonaka *et al.*, 2001b). However, the exact site at which taurine acts to relieve homocysteine-induced ER stress still remains unknown. Targets for drug discovery in the context of VSMCs and ER stress are not well studied and further experimental approaches, including *in vivo* tests of agents that target specifically VSMCs during ER stress will be beneficial.

11.2.2.4 Targeting oxidative stress

Oxidative protein folding in the ER stimulates the generation of reactive oxygen species. Oxidative stress has been implicated as a pro-apoptotic process in ER stress-induced cell death that promotes a feed-forward cycle of ER and additional oxidative stress (Malhotra and Kaufman, 2007). Recent studies using cultured macrophages relevant to advanced atherosclerosis have shown that saturated fatty acids (SFA), 7-keto-cholesterol, and oxidized phospholipids induce oxidative stress through a pathway requiring NADPH oxidase. This pathway is necessary for ER stress-induced macrophage apoptosis. Moreover, ER stress-induced apoptosis in macrophages can be partially suppressed by *N*- acetylcysteine (NAC), an anti-oxidant that reduces the ROS product of NADPH oxidase. *In vivo* work has shown that there are many sources of oxidative stress in atherosclerotic lesions, including peroxynitrite, homocyteine, and hyperglycemia, which independently have been shown to cause ER stress (Pacher and Szabo, 2006; Woo *et al.*, 1997). In one example, peroxynitrite, a potent oxidant generated by the reaction of nitric oxide with superoxide, was shown to be elevated in human atherosclerotic lesions (Ravalli *et al.*, 1997; Ravalli *et al.*, 1998). It has also been demonstrated that peroxynitrite induces ER stress in the vascular endothelium and that 3-nitrotyrosine (3-NT), a marker of peroxynitrite generation, and GRP78 staining are increased and colocalize in early atherosclerotic lesions from Apoe$^{-/-}$ mice (Dickhout *et al.*, 2005). This suggests that peroxynitrite contributes to atherogenesis through a mechanism involving ER stress. Despite convincing epidemiologic and mechanistic evidence, most clinical trials using Vitamin E have failed to demonstrate that anti-oxidant therapy in people who are at high risk for cardiovascular events exhibit a clear cardiovascular benefit (Yusuf *et al.*, 2000). One trial reported that this approach actually increased mortality (Lonn *et al.*, 2005). Thus, more selective compounds that specifically target ER stress-induced ROS formation in macrophages might be beneficial in the prevention of advanced atherosclerotic lesions.

11.2.3 Metabolic Risk Factors

The development of atherosclerosis in humans is affected by the presence of important risk factors, such as dyslipidemia, diabetes, and insulin resistance (IR) associated with obesity (Ginsberg and

Maccallum, 2009). In this regard, ER stress has been suggested to influence the course of atherosclerosis through affecting systemic risk factors. In one scenario, XBP-1 has been linked to lipid homeostasis in liver. Mice deficient in XBP-1 in liver exhibited a downregulation in the key lipogenic enzymes, including Acc2, Dgat2, and Scd1 (Lee *et al.*, 2008). In line with this observation, recent reports from different mouse models implicate connections between ER dysfunction and the regulation of lipid metabolism. This provides new opportunities to develop treatments for hyperlipidemia, which is an independent risk factor for atherosclerosis (Rutkowski *et al.*, 2008; Oyadomari *et al.*, 2008).

Atherosclerosis is the most important complication of type 2 diabetes characterized by IR (Reaven, 2002). IR has been implicated in the development of dyslipidemia and hyperglycemia, due to impaired suppression of hepatic glucose production. Both dyslipidemia and hyperglycemia are significant risk factors for atherosclerosis (Ginsberg and Maccallum, 2009; Biddinger *et al.*, 2008; Han *et al.*, 2009). In this context, activation of the UPR in liver and adipose tissues has been shown to contribute to the development of IR, at least in part through the IRE-1-dependent, JNK-1-mediated inhibition of insulin action (Ozcan *et al.*, 2004). Thus, pharmacological agents that specifically inhibit ER stress-induced IRE-1 dependent JNK activation may be beneficial in the treatment of type 2 diabetes and related atherosclerotic risk factors. Moreover, PBA and TUDCA have been shown to relieve ER stress in obesity, enhance insulin sensitivity, and maintain euglycemia in a severe mouse model of obesity (*ob/ob*) and type 2 diabetes (Ozcan *et al.*, 2006). Likewise, more recent work has shown that TUDCA therapy increases liver and muscle insulin sensitivity in obese, insulin-resistant subjects (Kars *et al.*, 2010). However, there was no change in ER stress markers in insulin sensitive tissues after TUDCA treatment, questioning its ER stress-relieving effect. Additional studies are needed to evaluate the exact mechanisms responsible for this improvement in insulin sensitivity. In line with this, macelignan, a natural compound isolated from myristica fragnans and a dual agonist of PPARα/γ, has also been shown to reduce ER stress parameters in liver and adipose tissue of *db/db* mice (Han *et al.*, 2008). However, it is not clear whether macelignan's beneficial effect on ER stress parameters is primarily related to its ER stress-relieving properties and further work needs to be done to support this.

Progression of T2D is also characterized by beta cell apoptosis that leads to impaired insulin secretion and marked hyperglycemia. In this context, recent studies document the relevance of chronic ER stress in promoting beta cell death, at least in part through UPR-induced CHOP upregulation (Song *et al.*, 2008b). In multiple mouse models of type 2 diabetes, CHOP gene ablation results in improved glycemic control and expanded beta cell mass through protecting against oxidative stress in response to ER stress. In the context of hyperglycemia, this can lead to endothelial dysfunction through oxidative stress and formation of advanced glycation end-products (AGEs). Interestingly, recent data suggest that hyperglycemia may exert some of its proatherogenic effects on ECs through Forkhead Box-O1 (FoxO1) and also through the induction of ER stress (Senokuchi *et al.*, 2008). Despite convincing epidemiologic evidence, some clinical trials have failed to demonstrate that aggressive glucose-lowering therapy in people with established, long-duration diabetes has a clear cardiovascular benefit (Gerstein *et al.*, 2008). However, currently available evidence also suggests that better glycemic control at the time of diagnosis has a long-term cardiovascular benefit (Holman *et al.*, 2008). Thus, strategies aimed at CHOP inhibition in beta cells under conditions of IR may serve as a potential drug target for beta cell dysfunction and resultant pro-atherogenic hyperglycemia.

Finally, recent work has shown that ER stress increases hepatic gluconeogenesis through a pathway involving ATF-6. ATF-6α was proposed to interfere with the induction of the gluconeogenic program through disrupting CREB–CRTC2 (CREB regulated transcription co-activator 2) interaction, thereby inhibiting CRTC2 occupancy over gluconeogenic genes (Wang *et al.*, 2009; Seo *et al.*, 2010). *In vivo* evidence has shown that ATF6α overexpression improves glucose balance by lowering gluconeogenic gene expression in *ob/ob* mice. Thus, small-molecule compounds that selectively induce ATF-6, without triggering the production of other UPR genes, in the setting of obesity, might have beneficial effects in the regulation of glucose homeostasis that is relevant to atherogenesis. Furthermore, recent studies have shown that IR is a potent inducer of the UPR in macrophages and that insulin resistant macrophages are more susceptible to ER stress-induced apoptosis. This is in part related to a failure to induce Akt activity (Han *et al.*, 2006). $Ldlr^{-/-}$ mice deficient in insulin receptor, specifically in macrophages, developed more plaque necrosis than control mice. In addition to macrophages, IR has been shown to promote endothelial dysfunction through impairing NO-mediated arterial responses, thereby promoting atherosclerosis. Therefore, studies aimed at relieving IR at the arterial wall may be beneficial. In addition to being an independent cardiovascular disease risk factor, obesity can affect atherosclerosis through increasing the incidence of other risk factors, notably diabetes, dyslipidemia, and the prothrombotic state. In line with these findings, ER stress has also been implicated in the development of leptin resistance and obesity (Ozcan *et al.*, 2009; Zhang *et al.*, 2008). Thus, targeting to relieve ER stress associated with obesity and leptin resistance may be beneficial.

11.3 Part II. Efferocytosis Therapy: Targeting Defective Efferocytosis in the Treatment of Advanced Atherosclerotic Plaque

11.3.1 Introduction to Defective Efferocytosis in Advanced Atherosclerosis

Macrophage apoptosis occurs throughout all stages of atherosclerosis, yet the consequences of this event vary in early versus aged atherosclerotic lesions (Tabas, 2005). This dichotomous setting implies that other factors downstream of pro-apoptotic signaling uniquely emerge in advanced lesions to impact the fate of dying cells. One such event is the phagocytic clearance of apoptotic cells, otherwise known as efferocytosis. Efferocytosis is a term coined by Peter Henson and colleagues (Vandivier *et al.*, 2006) that distinguishes apoptotic cell clearance from phagocytic uptake of foreign pathogens like bacteria. This is an important distinction as the mechanisms and downstream inflammatory consequences of pathogen uptake versus apoptotic cell engulfment are distinct. During early atherogenesis, efferocytosis is efficient (Tabas, 2007), and TUNEL-positive apoptotic nuclei are rarely detected. This is consistent with other non-diseased and macrophage-rich sites where high rates of cell turnover (Surh and Sprent, 1994) fail to exhibit significant accumulation of free apoptotic cells. Such efficiency of apoptotic cell clearance is critical for limiting inflammation that is associated with post apoptotic secondary necrosis. Thus, accelerated apoptosis in the context of defective efferocytosis is inflammatory and promotes increased leukocyte recruitment and lesion progression. In contrast, increased cell death combined with efficient and nonphlogistic clearance together act to reduce cell content and potentially limit lesion expansion. Consistent with efficient clearance of dying cells in early lesions, Arai *et al.* report reduced lesion size in mice with macrophages deficient for the survival protein known as AIM (apoptosis inhibitor expressed by macrophages), which *in vitro* accelerates macrophage death by oxidized LDL.

The consequences of apoptosis in advanced lesions are dissimilar to early lesions because efferocytosis is defective. In humans, this was first reported by Schrijvers *et al.* who found high levels of free and non-cleared apoptotic macrophages in human endaraterectomy specimens (Schrijvers *et al.*, 2005). Though the causes of this defective clearance remain a mystery, the cumulative effect is generation of the necrotic core. In concert with potentially pro-atherogenic effects of residual and inflammatory surviving macrophages, necrotic core expansion inhibits inflammation resolution and promotes plaque instability and thrombosis. Thus, the ability or lack thereof of lesional phagocytes to safely clear apoptotic cells may be an important determinant of acute atherothrombotic clinical events. This overall concept implicates efferocytosis pathways as potential therapeutic targets for the intervention of advanced atherosclerotic progression. Below we outline critical events that regulate atherosclerotic efferocytosis efficiency and discuss possible therapeutic targets for *in vivo* testing.

11.3.2 Candidate Efferocytosis Targets and Interventions

11.3.2.1 Alleviating cellular stress during clearance

A role for ER stress and ER associated calcium in efferocytosis? The first half of this review focused on ER stress signaling and its contribution to atherosclerotic progression. Much less is known about possible links between the UPR and apoptotic cell clearance, however a few intriguing clues warrant further study. For example, a recent report out of the Ravichandran group indicate that efferocytosis can be blocked by disabling ER calcium homeostasis with the SERCA inhibitor thapsigargin (Gronski *et al.*, 2009). Calcium plays a key role as a second messenger in many cell types, and extracellular and intracellular sources of Ca^{2+} are known to affect Fc-receptor mediated uptake of opsonized particles (Young *et al.*, 1984; Hackam *et al.*, 1997; Rosales and Brown, 1992; Zhang *et al.*, 2005). In macrophages, Ca^{2+} oscillations from intracellular stores can localize to periphagosomal regions (Marks and Maxfield, 1990). Extracellular Ca^{2+} may also play a role. Changes in extracellular Ca^{2+} concentration likely also affect the conformation and, therefore, capacity of phagocytic receptors to bind targets for engulfment. In addition to roles of ER calcium, the ER may play a more direct/physical role during efferocytosis regulation. For example, efferocytosis is inhibited after silencing of STIM-1 (Stromal interaction molecule), which localizes to ER-plasma membrane junctions (Gronski *et al.*, 2009). Moreover, the ER can contribute membrane surface area during large particle engulfment (Gagnon *et al.*, 2002; Becker *et al.*, 2005). Future work will be needed to address whether suppression of ER stress can lead to enhanced clearance in advanced lesions, which will be a challenging goal in the context of concomitant ER stress affects on cell survival.

Stresses on actin signaling. The engagement of apoptosis-associated ligands with cell surface receptors leads to transduction of extracellular signals into the cytosol. This culminates in the activation of low molecular weight GTPases and mobilization of cytoskeletal signaling pathways that are required for actin polymerization during apoptotic cell engulfment (May and Machesky, 2001). For example, apoptotic cell binding triggers mobilization of ELMO and DOCK180 as they cooperate as a guanine nucleotide exchange factor (GEF) to activate Rac and promote membrane ruffling (Lu and Ravichandran, 2006). In parallel, the small GTP-bound protein RhoA (i.e., RhoA-GTP) is inactivated. In general, Rac and Rho follow an inverse relationship during efferocytosis (Ravichandran and Lorenz, 2007). RhoA can be activated by the athero-relevant lysophosphatidic acid and appears to be involved in a number of cardiovascular related events (Loirand *et al.*, 2006). Interestingly, statins such as lovastatin have been shown to inhibit the activity of Rho and enhance efferocytosis *in vitro* by blocking farnesylation pathways that lead to Rho membrane translocation (Morimoto *et al.*, 2006). Downstream of RhoA is its effector kinsae ROCK. ROCK inhibitors have gained considerable attention in human clinical trials for their ability to alleviate a number of cardiovascular endpoints, including angina, hypertension, stroke, and heart failure. In preclinical animal models, the ROCK inhibitor fasudil has also shown promise for reducing vascular intimal hyperplasia, abdominal aortic aneurysm, and atherosclerotic lesion expansion. The effects of ROCK-inhibition/fasudil on advanced plaque parameters remain unknown.

Oxidative stress and cell survival. Numerous factors in atherosclerotic lesions have been identified that can negatively regulate the cytoskeletal signaling pathways described above. These include oxidant stress and superoxides such as 3-morpholinosydnonimine (SIN-1) (Schrijvers *et al.*, 2005). TNFα induces phospholipase 2 and arachidonic acid production, generating ROS production and modulation of Rho in mature macrophages (McPhillips *et al.*, 2007). Another oxidative insult may lie at the interface between macrophage and extracellular matrix (ECM). For example, oxidative stress can lead to reactive carbonyl modification of ECM and increased macrophage adhesion and decreased efferocytosis (Kirkham, 2007). In addition to oxidative stresses that directly impact clearance, efferocytosis itself leads to a NADPH-mediated oxidative burst that must be dampened soon after engulfment otherwise promoting phagocyte death (Yvan-Charvet *et al.*, 2010). Phagocyte survival is, of course, an important component of maintaining a pool of clearance-competent cells. Phagocytes are exposed to large amounts of cholesterol and lipid after the engulfment of dying cells. This is a stress that alters cellular homeostasis. Importantly, phagocytes induce compensatory cell survival signaling to offset these changes and ensure viability (Cui *et al.*, 2007). Thus, perturbations in engulfment-dependent cell survival signaling could lead to depletion of stores of phagocytes. Another relevant cellular stress is that which occurs in advanced age. For example, clearance of apoptotic cells is reduced in aged mice (Aprahamian *et al.*, 2008). The mechanisms of this defect are unknown but could be reproduced *in vitro* by exposure of macrophages from young mice to serum from old mice, suggesting the presence of an inhibitory factor or absence of a soluble efferocytosis effector in the aged serum.

11.3.3 Inflammatory Phagocyte Recruitment, Polarization, and Resolution

Recruiting the best efferocytes. Advanced atherosclerosis is characterized by a chronic maladaptive inflammatory response with continuous and progressive phagocyte recruitment from the nearby circulation (Swirski *et al.*, 2006). Recognition of adhesion molecules such as vascular cell adhesion molecule-1 (VCAM), intercellular adhesion molecule-1 (ICAM), and E-selectin (Frostegard *et al.*, 1991) lead to blood-borne monocyte infiltration through the endothelial layer and into the intima. Whether or not efferocytic efficiency is preprogrammed in monocyte macrophage precursors is unknown, however there is evidence that phagocytic efficiency certainly differs at the monocyte stage. For example, after injury, the heart mobilizes phagocytic Ly-6c^{HI} monocytes to help promote digestion of damaged tissue (Nahrendorf *et al.*, 2007). In addition, monocyte subsets differentially employ chemokine receptors to accumulate within atherosclerotic plaques (Tacke *et al.*, 2007). This suggests that selective recruitment of macrophage precursors with the potential for high efferocytosis efficiency is at least plausible. These findings in mice will, of course, need to be validated in humans. Human monocytes express two predominant monocytic subsets that are defined by their expression of CD16 and CD14 (Passlick *et al.*, 1989). Another strategy is to keep out poorly efficient or non-efferocytic myeloid cells. For example, apoptotic cells have been reported to secrete the *keep-out* signal lactoferrin, and thereby inhibit migration of granulocytes (Bournazou *et al.*, 2009). In addition, a number of soluble and potentially "drugable" extracellular *find-me* or *come-get-me* signals have been identified. These include thrombospondin, which is released by dying fibroblasts during wound healing (Moodley *et al.*, 2003), and other soluble factors released from apoptotic cells, including fractalkine (CX_3CL1) (Truman *et al.*, 2008) and lysophosphatidylcholine (Peter *et al.*, 2008). Furthermore, these *find-me* signals are only as useful as the ability of phagocytes to chemotax to the apoptotic cell (Lauber *et al.*, 2004). This strategy may be especially problematic in advanced lesions where flux in ECM production and degradation by metalloproteinases could impede directional chemotaxis (Gough *et al.*, 2006). Degradation of matrix, in combination with athero-relevant modulation of cytoskeletal signaling pathways, may combine to arrest directional phagocyte migration towards *find-me* signals. For example, Rho-GTPase mediated regulation of cytoskeletal chemotaxis can be impaired by increased phagocyte cholesterol loading (Nagao *et al.*, 2007).

Targeting cytokine-mediated polarization. In vitro, "alternatively" activated M2 macrophages preferentially clear apoptotic cells and are often characterized by secretion of anti-inflammatory cytokines such as TGFβ and IL-10 (Xu *et al.*, 2006). "Classically" activated M1 macrophages are characterized by the secretion of pro-inflammatory cytokines such as TNFα and IL-6. TNFα-induced reactive oxygen generation has been shown to suppress efferocytosis in mature macrophages, while interestingly leaving less differentiated monocytes unaffected (McPhillips *et al.*, 2007). With respect to immature monocyte phagocytes, Ly6C^{LO} subsets have shown a predilection to differentiation into immature CD11c^{HI} dendritic-like cells (Tacke *et al.*, 2007). Mature dendritic cells are characterized by reduced efferocytic efficiency. Interestingly IL-17 has been recently implicated in efferocytosis regulation. IL-17 was shown to promote murine macrophage clearance of aged neutrophils (Silverpil *et al.*, 2010). Delivery of nanoparticles that are targeted to advanced atheromata may also be a viable approach for delivery of cytokines that promote efferocytosis.

Promoting resolution through clearance. It is now clear that inflammation resolution is not simply a diminution of pro-inflammatory mediators but rather entails active processes that are driven by the biosynthesis and action of so-called pro-resolving factors (Serhan *et al.*, 2008). These factors include bioactive lipids such as lipoxins that are generated in place of arachidonic acid-derived prostaglandins and leukotrienes. Such pro-resolving pathways can be found downstream of cellular engulfment pathways. Therefore, the targeting of efferocytosis also holds potential to positively regulate pro-resolving factors. Lipoxins are eicosanoids that are produced through multicellular reactions involving the lipoxygenase pathway. Godson and colleagues showed that several members of this family, including LXA4, LXB4, aspirin-triggered 15-epi-LXB4, and their stable analogues promote efferocytosis of apoptotic neutrophils. Lipoxins promote apoptotic cell clearance through the lipoxin receptor and inhibition of protein kinase A. Importantly, these phenomena also occur *in vivo* as lipoxins stimulated the efferocytosis of neutrophils during peritonitis (Godson *et al.*, 2000).

11.3.3.1 Targeting and repairing the phagocytic synapse

The professional macrophage phagocyte is known to utilize a diverse array of cell-surface receptors that transduce extracellular signals leading to apoptotic cell engulfment (Platt *et al.*, 1998). In the case of other phagocytes such as dendritic cells, the full repertoire of receptors is just beginning to be elucidated in full detail. The diversity and number of receptors that are available imply multiple functions and combinatorial possibilities, depending on the local extracellular milieu. Though this assortment of receptors reflects the critical importance of fail-safe clearance mechanisms in maintaining tissue homeostasis, their diversity indicate they are not merely redundant. Structurally distinct receptor families are capable of recognizing unrelated ligands on apoptotic cell surfaces, leading to separable downstream pathways that modulate cytoskeletal signaling, cell survival, pro- and anti-inflammatory signaling, and metabolic processing of engulfed cells. Other receptors such as CD14 and CD31 contribute by aiding in the tethering of phagocyte and AC. Key apoptotic cell receptors include those that recognize phosphatidylserine, such as the newly implicated brain specific angiogenesis inhibitor 1 (BAI1) (Park *et al.*, 2007), T-cell immunoglobulin mucin receptors (Miyanishi *et al.*, 2007; Kobayashi *et al.*, 2007), and stabilin receptors. Candidate inhibitory mechanisms within atherosclerotic lesions include oxidized lipoproteins, which *in vitro* have been shown to directly interfere with efferocytosis by competitively binding apoptotic cell receptors on phagocytes. Specifically, both fully oxidized LDL as well as LDL that is only minimally oxidized, referred to as "minimally modified" LDL, have been shown to inhibit the engulfment of apoptotic cells by altering actin signaling through a pathway involving cell surface CD14 and TLR4 (Miller *et al.*, 2003). *In vivo*, much remains to be learned regarding the contribution of apoptotic cell receptors during the different stages of atherosclerosis. The majority of athero-relevant causative studies to date have focused on efferocytosis molecules at level of the apoptotic cell receptor. For example, during advanced atherosclerosis, a handful of receptors have been causally linked to apoptotic clearance and plaque necrosis. The cell-surface and protein cross-linking enzyme transglutaminase 2 (TG2), in cooperation with integrins, can engage lactadherin-opsonized apoptotic cells and promote engulfment (Toth *et al.*, 2009). *In vivo*, atherogenic *Ldlr*$^{-/-}$ mice engrafted with *Tg2*$^{-/-}$ bone marrow cells exhibit larger aortic root lesions and expanded necrotic cores relative to control (Boisvert *et al.*, 2006). Another interesting candidate is LRP1. Fazio and colleagues showed that efferocytosis of apoptotic macrophages was significantly reduced in LRP-1$^{-/-}$ macrophages relative to control. In addition, compared to wild-type macrophage lesions, LRP-1$^{-/-}$ lesions exhibited more necrotic core with more dead cells not associated with macrophages (Yancey *et al.*, 2010). Finally, another interesting candidate is the apoptotic cell receptor MERTK of the TAM receptor tyrosine kinase family. *In vitro*, macrophages engineered with a kinase dead form of MERTK fail to specifically engulf macrophages that have been rendered apoptotic by atherogenic stimuli (Li *et al.*, 2006). MERTK is a receptor on efferocytes for apoptotic cells; the kinase domain mutation renders the receptor non-functional. *In vivo*, mice deficient in MERTK exhibit reduced efferocytosis and increased plaque necrosis and inflammation and features of autoimmunity (Thorp *et al.*, 2008; Wallet *et al.*, 2008).

11.3.3.2 Metabolic risk factors and nuclear receptors

As introduced in the first half of this review, obesity and its associated metabolic disorders are intimately associated with the progression of cardiovascular disease. Therefore, cardiovascular therapies that target apoptotic cell clearance must consider both how these risk-factors directly affect clearance and the efficacy of potential therapeutic agents in the diseased milieu. In the setting of obesity, increases in SFA suppress efferocytosis in plaque. For example, defective efferocytosis in genetically obese mice is directly correlated to increased levels of saturated fatty acids. This leads to defective phosphatidyl inositol 3-kinase (PI3K) activation and reduced PIP3 in macrophage phagocytic cups (Li *et al.*, 2009c). Another link to metabolism is found at the level of nutrient sensing nuclear receptors. Ingestion of an apoptotic meal is recognized by nuclear receptor nutrient sensors such as Liver X receptors (LXRα and LXRβ) and peroxisome proliferator-activated receptors (PPAR). These transcriptional regulators can respond to increased cholesterol and lipid levels. LXRs recognize oxysterols (Peet *et al.*, 1998; Castrillo and Tontonoz, 2004), and PPARs bind fatty acids. Recent evidence highlights the role of nuclear receptors, including LXRs and PPARs, in directly regulating transcription of molecules required for apoptotic cell internalization. Efferocytosis activates LXR, which in turn leads to downstream expression of the apoptotic cell receptor MERTK (Gonzalez *et al.*, 2009). Transglutaminase 2 has also been described to be induced by LXR/RXR during efferocytosis (Rebe *et al.*, 2009). In the case of PPARs, PPARδ activates C1q to promote ingestion, a bridging molecule that links apoptotic cells to phagocytes (Mukundan *et al.*, 2009). The phagocytic receptor CD36 has a PPAR response element (PPRE) and is induced by thiazolidinediones to promote uptake (Majai *et al.*, 2007). PPARγ ligands have come under criticism for undesirable side effects and off-target effects. However, recent findings indicate that PPARγ ligands that were once thought to act solely on PPARγ also block recognition by upstream signaling partners (Choi *et al.*, 2010), opening the door for more specific strategies that selectively agonize PPAR-mediated clearance.

11.3.4 Potential Biomarkers of Defective Efferocytosis

In addition to such engineered tests of receptor causality, it is important to understand how receptor function naturally is regulated or compromised during the course of atherosclerotic lesion maturation. For example, variations in the expression, activity, or function of key apoptotic cell receptors, such as MERTK, may be affected by the heightened inflammatory milieu that is a hallmark of advanced plaque. This may be exacerbated by conditions that are closely tied to cardiovascular disease, including IR. For example, diabetic lesions exhibit increased inflammation and inflammation-associated proteases in conjunction with reduced levels of natural tissue protease inhibitors (Garcia-Touchard *et al.*, 2005; Cardellini *et al.*, 2009). Proteolytic-mediated cleavage of efferocytosis receptors has been implicated in impaired apoptotic cell clearance and exacerbated disease in cystic fibrosis (Krysko *et al.*, 2010) and bronchiectasis (Vandivier *et al.*, 2002), and proteases such as MMPs and ADAMs (A Disintegrin And Metalloprotease) have been found to be upregulated in advanced atherosclerosis (Canault *et al.*, 2006). *In vitro*, MERTK is proteolytically cleaved as a result of inflammatory stimuli such as LPS, and this leads to the generation of a solubilized MER that can act as a competitive inhibitor of uptake (Sather *et al.*, 2007). IL-17 was also shown to increase the soluble form of the phagocytic receptor, lectin-like oxidized low-density lipoprotein receptor-1 (Silverpil *et al.*, 2010).

11.4 Conclusions and Future Directions of ER Stress and Efferocytosis Therapy

Much needs to be done towards *in vivo* testing of therapeutics that target apoptosis and efferocytosis during efferocytosis. A key logistical requirement will be the availability and development of new mouse models that more closely mimic human atherothrombotic vascular disease. Recent advances in both areas indicate that we are on the precipice of finding agents that effectively target these key pathways.

With respect to the UPR, ER stress and activation of the UPR contribute to the pathogenesis of numerous diseases. Accumulating evidence supports that activation of the UPR promotes the progression of atherothrombotic vascular disease at multiple levels. Compelling work suggests that ER stress plays an important role in systemic atherosclerotic risk factors such as IR and hyperlipidemia and also macrophage and endothelial cell apoptosis at the level of arterial wall. For strategies to improve atherosclerosis, particularly targeting macrophages, through enhancing the ER folding capacity; several agents (See Table 11.1) such as PBA and TUDCA have emerged. However, their ER stress-relieving properties remain unknown and yet to be proven. In addition, such therapeutic targeting should also consider other cell types relevant to atherosclerosis, since the effect of ER stress in each individual cell may differ throughout atherosclerosis development. Moreover, given that ER stress affects the progression of multiple diseases, including cancer, careful work should be done in order to prevent a possible adverse affect. More studies are necessary to elucidate the contribution of each individual branch in the progression of atherosclerosis development and how to modulate these associated branches effectively to improve therapeutic strategies.

Table 11.1 List of pharmacological agents with published effects on ER stress

Drug	**Evidence for ER stress modulation**
PBA	Through ↓ macrophage ER stress (Erbay *et al.*, 2009b)
TUDCA	Through its suppressive effects on ER stress (Dong *et al.*, 2010)
JNK inhibitor	SP600125 through ↓ macrophage apoptosis (Ricci *et al.*, 2004)
Taurine	Reduces superoxide dismutase expression and secretion (Nonaka *et al.*, 2001a)
N-acetylcysteine	*N*-acetylcysteine through ↓ ROS formation (Li *et al.*, 2009a)

In the context of efferocytosis, the goal of enhancing efferocytosis may be approached by more general pro-efferocytosis strategies or by targeting specific processes that are defective in advanced atherosclerosis. An example of the former would be to consider the established concept that some macrophage subpopulations are more efficient at efferocytosis than others. A more specific approach would be to define mechanisms of defective efferocytosis in human lesions and from this formulate a therapeutic strategy. For example, the fact that MERTK is rendered inactive through sheddase-mediated cleavage (above) may provide a therapeutic opportunity. That is, if excess MERTK cleavage were a culprit in human advanced plaques, therapeutic inhibition of cleavage might suppress plaque necrosis.

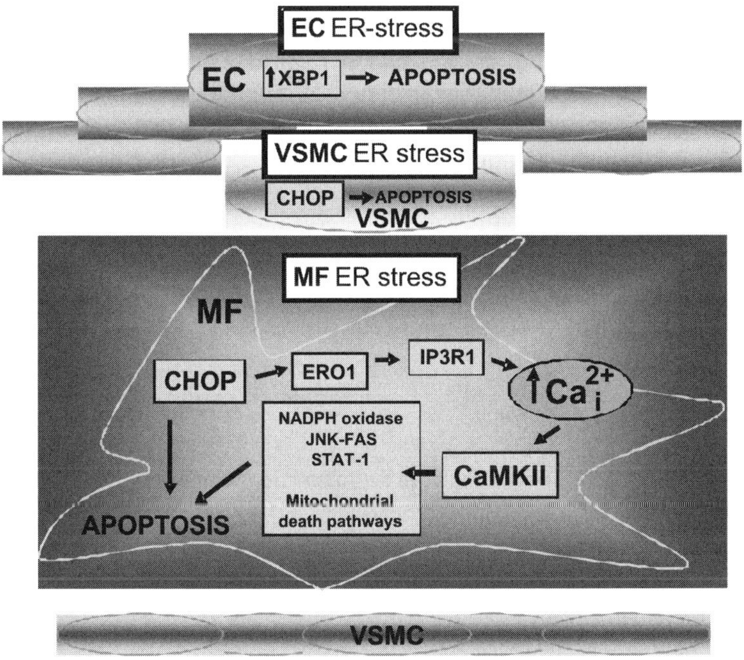

Figure 11.1 Potential targets for interfering with ER stress at the arterial wall.

In conclusion, advanced atherosclerotic progression that leads to plaque rupture and acute clinical events is a combination of multiple factors. Two prominent components of disease progression included UPR-mediated cell death and efferocytosis of dying cells. A thorough understanding of the mechanisms and consequences involved in these processes will be critical for translating our understanding of these pathways into novel therapeutic strategies. Potential therapies may in fact simultaneously combine both facets of UPR-mediated cell death and apoptotic cell clearance. As a proof of principle, this is already being achieved in cancer, where combinatorial therapy that promotes cellular death of lymphoma cells is combined with drugs that promote their clearance (Chao *et al.*, 2010).

There are many molecules and processes that are known to induce ER stress in advanced lesions. Activation of the UPR in macrophages (MFs) leads to induction of CHOP, which leads to elevation of cytoplasmic calcium through a pathway involving ERO-1 and IP3R-mediated ER calcium release. Accumulation of cytosolic calcium activates calcium/calmodulin dependent protein kinase II (CaMKII), which triggers apoptosis through at least 4 pathways: JNK-mediated Fas induction, activation of a proapoptotic signal transducer, STAT1, NADPH oxidase activation and subsequent reactive oxygen species generation, and activation of mitochondrial apoptotic pathways. In addition to macrophages, prolonged activation of UPR in ECs leads to elevated levels of XBP-1, which promotes apoptosis. In the case of VSMCs, the exact mechanisms of how ER stress leads to VSMC dysfunction are not well studied, however *in vitro* work has shown that induction of CHOP triggers death of VSMCs.

Table 11.2 List of potential pharmacological agents with reported enhancing effects on efferocytosis

Drug	Evidence for efferocytosis enhancement
IL-10	Correlated with ↑ CD14 (Lingnau *et al.*, 2007)
MFGE8	Via direct injection of exosomes (Miksa *et al.*, 2006)
Lipoxins	Through PKA (Serhan *et al.*, 2008)
LXR-agonist	Through upregulation of MERTK (Gonzalez *et al.*, 2009)
Statins	Lovastatin through ↓ RhoA (Morimoto *et al.*, 2006)
TZDs	PPARγ through ↑ CD36 (Majai *et al.*, 2007)

Numerous steps before, during and after engulfment may regulate and therefore be targeted for regulation of the efficiency of apoptotic cell clearance in plaque. These include recruitment, chemotaxis, engulfment, and downstream metabolic processing and inflammatory signaling.

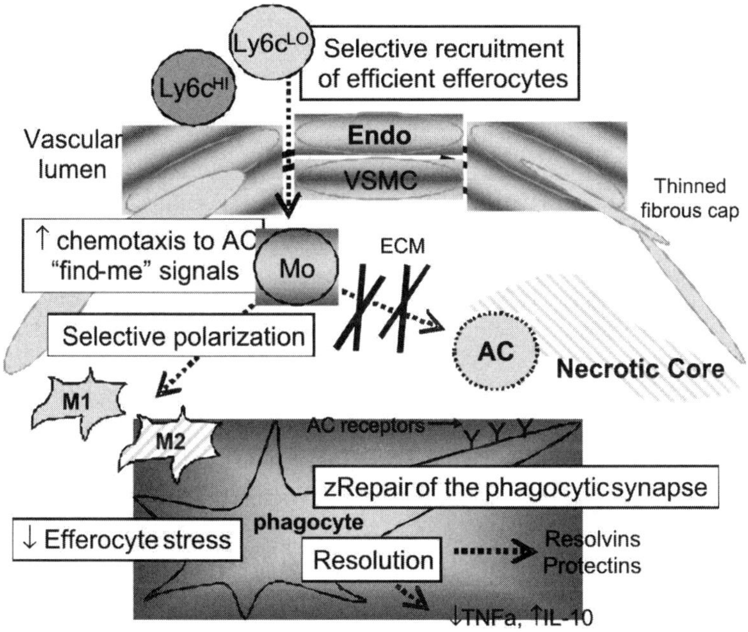

Figure 11.2 Potential targets for rescuing and enhancing efferocytosis in advanced atherosclerosis.

References

Aprahamian, T., Takemura, Y., Goukassian, D., and Walsh, K. (2008). Ageing is associated with diminished apoptotic cell clearance *in vivo*. *Clin. Exp. Immunol.* 152, 448–455.

Ball, R.Y., Stowers, E.C., Burton, J.H., Cary, N.R., Skepper, J.N., and Mitchinson, M.J. (1995). Evidence that the death of macrophage foam cells contributes to the lipid core of atheroma. *Atherosclerosis.* 114, 45–54.

Becker, T., Volchuk, A., and Rothman, J.E. (2005). Differential use of endoplasmic reticulum membrane for phagocytosis in J774 macrophages. *Proc. Natl. Acad. Sci. U. S. A.* 102, 4022–4026.

Biddinger, S.B., Hernandez-Ono, A., Rask-Madsen, C., Haas, J.T., Aleman, J.O., Suzuki, R., Scapa, E.F., Agarwal, C., Carey, M.C., Stephanopoulos, G., Cohen, D.E., King, G.L., Ginsberg, H.N., and Kahn, C.R. (2008). Hepatic insulin resistance is sufficient to produce dyslipidemia and susceptibility to atherosclerosis. *Cell Metab.* 7, 125–134.

Boisvert, W.A., Rose, D.M., Boullier, A., Quehenberger, O., Sydlaske, A., Johnson, K.A., Curtiss, L.K., and Terkeltaub, R. (2006). Leukocyte transglutaminase 2 expression limits atherosclerotic lesion size. *Arterioscler. Thromb. Vasc. Biol.* 26, 563–569.

Bournazou, I., Pound, J.D., Duffin, R., Bournazos, S., Melville, L.A., Brown, S.B., Rossi, A.G., and Gregory, C.D. (2009). Apoptotic human cells inhibit migration of granulocytes via release of lactoferrin. *J. Clin. Invest.* 119, 20–32.

Canault, M., Peiretti, F., Kopp, F., Bonardo, B., Bonzi, M.F., Coudeyre, J.C., Alessi, M.C., Juhan-Vague, I., and Nalbone, G. (2006). The TNF alpha converting enzyme (TACE/ADAM17) is expressed in the atherosclerotic lesions of apolipoprotein E-deficient mice: possible contribution to elevated plasma levels of soluble TNF alpha receptors. *Atherosclerosis.* 187, 82–91.

Cardellini, M., Menghini, R., Martelli, E., Casagrande, V., Marino, A., Rizza, S., Porzio, O., Mauriello, A., Solini, A., Ippoliti, A., Lauro, R., Folli, F., and Federici, M. (2009). TIMP3 is reduced in atherosclerotic plaques from subjects with type 2 diabetes and increased by SirT1. *Diabetes.* 58, 2396–2401.

Castrillo, A., and Tontonoz, P. (2004). Nuclear receptors in macrophage biology: at the crossroads of lipid metabolism and inflammation. *Annu. Rev. Cell Dev. Biol.* 20:455-80., 455–480.

Chami, M., Oules, B., Szabadkai, G., Tacine, R., Rizzuto, R., and Paterlini-Brechot, P. (2008). Role of SERCA1 truncated isoform in the proapoptotic calcium transfer from ER to mitochondria during ER stress. *Mol. Cell.* 32, 641–651.

Chao, M.P., Alizadeh, A.A., Tang, C., Myklebust, J.H., Varghese, B., Gill, S., Jan, M., Cha, A.C., Chan, C.K., Tan, B.T., Park, C.Y., Zhao, F., Kohrt, H.E., Malumbres, R., Briones, J., Gascoyne, R.D., Lossos, I.S., Levy, R., Weissman, I.L., and Majeti, R. (2010). Anti-CD47 Antibody synergizes with rituximab to promote phagocytosis and eradicate non-hodgkin lymphoma. *Cell.* 142, 699–713.

Choi, J.H., Banks, A.S., Estall, J.L., Kajimura, S., Bostrom, P., Laznik, D., Ruas, J.L., Chalmers, M.J., Kamenecka, T.M., Bluher, M., Griffin, P.R., and Spiegelman, B.M. (2010). Anti-diabetic drugs inhibit obesity-linked phosphorylation of PPARgamma by Cdk5. *Nature.* 466, 451–456.

Civelek, M., Manduchi, E., Riley, R.J., Stoeckert, C.J., Jr., and Davies, P.F. (2009). Chronic endoplasmic reticulum stress activates unfolded protein response in arterial endothelium in regions of susceptibility to atherosclerosis. *Circ. Res.* 105, 453–461.

Cui, D., Thorp, E., Li, Y., Wang, N., Yvan-Charvet, L., Tall, A.R., and Tabas, I. (2007). Pivotal advance: macrophages become resistant to cholesterol-induced death after phagocytosis of apoptotic cells. *J. Leukoc. Biol.* 82, 1040–1050.

De Almeida, S.F., Picarote, G., Fleming, J.V., Carmo-Fonseca, M., Azevedo, J.E., and de, S.M. (2007). Chemical chaperones reduce endoplasmic reticulum stress and prevent mutant HFE aggregate formation. *J. Biol. Chem.* 282, 27905–27912.

DeVries-Seimon, T., Li, Y., Yao, P.M., Stone, E., Wang, Y., Davis, R.J., Flavell, R., and Tabas, I. (2005). Cholesterol-induced macrophage apoptosis requires ER stress pathways and engagement of the type A scavenger receptor. *J. Cell Biol.* 171, 61–73.

Dickhout, J.G., Hossain, G.S., Pozza, L.M., Zhou, J., Lhotak, S., and Austin, R.C. (2005). Peroxynitrite causes endoplasmic reticulum stress and apoptosis in human vascular endothelium: implications in atherogenesis. *Arterioscler. Thromb. Vasc. Biol.* 25, 2623–2629.

Dickhout, J.G., Sood, S.K., and Austin, R.C. (2007). Role of endoplasmic reticulum calcium disequilibria in the mechanism of homocysteine-induced ER stress. *Antioxid. Redox. Signal.* 9, 1863–1873.

Dong, Y., Zhang, M., Liang, B., Xie, Z., Zhao, Z., Asfa, S., Choi, H.C., and Zou, M.H. (2010). Reduction of AMP-activated protein kinase alpha2 increases endoplasmic reticulum stress and atherosclerosis *in vivo*. *Circulation.* 121, 792–803.

Erbay, E., Babaev, V.R., Mayers, J.R., Makowski, L., Charles, K.N., Snitow, M.E., Fazio, S., Wiest, M.M., Watkins, S.M., Linton, M.F., and Hotamisligil, G.S. (2009b). Reducing endoplasmic reticulum stress through a macrophage lipid chaperone alleviates atherosclerosis 303. *Nat. Med.* 15, 1383–1391.

Erbay, E., Babaev, V.R., Mayers, J.R., Makowski, L., Charles, K.N., Snitow, M.E., Fazio, S., Wiest, M.M., Watkins, S.M., Linton, M.F., and Hotamisligil, G.S. (2009a). Reducing endoplasmic reticulum stress through a macrophage lipid chaperone alleviates atherosclerosis. *Nat. Med.* 15, 1383–1391.

Feaver, R.E., Hastings, N.E., Pryor, A., and Blackman, B.R. (2008). GRP78 upregulation by atheroprone shear stress via p38-, alpha2beta1-dependent mechanism in endothelial cells. *Arterioscler. Thromb. Vasc. Biol.* 28, 1534–1541.

Feng, B., Yao, P.M., Li, Y., Devlin, C.M., Zhang, D., Harding, H.P., Sweeney, M., Rong, J.X., Kuriakose, G., Fisher, E.A., Marks, A.R., Ron, D., and Tabas, I. (2003a). The endoplasmic reticulum is the site of cholesterol-induced cytotoxicity in macrophages. *Nat. Cell Biol.* 5, 781–792.

Feng, B., Zhang, D., Kuriakose, G., Devlin, C.M., Kockx, M., and Tabas, I. (2003b). Niemann-Pick C heterozygosity confers resistance to lesional necrosis and macrophage apoptosis in murine atherosclerosis. *Proc. Natl. Acad. Sci. U. S. A.* 100, 10423–10428.

Frostegard, J., Haegerstrand, A., Gidlund, M., and Nilsson, J. (1991). Biologically modified LDL increases the adhesive properties of endothelial cells. *Atherosclerosis.* 90, 119–126.

Gagnon, E., Duclos, S., Rondeau, C., Chevet, E., Cameron, P.H., Steele-Mortimer, O., Paiement, J., Bergeron, J.J., and Desjardins, M. (2002). Endoplasmic reticulum-mediated phagocytosis is a mechanism of entry into macrophages. *Cell.* 110, 119–131.

Garcia-Touchard, A., Henry, T.D., Sangiorgi, G., Spagnoli, L.G., Mauriello, A., Conover, C., and Schwartz, R.S. (2005). Extracellular proteases in atherosclerosis and restenosis. *Arterioscler. Thromb. Vasc. Biol.* 25, 1119–1127.

Gargalovic, P.S., Gharavi, N.M., Clark, M.J., Pagnon, J., Yang, W.P., He, A., Truong, A., Baruch-Oren, T., Berliner, J.A., Kirchgessner, T.G., and Lusis, A.J. (2006). The unfolded protein response is an important regulator of inflammatory genes in endothelial cells. *Arterioscler. Thromb. Vasc. Biol.* 26, 2490–2496.

Geng, Y.J., and Libby, P. (2002). Progression of atheroma: a struggle between death and procreation. *Arterioscler. Thromb. Vasc. Biol.* 22, 1370–1380.

Gerstein, H.C., Miller, M.E., Byington, R.P., Goff, D.C., Jr., Bigger, J.T., Buse, J.B., Cushman, W.C., Genuth, S., Ismail-Beigi, F., Grimm, R.H., Jr., Probstfield, J.L., Simons-Morton, D.G., and Friedewald, W.T. (2008). Effects of intensive glucose lowering in type 2 diabetes. *N. Engl. J. Med.* 358, 2545–2559.

Gharavi, N.M., Gargalovic, P.S., Chang, I., Araujo, J.A., Clark, M.J., Szeto, W.L., Watson, A.D., Lusis, A.J., and Berliner, J.A. (2007). High-density lipoprotein modulates oxidized phospholipid signaling in human endothelial cells from proinflammatory to anti-inflammatory. *Arterioscler. Thromb. Vasc. Biol.* 27, 1346–1353.

Ginsberg, H.N., and Maccallum, P.R. (2009). The obesity, metabolic syndrome, and type 2 diabetes mellitus pandemic: part I. Increased cardiovascular disease risk and the importance of atherogenic dyslipidemia in persons with the metabolic syndrome and type 2 diabetes mellitus. *J. Cardiometab. Syndr.* 4, 113–119.

Giorgi, C., De, S.D., Bononi, A., Rizzuto, R., and Pinton, P. (2009). Structural and functional link between the mitochondrial network and the endoplasmic reticulum. *Int. J. Biochem. Cell Biol.* 41, 1817–1827.

Glimcher, L.H. (2010). XBP1: the last two decades. *Ann. Rheum. Dis.* 69 *Suppl* 1, i67-i71.

Godson, C., Mitchell, S., Harvey, K., Petasis, N.A., Hogg, N., and Brady, H.R. (2000). Cutting edge: lipoxins rapidly stimulate nonphlogistic phagocytosis of apoptotic neutrophils by monocyte-derived macrophages. *J. Immunol.* 164, 1663–1667.

Gonzalez, N., Bensinger, S.J., Hong, C., Beceiro, S., Bradley, M.N., Zelcer, N., Deniz, J., Ramirez, C., Diaz, M., Gallardo, G., de Galarreta, C.R., Salazar, J., Lopez, F., Edwards, P., Parks, J., Andujar, M., Tontonoz, P., and Castrillo, A. (2009). Apoptotic cells promote their own clearance and immune tolerance through activation of the nuclear receptor LXR. *Immunity.* 31, 245–258.

Gough, P.J., Gomez, I.G., Wille, P.T., and Raines, E.W. (2006). Macrophage expression of active MMP-9 induces acute plaque disruption in apoE-deficient mice. *J. Clin. Invest.* 116, 59–69.

Gronski, M.A., Kinchen, J.M., Juncadella, I.J., Franc, N.C., and Ravichandran, K.S. (2009). An essential role for calcium flux in phagocytes for apoptotic cell engulfment and the anti-inflammatory response. *Cell Death. Differ.* 16, 1323–1331.

Hackam, D.J., Rotstein, O.D., Schreiber, A., Zhang, W., and Grinstein, S. (1997). Rho is required for the initiation of calcium signaling and phagocytosis by Fcgamma receptors in macrophages. *J. Exp. Med.* 186, 955–966.

Han, K.L., Choi, J.S., Lee, J.Y., Song, J., Joe, M.K., Jung, M.H., and Hwang, J.K. (2008). Therapeutic potential of peroxisome proliferators--activated receptor-alpha/gamma dual agonist with alleviation of endoplasmic reticulum stress for the treatment of diabetes. *Diabetes.* 57, 737–745.

Han, S., Liang, C.P., Vries-Seimon, T., Ranalletta, M., Welch, C.L., Collins-Fletcher, K., Accili, D., Tabas, I., and Tall, A.R. (2006). Macrophage insulin receptor deficiency increases ER stress-induced apoptosis and necrotic core formation in advanced atherosclerotic lesions. *Cell Metab.* 3, 257–266.

Han, S., Liang, C.P., Westerterp, M., Senokuchi, T., Welch, C.L., Wang, Q., Matsumoto, M., Accili, D., and Tall, A.R. (2009). Hepatic insulin signaling regulates VLDL secretion and atherogenesis in mice. *J. Clin. Invest.* 119, 1029–1041.

Hayashi, T., and Su, T.P. (2007). Sigma-1 receptor chaperones at the ER-mitochondrion interface regulate Ca^{2+} signaling and cell survival. *Cell.* 131, 596–610.

Holman, R.R., Paul, S.K., Bethel, M.A., Matthews, D.R., and Neil, H.A. (2008). 10-year follow-up of intensive glucose control in type 2 diabetes. *N. Engl. J. Med.* 359, 1577–1589.

Hossain, G.S., Van Thienen, J.V., Werstuck, G.H., Zhou, J., Sood, S.K., Dickhout, J.G., De Koning, A.B., Tang, D., Wu, D., Falk, E., Poddar, R., Jacobsen, D.W., Zhang, K., Kaufman, R.J., and Austin, R.C. (2003). TDAG51 is induced by homocysteine, promotes detachment-mediated programmed cell death, and contributes to the cevelopment of atherosclerosis in hyperhomocysteinemia. *J. Biol. Chem.* 278, 30317–30327.

Kars, M., Yang, L., Gregor, M.F., Mohammed, B.S., Pietka, T.A., Finck, B.N., Patterson, B.W., Horton, J.D., Mittendorfer, B., Hotamisligil, G.S., and Klein, S. (2010). Tauroursodeoxycholic Acid may improve liver and muscle but not adipose tissue insulin sensitivity in obese men and women. *Diabetes.* 59, 1899–1905.

Kedi, X., Ming, Y., Yongping, W., Yi, Y., and Xiaoxiang, Z. (2009a). Free cholesterol overloading induced smooth muscle cells death and activated both ER- and mitochondrial-dependent death pathway. *Atherosclerosis.* 207, 123–130.

Kedi, X., Ming, Y., Yongping, W., Yi, Y., and Xiaoxiang, Z. (2009b). Free cholesterol overloading induced smooth muscle cells death and activated both ER- and mitochondrial-dependent death pathway. *Atherosclerosis.* 207, 123–130.

Khan, M.I., Pichna, B.A., Shi, Y., Bowes, A.J., and Werstuck, G.H. (2009). Evidence supporting a role for endoplasmic reticulum stress in the development of atherosclerosis in a hyperglycaemic mouse model. *Antioxid. Redox. Signal.* 11, 2289–2298.

Kirkham, P. (2007). Oxidative stress and macrophage function: a failure to resolve the inflammatory response. *Biochem. Soc. Trans.* 35, 284–287.

Kobayashi, N., Karisola, P., Pena-Cruz, V., Dorfman, D.M., Jinushi, M., Umetsu, S.E., Butte, M.J., Nagumo, H., Chernova, I., Zhu, B., Sharpe, A.H., Ito, S., Dranoff, G., Kaplan, G.G., Casasnovas, J.M., Umetsu, D.T., Dekruyff, R.H., and Freeman, G.J. (2007). TIM-1 and TIM-4 glycoproteins bind phosphatidylserine and mediate uptake of apoptotic cells. *Immunity.* 27, 927–940.

Kornmann, B., Currie, E., Collins, S.R., Schuldiner, M., Nunnari, J., Weissman, J.S., and Walter, P. (2009). An ER-mitochondria tethering complex revealed by a synthetic biology screen. *Science.* 325, 477–481.

Kurokawa, M., Hideshima, M., Ishii, Y., Kyuwa, S., and Yoshikawa, Y. (2009). Aortic ER stress in streptozotocin-induced diabetes mellitus in APA hamsters. *Exp. Anim.* 58, 113–121.

Lauber, K., Blumenthal, S.G., Waibel, M., and Wesselborg, S. (2004). Clearance of apoptotic cells: getting rid of the corpses. *Mol. Cell.* 14, 277–287.

Lee, A.H., Scapa, E.F., Cohen, D.E., and Glimcher, L.H. (2008). Regulation of hepatic lipogenesis by the transcription factor XBP1. *Science.* 320, 1492–1496.

Lei, K., and Davis, R.J. (2003). JNK phosphorylation of Bim-related members of the Bcl2 family induces Bax-dependent apoptosis. *Proc. Natl. Acad. Sci. U. S. A* 100, 2432–2437.

Li, G., Mongillo, M., Chin, K.T., Harding, H., Ron, D., Marks, A.R., and Tabas, I. (2009b). Role of ERO1-alpha-mediated stimulation of inositol 1,4,5-triphosphate receptor activity in endoplasmic reticulum stress-induced apoptosis. *J. Cell Biol.* 186, 783–792.

Li, G., Mongillo, M., Chin, K.T., Harding, H., Ron, D., Marks, A.R., and Tabas, I. (2009a). Role of ERO1-alpha-mediated stimulation of inositol 1,4,5-triphosphate receptor activity in endoplasmic reticulum stress-induced apoptosis. *J. Cell Biol.* 186, 783–792.

Li, S., Sun, Y., Liang, C.P., Thorp, E.B., Han, S., Jehle, A.W., Saraswathi, V., Pridgen, B., Kanter, J.E., Li, R., Welch, C.L., Hasty, A.H., Bornfeldt, K.E., Breslow, J.L., Tabas, I., and Tall, A.R. (2009c). Defective phagocytosis of apoptotic cells by macrophages in atherosclerotic lesions of ob/ob mice and reversal by a fish oil diet. *Circ. Res.* 105, 1072–1082.

Li, Y., Gerbod-Giannone, M.C., Seitz, H., Cui, D., Thorp, E., Tall, A.R., Matsushima, G.K., and Tabas, I. (2006). Cholesterol-induced apoptotic macrophages elicit an inflammatory response in phagocytes, which is partially attenuated by the mer receptor. *J. Biol. Chem.* 281, 6707–6717.

Lim, W.S., Timmins, J.M., Seimon, T.A., Sadler, A., Kolodgie, F.D., Virmani, R., and Tabas, I. (2008). Signal transducer and activator of transcription-1 is critical for apoptosis in macrophages subjected to endoplasmic reticulum stress in vitro and in advanced atherosclerotic lesions *in vivo. Circulation.* 19;117, 940–951.

Lingnau, M., Hoflich, C., Volk, H.D., Sabat, R., and Docke, W.D. (2007). Interleukin-10 enhances the CD14-dependent phagocytosis of bacteria and apoptotic cells by human monocytes. *Hum. Immunol.* 68, 730–738.

Loirand, G., Guerin, P., and Pacaud, P. (2006). Rho kinases in cardiovascular physiology and pathophysiology. *Circ. Res.* 98, 322–334.

Lonn, E., Bosch, J., Yusuf, S., Sheridan, P., Pogue, J., Arnold, J.M., Ross, C., Arnold, A., Sleight, P., Probstfield, J., and Dagenais, G.R. (2005). Effects of long-term vitamin E supplementation on cardiovascular events and cancer: a randomized controlled trial. *JAMA*. 293, 1338–1347.

Loo, T.W., and Clarke, D.M. (2007). Chemical and pharmacological chaperones as new therapeutic agents. *Expert. Rev. Mol. Med.* 9, 1–18.

Lu, M., and Ravichandran, K.S. (2006). Dock180-ELMO cooperation in Rac activation. *Methods Enzymol.* 406:388–402., 388–402.

Luo, D., He, Y., Zhang, H., Yu, L., Chen, H., Xu, Z., Tang, S., Urano, F., and Min, W. (2008). AIP1 is critical in transducing IRE1-mediated endoplasmic reticulum stress response. *J. Biol. Chem.* 283, 11905–11912.

Lusis, A.J. (2000). Atherosclerosis. *Nature*. 407, 233–241.

Majai, G., Sarang, Z., Csomos, K., Zahuczky, G., and Fesus, L. (2007). PPARgamma-dependent regulation of human macrophages in phagocytosis of apoptotic cells. *Eur. J. Immunol.* 37, 1343–1354.

Malhotra, J.D., and Kaufman, R.J. (2007). The endoplasmic reticulum and the unfolded protein response. Semin. *Cell Dev. Biol.* 18, 716–731.

Marciniak, S.J., and Ron, D. (2006). Endoplasmic reticulum stress signaling in disease. *Physiol Rev.* 86, 1133–1149.

Marciniak, S.J., Yun, C.Y., Oyadomari, S., Novoa, I., Zhang, Y., Jungreis, R., Nagata, K., Harding, H.P., and Ron, D. (2004). CHOP induces death by promoting protein synthesis and oxidation in the stressed endoplasmic reticulum. *Genes Dev.* 18, 3066–3077.

Marks, P.W., and Maxfield, F.R. (1990). Local and global changes in cytosolic free calcium in neutrophils during chemotaxis and phagocytosis. *Cell Calcium* 11, 181–190.

May, R.C., and Machesky, L.M. (2001). Phagocytosis and the actin cytoskeleton. *J. Cell Sci.* 114, 1061–1077.

McPhillips, K., Janssen, W.J., Ghosh, M., Byrne, A., Gardai, S., Remigio, L., Bratton, D.L., Kang, J.L., and Henson, P. (2007). TNF-alpha inhibits macrophage clearance of apoptotic cells via cytosolic phospholipase A2 and oxidant-dependent mechanisms. *J. Immunol.* 178, 8117–8126.

Miksa, M., Wu, R., Dong, W., Das, P., Yang, D., and Wang, P. (2006). Dendritic cell-derived exosomes containing milk fat globule epidermal growth factor-factor VIII attenuate proinflammatory responses in sepsis. *Shock*. 25, 586–593.

Miller, Y.I., Viriyakosol, S., Binder, C.J., Feramisco, J.R., Kirkland, T.N., and Witztum, J.L. (2003). Minimally modified LDL binds to CD14, induces macrophage spreading via TLR4/MD-2, and inhibits phagocytosis of apoptotic cells. *J. Biol. Chem.* 278, 1561–1568.

Miyanishi, M., Tada, K., Koike, M., Uchiyama, Y., Kitamura, T., and Nagata, S. (2007). Identification of Tim4 as a phosphatidylserine receptor. *Nature.* 450, 435–439.

Moodley, Y., Rigby, P., Bundell, C., Bunt, S., Hayashi, H., Misso, N., McAnulty, R., Laurent, G., Scaffidi, A., Thompson, P., and Knight, D. (2003). Macrophage recognition and phagocytosis of apoptotic fibroblasts is critically dependent on fibroblast-derived thrombospondin 1 and CD36. *Am. J. Pathol.* 162, 771–779.

Morimoto, K., Janssen, W.J., Fessler, M.B., McPhillips, K.A., Borges, V.M., Bowler, R.P., Xiao, Y.Q., Kench, J.A., Henson, P.M., and Vandivier, R.W. (2006). Lovastatin enhances clearance of apoptotic cells (efferocytosis) with implications for chronic obstructive pulmonary disease. *J. Immunol.* 176, 7657–7665.

Mukundan, L., Odegaard, J.I., Morel, C.R., Heredia, J.E., Mwangi, J.W., Ricardo-Gonzalez, R.R., Goh, Y.P., Eagle, A.R., Dunn, S.E., Awakuni, J.U., Nguyen, K.D., Steinman, L., Michie, S.A., and Chawla, A. (2009). PPAR-delta senses and orchestrates clearance of apoptotic cells to promote tolerance. *Nat. Med.* 15(11):1266–1272.

Myoishi, M., Hao, H., Minamino, T., Watanabe, K., Nishihira, K., Hatakeyama, K., Asada, Y., Okada, K., Ishibashi-Ueda, H., Gabbiani, G., Bochaton-Piallat, M.L., Mochizuki, N., and Kitakaze, M. (2007). Increased endoplasmic reticulum stress in atherosclerotic plaques associated with acute coronary syndrome. *Circulation.* 116, 1226–1233.

Nagao, T., Qin, C., Grosheva, I., Maxfield, F.R., and Pierini, L.M. (2007). Elevated cholesterol levels in the plasma membranes of macrophages inhibit migration by disrupting RhoA regulation. *Arterioscler. Thromb. Vasc. Biol.* 27, 1596–1602.

Nahrendorf, M., Swirski, F.K., Aikawa, E., Stangenberg, L., Wurdinger, T., Figueiredo, J.L., Libby, P., Weissleder, R., and Pittet, M.J. (2007). The healing myocardium sequentially mobilizes two monocyte subsets with divergent and complementary functions. *J. Exp. Med.* 204, 3037–3047.

Nakagawa, T., Zhu, H., Morishima, N., Li, E., Xu, J., Yankner, B.A., and Yuan, J. (2000). Caspase-12 mediates endoplasmic-reticulum-specific apoptosis and cytotoxicity by amyloid-beta. *Nature.* 403, 98–103.

Nakano, T., Watanabe, H., Ozeki, M., Asai, M., Katoh, H., Satoh, H., and Hayashi, H. (2006). Endoplasmic reticulum Ca^{2+} depletion induces endothelial cell apoptosis independently of caspase-12. *Cardiovasc. Res.* 69, 908–915.

Nonaka, H., Tsujino, T., Watari, Y., Emoto, N., and Yokoyama, M. (2001b). Taurine prevents the decrease in expression and secretion of extracellular superoxide dismutase induced by homocysteine: amelioration of homocysteine-induced endoplasmic reticulum stress by taurine. *Circulation.* 104, 1165–1170.

Nonaka, H., Tsujino, T., Watari, Y., Emoto, N., and Yokoyama, M. (2001a). Taurine prevents the decrease in expression and secretion of extracellular superoxide dismutase induced by homocysteine: amelioration of homocysteine-induced endoplasmic reticulum stress by taurine. *Circulation.* 104, 1165–1170.

O Krysko, P Vandenabeele, DV Krysko, and C Bachert (2010). Impairment of phagocytosis of apoptotic cells and its role in chronic airway diseases. *Apoptosis.* 15(9):1137–1146.

Outinen, P.A., Sood, S.K., Pfeifer, S.I., Pamidi, S., Podor, T.J., Li, J., Weitz, J.I., and Austin, R.C. (1999). Homocysteine-induced endoplasmic reticulum stress and growth arrest leads to specific changes in gene expression in human vascular endothelial cells. *Blood.* 94, 959–967.

Oyadomari, S., Harding, H.P., Zhang, Y., Oyadomari, M., and Ron, D. (2008). Dephosphorylation of translation initiation factor 2alpha enhances glucose tolerance and attenuates hepatosteatosis in mice. *Cell Metab.* 7, 520–532.

Oyadomari, S., Koizumi, A., Takeda, K., Gotoh, T., Akira, S., Araki, E., and Mori, M. (2002). Targeted disruption of the Chop gene delays endoplasmic reticulum stress-mediated diabetes. *J. Clin. Invest.* 109, 525–532.

Ozcan, L., Ergin, A.S., Lu, A., Chung, J., Sarkar, S., Nie, D., Myers, M.G., Jr., and Ozcan, U. (2009). Endoplasmic reticulum stress plays a central role in development of leptin resistance. *Cell Metab.* 9, 35–51.

Ozcan, L., and Tabas, I. (2010). Pivotal role of calcium/calmodulin-dependent protein kinase II in ER stress-induced apoptosis. *Cell Cycle.* 9, 223–224.

Ozcan, U., Cao, Q., Yilmaz, E., Lee, A.H., Iwakoshi, N.N., Ozdelen, E., Tuncman, G., Gorgun, C., Glimcher, L.H., and Hotamisligil, G.S. (2004). Endoplasmic reticulum stress links obesity, insulin action, and type 2 diabetes. *Science.* 306, 457–461.

Ozcan, U., Yilmaz, E., Ozcan, L., Furuhashi, M., Vaillancourt, E., Smith, R.O., Gorgun, C.Z., and Hotamisligil, G.S. (2006). Chemical chaperones reduce ER stress and restore glucose homeostasis in a mouse model of type 2 diabetes. *Science.* 313, 1137–1140.

Pacher, P., and Szabo, C. (2006). Role of peroxynitrite in the pathogenesis of cardiovascular complications of diabetes. *Curr. Opin. Pharmacol.* 6, 136–141.

Park, D., Tosello-Trampont, A.C., Elliott, M.R., Lu, M., Haney, L.B., Ma, Z., Klibanov, A.L., Mandell, J.W., and Ravichandran, K.S. (2007). BAI1 is an engulfment receptor for apoptotic cells upstream of the ELMO/Dock180/Rac module. *Nature.* 450, 430–434.

Passlick, B., Flieger, D., and Ziegler-Heitbrock, H.W. (1989). Identification and characterization of a novel monocyte subpopulation in human peripheral blood. *Blood.* 74, 2527–2534.

Pedruzzi, E., Guichard, C., Ollivier, V., Driss, F., Fay, M., Prunet, C., Marie, J.C., Pouzet, C., Samadi, M., Elbim, C., O'dowd, Y., Bens, M., Vandewalle, A., Gougerot-Pocidalo, M.A., Lizard, G., and Ogier-Denis, E. (2004). NAD(P)H oxidase Nox-4 mediates 7-ketocholesterol-induced endoplasmic reticulum stress and apoptosis in human aortic smooth muscle cells. *Mol. Cell Biol.* 24, 10703–10717.

Peet, D.J., Turley, S.D., Ma, W., Janowski, B.A., Lobaccaro, J.M., Hammer, R.E., and Mangelsdorf, D.J. (1998). Cholesterol and bile acid metabolism are impaired in mice lacking the nuclear oxysterol receptor LXR alpha. *Cell.* 93, 693–704.

Peter, C., Waibel, M., Radu, C.G., Yang, L.V., Witte, O.N., Schulze-Osthoff, K., Wesselborg, S., and Lauber, K. (2008). Migration to apoptotic "find-me" signals is mediated via the phagocyte receptor G2A. *J. Biol. Chem.* 283, 5296–5305.

Platt, N., da Silva, R.P., and Gordon, S. (1998). Recognizing death: the phagocytosis of apoptotic cells. *Trends Cell Biol.* 8, 365–372.

Putcha, G.V., Le, S., Frank, S., Besirli, C.G., Clark, K., Chu, B., Alix, S., Youle, R.J., LaMarche, A., Maroney, A.C., and Johnson, E.M., Jr. (2003). JNK-mediated BIM phosphorylation potentiates BAX-dependent apoptosis. *Neuron.* 38, 899–914.

Ravalli, S., Albala, A., Ming, M., Szabolcs, M., Barbone, A., Michler, R.E., and Cannon, P.J. (1998). Inducible nitric oxide synthase expression in smooth muscle cells and macrophages of human transplant coronary artery disease. *Circulation.* 97, 2338–2345.

Ravalli, S., Szabolcs, M., Barbone, A., Albala, A., Michler, R.E., and Cannon, P.J. (1997). Inducible nitric oxide synthase is upregulated in human transplant coronary artery disease. *Transplant. Proc.* 29, 2579–2580.

Ravichandran, K.S., and Lorenz, U. (2007). Engulfment of apoptotic cells: signals for a good meal. *Nat. Rev. Immunol.* 7, 964–974.

Reaven, G. (2002). Metabolic syndrome: pathophysiology and implications for management of cardiovascular disease. *Circulation.* 106, 286–288.

Rebe, C., Raveneau, M., Chevriaux, A., Lakomy, D., Sberna, A.L., Costa, A., Bessede, G., Athias, A., Steinmetz, E., Lobaccaro, J.M., Alves, G., Menicacci, A., Vachenc, S., Solary, E., Gambert, P., and Masson, D. (2009). Induction of transglutaminase 2 by a liver X receptor/retinoic acid receptor alpha pathway increases the clearance of apoptotic cells by human macrophages. *Circ. Res.* 105, 393–401.

Ricci, R., Sumara, G., Sumara, I., Rozenberg, I., Kurrer, M., Akhmedov, A., Hersberger, M., Eriksson, U., Eberli, F.R., Becher, B., Boren, J., Chen, M., Cybulsky, M.I., Moore, K.J., Freeman, M.W., Wagner, E.F., Matter, C.M., and Luscher, T.F. (2004). Requirement of JNK2 for scavenger receptor A-mediated foam cell formation in atherogenesis. *Science.* 306, 1558–1561.

Ron, D., and Walter, P. (2007a). Signal integration in the endoplasmic reticulum unfolded protein response. *Nat. Rev. Mol. Cell Biol.* 8, 519–529.

Ron, D., and Walter, P. (2007b). Signal integration in the endoplasmic reticulum unfolded protein response. *Nat. Rev. Mol. Cell Biol.* 8, 519–529.

Rosales, C., and Brown, E.J. (1992). Signal transduction by neutrophil immunoglobulin G Fc receptors. Dissociation of intracytoplasmic calcium concentration rise from inositol 1,4,5-trisphosphate. *J. Biol. Chem.* 267, 5265–5271.

Rutkowski, D.T., and Kaufman, R.J. (2004). A trip to the ER: coping with stress. *Trends Cell Biol.* 14, 20–28.

Rutkowski, D.T., Wu, J., Back, S.H., Callaghan, M.U., Ferris, S.P., Iqbal, J., Clark, R., Miao, H., Hassler, J.R., Fornek, J., Katze, M.G., Hussain, M.M., Song, B., Swathirajan, J., Wang, J., Yau, G.D., and Kaufman, R.J. (2008). UPR pathways combine to prevent hepatic steatosis caused by ER stress-mediated suppression of transcriptional master regulators. *Dev. Cell.* 15, 829–840.

Sanson, M., Auge, N., Vindis, C., Muller, C., Bando, Y., Thiers, J.C., Marachet, M.A., Zarkovic, K., Sawa, Y., Salvayre, R., and Negre-Salvayre, A. (2009). Oxidized low-density lipoproteins trigger endoplasmic reticulum stress in vascular cells: prevention by oxygen-regulated protein 150 expression. *Circ. Res.* 104, 328–336.

Sather, S., Kenyon, K.D., Lefkowitz, J.B., Liang, X., Varnum, B.C., Henson, P.M., and Graham, D.K. (2007). A soluble form of the Mer receptor tyrosine kinase inhibits macrophage clearance of apoptotic cells and platelet aggregation. *Blood.* 109, 1026–1033.

Schrijvers, D.M., De Meyer, G.R., Kockx, M.M., Herman, A.G., and Martinet, W. (2005). Phagocytosis of apoptotic cells by macrophages is impaired in atherosclerosis. *Arterioscler. Thromb. Vasc. Biol.* 25, 1256–1261.

Seimon, T., and Tabas, I. (2009). Mechanisms and consequences of macrophage apoptosis in atherosclerosis. *J. Lipid Res.* 50 Suppl:S382–S387. Epub;2008 Oct 25., S382–S387.

Seimon, T.A., Obstfeld, A., Moore, K.J., Golenbock, D.T., and Tabas, I. (2006). Combinatorial pattern recognition receptor signaling alters the balance of life and death in macrophages. *Proc. Natl. Acad. Sci. U. S. A.* 103, 19794–19799.

Senokuchi, T., Liang, C.P., Seimon, T.A., Han, S., Matsumoto, M., Banks, A.S., Paik, J.H., Depinho, R.A., Accili, D., Tabas, I., and Tall, A.R. (2008). Forkhead transcription factors (FoxOs) promote apoptosis of insulin-resistant macrophages during cholesterol-induced endoplasmic reticulum stress. *Diabetes.* 57, 2967–2976.

Seo, H.Y., Kim, M.K., Min, A.K., Kim, H.S., Ryu, S.Y., Kim, N.K., Lee, K.M., Kim, H.J., Choi, H.S., Lee, K.U., Park, K.G., and Lee, I.K. (2010). Endoplasmic reticulum stress-induced activation of activating transcription factor 6 decreases cAMP-stimulated hepatic gluconeogenesis via inhibition of CREB. *Endocrinology.* 151, 561–568.

Serhan, C.N., Chiang, N., and Van Dyke, T.E. (2008). Resolving inflammation: dual anti-inflammatory and pro-resolution lipid mediators. *Nat. Rev. Immunol.* 8, 349–361.

Silverpil E, Glader P, Hansson M, Lindén A. Impact of interleukin-17 on macrophage phagocytosis of apoptotic neutrophils and particles. Inflammation. 2011 Feb;34(1):1-9. *PubMed PMID*: 20339909.

Song, B., Scheuner, D., Ron, D., Pennathur, S., and Kaufman, R.J. (2008a). Chop deletion reduces oxidative stress, improves beta cell function, and promotes cell survival in multiple mouse models of diabetes. *J. Clin. Invest.* 118, 3378–3389.

Song, B., Scheuner, D., Ron, D., Pennathur, S., and Kaufman, R.J. (2008b). Chop deletion reduces oxidative stress, improves beta cell function, and promotes cell survival in multiple mouse models of diabetes. *J. Clin. Invest.* 118, 3378–3389.

Surh, C.D., and Sprent, J. (1994). T-cell apoptosis detected *in situ* during positive and negative selection in the thymus. *Nature.* 372, 100–103.

Swirski, F.K., Pittet, M.J., Kircher, M.F., Aikawa, E., Jaffer, F.A., Libby, P., and Weissleder, R. (2006). Monocyte accumulation in mouse atherogenesis is progressive and proportional to extent of disease. *Proc. Natl. Acad. Sci. U. S. A.* 103, 10340–10345.

Szegezdi, E., Logue, S.E., Gorman, A.M., and Samali, A. (2006). Mediators of endoplasmic reticulum stress-induced apoptosis. *EMBO Rep.* 7, 880–885.

Tabas, I. (2007). Apoptosis and efferocytosis in mouse models of atherosclerosis. *Curr. Drug Targets.* 8, 1288–1296.

Tabas, I. (2009). Macrophage apoptosis in atherosclerosis: consequences on plaque progression and the role of endoplasmic reticulum stress. *Antioxid. Redox. Signal.* 11, 2333–2339.

Tabas, I. (2010). Macrophage death and defective inflammation resolution in atherosclerosis. *Nat. Rev. Immunol.* 10, 36–46.

Tabas, I. (2005). Consequences and therapeutic implications of macrophage apoptosis in atherosclerosis: the importance of lesion stage and phagocytic efficiency. *Arterioscler. Thromb. Vasc. Biol.* 25, 2255–2264.

Tabas, I., Seimon, T., Timmins, J., Li, G., and Lim, W. (2009). Macrophage apoptosis in advanced atherosclerosis. *Ann. N. Y. Acad. Sci.* 1173 Suppl 1:E40–E45., E40–E45.

Tacke, F., Alvarez, D., Kaplan, T.J., Jakubzick, C., Spanbroek, R., Llodra, J., Garin, A., Liu, J., Mack, M., van Rooijen, N., Lira, S.A., Habenicht, A.J., and Randolph, G.J. (2007). Monocyte subsets differentially employ CCR2, CCR5, and CX3CR1 to accumulate within atherosclerotic plaques. *J. Clin. Invest.* 117, 185–194.

Tamaki, N., Hatano, E., Taura, K., Tada, M., Kodama, Y., Nitta, T., Iwaisako, K., Seo, S., Nakajima, A., Ikai, I., and Uemoto, S. (2008). CHOP deficiency attenuates cholestasis-induced liver fibrosis by reduction of hepatocyte injury. *Am. J. Physiol Gastrointest. Liver Physiol.* 294, G498–G505.

Tatzelt, J., Prusiner, S.B., and Welch, W.J. (1996). Chemical chaperones interfere with the formation of scrapie prion protein. *EMBO J.* 15, 6363–6373.

Thorp, E., Cui, D., Schrijvers, D.M., Kuriakose, G., and Tabas, I. (2008). Mertk receptor mutation reduces efferocytosis efficiency and promotes apoptotic cell accumulation and plaque necrosis in atherosclerotic lesions of apoe-/- mice. *Arterioscler. Thromb. Vasc. Biol.* 28, 1421–1428.

Thorp, E., Li, G., Seimon, T.A., Kuriakose, G., Ron, D., and Tabas, I. (2009). Reduced apoptosis and plaque necrosis in advanced atherosclerotic lesions of Apoe-/- and Ldlr-/- mice lacking CHOP. *Cell Metab.* 9, 474–481.

Timmins, J.M., Ozcan, L., Seimon, T.A., Li, G., Malagelada, C., Backs, J., Backs, T., Bassel-Duby, R., Olson, E.N., Anderson, M.E., and Tabas, I. (2009). Calcium/calmodulin-dependent protein kinase II links ER stress with Fas and mitochondrial apoptosis pathways. *J. Clin. Invest.* 119, 2925–2941.

Toth, B., Garabuczi, E., Sarang, Z., Vereb, G., Vamosi, G., Aeschlimann, D., Blasko, B., Becsi, B., Erdodi, F., Lacy-Hulbert, A., Zhang, A., Falasca, L., Birge, R.B., Balajthy, Z., Melino, G., Fesus, L., and Szondy, Z. (2009). Transglutaminase 2 is needed for the formation of an efficient phagocyte portal in macrophages engulfing apoptotic cells. *J. Immunol.* 182, 2084–2092.

Truman, L.A., Ford, C.A., Pasikowska, M., Pound, J.D., Wilkinson, S.J., Dumitriu, I.E., Melville, L., Melrose, L.A., Ogden, C.A., Nibbs, R., Graham, G., Combadiere, C., and Gregory, C.D. (2008). CX3CL1/fractalkine is released from apoptotic lymphocytes to stimulate macrophage chemotaxis. *Blood.* 112, 5026–5036.

Tsukamoto, Y., Kuwabara, K., Hirota, S., Ikeda, J., Stern, D., Yanagi, H., Matsumoto, M., Ogawa, S., and Kitamura, Y. (1996). 150-kD oxygen-regulated protein is expressed in human atherosclerotic plaques and allows mononuclear phagocytes to withstand cellular stress on exposure to hypoxia and modified low density lipoprotein. *J. Clin. Invest.* 98, 1930–1941.

Tsukano, H., Gotoh, T., Endo, M., Miyata, K., Tazume, H., Kadomatsu, T., Yano, M., Iwawaki, T., Kohno, K., Araki, K., Mizuta, H., and Oike, Y. (2010). The endoplasmic reticulum stress- choppathway-mediated apoptosis in macrophages contributes to the instability of atherosclerotic plaques. *Arterioscler. Thromb. Vasc. Biol.* 30(10):1925-1932.

Urano, F., Wang, X., Bertolotti, A., Zhang, Y., Chung, P., Harding, H.P., and Ron, D. (2000). Coupling of stress in the ER to activation of JNK protein kinases by transmembrane protein kinase IRE1. *Science.* 287, 664–666.

Vandivier, R.W., Fadok, V.A., Hoffmann, P.R., Bratton, D.L., Penvari, C., Brown, K.K., Brain, J.D., Accurso, F.J., and Henson, P.M. (2002). Elastase-mediated phosphatidylserine receptor cleavage impairs apoptotic cell clearance in cystic fibrosis and bronchiectasis. *J. Clin. Invest.* 109, 661–670.

Vandivier, R.W., Henson, P.M., and Douglas, I.S. (2006). Burying the dead: the impact of failed apoptotic cell removal (efferocytosis) on chronic inflammatory lung disease. *Chest.* 129, 1673–1682.

Vilatoba, M., Eckstein, C., Bilbao, G., Smyth, C.A., Jenkins, S., Thompson, J.A., Eckhoff, D.E., and Contreras, J.L. (2005). Sodium 4-phenylbutyrate protects against liver ischemia reperfusion injury by inhibition of endoplasmic reticulum-stress mediated apoptosis. *Surgery.* 138, 342–351.

Wallet, M.A., Sen, P., Flores, R.R., Wang, Y., Yi, Z., Huang, Y., Mathews, C.E., Earp, H.S., Matsushima, G., Wang, B., and Tisch, R. (2008). MerTK is required for apoptotic cell-induced T cell tolerance. *J. Exp. Med.* 205, 219–232.

Wang, Y., Vera, L., Fischer, W.H., and Montminy, M. (2009). The CREB coactivator CRTC2 links hepatic ER stress and fasting gluconeogenesis. *Nature.* 460, 534–537.

Werstuck, G.H., Khan, M.I., Femia, G., Kim, A.J., Tedesco, V., Trigatti, B., and Shi, Y. (2006). Glucosamine-induced endoplasmic reticulum dysfunction is associated with accelerated atherosclerosis in a hyperglycemic mouse model. *Diabetes.* 55, 93–101.

Williams, K.J., and Tabas, I. (1995). The response-to-retention hypothesis of early atherogenesis. *Arterioscler. Thromb. Vasc. Biol.* 15, 551–561.

Woo, K.S., Chook, P., Lolin, Y.I., Cheung, A.S., Chan, L.T., Sun, Y.Y., Sanderson, J.E., Metreweli, C., and Celermajer, D.S. (1997). Hyperhomocyst(e) inemia is a risk factor for arterial endothelial dysfunction in humans. *Circulation.* 96, 2542–2544.

Wu, J., and Kaufman, R.J. (2006). From acute ER stress to physiological roles of the unfolded protein response. *Cell Death Differ.* 13, 374–384.

Xu, W., Roos, A., Schlagwein, N., Woltman, A.M., Daha, M.R., and Van Kooten, C. (2006). IL-10-producing macrophages preferentially clear early apoptotic cells. *Blood.* 107, 4930–4937.

Yancey, P.G., Blakemore, J., Ding, L., Fan, D., Overton, C.D., Zhang, Y., Linton, M.F., and Fazio, S. (2010). Macrophage LRP-1 controls plaque cellularity by regulating efferocytosis and Akt activation. *Arterioscler. Thromb. Vasc. Biol.* 30, 787–795.

Young, J.D., Ko, S.S., and Cohn, Z.A. (1984). The increase in intracellular free calcium associated with IgG gamma 2b/gamma 1 Fc receptor-ligand interactions: role in phagocytosis. *Proc. Natl. Acad. Sci. U. S. A.* 81, 5430–5434.

Yusuf, S., Dagenais, G., Pogue, J., Bosch, J., and Sleight, P. (2000). Vitamin E supplementation and cardiovascular events in high-risk patients. The heart outcomes prevention evaluation study investigators. *N. Engl. J. Med.* 342, 154–160.

Yvan-Charvet, L., Pagler, T.A., Seimon, T.A., Thorp, E., Welch, C.L., Witztum, J.L., Tabas, I., and Tall, A.R. (2010). ABCA1 and ABCG1 protect against oxidative stress-induced macrophage apoptosis during efferocytosis. *Circ. Res.* 106, 1861–1869.

Zeng, L., Zampetaki, A., Margariti, A., Pepe, A.E., Alam, S., Martin, D., Xiao, Q., Wang, W., Jin, Z.G., Cockerill, G., Mori, K., Li, Y.S., Hu, Y., Chien, S., and Xu, Q. (2009). Sustained activation of XBP1 splicing leads to endothelial apoptosis and atherosclerosis development in response to disturbed flow. *Proc. Natl. Acad. Sci. U. S. A.* 106, 8326–8331.

Zhang, C., Cai, Y., Adachi, M.T., Oshiro, S., Aso, T., Kaufman, R.J., and Kitajima, S. (2001a). Homocysteine induces programmed cell death in human vascular endothelial cells through activation of the unfolded protein response. *J. Biol. Chem.* 276, 35867–35874.

Zhang, C., Kawauchi, J., Adachi, M.T., Hashimoto, Y., Oshiro, S., Aso, T., and Kitajima, S. (2001b). Activation of JNK and transcriptional repressor ATF3/LRF1 through the IRE1/TRAF2 pathway is implicated in human vascular endothelial cell death by homocysteine. *Biochem. Biophys. Res. Commun.* 289, 718–724.

Zhang, J., Guo, J., Dzhagalov, I., and He, Y.W. (2005). An essential function for the calcium-promoted Ras inactivator in Fcgamma receptor-mediated phagocytosis. *Nat. Immunol.* 6, 911–919.

Zhang, X., Zhang, G., Zhang, H., Karin, M., Bai, H., and Cai, D. (2008). Hypothalamic IKKbeta/NF-kappaB and ER stress link overnutrition to energy imbalance and obesity. *Cell.* 135, 61–73.

Zinszner, H., Kuroda, M., Wang, X., Batchvarova, N., Lightfoot, R.T., Remotti, H., Stevens, J.L., and Ron, D. (1998). CHOP is implicated in programmed cell death in response to impaired function of the endoplasmic reticulum. *Genes Dev.* 12, 982–995.

Chapter 12

MicroRNAs in the Pathogenesis and Therapy of Atherosclerotic Vascular Disease

Andreas Schober[a] **and Mihail Hristov**[b]
[a] *Institute for Molecular Cardiovascular Research (IMCAR), RWTH Aachen University, Pauwelsstraße 30, 52074 Aachen, Germany*
[b] *Institute for Cardiovascular Prevention, Ludwig-Maximilians-University Munich Pettenkoferstraße 9, 80336 Munich, Germany*
aschober@ukaachen.de, mihail.hristov@med.uni-muenchen.de

12.1 Introduction

The non-coding, small RNAs (~22 nt) regulate gene expression on a post-transcriptional level through translational repression or mRNA decay [1]. Specific sets of these microRNAs (miRs) play key roles in determining cell fate and tissue homeostasis [2, 3]. In various disease states, distinct changes in the miR expression patterns have been identified which can drive or limit the disease process *in vivo* [4]. The fact that each miR can target hundreds of mRNAs, some of them with similar functions, enables the modification of specific cellular functions at different levels [5]. On the other side, a single mRNA target can be regulated by multiple miRs either by repression

Atherosclerosis: Treatment and Prevention
Edited by Christian Weber and Oliver Soehnlein

ISBN 978-981-4316-26-2 (Hardcover), ISBN 978-981-4364-26-3 (eBook)
www.panstanford.com

or by de-repression depending on whether the individual miR is up- or down-regulated [6, 7]. Identification of atherosclerosis-specific miRs promises to become a completely new class of targets in the treatment and prevention of atherosclerosis. Furthermore, unique patterns of circulating miR levels have been described in different disease states implicating a unexpected high stability of miRs in the circulation and the suitability as a biomarker to diagnose the presence and extend of a specific disease process [8].

12.2 MicroRNAs: Biogenesis and Function

In humans, approximately 1000 different miRs have been annotated, although experimental verification for most of them is still required. In mammals, miRs are predicted to directly regulate the expression of 50% of all protein-coding genes [9].

MiRs genes are located either in genomic regions distinct from known transcription units (intergenic), in the introns of annotated genes (intronic), or more rarely exonic [10]. Intergenic miRs can be monocistronic with their own promoter or polycistronic with several miRs transcribed as a cluster or primary transcripts with a shared promoter. Intronic miRs can be found as a single miR or as a cluster of several miRs and are thought to be transcribed from the same promoter as their host gene and processed from the introns of host gene transcripts [10]. Intronic miRs tend to be regulated by the same promoter as the host gene, resulting in a similar expression profile of the "host" transcript and the miR. Moreover, some mature miRs are transcribed from multiple genomic loci with different miR hairpins and, therefore, different miR* strands [11]. The majority of miR genes are transcribed by RNA polymerase II into primary miRNA transcripts [12] which are usually several kilobases long and consists of an imperfectly paired stem of ~33 bp with a terminal loop and flanking segments [13–15].

The transcription of the miR genes is regulated by transcription factors, which also control the expression of protein-coding genes, such as c-myc and p53, via binding to typical promoter sequences or by epigenetic alterations [16]. The pri-miRs bear a 7-methylguanylate cap at the 5′-end and a poly (A) tail at the 3′-end like mRNAs [16, 17]. The hairpin structure of the pri-miR is the substrate for two endonucleases from the RNase III enzyme family, Drosha and Dicer.

In a first step, a Microprocessor complex consisting at least in Drosha and the dsRNA binding protein DGRC8 cleave both strands of the pri-miR near the base of the stem loop with a 2 nt overhang at the 3′-end. This results in the generation of a ~60–70 nt miR precursor (pre-miR) which is actively transported to the cytoplasm. The second processing step by Dicer-mediated cleavage near the terminal loop results in ~22 nt miR duplexes [18] and requires the assembly of a multi-protein complex composed of Dicer, TRBP (Tar RNA binding protein), PACT (protein activator of PKR), and Argonaute-2 (Ago-2). This complex is involved in the subsequent selection and loading of one strand of the duplex into the miR-induced silencing complex (RISC). Argonaut proteins characteristically share a PAZ domain, which recognizes the 2 nt overhang of the 3′ end of the miR duplexes, and a PIWI domain, which is thought to mediate the enodnuclease activity of cleavage-competent Ago proteins, like Ago2 [19, 20]. All four different mouse Ago proteins have been shown to redundantly mediate miR-induced gene silencing, indicating the vital role of the miRs in mammalian species [21].

Although either strand can be stably associated with an Argonaut family protein, the core component of the RISC, preferential loading of a specific strand (guide strand) is common. The strand that is not loaded into the RISC, known as the passenger strand or miR*, is generally degraded [14]. Which strand is ultimately sorted to the RISC is tissue-specific and the accumulation of both strands, suggesting that both strands separately enter the silencing complex, has been described [11, 22]. Furthermore, the regulatory activity of miR* has been confirmed [23, 24], which supports the hypothesis that each pre-miR targets two sets of genes through the 5′ and the sister 3′-strand [11]. Therefore, the regulation of the strand selection process significantly contributes to miR induced silencing. The miR strand guides the RISC to the target mRNA via partially complementary binding to a recognition element primarily located in the 3′-UTR. The nucleotides 2–7 at the 5′ end of the miR, the so-called seed sequence, and the evolutionary conservation of the miR target are of crucial importance for the prediction of target [25, 26]. In addition, supplementary and compensatory sites were described, e.g., in the 3′ region of the miR, increasing the specificity and affinity of the pairing, although the nucleotides 9–12 generally bulge out, which prevents cleavage by Ago2. The terminal 5′ nucleotide of the miR, however, is not involved in seed pairing.

MiR-mediated repression can be due to degradation or translational inhibition of the mRNA [1]. Although translational repression has been thought to prevail in animals compared with plants, because of a more incomplete seed match, recent evidence indicates, however, that the miR-induced decay of transcripts also dominates in mammalian cells [27]. Translational repression has been shown to occur at initiation through competitive binding of Ago protein to the 7-methyl-guanine cap of the mRNA instead of eIF4E or inhibition of ribosomal subunit joining Ago protein-mediated recruitment of eIF6 [28, 29]. Furthermore, post-initiation mechanisms have been suggested like a premature dissociation of ribosomes or co-translational proteolysis [28]. MiR target degradation is directed by the association of TNRC6A and PAPBC with the Ago protein in the miRISC which triggers de-adenylation of the mRNA [1]. In animal cells, de-adenylated mRNA is ultimately decapped and degraded by the 5′-to-3′ exonuclease XRN1 [1].

12.3 miRs Drive Smooth Muscle Cell Function in Atherosclerosis

Smooth muscle cells (SMCs) are a typical feature of advanced atherosclerotic plaques, and active contribution of this cell type to lesion growth mainly through pro-inflammatory features has been suggested [30–32]. The role of SMCs in atherosclerosis, however, appears to be more complex, since SMCs contribute to the fibrous cap formation and SMC apoptosis which results in an unstable plaque phenotype [33]. Furthermore, SMCs show a remarkable plasticity under various disease conditions between a contractile and synthetic phenotype, although the specific impact of the separate phenotypes to vascular diseases is unclear [31]. Synthetic SMCs are characterized by a reduced content of contractile proteins, an increased proliferation rate, and an increased secretion of extracellular matrix proteins and cytokines [30]. Vascular injury models, although associated with differing lesion morphology compared with native atherosclerosis especially in normolipidemic animals, serve as a tool to study the functions of SMCs in atherogenesis.

Following balloon injury in rat carotid arteries, more than 100 out of 140 miRs were differentially regulated in the course of neointimal formation [34]. Among those, miR-21 was highly upregulated after 7 days and mediated the neointima formation through increased proliferation and reduced apoptosis as determined by local administration of the antisense oligonucleotide 2′OMe-miR-21 [34]. Mir-21-mediated decrease of PTEN and the up-regulation of Bcl-2 expression in SMCs were identified as the molecular targets [34]. Interestingly, miR-21 is induced by BMP4 and TGF-β and increases the biosynthesis of contractile proteins in SMCs through suppression of *programmed cell death 4* (PDCD4) [35]. In addition to miR-21, the proliferation of SMCs is enhanced after vascular injury redundantly through miR-221 and miR-222 which target the tumor suppressors and cell cycle inhibitors p27(Kip1) and p57(Kip2) [36]. Treatment with an miR inhibitor against miR-221 and miR-222 after balloon-injury reduced neointimal formation most likely due to reduced expression of p27(Kip1) and p57(Kip2) [36]. In addition to proliferation, *platelet-derived growth factor* (PDGF) induced dedifferentiation is mediated by repression of c-kit and p27(Kip1) through miR-221 [37].

The SMC-specific expression of miR-145 and miR-143, derived from a common bicistronic precursor, is regulated by myocardin, the serum response factor (SRF), and Nkx2-5. Reduced expression of miR-145/-143 in SMCs after vascular injury is associated with the down-regulation of contractile proteins [38, 39]. In early atherosclerotic lesions of hyperlipidemic ApoE$^{-/-}$ mice, however, only the expression of miR-145 is decreased to almost undetectable levels [39]. Over-expression of miR-145 in injured arteries by adenoviral transduction inhibited the dedifferentiation of the SMCs and reduced neointimal hyperplasia [38]. Similarly, miR-145 reconstitution in ligated murine carotid arteries increased the expression of SMC-specific proteins [39]. Cordes et al. described an analogous effect of miR-145 on the SMC phenotype; for instance, the myocardin-induced reprogramming of fibroblasts towards a SMC fate is augmented by miR-145, but not by miR-143 [39]. Interestingly, this was associated with increased translation of myocardin through binding of miR-145 to a specific recognition element in the 3′UTR of the myocardin mRNA [39]. The activation of translation has been reported for a small set of miRs in non-proliferating cells by recruiting microRNP-related proteins to AU-rich-elements [40]. In miR-145$^{-/-}$ and miR-143/145$^{-/-}$ mice, however, neointima formation after carotid ligation was nearly absent and miR-143 deficiency reduced the lesion area by 60% [41]. Moreover, aged miR-143/145$^{-/-}$ mice spontaneously develop neointimal lesions even in the absence of vascular injury or hyperlipidemia [42]. The presence of macrophages in these lesions indicates an inflammatory response elicited by the absence of miR-143 and miR-145. Although the molecular mechanism of this type of lesion formation is not completely understood, angiotensin converting enzyme (ACE) was found to be increased in miR-143/145 deficient mice. This might contribute to plaque formation via increased angiotensin II generation, which is known to exacerbate atherogenesis [42]. These findings were derived from different sets of miR-143/145−/− mice independently generated from two groups, which already differ in the phenotype of the vascular SMCs. Whereas Boettger et al. report a shift towards a synthetic phenotype in the normal arteries of miR-143/145−/− mice, Xin et al. found no difference in the expression of contractile proteins in SMCs but a reduction of stress fibers indicating disturbed actin cytoskeleton dynamics [41, 42]. Thinning of the arterial wall and reduced blood pressure, however, was described in both types of miR-143/145−/− mice [41, 42]. Mechanistically, the effect of miR-145 on SMCs appears to be mediate at least in part by targeting of Kruppel-like factor 5 (KLF5), which suppresses the master-regulator of SMC differentiation, Myocardin [38, 41]. Furthermore, down-regulation of miR-145 is involved in the PDGF-mediated dedifferentiation of SMCs by induction of KLF5 [38]. Of note, the myocardin-related transcription factor (MRTF)-B is negatively regulated by both miR-145 and miR-143, which may have an effect on myocardin function as transcriptional co-activator [41, 43]. In addition, miR-145 represses Kruppel-like factor 4 (KLF4) and Calmodulin kinase II-δ, which play a central role in SMC homeostasis and neointimal formation [39, 41]. Apart from phenotypic modulation, treatment with miR-145 mimics inhibits the PDGF-induced proliferation of SMCs *in vitro* demonstrating an important role of PDGF-mediated suppression of miR-145 in the proliferative response [38, 39]. The molecular mechanism of this miR-145 effect is uncertain. In contrast to miR-145, inhibition of miR-143 increased the proliferation rate of SMCs probably through the up-regulation of Elk-1, which has been found to reduce SMC-restricted gene expression and to enforce SMC proliferation [39].

MiR-1 has been primarily found in skeletal and cardiac muscle and is down-regulated in cardiac hypertrophy [44]. However, miR-1 is also induced during SMC differentiation and increases the expression of SMC-specific contractile proteins by targeting KLF4 [45, 46]. Furthermore, myocardin-induced miR-1 expression is centrally involved in the myocardin-dependent SMC marker synthesis, contractility, and proliferation [45, 47]. The oncogenic serine/threonine kinase Pim-1, which is suppressed by miR-1 in lung cancer cells, was found to be a direct target of miR-1 in SMCs [47]. Accordingly, miR-1 is down-regulated, and Pim-1 is increased in neointimal lesions of ligated carotid arteries [47]. It remains to be resolved, however, whether Pim-1 mediates the miR-1 effects on SMC proliferation and how the reduced expression of miR-1 affects neointima formation.

12.4 miRs Modulate Endothelial Function in Atherosclerosis

Leukocyte capture and influx at sites of atherosclerotic lesion formation is mediated by adhesion molecules expressed on activated endothelial cells [48]. The expression of the cytokine-inducible vascular cell adhesion molecule (VCAM)-1 on arterial endothelial cells, which plays a key role in mediating inflammatory arrest of monocytes and T-cells under atherogenic conditions, is regulated by endothelial miR-126 [49]. The pri-miR-126 is encoded in intron 7 of the egfl7 (epidermal growth factor-like domain 7) gene. EGFL7 is secreted primarily from endothelial cells during development and induces angiogenesis through inhibition of Notch signaling [50]. The transcription factors Ets-1 and -2 have been found to regulate the expression of egfl7/miR-126 [51]. Whereas Ets-1 mediates the angiotensin II-induced vascular inflammation through up-regulation of VCAM-1 and MCP-1 *in vivo* [52], silencing of Ets-1 and -2 after TNF-stimulation enhanced the expression of VCAM-1, which might be due to reduced miR-126 [51]. While over-expression of the miR-126 precursor inhibited VCAM-1 expression, decreasing endogenous miR-126 levels promoted VCAM-1 induction and leukocyte adhesion to endothelial cells, suggesting that it may critically control vascular inflammation [49]. In addition, miR-126 governs vascular integrity and angiogenesis by regulating endothelial cell responses to VEGF, e.g., by repressing SPRED1, which is an intracellular inhibitor of angiogenic kinase signaling, or a regulatory subunit of the PIK3 kinase (PIK3R2) [53, 54]. Moreover, targeted deletion or knock-down of miR-126 causes vascular leakage during embryonic development, which might also increase permeability and vascular deposition of lipids parallel to impaired neovascularization after infarction due to defects in endothelial cell function.

A recent study further unraveled a novel mechanism, by which endothelial cell-derived apoptotic bodies transfer miR-126 as a messenger signal to induce secretion of the chemokine CXCL12 [55]. This involves the repression of the negative regulator RGS16, which "unlocks" CXCR4 and, thus, drives the expression and secretion of CXCL12 in an autoregulatory, self amplifying feedback loop through CXCR4. Apoptotic bodies carrying miR-126 or local transfer of miR-126 also repressed arterial expression of RGS16 and reduced macrophage and apoptotic cell content, while increasing CXCL12 expression, progenitor influx and SMC content in atherosclerotic plaque, thereby conferring a more stable plaque phenotype [55]. This mechanism might be of particular importance also at the early stage of atherosclerotic lesion formation, with endothelial cell apoptosis preceding the development of atherosclerotic plaques. This would be in accordance with the finding that miR-126 plasma levels are lower in patients with coronary atherosclerosis as compared to healthy volunteers [83]. In patients with prevalent and manifest Diabetes mellitus type 2, the miR-126 plasma levels were significantly reduced due to a diminished miR-126 content in endothelial microvesicles [56]. This would be compatible with a main role of miR-126 in accelerated plaque formation typically found in diabetic atherosclerosis. The release of small membrane vesicles, also called exosomes, is triggered by ceramide [57]. Inhibition of the ceramide-generating enzyme neutral sphingomyelinase 2 (nSMase2) greatly reduces the secretion of miRs [57]. Interestingly, nSMase2 is also critical for the scavenger receptor class B type I-dependent miR transfer by HDL particles [58]. Hypercholesterolemia changes the miR profile in HDL, which induces differential gene expression in hepatocytes [58]. Whether this contributes to the protective effect of HDL in atherosclerosis remains to be determined. In addition to the transportation of miRs in microvesicles and HDL, substantial amounts of circulating miRs are bound to Argonaute2 containing protein complexes, which protects miRs from extracellular degradation [59].

Low endothelial shear stress promotes the activation of endothelial cells to a proatherogenic phenotype and constitutes a main reason for the formation of atherosclerotic plaques at predilection sites like bifurcations or curvatures [60]. MiR expression has been found to be regulated by shear stress and may, thus, contribute to the lesion formation [61]. *In vitro*, miR-663 is up-regulated by oscillatory shear stress in human endothelial cells and enhances the endothelial adhesion of monocytes [62]. In contrast, high shear stress induces miR-21 in endothelial cells, which increases the athero-protective NO production [63]. Furthermore, miR-10a is down-regulated in endothelial cells from athero-susceptible regions of the aortic arch and aorto-renal branches [64]. Two regulators of IκBα degradation, MAP3K7 and βTRC, were targeted by miR-10a [64]. This may explain the activated NFκB pathway in endothelial cells after miR-10a knockdown, which results in pro-inflammatory activation with increased production CCL2, IL-6, IL-8, VCAM-1, and E-selectin [64]. Along these lines, ageing is one major risk factor for the development of atherosclerosis. By inducing a premature senescence-like phenotype with impaired NO synthase acetylation in endothelial cells via inhibition of the deacetylase silent information regulator 1/ sirtuin type 1 (SirT1), miR-217 might further aggravate endothelial dysfunction. Importantly, miR-217 was found to be expressed in human atherosclerotic lesions, and impairing endothelial integrity may contribute to the development of atherosclerosis [65].

12.5 miRs in Atherogenic Macrophage Function

Chronic inflammation of the vessel wall with infiltration of various types of leukocytes, especially monocytes/macrophages and also T cells, dendritic cells, and neutrophils, is the hallmark of atherosclerosis [48]. The differentiation and function of these leukocyte subtypes is strictly regulated by a specific set of miRs. Thus, miRs play an important role in the regulation of the immune system [66]. Although direct evidence for leukocyte-derived miRs involved in the inflammatory response of atherosclerotic vessels is currently scarce, the identification of miR function in leukocyte homeostasis and activation indicates a central role also in atherogenesis [67–69]. Macrophages derived from circulating monocytes accumulate in the subintimal space and transform into lipid-laden foam cells upon uptake of modified LDL particles. Furthermore, modified LDL can activate TLR4 signaling, which induces the expression of pro-inflammatory cytokines. The macrophage inflammatory response to infectious stimuli, for example, is characterized by the up-regulation of an array of miRs, such as miR-155, miR-146, miR-147, miR-21, and miR-9 [66].

The miR-155 gene is located on chromosome 21 in the exon of a non-coding RNA transcribed from the *B-cell Integration Cluster* (BIC). miR-155 is constitutively expressed in endothelial cells and SMCs *in vitro* and targets the angiotensin II type 1 receptor and the pro-inflammatory transcription factor ETS-1 [70, 71]. In macrophages, miR-155 is strongly up-regulated by activation of TLR-2 (P3C), TLR-3 (poly(I:C)), TLR-4 (LPS), TLR-9 (CpG) via either MyDD88- or TRIF-dependent signaling pathways [72]. In addition, IFN-β and -γ induce macrophage miR-155 through TNF-α [72]. At least TLR3 and TNF-α mediated up-regulation of miR-155 depends on the JNK pathway, which activates AP-1 [72]. The RNA-binding protein KSRP binds to the terminal loop of the miR-155 precursor and appears to promote the maturation of miR-155 in LPS-stimulated macrophages [73]. TLR4-induced miR-155 expression can be inhibited by IL-10 [74]. The evidence for the functional role of miR-155 in the pro-inflammatory activation of the macrophage lineage is conflicting. In monocyte-derived dendritic cells, miR-155 inhibits the production of IL-1β upon LPS stimulation and modulates the TLR/IL-1 signaling cascade by directly targeting TAB2, an intermediate in the IL-1 pathway, which also activates JNK, p38, and NF-κB [75]. Similarly, Ruggerio and co-workers reported that the inhibition of miR-155 was primarily associated with the up-regulation of pro-inflammatory mediators, such as IL1β, CCL5, and IL12. However, molecules with anti-inflammatory functions, like IL-10 or SOCS3, were also increased following miR-155 inhibition [73]. Further evidence for a pro-inflammatory role of miR-155 has been provided by the identification of SHIP1, an important negative regulator of PI3K/Akt pathway and TLR4 signaling, as a direct miR-155 target in macrophages [76]. Accordingly, Androulidaki and co-workers reported that inhibition of miR-155 reduced the expression of TNF-α, IL-6, IL-17, IP-10, and MCP-1 in LPS-stimulated macrophages through targeting of SOCS1 [77]. Interestingly, Akt activation negatively regulated miR-155 expression, which appears to be required for endotoxin tolerance *in vivo* [77]. Furthermore, miR-155 represses the IL13 receptor alpha1, resulting in reduced expression of IL-13-dependent genes, such as SOCS1, CCL18, and CD23, which are involved in the establishment of an M2 phenotype in macrophages [78]. The TGF-β signaling pathway in macrophages is also affected by miR-155 through repression of SMAD2 [79]. This leads to a reduced expression of IL-1β, MMP9, VEGF, ICAM-1, and DC-SIGN upon TGF-β stimulation [79]. Of note, even the basal levels of IL-1β expression were reduced by knock-down of miR-155 in this study. In mitogen-activated protein kinase phosphatase-1 (MKP-1) deficient macrophages, miR-155 expression is up-regulated, which leads to a increased STAT1 activation and enhanced iNOS expression following LPS stimulation due to repression of SOCS-1 [80]. In primary human monocytes, miR-155 is also induced along with miR-146a, miR-146b, miR-9, and miR-125a by stimulation with oxidized LDL [81]. In macrophages, the silencing of oxidized LDL-induced miR-155 enhanced the lipid uptake, activated the NF-κB pathway, increased the expression of scavenger receptors, and promoted the secretion of several pro-inflammatory cytokines, such as IL-6, IL-9, and TNF-α, which indicates a negative feedback regulation by miR-155 [82]. Interestingly, the levels of circulating miR-155 were significantly reduced in patients with coronary heart disease [83]. Moreover, miR-155 plasma levels decline with age and are significantly higher in females compared with males [83]. Taken together, miR-155 is centrally involved in the fine-tuning of the macrophage inflammatory response, although the net effect might dependent on the disease context.

MiR-146a and -146b differ only in two nucleotides and although the respective genes are located on different chromosomes stimulation of TLR-2, TLR-4, and TLR-5, but not by TLR-3, TLR-7, and TLR-9 in macrophages strongly induces both miRs [84]. In addition, TNF-α and IL-1β modestly increase the miR-146 expression, whereas CD40L had no effect [84]. Human mir-146a resides in the second exon of the LOC285628 gene on chromosome 5, which is transcribed into a probably non-coding RNA [84]. A promoter region of the miR-146a has been characterized, which contains NF-κB binding sites that are required for the LPS responsiveness [84]. Functionally, miR-146a/b base-pairs with the MRE in the 3′UTR of the predicted targets IL-1 receptor-associated kinase 1 and TNF-receptor-associated factor 6, indicating a negative feedback loop that limits the inflammatory Toll-like and cytokine signaling [84]. This mechanism has been confirmed for miR-146a to be relevant in LPS tolerance of monocytes through reduced expression of TNF-α, IL-1β, and IL-6 [85]. Both miR-146a and –b were up-regulated after stimulation with oxidized LDL in primary human monocytes [81]. In macrophages, however, oxLDL treatment suppressed the expression of miR-146a [86]. This appears to be critical for lipid accumulation and cytokine secretion from macrophages stimulated with oxLDL, since treatment with miR-146a mimics reduced the intracellular lipid content and the release of IL-6, IL-8, CCL2, and MMP9 [86]. In this study, miR-146a has been shown to directly target the TLR4, which may account for the observed effect of miR-146a mimics on oxLDL-stimulated macrophages [86].

Similar to miR-146, miR-147 also limits the macrophage inflammatory response following TLR stimulation [87]. Of note, activation of TLR4 resulted in a much stronger induction of miR-147 than stimulation of TLR-2 or TLR3. Analysis of the miR-147 promoter region revealed functional binding sites for NF-κB and a GAS element required for LPS-induced miR-147 expression [87]. TLR4 stimulation induces NF-κB and STAT1 binding to the miR-147 promoter via MyD88 and TRIF [87]. Inhibition of TLR-induced miR-147 reduced the secretion of inflammatory cytokines, such as TNF-α and IL-6, from macrophages [87]. This negative regulation of stimulated monocytes/macrophages might explain the finding that peripheral monocytes from patients with coronary artery disease (CAD) have reduced levels of miR-147, which might exacerbate the vascular inflammation during atherogenesis [88].

In addition, ox-LDL up-regulates miR-125a-5p in primary human monocytes and inhibition of miR-125a-5p increased the lipid accumulation probably due to enhanced expression of the scavenger receptors LOX-1 and CD68. Moreover, miR-125a-5p inhibitors increased the secretion of IL-6, TNF-α, IL-2, and TGF-β from oxLDL treated THP-1 cells [81]. The oxysterol-binding protein ORP9 has been found to be a direct target of miR-125a-5p in monocytes/macrophages. The functional role of miR-125a-5p-dependent regulation of ORP9 in oxLDL-stimulated monocytes, however, is unclear [81].

In analogy to endothelial cells, miRs can be enriched in microvesicles derived from monocytes, especially miR-150, upon stimulation, e.g., with LPS or H_2O_2. This active secretion in microvesicles contributes to increased miR-150 plasma levels and results in transfer of miR-150 to endothelial cells [89]. The exogenous miR-150 targets c-myb and enhances endothelial cell migration [89].

Furthermore, patients with atherosclerosis have increased miR-150 content in circulating microvesicles [89]. Interestingly, microvesicles were also released from monocytes/macrophages by cholesterol enrichment, which may result in increased levels of circulating microvesicles under hyperlipidemia [90].

Given the importance of a delicately orchestrated immune response in atherosclerosis, these findings strongly predict that the above miRs will exert profound effects during the evolution of lesion formation.

12.6 miR in Angiogenesis and Cardiovascular Medicine

Angiogenesis as a multi-step process of capillary network formation by sprouting of pre-existing endothelial cells is finely controlled by distinct angiogenic growth factors [20]. MiRs are differentially involved in the regulation of angiogenesis by modulating the release of these soluble growth factors. For instance, pro-angiogenic properties have been described for miR-18a and miR-19a in cancer cells [61]. Likewise, miR-132 was shown to induce angiogenesis and blocking miR-132 by respective antagomirs substantially suppressed tumor progression *in vivo* [11]. Recent data further revealed that miR-92a and miR-100 are instrumental in angiogenesis and tissue regeneration in mouse models of limb ischemia and myocardial infarction [8, 73]. Though, forced over-expression of miR-92a inhibited angiogenesis while suppression of miR-92a by antagomirs-enhanced vessel growth and recovery of ischemic tissue [73]. Similarly, miR-100 retains anti-angiogenic function and blocking miR-100 by specific antagomirs-stimulated angiogenesis and functional improvement of ischemic limbs in mice [8]. Beside miR-18a, miR-19a, miR-92a, and miR-132, other miRs such as miR-21, miR-222, miR-130a, and miR-126 have been reported to control endothelial cell function and capillary tube formation [3, 5].

Some miRs are closely associated with cardiovascular disease. In particular, the significance of circulating miRs as possible novel prognostic biomarker for CAD has been recently addressed [21, 84]. So far, clinical results reported about significant down-regulation of vascular and inflammation-related miRs (miR-126, miR-92a, miR-17, and miR-155) in blood of patients with CAD versus healthy volunteers [84]. Moreover, risk factors for CAD such as type 2 diabetes mellitus associated with altered plasma levels of miR-126 [69]. MiR-126 was also shown to be down-regulated in blood samples of stroke patients [40]. As outlined above, the transfer and incorporation of miR-126 have been mechanistically associated with increased production of CXCL12 and plaque stabilization in a mouse model of atherosclerosis, thus bearing even protective effects on the vasculature [55]. Hence, reduced levels of plasma miR-126 might be predictive for vascular dysfunction. Very recent results further revealed reduced levels of miR-126 but elevated levels of miR-221, miR-222, and miR92a in angiogenic cells cultured from peripheral blood of CAD patients as compared to healthy controls [58]. Such a dysregulation of the miR profile might contribute to impaired function of angiogenic cells and might, thus, represent a valuable cue towards specific therapeutic interference or reconstitution.

12.7 Concluding Remarks

It is more than evident that miRs critically affect relevant pro-and anti-atherogenic functions of major cell types involved in atherogenesis. Surprisingly, data on the role of miRs in atherosclerosis models are still scarce. This is required, however, to gain further insights into miR-dependent atherogenesis. The availability of highly effective miRs inhibitors *in vivo* promises already the introduction of a new class of therapeutics for cardiovascular diseases by targeting pro-atherogenic miRs. In addition, many miRs appear to have actually anti-atherogenic properties, such as miR-126. Thus, the therapeutic application of miRs, e.g., loaded in microvesicles for better transfer, might be of even greater importance in the future. An improved understanding of the exceptional plasma stability and cell-targeted delivering strategies would greatly assist in this approach.

References

1. Huntzinger, E., and Izaurralde, E. (2011). Gene silencing by microRNAs: Contributions of translational repression and mrna decay. *Nat Rev Genet.* **12**, pp. 99–110.

2. Fazi, F., and Nervi, C. (2008). MicroRNA: Basic mechanisms and transcriptional regulatory networks for cell fate determination. *Cardiovasc Res.* **79**, pp. 553–561.

3. Small, E. M., and Olson, E. N. (2011). Pervasive roles of microRNAs in cardiovascular biology. *Nature.* **469**, pp. 336-342.

4. Drakaki, A., and Iliopoulos, D. (2009). MicroRNA gene networks in oncogenesis. *Curr Genomics.* **10**, pp. 35–41.

5. Selbach, M., Schwanhäusser, B., Thierfelder, N., Fang, Z., Khanin, R., and Rajewsky, N. (2008). Widespread changes in protein synthesis induced by microRNAs. *Nature.* **455**, pp. 58–63.

6. Hua, Z., Lv, Q., Ye, W., Wong, C. K., Cai, G., Gu, D., Ji, Y., Zhao, C., Wang, J., Yang, B. B., and Zhang, Y. (2006). Mirna-directed regulation of VEGF and other angiogenic factors under hypoxia. *PLoS ONE.* **1**, pp. e116. doi:10.1371/journal.pone.0000116.

7. Krek, A., Grun, D., Poy, M. N., Wolf, R., Rosenberg, L., Epstein, E. J., MacMenamin, P., da Piedade, I., Gunsalus, K. C., Stoffel, M., and Rajewsky, N. (2005). Combinatorial microRNA target predictions. *Nat Genet.* **37**, pp. 495–500.

8. Scholer, N., Langer, C., Dohner, H., Buske, C., and Kuchenbauer, F. (2010). Serum microRNAs as a novel class of biomarkers: A comprehensive review of the literature. *Exp Hematol.* **38**, pp. 1126–1130.

9. Krol, J., Loedige, I., and Filipowicz, W. (2010). The widespread regulation of microRNA biogenesis, function and decay. *Nat Rev Genet.* **11**, pp. 597–610.

10. Olena, A. F., and Patton, J. G. (2009). Genomic organization of microRNAmicroRNAs. *J Cell Physiol.* **222**, pp. 540–545.

11. Ro, S., Park, C., Young, D., Sanders, K. M., and Yan, W. (2007). Tissue-dependent paired expression of mirnas. *Nucleic Acids Res.* **35**, pp. 5944–5953.

12. Winter, J., Jung, S., Keller, S., Gregory, R. I., and Diederichs, S. (2009). Many roads to maturity: MicroRNA biogenesis pathways and their regulation. *Nat Cell Biol.* **11**, pp. 228–234.

13. Bartel, D. P. (2004). MicroRNAs: Genomics, biogenesis, mechanism, and function. *Cell.* **116**, pp. 281–297.

14. Carthew, R. W. and Sontheimer, E. J. (2009). Origins and mechanisms of mirnas and sirnas. *Cell.* **136**, pp. 642–655.

15. Kim, V. N. (2005). MicroRNA biogenesis: Coordinated cropping and dicing. *Nat Rev Mole Cell Biol.* **6**, pp. 376–385.

16. Davis, B. N., and Hata, A. (2010). Mechanisms of control of microRNA biogenesis. *J Biochem.* **148**, pp. 381–392.

17. Kim, V., and Nam, J. (2006). Genomics of microRNA. *Trends Genet.* **22**, pp. 165–173.

18. Kim, V. N., Han, J., and Siomi, M. C. (2009). Biogenesis of small rnas in animals. *Nat Rev Mol Cell Biol.* **10**, pp. 126–139.

19. Czech, B., and Hannon, G. J. (2010). Small rna sorting: Matchmaking for argonautes. *Nat Rev Genet.* **12**, pp. 19–31.

20. Peters, L., and Meister, G. (2007). Argonaute proteins: Mediators of RNA silencing. *Mol Cell.* **26**, pp. 611–623.

21. Su, H., Trombly, M. I., Chen, J., and Wang, X. (2009). Essential and overlapping functions for mammalian argonautes in microRNA silencing. *Genes Dev.* **23**, pp. 304–317.

22. Chiang, H. R., Schoenfeld, L. W., Ruby, J. G., Auyeung, V. C., Spies, N., Baek, D., Johnston, W. K., Russ, C., Luo, S., Babiarz, J. E., Blelloch, R., Schroth, G. P., Nusbaum, C., and Bartel, D. P. (2010). Mammalian microRNAs: Experimental evaluation of novel and previously annotated genes. *Genes Dev.* **24**, pp. 992–1009.

23. Okamura, K., Phillips, M. D., Tyler, D. M., Duan, H., Chou, Y.-t., and Lai, E. C. (2008). The regulatory activity of microRNA* species has substantial influence on microRNA and 3′ utr evolution. *Nat Struct &; Mol Biol.* **15**, pp. 354–363.

24. Yang, J. S., Phillips, M. D., Betel, D., Mu, P., Ventura, A., Siepel, A. C., Chen, K. C., and Lai, E. C. (2010). Widespread regulatory activity of vertebrate microRNA* species. *RNA,* New York, N.Y. doi: 10.1261/rna.2537911.

25. Bartel, D. P. (2009). MicroRNAs: Target recognition and regulatory functions. *Cell.* **136**, pp. 215–233.

26. Lewis, B. P., Shih, I. H., Jones-Rhoades, M. W., Bartel, D. P., and Burge, C. B. (2003). Prediction of mammalian microRNA targets. *Cell.* **115**, pp. 787–798.

27. Guo, H., Ingolia, N. T., Weissman, J. S., and Bartel, D. P. (2010). Mammalian microRNAs predominantly act to decrease target mrna levels. *Nature.* **466**, pp. 835–840.

28. Eulalio, A., Huntzinger, E., and Izaurralde, E. (2008). Getting to the root of mirna-mediated gene silencing. *Cell.* **132**, pp. 9–14.

29. Lloyd-Jones, D. M. (2010). Cardiovascular risk prediction: Basic concepts, current status, and future directions. *Circulation.* **121**, pp. 1768–1777.

30. Doran, A. C., Meller, N., and McNamara, C. A. (2008). Role of smooth muscle cells in the initiation and early progression of atherosclerosis. *Arterioscler Thromb Vasc Biol.* **28**, pp. 812–819.

31. Owens, G. K., Kumar, M. S., and Wamhoff, B. R. (2004). Molecular regulation of vascular smooth muscle cell differentiation in development and disease. *Physiol Rev.* **84**, pp. 767–801.

32. Zeiffer, U., Schober, A., Lietz, M., Liehn, E. A., Erl, W., Emans, N., Yan, Z. Q., and Weber, C. (2004). Neointimal smooth muscle cells display a proinflammatory phenotype resulting in increased leukocyte recruitment mediated by p-selectin and chemokines. *Circ Res.* 94, pp. 776–784.

33. Clarke, M. C., Figg, N., Maguire, J. J., Davenport, A. P., Goddard, M., Littlewood, T. D., and Bennett, M. R. (2006). Apoptosis of vascular smooth muscle cells induces features of plaque vulnerability in atherosclerosis. *Nat Med.* **12**, pp. 1075–1080.

34. Ji, R., Cheng, Y., Yue, J., Yang, J., Liu, X., Chen, H., Dean, D. B., and Zhang, C. (2007). MicroRNA expression signature and antisense-mediated depletion reveal an essential role of microRNA in vascular neointimal lesion formation. *Circ Res.* **100**, pp. 1579–1588.

35. Davis, B. N., Hilyard, A. C., Lagna, G., and Hata, A. (2008). Smad proteins control drosha-mediated microRNA maturation. *Nature.* **454**, pp. 56–61.

36. Liu, X., Cheng, Y., Zhang, S., Lin, Y., Yang, J., and Zhang, C. (2009). A necessary role of mir-221 and mir-222 in vascular smooth muscle cell proliferation and neointimal hyperplasia. *Circ Res.* **104**, pp. 476–487.

37. Davis, B. N., Hilyard, A. C., Nguyen, P. H., Lagna, G., and Hata, A. (2009). Induction of microRNA-221 by platelet-derived growth factor signaling is critical for modulation of vascular smooth muscle phenotype. *J Biol Chem.* **284**, pp. 3728–3738.

38. Cheng, Y., Liu, X., Yang, J., Lin, Y., Xu, D. Z., Lu, Q., Deitch, E. A., Huo, Y., Delphin, E. S., and Zhang, C. (2009). MicroRNA-145, a novel smooth muscle cell phenotypic marker and modulator, controls vascular neointimal lesion formation. *Circ Res.* **105**, pp. 158–166.

39. Cordes, K. R., Sheehy, N. T., White, M. P., Berry, E. C., Morton, S. U., Muth, A. N., Lee, T. H., Miano, J. M., Ivey, K. N., and Srivastava, D. (2009). Mir-145 and mir-143 regulate smooth muscle cell fate and plasticity. *Nature.* **460**, pp. 705–710.

40. Vasudevan, S., Tong, Y., and Steitz, J. A. (2007). Switching from repression to activation: MicroRNAs can up-regulate translation. *Science.* **318**, pp. 1931–1934.

41. Xin, M., Small, E. M., Sutherland, L. B., Qi, X., McAnally, J., Plato, C. F., Richardson, J. A., Bassel-Duby, R., and Olson, E. N. (2009). MicroRNAs mir-143 and mir-145 modulate cytoskeletal dynamics and responsiveness of smooth muscle cells to injury. *Genes Dev.* **23**, pp. 2166–2178.

42. Boettger, T., Beetz, N., Kostin, S., Schneider, J., Kruger, M., Hein, L., and Braun, T. (2009). Acquisition of the contractile phenotype by murine arterial smooth muscle cells depends on the mir143/145 gene cluster. *J Clin Invest.* **119**, pp. 2634–2647.

43. Parmacek, M. S. (2007). Myocardin-related transcription factors: Critical coactivators regulating cardiovascular development and adaptation. *Circ Res.* **100**, pp. 633–644.

44. Han, M., Toli, J., and Abdellatif, M. (2011). MicroRNAs in the cardiovascular system. *Curr Opin Cardiol.* **26**, pp. 181–189.

45. Jiang, Y., Yin, H., and Zheng, X.-L. (2010). MicroRNA-1 inhibits myocardin-induced contractility of human vascular smooth muscle cells. *J Cell Physiol.* **225**, pp. 506–511.

46. Xie, C., Huang, H., Sun, X., Guo, Y., Hamblin, M., Ritchie, R. P., Garcia-Barrio, M. T., Zhang, J., and Chen, Y. E. (2011). MicroRNA-1 regulates smooth muscle cell differentiation by repressing kruppel-like factor 4. *Stem Cells Dev.* **20**, pp. 205–210.

47. Chen, J., Yin, H., Jiang, Y., Radhakrishnan, S. K., Huang, Z. P., Li, J., Shi, Z., Kilsdonk, E. P. C., Gui, Y., Wang, D. Z., and Zheng, X. L. (2010). Induction of microRNA-1 by myocardin in smooth muscle cells inhibits cell proliferation. *Arterioscler Thromb Vasc Biol.* **31**, pp. 368–375.

48. Weber, C., Zernecke, A., and Libby, P. (2008). The multifaceted contributions of leukocyte subsets to atherosclerosis: Lessons from mouse models. *Nat Rev Immunol.* **8**, pp. 802–815.

49. Harris, T. A., Yamakuchi, M., Ferlito, M., Mendell, J. T., and Lowenstein, C. J. (2008). MicroRNA-126 regulates endothelial expression of vascular

cell adhesion molecule 1. *Proc Natl Acad Sci U S A.* **105**, pp. 1516–1521.

50. Nichol, D., Shawber, C., Fitch, M. J., Bambino, K., Sharma, A., Kitajewski, J., and Stuhlmann, H. (2010). Impaired angiogenesis and altered notch signaling in mice overexpressing endothelial egfl7. *Blood.* **116**, pp. 6133–6143.
51. Harris, T. A., Yamakuchi, M., Kondo, M., Oettgen, P., and Lowenstein, C. J. (2010). Ets-1 and ets-2 regulate the expression of microRNA-126 in endothelial cells. *Arterioscler Thromb Vasc Biol.* 30, pp. 1990-1997.
52. Zhan, Y., Brown, C., Maynard, E., Anshelevich, A., Ni, W., Ho, I. C., and Oettgen, P. (2005). Ets-1 is a critical regulator of ang II-mediated vascular inflammation and remodeling. *J Clin Invest.* **115**, pp. 2508–2516.
53. Fish, J. E., Santoro, M. M., Morton, S. U., Yu, S., Yeh, R. F., Wythe, J. D., Ivey, K. N., Bruneau, B. G., Stainier, D. Y., and Srivastava, D. (2008). Mir-126 regulates angiogenic signaling and vascular integrity. *Dev Cell.* **15**, pp. 272–284.
54. Wang, S., Aurora, A. B., Johnson, B. A., Qi, X., McAnally, J., Hill, J. A., Richardson, J. A., Bassel-Duby, R., and Olson, E. N. (2008). The endothelial-specific microRNA mir-126 governs vascular integrity and angiogenesis. *Dev Cell.* **15**, pp. 261–271.
55. Zernecke, A., Bidzhekov, K., Noels, H., Shagdarsuren, E., Gan, L., Denecke, B., Hristov, M., Koppel, T., Jahantigh, M. N., Lutgens, E., Wang, S., Olson, E. N., Schober, A., and Weber, C. (2009). Delivery of microRNA-126 by apoptotic bodies induces cxcl12-dependent vascular protection. *Sci Signal.* **2**, pp. ra81.
56. Zampetaki, A., Kiechl, S., Drozdov, I., Willeit, P., Mayr, U., Prokopi, M., Mayr, A., Weger, S., Oberhollenzer, F., Bonora, E., Shah, A., Willeit, J., and Mayr, M. (2010). Plasma microRNA profiling reveals loss of endothelial mir-126 and other microRNAs in type 2 diabetes. *Circ Res.* **107**, pp. 810–817.
57. Kosaka, N., Iguchi, H., Yoshioka, Y., Takeshita, F., Matsuki, Y., and Ochiya, T. (2010). Secretory mechanisms and intercellular transfer of microRNAs in living cells. *J Biol Chem.* **285**, pp. 17442–17452.
58. Vickers, K. C., Palmisano, B. T., Shoucri, B. M., Shamburek, R. D., and Remaley, A. T. (2011). MicroRNAs are transported in plasma and delivered to recipient cells by high-density lipoproteins. *Nat Cell Biol,* **13**, pp.423–33.

59. Arroyo, J. D., Chevillet, J. R., Kroh, E. M., Ruf, I. K., Pritchard, C. C., Gibson, D. F., Mitchell, P. S., Bennett, C. F., Pogosova-Agadjanyan, E. L., Stirewalt, D. L., Tait, J. F., and Tewari, M. (2011). Argonaute2 complexes carry a population of circulating microRNAs independent of vesicles in human plasma. *Proc Natl Acad Sci U S A.* **108**(12): pp. 5003-5008.

60. Chatzizisis, Y. S., Coskun, A. U., Jonas, M., Edelman, E. R., Feldman, C. L., and Stone, P. H. (2007). Role of endothelial shear stress in the natural history of coronary atherosclerosis and vascular remodelingmolecular, cellular, and vascular behavior. *J AmColl Cardiol.* **49**, pp. 2379–2393.

61. Qin, X., Wang, X., Wang, Y., Tang, Z., Cui, Q., Xi, J., Li, Y. S., Chien, S., and Wang, N. (2010). MicroRNA-19a mediates the suppressive effect of laminar flow on cyclin d1 expression in human umbilical vein endothelial cells. *Proc Natl Acad Sci U S A.* **107**, pp. 3240–3244.

62. Ni, C. W., Qiu, H., and Jo, H. (2011). MicroRNA-663 upregulated by oscillatory shear stress plays a role in inflammatory response of endothelial cells. *Am J Physiol Heart Circ Physiol.* **300**(5), pp. H1762–H17629.

63. Weber, M., Baker, M. B., Moore, J. P., and Searles, C. D. (2010). Mir-21 is induced in endothelial cells by shear stress and modulates apoptosis and eNOS activity. *Biochem Biophys Res Commun.* **393**, pp. 643–648.

64. Fang, Y., Shi, C., Manduchi, E., Civelek, M., and Davies, P. F. (2010). MicroRNA-10a regulation of proinflammatory phenotype in athero-susceptible endothelium *in vivo* and *in vitro. Proc Natl Acad Sci U S A.* **107**, pp. 13450–13455.

65. Menghini, R., Casagrande, V., Cardellini, M., Martelli, E., Terrinoni, A., Amati, F., Vasa-Nicotera, M., Ippoliti, A., Novelli, G., Melino, G., Lauro, R., and Federici, M. (2009). MicroRNA 217 modulates endothelial cell senescence via silent information regulator 1. *Circulation.* **120**, pp. 1524–1532.

66. O'Connell, R. M., Rao, D. S., Chaudhuri, A. A., and Baltimore, D. (2010). Physiological and pathological roles for microRNAs in the immune system. *Nat Rev Immunol.* **10**, pp. 111–122.

67. Baltimore, D., Boldin, M. P., O'Connell, R. M., Rao, D. S., and Taganov, K. D. (2008). MicroRNAs: New regulators of immune cell development and function. *Nat Immunol.* **9**, pp. 839–845.

68. Bi, Y., Liu, G., and Yang, R. (2009). MicroRNAs: Novel regulators during the immune response. *J Cell Physiol.* **218**, pp. 467–472.

69. Tsitsiou, E., and Lindsay, M. A. (2009). MicroRNAs and the immune response. *Curr Opin Pharmacol.* **9**, pp. 514–520.

70. Martin, M. M., Buckenberger, J. A., Jiang, J., Malana, G. E., Nuovo, G. J., Chotani, M., Feldman, D. S., Schmittgen, T. D., and Elton, T. S. (2007). The human angiotensin II type 1 receptor +1166 a/c polymorphism attenuates microRNA-155 binding. *J Biol Chem.* **282**, pp. 24262–24269.

71. Zhu, N., Zhang, D., Chen, S., Liu, X., Lin, L., Huang, X., Guo, Z., Liu, J., Wang, Y., Yuan, W., and Qin, Y. (2011). Endothelial enriched microRNAs regulate angiotensin II-induced endothelial inflammation and migration. *Atherosclerosis.* **215**, pp. 286–293.

72. O'Connell, R. M., Taganov, K. D., Boldin, M. P., Cheng, G., and Baltimore, D. (2007). MicroRNA-155 is induced during the macrophage inflammatory response. *Proc Natl Acad Sci U S A.* **104**, pp. 1604–1609.

73. Ruggiero, T., Trabucchi, M., De Santa, F., Zupo, S., Harfe, B. D., McManus, M. T., Rosenfeld, M. G., Briata, P., and Gherzi, R. (2009). Lps induces kh-type splicing regulatory protein-dependent processing of microRNA-155 precursors in macrophages. *FASEB J.* **23**, pp. 2898–2908.

74. McCoy, C. E., Sheedy, F. J., Qualls, J. E., Doyle, S. L., Quinn, S. R., Murray, P. J., and O'Neill, L. A. J. (2010). Il-10 inhibits mir-155 induction by toll-like receptors. *J Biol Chem.* **285**, pp. 20492–20498.

75. Ceppi, M., Pereira, P. M., Dunand-Sauthier, I., Barras, E., Reith, W., Santos, M. A., and Pierre, P. (2009). MicroRNA-155 modulates the interleukin-1 signaling pathway in activated human monocyte-derived dendritic cells. *Proc Natl Acad Sci U S A.* **106**, pp. 2735–2740.

76. O'Connell, R. M., Chaudhuri, A. A., Rao, D. S., and Baltimore, D. (2009). Inositol phosphatase ship1 is a primary target of mir-155. *Proc Natl Acad Sci U S A.* **106**, pp. 7113–7118.

77. Androulidaki, A., Iliopoulos, D., Arranz, A., Doxaki, C., Schworer, S., Zacharioudaki, V., Margioris, A. N., Tsichlis, P. N., and Tsatsanis, C. (2009). The kinase akt1 controls macrophage response to lipopolysaccharide by regulating microRNAs. *Immunity.* **31**, pp. 220–231.

78. Martinez-Nunez, R. T., Louafi, F., and Sanchez-Elsner, T. (2010). The interleukin 13 (il-13) pathway in human macrophages is modulated by microRNA-155 via direct targeting of interleukin 13 receptor 1 (il13r 1). *J Biol Chem.* **286**, pp. 1786–1794.

79. Louafi, F., Martinez-Nunez, R. T., and Sanchez-Elsner, T. (2010). MicroRNA-155 targets smad2 and modulates the response of

macrophages to transforming growth factor. *J Biol Chem.* **285**, pp. 41328–41336.

80. Wang, X., Zhao, Q., Matta, R., Meng, X., Liu, X., Liu, C. G., Nelin, L. D., and Liu, Y. (2009). Inducible nitric-oxide synthase expression is regulated by mitogen-activated protein kinase phosphatase-1. *J Biol Chem.* **284**, pp. 27123–27134.
81. Chen, T., Huang, Z., Wang, L., Wang, Y., Wu, F., Meng, S., and Wang, C. (2009). MicroRNA-125a-5p partly regulates the inflammatory response, lipid uptake, and orp9 expression in oxldl-stimulated monocyte/macrophages. *Cardiovasc Res.* **83**, pp. 131–139.
82. Huang, R. S., Hu, G. Q., Lin, B., Lin, Z. Y., and Sun, C. C. (2010). MicroRNA-155 silencing enhances inflammatory response and lipid uptake in oxidized low-density lipoprotein-stimulated human thp-1 macrophages. *J Investig Med.* **58**, pp. 961–967.
83. Fichtlscherer, S., De Rosa, S., Fox, H., Schwietz, T., Fischer, A., Liebetrau, C., Weber, M., Hamm, C. W., Roxe, T., Muller-Ardogan, M., Bonauer, A., Zeiher, A. M., and Dimmeler, S. (2010). Circulating microRNAs in patients with coronary artery disease. *Circ Res.* **107**, pp. 677–684.
84. Taganov, K. D., Boldin, M. P., Chang, K. J., and Baltimore, D. (2006). Nf-kappab-dependent induction of microRNA mir-146, an inhibitor targeted to signaling proteins of innate immune responses. *Proc Natl Acad Sci U S A.* **103**, pp. 12481–12486.
85. Nahid, M. A., Pauley, K. M., Satoh, M., and Chan, E. K. L. (2009). Mir-146a is critical for endotoxin-induced tolerance: Implication in innate immunity. *J Biol Chem.* **284**, pp. 34590–34599.
86. Yang, K., He, Y. S., Wang, X. Q., Lu, L., Chen, Q. J., Liu, J., Sun, Z., and Shen, W. F. (2011). Mir-146a inhibits oxidized low-density lipoprotein-induced lipid accumulation and inflammatory response via targeting toll-like receptor 4. *FEBS Lett.* **585**, pp. 854–860.
87. Liu, G., Friggeri, A., Yang, Y., Park, Y. J., Tsuruta, Y., and Abraham, E. (2009). Mir-147, a microRNA that is induced upon toll-like receptor stimulation, regulates murine macrophage inflammatory responses. *Proc Natl Acad Sci U S A.* **106**, pp. 15819–15824.
88. Hoekstra, M., van der Lans, C. A. C., Halvorsen, B., Gullestad, L., Kuiper, J., Aukrust, P., van Berkel, T. J. C., and Biessen, E. A. L. (2010). The peripheral blood mononuclear cell microRNA signature of coronary artery disease. *Biochem Biophys Res Commun.* **394**, pp. 792–797.

89. Zhang, Y., Liu, D., Chen, X., Li, J., Li, L., Bian, Z., Sun, F., Lu, J., Yin, Y., and Cai, X. (2010). Secreted monocytic mir-150 enhances targeted endothelial cell migration. *Mol Cell.* **39**, pp. 133–144.

90. Liu, M. L., Reilly, M. P., Casasanto, P., McKenzie, S. E., and Williams, K. J. (2007). Cholesterol enrichment of human monocyte/macrophages induces surface exposure of phosphatidylserine and the release of biologically-active tissue factor-positive microvesicles. *Arterioscler Thromb Vasc Biol.* **27**, pp. 430–435.

Chapter 13

Neutrophilic Granulocytes in the Treatment of Atherosclerosis

Oliver Soehnlein and Christian Weber
Institute for Cardiovascular Prevention, Ludwig-Maximilians-Universität, Munich, Germany
oliver.soehnlein@med.uni-muenchen.de

Polymorphonuclear leukocytes (PMN) have so far rarely been associated with atherosclerosis and its complications. Just now, studies are evolving that highlight mechanisms by which PMN control inflammatory process in atherosclerosis. Due to the restricted knowledge on the impact of PMN in atherosclerosis lesion formation, progression, and rupture, little therapeutic strategies specifically targeting the PMN have been developed. Hence, we here describe mechanisms by which PMN might promote atherosclerotic lesion formation. Potential targets detailed here, primarily derive from microvascular studies.

Atherosclerosis: Treatment and Prevention
Edited by Christian Weber and Oliver Soehnlein

ISBN 978-981-4316-26-2 (Hardcover), ISBN 978-981-4364-26-3 (eBook)
www.panstanford.com

13.1 Neutrophils Contribute to Atherosclerosis: Evidence from Human and Murine Studies

Atherosclerosis is looked upon as a chronic inflammatory disease of the arterial vessel wall with prominent roles for endothelial cells, T lymphocytes, and monocyte-derived cells (1,2). In contrast to lymphocytes and monocytes/macrophages, PMN are not detected in high numbers in atherosclerotic lesions and have, therefore, been neglected players in the pathophysiology of atherosclerosis. The rare detection of PMN in atherosclerosis may be due to inefficient recruitment of these cells or, more likely, due to their short life span in the tissue. While macrophages and T-lymphocytes reside for a long time within the lesion, PMN undergo rapid apoptosis and phagocytic clearance (3). Hence, even low PMN numbers detected in atherosclerotic plaques might indicate a significant recruitment and turnover in lesions. In addition, due to phenotypic changes of PMN hence appearing like macrophages or dendritic cells (4) and inadequate detection methods, attempts have failed to detect PMN in the plaque in high numbers. Over the past years, however, refined staining techniques allowed for sensitive detection of PMN in murine and human atherosclerotic plaque specimens. The use of antibodies to Ly6G specifically expressed on mouse PMN enabled detection of PMN in rupture prone atherosclerotic lesions (5). Similarly, utilization of $Apoe^{-/-}/Lysm^{egfp/egfp}$ mice (6) allowed for sensitive detection of PMN within plaques. Therein, the accumulation of PMN within atherosclerotic lesions was more prominent in regions of high inflammatory activity. Application of these mice also revealed that the majority of leukocytes rolling along atherosclerotic endothelium are PMN (7).

Equally important, histological observations indicate that PMN are prominent in human lesions. Just recently, Ionita *et al.* proved the intraplaque localization of PMN to be heterogeneous (8). PMN were found infiltrated in the cap, in the shoulder, and in areas toward the media. In the latter, PMN were primarily found around microvessels, while in the cap, PMN were also observed underneath the luminal endothelium. These may represent two distinct routes by which PMN infiltrate into the plaque. In addition, PMN were observed in areas with intraplaque hemorrhaging, this being a third possible route by which PMN come into the plaque. High PMN numbers were primarily found in plaques with features of rupture-prone lesions (bigger lipid core, heavy macrophage influx, and minor collagen and smooth muscle cells). However, it remains unclear if the accumulation of PMN in plaques with an unstable phenotype is cause or consequence. In addition, specimens from ruptured or eroded human plaques show distinct infiltrations with PMN. In line, Leclercq *et al.*, in carotid arteries, and Naruko *et al.*, in coronary arteries, reported the localization of PMN in the vicinity of intraplaque vessels (9,10). The latter study showed the presence of PMN in coronary lesions obtained at autopsy from patients with acute myocardial infarction and in atherectomy specimens from patients with unstable angina. In this study, all culprit lesions of patients who had died of acute myocardial infarction had PMN within the plaques, although at a variable extent, while PMN were extremely rare in coronary lesions obtained from patients who had died of non-cardiovascular diseases. Similarly, the number of PMN in the culprit lesions in patients with unstable angina was significantly higher than in patients with stable disease. More recently, a histological analysis of human carotid endarterectomy specimens suggested that intraplaque hemorrhage could convey PMN into the atherosclerotic lesion, leading to its enrichment in neutrophil proteases, which established a potential link between intraplaque hemorrhage, PMN infiltration, and plaque fragility (9).

13.2 Potential Mechanisms of Neutrophil-Mediated Atherosclerosis and Means of Interference

Although there is a great deal of data on the presence of PMN in human and murine plaque specimens at different disease stages, there are little data available elucidating mechanisms of PMN-driven atheroprogression. Many data provided in this section stem from microvascular inflammatory models and are extrapolated to atherosclerosis.

13.3 Neutrophil Priming and Induction of Neutrophilia by Hypercholesterolemia

Hyperlipidemia, especially hypercholesterolemia, is regarded as an independent risk factor in the development of ischemic heart disease, including myocardial infarction. Epidemiological studies showed that there is a strong relationship between the elevation of serum total cholesterol concentration and the morbidity and mortality of myocardial infarction (11,12). Apart from these significant studies, several additional findings point at the importance of hypercholesterolemia in atherosclerosis. Animals, with some rare exceptions, do not spontaneously develop atherosclerosis. The LDL level in most animals is 50 mg/dl or even less as compared to an average range of 130–160 mg/dl in humans (13). In addition, in Japan in the 1960s, LDL levels were only about 100 mg/dl. This was associated with a mortality from cardiovascular diseases that was about 10% of that in the United States and the rest of the developed countries. This was true despite the fact that the Japanese held the world record for the average nicotine consumption per day, a higher incidence of hypertension, and a prevalence of diabetes similar to that in other developed countries. More solid support stems from randomized clinical trials of lipid-lowering therapy. These have produced up to 30% reduction of major coronary events, thereby firmly vindicating the significance of high lipid levels as major contributing risk factor in atherosclerosis (14).

The presence of primed PMN in hyperlipidemia has been reported by Araujo *et al.* They show a positive correlation between plasma triglycerides and LDL and PMN ROS formation (15). In a more recent study, Mazor *et al.* found an increased rate of superoxide release and CD11b surface expression positively correlating with the severity of hyperlipidemia (16). In addition, circulating PMN contained less MPO, while plasma MPO levels were elevated, indicative of granule discharge from PMN in patients with hyperlipidemia. Finally, the authors showed that hyperlipidemia resulted in a slight (non-significant) increase in circulating PMN counts associated with enhanced levels of PMN apoptosis suggesting a higher turnover of PMN. Taken together these studies indicate a priming of PMN in hyperlipidemia.

OxLDL in the vessel wall may further activate PMN, thus modulating PMN-mediated pro-inflammatory effects. As for monocytes, oxLDL was shown to stimulate PMN adhesion (17,18) and transendothelial migration (19). Increased adhesion may be due to enhanced β_2-integrin mobilization from intracellular stores (18), thus allowing for firm arrest. As indicated above, major pro-inflammatory tools of PMN are granule proteins and reactive oxygen species. Therefore, it is of interest that oxLDL was shown to induce release of secondary and primary granules as indicated by discharge of lactoferrin and MPO, respectively (19). Similarly, oxLDL, but not native LDL, evoked a clear-cut increase in production and release of superoxide by PMN. This increase was preceded by a rapid rise in intracellular Ca^{2+}. Interestingly, both the transient Ca^{2+} increase and the superoxide production were abolished by presence of fucoidan, an unspecific scavenger receptor antagonist (20). Thus, these data suggest that PMN, contrary to common believe, may possess biological active scavenger receptors.

Hyperlipidemia exhibits apparent effects on homeostasis of bone marrow-derived cells, with increases in circulating numbers of lymphocytes, platelets, monocytes, and progenitor cells (21–23). In most cases, hyperlipidemia-induced perturbations in leukocyte homeostasis are multifactorial. For instance, hypercholesterolemia-associated monocytosis resulted from continued bone marrow production of inflammatory monocytes, increased survival of these cells in the periphery, and impaired conversion to resident monocytes (22,24). Clinical studies provide evidence for a positive correlation between circulating PMN counts and the risk for cardiovascular events (25,26). Recently it has been shown that hypercholesterolemia induces neutrophilia in mice which positively associates with atherosclerotic plaque burden (27). PMN homeostasis is regulated at various levels, including production, mobilization, and clearance, much of which is regulated by an equilibrium of chemokines, cytokines, and growth factors. Our study shows that hypercholesterolemia induces G-CSF, the key cytokine in regulating granulopoiesis. G-CSF itself is primarily induced by increased levels of TNF and IL-17, the latter of which is the effector of a PMN clearance feed-back loop (28). Interestingly, both cytokines are enhanced in the plasma of atherosclerotic mice. G-CSF not just stimulates proliferation of myeloid precursors but also reduces bone marrow CXCL12 levels, hence reducing clearance of aged PMN (29,30). Finally, hypercholesterolemia enhances serum CXCL1 levels, which promotes PMN mobilization via CXCR2. Hence, hyperlipidemia disturbs the tightly-regulated cytokine system controlling PMN homeostasis at various levels ultimately increasing peripheral PMN counts.

The statins form a class of hypolipidemic drugs used to lower cholesterol levels in dyslipidemic subjects; they act by inhibiting the enzyme HMG-CoA reductase, which is the rate-limiting enzyme of the mevalonate pathway of cholesterol synthesis (14). The clinical benefits of statins are strongly related to their lipid-lowering properties. However, because mevalonate is the precursor not only of cholesterol but also of non-steroidal isoprenoid compounds, the inhibition of HMG-CoA reductase may result in pleiotropic effects, independent of their hypocholesterolemic properties (14). Evidence from clinical studies suggests that statins reduced PMN priming in hyperlipidemic patients independently of lowering lipid levels. In this context, Sugano *et al.* showed that *ex vivo* endothelial adhesiveness of PMN obtained from individuals with hypercholesterolemia was increased compared to control subjects, and that it was attenuated by a 3 month treatment with fluvastatin (20 mg/day), independently of LDL reduction (31). Chello *et al.* reported that simvastatin (40 mg/day) and atorvastatin (20 mg/day), administered for 3 weeks prior to cardiopulmonary bypass, significantly reduced PMN CD11b expression and neutrophil-endothelial adhesion, irrespective of their efficacy at lowering cholesterol concentration (32,33). Similarly, van Oostrom *et al.* showed that rosuvastatin treatment (20 mg/day for 1 month, followed by 40 mg/day for 1 further month) blunted the postprandial increment of PMN migration towards different chemoattractants in mildly hyperlipidemic patients with premature coronary artery disease, through an effect that was unrelated to the improvement of lipoprotein metabolism (34). Finally, Guasti *et al.* and Marino *et al.* compared PMN obtained from dyslipidemic patients at a moderately increased risk of cardiovascular events with PMN obtained from matched healthy controls (35–37). They demonstrated an activation of PMN from patients at increased vascular risk, consisting in higher resting and stimulated IL-8 production, higher levels of angiotensin II type 1 receptor (AT_1R) messenger ribonucleic acid (mRNA), and increased reactive oxygen species (ROS) generation. In these patients, a 30 day treatment with simvastatin 20 mg daily had no influence on PMN count and ROS generation but reduced resting and stimulated IL-8 production and AT_1R mRNA to the level of healthy controls (35,36). Furthermore, treatment with simvastatin decreased PMN chemotaxis in response to fMLP (37). Importantly, the modulation of PMN function in dyslipidemic patients persisted in the 1-year follow-up, indicating that statin therapy is consistently associated with the reversion of the dysregulated PMN function associated with dyslipidemia (37).

In addition to such clinical data pointing at the inhibition of PMN priming by statins, data from *in vitro* experiments indicate that statins reduce PMN adhesion and migration. In this context, Dunzendorfer *et al.* demonstrated that incubation of PMN obtained from the peripheral blood of healthy volunteers with pravastatin or cerivastatin inhibits PMN transendothelial migration and chemotaxis, through an effect related to inhibition of the mevalonate synthesis (38,39). Furthermore, Eccles *et al.* showed that simvastatin and fluvastatin selectively reduce P- and E-selectin mediated interaction between human endothelial cells and human PMN *in vitro*, by blocking cell surface expression of both selectins in an HMG-CoA-dependent manner (40). Also, several findings indicate that statins may modulate the endothelial production of various chemokines that attract and activate PMN, such as CXCL5 (epithelial neutrophil-activating peptide or ENA-78) (40) and CXCL8 (interleukin-8 or IL-8) (41,42), through pathways involving HMG-CoA reductase and protein prenylation. Altogether, *in vitro* observations suggest that statins may directly or indirectly prevent neutrophil-mediated inflammatory reactions in the arterial wall. This hypothesis is supported by the recent findings from Nakamura *et al.* who investigated the effect of short-term fluvastatin administration in apolipoprotein E-deficient mice subjected to ligation of the common carotid artery, followed by collar positioning. In this study, fluvastatin treatment (10 mg/kg per day given orally) was found to attenuate PMN infiltration in neointimal carotid lesions, independent of plasma cholesterol lowering (42).

13.4 Neutrophil Recruitment in Atherosclerosis

PMN extravasation involves the coordinated and well-regulated interaction of selectins, cell adhesion molecules, and chemokines. It has previously been reported that the majority of transient leukocyte endothelial contacts in atherosclerosis is attributable to PMN, which interact with endothelial selectins (7,43). We recently extended these observations, describing that PMN adhere to the lumen of large arteries at early stages of atherosclerosis. The importance of molecules, such as P-selectin, β_2-integrins, and ICAM-1 in PMN adhesion and recruitment is without doubt. Hence, the vast reduction of atherosclerotic lesions in mice lacking P-selectin (44), the common β_2-integrin chain CD18 (45), or its counter receptor

ICAM-1 (46) may at least in part be explained by reduced PMN extravasation. In addition, leukotriene B4 is a potent chemoattractant for PMN, and deletion of its high affinity receptor BLT1 reduces atheroslerosis specifically at early stages of atherosclerosis (47). This is in agreement with a recent study attributing an important role to PMN during initial phases of atherosclerotic lesion formation. In addition, deletion of chemokine receptors CCR2 and CXCR2 results in reduced atherosclerotic burden (48). Given the importance of both these receptors in transmitting chemotactic signals for PMN, the atherosclerotic phenotype in these mice may in part be due to diminished arterial PMN infiltration. In addition and in contrast to PMN extravasation in the microcirculation, PMN extravasation in large arteries seems to require CCR1 and CCR5. It has previously been shown that the utilization of monocytic CCR1 and CCR5 in arterial recruitment is partially due to chemokines that are deposited by activated platelets (49,50). This mechanism is primarily important in early stages of atherosclerosis (51) and, hence, led to the investigation of the importance of platelet-derived chemokines in PMN adhesion and recruitment. In line, it has recently been found that CCL5 deposited by activated platelets induces PMN adhesion through engagement of CCR1 and CCR5 (27). The contribution of CCR1 and CCR5 to the extent of lesion formation, however, may differ, as a prevailing role of CCR5 in atherosclerosis has been reported (52). Deficiency of CXCR4, on the other hand, goes along with increased circulating PMN counts, which hence results in higher numbers of PMN in atherosclerotic lesions.

PMN recruitment into inflamed tissues is dependent on various cell adhesion molecules such as ICAM-1 and VCAM-1, selectins and integrins as well as chemokines. Despite reduced lesion sizes in mice lacking cell adhesion molecules, selectins, or integrins, these molecules may not be suited as therapeutic targets in atherosclerosis as long term interference may also hamper host defense mechanisms (53). In contrast, chemokines and their receptors have evolved as potential targets for infiltration of monocytes and PMN in atherosclerosis (54). PMN are commonly recruited by chemokines of the Glu-Leu-Arg $(ELR)^+$ CXC subfamily, including CXCL1, 2, 3, 5 (ligands of CXCR2) and CXCL 6–8 (ligands of both CXCR1 and CXCR2) (55). Several small molecule CXCR2 and dual CXCR1/CXCR2 antagonists have been successfully identified, some of which have been progressed into clinical trials for non-cardiovascular inflammatory disorders

(55). Reparixin, also known as repertaxin, inhibits CXCL8-induced PMN chemotaxis with an IC_{50} value of 1 nM and has been shown to decrease PMN infiltrates in a number of disease models, including cerebral ischemia-reperfusion injury (54,55). SB 656933 is a potent CXCR2 inhibitor which has been shown to inhibit PMN CD11b upregulation and shape change in response to CXCL1 and CXCL8. It has reportedly entered Phase I clinical trials for the treatment of chronic obstructive pulmonary disease and cystic fibrosis, and it is now entering Phase II clinical trials for ulcerative colitis and cystic fibrosis. At present, none of these compounds is reported to be under clinical investigation for atherosclerosis-related cardiovascular diseases. In contrast, the CXCR2 antagonist SB-517785-M was shown to reduce angiotensin II-induced leukocyte recruitment in rat arterioles. (56) However, data from clinical studies are not available at this point. In addition to CXCR2, CC chemokine receptors were shown to be important in recruitment of PMN to the artery. A Phase II, double-Blind, randomized, placebo-controlled trial in has been disclosed for MLN 1202, a humanized monoclonal antibody with high specificity to CCR2 (54). In addition, CCX140 targeting CCR2 is in Phase I clinical trial for restenosis after percutaneous intervention. A recent study indicates the importance of CCR1 and CCR5 in arterial but not microcirculatory recruitment of PMN (27). Hence, targeting of these two receptors may harbor options for treatment of atheroprogression without suppressing host-defense. Indeed, antagonists to CCR5 such as TAK779 or NBI-74330 were shown to markedly reduce atherosclerosis formation in mouse models (57,58). However, due to their poor oral bioavailability, these antagonists have not reached clinical testing for atherosclerosis. Nevertheless, CCR5-dependent recruitment can be tackled in yet another way. CCL5, a ligand of CCR5, forms heteromers with CXCL4, thereby enhancing leukocyte adhesion (59). Recent data have shown that disruption of CCL5-CXCL4 heteromers reduces atherosclerosis formation and leukocyte adhesion in mice (60).

13.5 Monocyte and Macrophage Activation by PMN Granule Proteins

While the PMN is traditionally looked upon as a leukocyte that crawls along the endothelium, escapes from the circulation, digests bacteria, and produces oxygen radicals, it also is a cell that has emerged as an initiator of the immune response (61). Much of this ability is mediated via release of preformed granule proteins which act to alarm neighbouring cells, such as endothelial cells, macrophages, and dendritic cells (62,63). Prominent members of the set of PMN-derived alarmins are LL-37 (64), α-defensins (human neutrophil peptides, HNPs) (65), HBP (azurocidin, CAP37) (66) as well as the serprocidins (elastase, cathepsin G, proteinase-3) (67). Interestingly, all of these proteins have been identified in the atherosclerotic lesion. Much of these proteins are found at the luminal site of the endothelium (68), suggesting their deposition by PMN. In this location, these proteins may activate monocytes in flow and induce adhesion (69). A similar mechanism has previously been shown for platelets which seed the arrest chemokine RANTES resulting in enhanced monocyte adhesion (70). Besides the endothelial location, PMN granule proteins are also detected in the subendothelial space where they may act to attract inflammatory monocytes by engagement of formyl-peptide receptors (50). In line, it has recently been shown that aortic lesions of neutropenic mice contain lower numbers of inflammatory monocytes as well as macrophages (27). Moreover, proteolytic modification of chemokines enhances or decreases their biological activity (67,71). Thus, N-terminal cleavage of IL-8 by proteinase-3 and epithelial neutrophil-activating protein 78 (ENA-78) by cathepsin G releases truncated forms of these chemokines that have higher chemotactic activity than the full-length molecules (72–74). Similarly, N-terminal modification of MIP-1δ by cathepsin G increased its monocyte-chemotactic activity many fold (74). Recently, it has been shown that activation of chemerin, which is known to attract antigen-presenting cells, can be mediated by neutrophil elastase and cathepsin G through the proteolytic removal of a C-terminal peptide (75). However, N-terminal truncation of a chemokine through proteolysis does not always lead to increased cellular activation. Processing of stromal cell-derived factor-1α (SDF-1α) by neutrophil elastase and proteolysis of MIP-1α isoforms by all three neutrophil serine proteases results in loss of chemotactic activity (76,77).

Neutrophil granule proteins may also activate macrophages to produce and release proinflammatory cytokines such as TNF and IL-6 (78,79). The activation of monocytes and macrophages by granule proteins is mediated via surface receptors such as β_2-integrins

(78,80), TLR-4 (81), and PARs (82). Mice deficient in these receptors show reduced lesion formation and have a tendency for more stable plaques (45,46,83). Although these receptors are promiscuous and PMN granule proteins are likely not their major ligands, these findings further point at the importance of PMN in atherosclerosis.

Formyl-peptide receptors play an important role in PMN biology. PMN express FPR1 and FPR2. Ligation of these receptors induces intracellular Ca^{2+} mobilization, chemotactic migration, and release of PMN granule proteins. As described above, granule proteins such as LL-37, azurocidin, and cathepsin G activate formyl-peptide receptors on inflammatory monocytes, thereby inducing recruitment of these cells (63,84). Hence, targeting formyl-peptide receptors might directly interfere with PMN accumulation and activation as well as with PMN-dependent monocyte recruitment. Early studies showed that replacing the formyl group of the classical FPR agonist fMLF with tertiary butyloxycarbonyl group (*t*-Boc) renders the peptide antagonistic (85). *t*-Boc-Met-Leu-Phe (Boc1) and *t*-Boc-Phe-d-Leu-Phe-d-Leu-Phe (Boc2) are two frequently used antagonists for FPR1. In several recent studies, Boc2 was used at high concentrations (e.g., 100 μM) for inhibition of FPR2 (86,87). A recent study has shown that when used at low micromolar concentrations, both Boc1 and Boc2 are selective antagonists for FPR1. At high micromolar concentrations, Boc2 partially inhibits FPR2 in addition to FPR1 (88). Therefore, the antagonistic effect of Boc2 at high concentrations is not specific for FPR2. In another ligand screen, the peptide WRWWWW was identified as a highly selective antagonist for FPR2/ALX (89), with a pIC_{50} of 6.64 in calcium flux assay. As an antagonist, WRWWWW is more selective at FPR2 than Boc2 (88). Cyclosporin H (CsH) produced by fungi is an isomer of the immunosuppressant CsA. CsH lacks immunosuppressive activity but displays selective antagonistic activity at human FPR1 (90). Studies have shown that CsH is 14-fold more potent than Boc2 in FPR1 binding assays, and approximately 5-fold more potent than Boc2 in the inhibition of fMLF-induced calcium flux and enzyme release (91). Both Boc2 and CsH competitively displace FPR1-bound [^{3}H]fMLF, indicating that its antagonistic activity is mediated through inhibition of fMLF binding. Two types of endogenous FPR1 antagonists have been identified. Spinorphin (LVVYPWT), an opioid, is an endogenous peptide antagonist for FPR1 (92,93). The bile acids deoxycholic acid (DCA) and chenodeoxycholic acid (CDCA) are two other identified antagonists for FPR1 (94,95). The physiological functions of DCA- and CDCA-mediated FPR1 antagonism have not been fully understood. Chemotaxis inhibitory protein of *S. aureus* (CHIPS) is a bacteria-derived protein of 14.1 kDa found in more than half of the clinical strains of *S. aureus*. CHIPS has antagonistic activity for FPR1 and C5aR. An N-terminal peptide (FTFEPFPTNEEIESN) derived from CHIPS is a selective antagonist for FPR1 but not C5aR (96). Iodinated CHIPS exhibits a pK_d of 7.46 at FPR1, which is by far the most potent peptide antagonist for this receptor. The identification of a bacteria-derived FPR1 antagonist suggests a mechanism used by microorganisms to thwart host defenses. In a subsequent study, the same group reported the identification from *S. aureus* of a 105-amino acid protein, termed FPRL1 inhibitory protein (FLIPr), that selectively inhibits the binding of and activation by FPR2 agonists, including MMK-1, WKYMVM, the prion fragement $PrP_{106-126}$, and amyloid peptide Aβ1–42 (97). At higher concentrations, FLIPr also inhibits fMLF binding to FPR1. FLIPr was found to bind directly to FPR2 and FPR1, but not to FPR3 and C5aR. It does not interfere with LXA4 activity on LTB4. The biological function of this inhibition has not been identified. Quin-C7 is a synthetic, nonpeptide antagonist of FPR2, developed through chemical modification of the FPR2 agonist Quin-C1 (98). In binding assays, Quin-C7 inhibited iodinated WKYMVm binding to FPR2 with a pK_i of 5.18. This antagonist is highly selective for FPR2/ALX, as it does not affect the binding of [^{3}H]fMLF to transfected cells expressing FPR1 (98).

In summary, several FPR1 and FPR2 antagonists have been identified and characterized. However, to our knowledge none of these antagonists is currently being tested in clinical settings or in atherosclerosis-related pre-clinical studies. Nevertheless, antagonists to FPR1 or FPR2 could emerge as potential players in targeting atherosclerosis-related inflammatory processes.

13.6 Production of Reactive Oxygen Species

Besides granule proteins, which are readily released upon PMN activation, oxygen radicals are yet another weapon that is at the PMN's immediate demand. PMN produce large amounts of oxygen radicals via myeloperoxidase, lipoxygenases, and NADPH oxidase. Much of the oxygen radicals are secreted extracellularily, where they have been proposed to be key mediators in atherosclerosis resulting in the oxidative modification hypothesis (99). Increased ROS are involved in the development of atherosclerosis in various aspects. First, endothelial dysfunction is an early key event in atherosclerosis (100–102). It has been thought that ROS are involved in the progression of endothelial cell dysfunction, which is accompanied by inactivation of endothelial nitric oxide synthase (eNOS) and decrease of nitric oxide (NO) levels (103). Second, ROS also induce expression of adhesion molecules such as intercellular adhesion molecule-1 (ICAM-1) and vascular adhesion molecule-1 (VCAM-1), which facilitates inflammatory cell recruitment and lipid deposition in the intimal layer. The subsequent ingestion of excess oxidized low-density lipoprotein (LDL) particles by macrophages and monocytes leads to release of various inflammatory cytokines and growth factors. Finally, proliferation of vascular smooth muscle cells (VSMCs) is a key step in the development of atherosclerosis. It has been suggested that ROS regulate expression of various growth factors and several growth-related protooncogenes such as c-Myc, c-Fos, and c-Jun (103,104). Clinical mass studies have also provided support for the significance of ROS in the development of atherosclerosis (105,106).

The central role of oxidative stress in the atherosclerotic process has been studied in numerous epidemiological and experimental studies. Although a wealth of evidence exists to support the correlation between increased oxidative stress and various vascular diseases, the findings from antioxidant administration for the prevention of cardiovascular diseases are controversial (107,108). The initial hypothesis for the use of antioxidants is that since they interfere in the LDL oxidation they should reduce the level of atherosclerotic lesions at the clinical level. This hypothesis led to clinical trials for the examination of their action in cardiovascular diseases (109,110). It is already known that there are numerous cardiovascular agents that have antioxidant properties, such as carvedilol (a non-specific β-blocker that also acts as an α-blocker), nebivolol, which reduces oxidative stress in hypertensive patients and increases NO production, Ca^{2+} channel blockers, and aspirin, whose action is related to the improvement of endothelial function (111). Furthermore, inhibition of the renin-angiotensin system by angiotensin converting enzyme inhibitors (ramipril-SECURE study) or angiotensin II receptor antagonists (losartan-LIFE study) has been proved to reduce the activity of NAD(P)H oxidase, improve endothelial dysfunction, and lead to reduction of cardiovascular events in experimental models with arterial hypertension and hypercholesterolemia, as well as in high risk patients (112,113). According to experimental data, statins, through the increase of catalase and BH4 levels, lead to an increase of NO production and inhibit LDL oxidation, while at the same time restoring vitamin C and E levels and endogenous antioxidants such as ubiquinone and glutathione. Vitamins C and E are also antioxidants that can inhibit the oxidative process for the prevention of atherosclerotic lesions. It has been proved in experimental models with atheromatosis that vitamin C stimulates the increase of BH4 levels and the activity of NO synthase and improves endothelial dysfunction (114). In addition, according to clinical studies, vitamin C administration in patients with coronary syndromes, arterial hypertension, and hypercholesterolemia increases NO bioavailability (115–117). Similar data arise from vitamin E administration, which reduces LDL oxidation and improves NO bioactivity and endothelial dysfunction owing to malnutrition. Co-administration of vitamin C and E seems to improve endothelial function in hyperlipidemic patients (118). Laboratory studies have shown that antioxidant vitamins can restore a deficiency of antioxidant enzymes, which are reduced in various cardiovascular diseases (119). Glutathione superoxidase is significantly reduced in patients with coronary syndromes. Therefore, as the levels of this enzyme are negatively related to the risk of coronary syndromes, this could be used as a new marker of oxidative stress (120). In patients with coronary syndromes a reduction of superoxide dismutase has also been observed, an event that contributes to endothelial dysfunction. In addition, there are experimental studies showing that overexpression of this enzyme reduces LDL oxidation and apoptosis. Studies in human cells have proved that vitamin C can replace absent glutathione, while the combination of C and E increases paraoxonase activity, which is reduced in cardiovascular diseases. Natural antioxidants such as polyphenols, which are found in fruits and vegetables, seem to be extremely useful, can improve lipid metabolism, and reduce oxLDL (121,122). Their combination seems to be better than monotherapy.

13.7 Concluding Remarks

As little is known about the role of PMN in atherosclerosis, only limited work is available on targeting PMN-derived proinflammatory activities. Potential targets are the inhibition of neutrophil priming, prevention of risk factor-induced neutrophilia, interference with arterial recruitment, and blockade of neutrophil-mediated activation of neighbouring cells. However, as PMN are vital in immune responses, it is a balancing act between targeting PMN activity in atherosclerosis while not negatively affecting host defence.

References

1. Weber, C., Zernecke, A., and Libby, P. (2008) The multifaceted contributions of leukocyte subsets to atherosclerosis: lessons from mouse models. *Nat Rev Immunol* **8**, pp. 802–815.
2. Hansson, G.K., and Hermansson, A. (2011) The immune system in atherosclerosis. *Nat Immunol* **12**, pp. 204–212.
3. Soehnlein, O., and Lindbom, L. (2010) Phagocyte partnership during the onset and resolution of inflammation. *Nat Rev Immunol* **10**, pp. 427–439.
4. Galligan, C., and Yoshimura, T. (2003) Phenotypic and functional changes of cytokine-activated neutrophils. *Chem Immunol Allergy* **83**, pp. 24–44.
5. Van Leeuwen, M., Gijbels, M.J., Duijvestijn, A., Smook, M., van de Gaar, M.J., Heeringa, P., de Winther, M.P., and Tervaert, J.W. (2008) Accumulation of myeloperoxidase-positive neutrophils in atherosclerotic lesions in LDLR-/- mice. *Arterioscler Thromb Vasc Biol* **28**, pp. 84–89.
6. Rotzius, P., Soehnlein, O., Kenne, E., Lindbom, L., Nystrom, K., Thams, S., and Eriksson, E.E. (2009) ApoE(-/-)/lysozyme M(EGFP/EGFP) mice as a versatile model to study monocyte and neutrophil trafficking in atherosclerosis. *Atherosclerosis* **202**, pp. 1111–1118.
7. Rotzius, P., Thams, S., Soehnlein, O., Kenne, E., Tseng, C.N., Björkström, N.K., Malmberg, K.J., Lindbom, L., and Eriksson, E.E. (2010) Distinct infiltration of neutrophils in lesion shoulders in ApoE-/- mice. *Am J Pathol* **177**, pp. 493–500.
8. Ionita, M.G., van den Borne, P., Catanzariti, L.M., Moll, F.L., de Vries, J.P., Pasterkamp, G., Vink, A., and de Kleijn, D.P. (2010) High neutrophil numbers in human carotid atherosclerotic plaques are associated with

characteristics of rupture-prone lesions. *Arterioscler Thromb Vasc Biol* **30**, pp. 1842–1848.

9. Leclercq, A., Houard, X., Philippe, M., Ollivier, V., Sebbag, U., Meilhac, O., and Michel, J.B. (2007) Involvement of intraplaque hemorrhage in atherothrombosis evolution via neutrophil protease enrichment. *J Leukoc Biol* **82**, pp. 1420–1429.
10. Naruko, T., Ueda, M., Haze, K., van der Wal, A.C., van der Loos, C.M., Itoh, A., Komatsu, R., Ikura, Y., Ogami, M., Shimada, Y., Ehara, S., Yoshiyama, M., Takeuchi, K., Yoshikawa, J., and Becker, A.E. (2002) Neutrophil infiltration of culprit lesions in acute coronary syndromes. *Circulation* **106**, pp. 2894–2900.
11. Thomas, H.E. Jr., Kannel, W.B., Dawber, T.R., and McNamara, P.M. (1996) Cholesterol-phospholipid ratio in the prediction of coronary heart disease. The Framingham study. *N Engl J Med* **274**, pp. 701–705.
12. Houterman, S., Verschuren, W.M., Hofman, A., and Witteman, J.C. (1999) Serum cholesterol is a risk factor for myocardial infarction in elderly men and women: the Rotterdam Study. *J Intern Med* **246**, pp. 25–33.
13. Mills, G.L., and Taylaur, C.E. (1971) The distribution and composition of serum lipoproteins in eighteen animals. *Comp Biochem Physiol B.* **40**, pp. 489–501.
14. Montecucco, F., and Mach, F. (2009) Update on statin-mediated anti-inflammatory activities in atherosclerosis. *Semin Immunopathol* **31**, pp. 127–142.
15. Araujo, F.B., Barbosa, D.S., Hsin, C.Y., Maranhão, R.C., and Abdalla, D.S. (1995) Evaluation of oxidative stress in patients with hyperlipidemia. *Atherosclerosis* **117**, pp. 61–71.
16. Mazor, R., Shurtz-Swirski, R., Farah, R., Kristal, B., Shapiro, G., Dorlechter, F., Cohen-Mazor, M., Meilin, E., Tamara, S., and Sela, S. (2008) Primed polymorphonuclear leukocytes constitute a possible link between inflammation and oxidative stress in hyperlipidemic patients. *Atherosclerosis* **197**, pp. 937–943.
17. Fontana, L., Giagulli, C., Cominacini, L., Pasini, A.F., Minuz, P., Lechi, A., Sala, A., and Laudanna, C. (2002) Beta2 integrin-dependent neutrophil adhesion induced by minimally modified low-density lipoproteins is mainly mediated by F2-isoprostanes. *Circulation* **106**, pp. 2434–2441.
18. Lehr, H.A., Krombach, F., Münzing, S., Bodlaj, R., Glaubitt, S.I., Seiffge, D., Hübner, C., von Andrian, U.H., and Messmer, K. (1995) *In vitro* effects of oxidized low density lipoprotein on CD11b/CD18 and L-selectin presentation on neutrophils and monocytes with relevance for the *in vivo* situation. *Am J Pathol* **146**, pp. 218–227.

19. Sedgwick, J.B., Hwang, Y.S., Gerbyshak, H.A., Kita, H., and Busse, W.W. (2003) Oxidized low-density lipoprotein activates migration and degranulation of human granulocytes. *Am J Respir Cell Mol Biol* **29**, pp. 702–709.

20. Van Tits, L.J., Hak-Lemmers, H.L., Demacker, P.N., Stalenhoef, A.F., and Willems, P.H. (2000) Oxidized low-density lipoprotein induces calcium influx in polymorphonuclear leukocytes. *Free Radic Biol Med* **29**, pp. 747–755.

21. Soehnlein, O., Drechsler, M., Hristov, M., and Weber, C. (2009) Functional alterations of myeloid cell subsets in hyperlipidaemia: relevance for atherosclerosis. *J Cell Mol Med* **13**, pp. 4293–4303.

22. Swirski, F.K., Libby, P., Aikawa, E., Alcaide, P., Luscinskas, F.W., Weissleder, R., and Pittet, M.J. (2007) Ly-6Chi monocytes dominate hypercholesterolemia-associated monocytosis and give rise to macrophages in atheromata. *J Clin Invest* **117**, pp. 195–205.

23. Gomes, A.L., Carvalho, T., Serpa, J., Torre, C., and Dias, S. Hypercholesterolemia promotes bone marrow cell mobilization by perturbing the SDF-1:CXCR4 axis. *Blood* **115**, pp. 3886–3894.

24. Landsman, L., Bar-On, L., Zernecke, A., Kim, K.W., Krauthgamer, R., Shagdarsuren, E., Lira, S.A., Weissman, I.L., Weber, C., and Jung, S. CX3CR1 is required for monocyte homeostasis and atherogenesis by promoting cell survival. *Blood* **113**, pp. 963–972.

25. Friedman, G.D., Klatsky, A.L., and Siegelaub, A.B. (1974) The leukocyte count as a predictor of myocardial infarction. *N Engl J Med* **290**, pp. 1275–1278.

26. Giugliano, G., Brevetti, G., Lanero, S., Schiano, V., Laurenzano, E., and Chiariello, M. (2010) Leukocyte count in peripheral arterial disease: a simple, reliable, inexpensive approach to cardiovascular risk prediction. *Atherosclerosis* **210**, pp. 288–293.

27. Drechsler, M., Megens, R.T., van Zandvoort, M., Weber, C., and Soehnlein, O. (2010) Hyperlipidemia-triggered neutrophilia promotes early atherosclerosis. *Circulation* **122**, pp. 1837–1845.

28. Stark, M.A., Huo, Y., Burcin, T.L., Morris, M.A., Olson, T.S., and Ley, K. (2005) Phagocytosis of apoptotic neutrophils regulates granulopoiesis via IL-23 and IL-17. *Immunity* **22**, pp. 285–294.

29. Christopher, M.J., and Link, D.C. (2007) Regulation of neutrophil homeostasis. *Curr Opin Hematol* **14**, pp. 3–8.

30. Martin, C., Burdon, P.C., Bridger, G., Gutierrez-Ramos, J.C., Williams, T.J., and Rankin, S.M. (2003) Chemokines acting via CXCR2 and CXCR4

control the release of neutrophils from the bone marrow and their return following senescence. *Immunity* **19**, pp. 583–593.

31. Sugano, R., Matsuoka, H., Haramaki, N., Umei, H., Murase, E., Fukami, K., Iida, S., Ikeda, H., and Imaizumi, T. (2005) Polymorphonuclear leukocytes may impair endothelial function: results of crossover randomized study of lipid-lowering therapies. *Arterioscler Thromb Vasc Biol* **25**, pp. 1262–1267.
32. Chello, M., Patti, G., Candura, D., Mastrobuoni, S., Di Sciascio, G., Agrò, F., Carassiti, M., and Covino, E. (2006) Effects of atorvastatin on systemic inflammatory response after coronary bypass surgery. *Crit Care Med* **34**, pp. 660–667.
33. Chello, M., Anselmi, A., Spadaccio, C., Patti, G., Goffredo, C., Di Sciascio, G., and Covino, E. (2007) Simvastatin increases neutrophil apoptosis and reduces inflammatory reaction after coronary surgery. *Ann Thorac Surg* **83**, pp. 1374–1380.
34. Van Oostrom, A.J., Plokker, H.W., van Asbeck, B.S., Rabelink, T.J., van Kessel, K.P., Jansen, E.H., Stehouwer, C.D., and Cabezas, M.C. (2006) Effects of rosuvastatin on postprandial leukocytes in mildly hyperlipidemic patients with premature coronary sclerosis. *Atherosclerosis* **185**, pp. 331–339.
35. Guasti, L., Marino, F., Cosentino, M., Cimpanelli, M., Maio, R.C., Klersy, C., Crespi, C., Restelli, D., Simoni, C., Franzetti, I., Gaudio, G., Marnini, P., Grandi, A.M., Lecchini, S., and Venco, A. (2006) Simvastatin treatment modifies polymorphonuclear leukocyte function in high-risk individuals: a longitudinal study. *J Hypertens* **24**, pp. 2423–2430.
36. Marino, F., Guasti, L., Cosentino, M., Ferrari, M., Rasini, E., Maio, R.C., Cimpanelli, M.G., Cereda, E., Crespi, C., Simoni, C., Restelli, D., Venco, A., and Lecchini, S. (2007) Angiotensin II type 1 receptor expression in polymorphonuclear leukocytes from high-risk subjects: changes after treatment with simvastatin. *J Cardiovasc Pharmacol* **49**, pp. 299–305.
37. Guasti, L., Marino, F., Cosentino, M., Maio, R.C., Rasini, E., Ferrari, M., Castiglioni, L., Klersy, C., Gaudio, G., Grandi, A.M., Lecchini, S., and Venco, A. (2008) Prolonged statin-associated reduction in neutrophil reactive oxygen species and angiotensin II type 1 receptor expression: 1-year follow-up. *Eur Heart J* **29**, pp. 1118–1126.
38. Dunzendorfer, S., Rothbucher, D., Schratzberger, P., Reinisch, N., Kähler, C.M., and Wiedermann, C.J. (1997) Mevalonate-dependent inhibition of transendothelial migration and chemotaxis of human peripheral blood neutrophils by pravastatin. *Circ Res* **81**, pp. 963–969.

39. Kaneider, N.C., Reinisch, C.M., Dunzendorfer, S., Meierhofer, C., Djanani, A., Wiedermann, C.J. (2001) Induction of apoptosis and inhibition of migration of inflammatory and vascular wall cells by cerivastatin. *Atherosclerosis* **158**, pp. 23–33.

40. Eccles, K.A., Sowden, H., Porter, K.E., Parkin, S.M., Homer-Vanniasinkam, S., and Graham, A.M. (2008) Simvastatin alters human endothelial cell adhesion molecule expression and inhibits leukocyte adhesion under flow. *Atherosclerosis* **200**, pp. 69–79.

41. Takata, M., Urakaze, M., Temaru, R., Yamazaki, K., Nakamura, N., Nobata, Y., Kishida, M., Sato, A., and Kobayashi, M. (2001) Pravastatin suppresses the interleukin-8 production induced by thrombin in human aortic endothelial cells cultured with high glucose by inhibiting the p44/42 mitogen activated protein kinase. *Br J Pharmacol* **134**, pp. 753–762.

43. Nakamura, K., Sasaki, T., Cheng, X.W., Iguchi, A., Sato, K., and Kuzuya, M. Statin prevents plaque disruption in apoE-knockout mouse model through pleiotropic effect on acute inflammation. *Atherosclerosis* **206**, pp. 355–361.

44. Eriksson, E.E., Xie, X., Werr, J., Thoren, P., and Lindbom, L. (2001) Direct viewing of atherosclerosis *in vivo*: plaque invasion by leukocytes is initiated by the endothelial selectins. *FASEB J* **15**, pp. 1149–1157.

45. Johnson, R.C., Chapman, S.M., Dong, Z.M., Ordovas, J.M., Mayadas, T.N., Herz, J., Hynes, R.O., Schaefer, E.J., and Wagner, D.D. (1997) Absence of P-selectin delays fatty streak formation in mice. *J Clin Invest* **99**, pp. 1037–1043.

46. Nageh, M.F., Sandberg, E.T., Marotti, K.R., Lin, A.H., Melchior, E.P., Bullard, D.C., and Beaudet, A.L. (1997) Deficiency of inflammatory cell adhesion molecules protects against atherosclerosis in mice. *Arterioscler Thromb Vasc Biol* **17**, pp. 1517–1520.

47. Collins, R.G., Velji, R., Guevara, N.V., Hicks, M.J., Chan, L., and Beaudet, A.L. P-Selectin or intercellular adhesion molecule (ICAM)-1 deficiency substantially protects against atherosclerosis in apolipoprotein E-deficient mice. *J Exp Med* **191**, pp. 189–194.

48. Subbarao, K., Jala, V.R., Mathis, S., Suttles, J., Zacharias, W., Ahamed, J., Ali, H., Tseng, M.T., and Haribabu, B. (2004) Role of leukotriene B4 receptors in the development of atherosclerosis: potential mechanisms. *Arterioscler Thromb Vasc Biol* **24**, pp. 369–375.

49. Zernecke, A., and Weber, C. (2010) Chemokines in the vascular inflammatory response of atherosclerosis. *Cardiovasc Res* **86**, pp. 192–201.

50. Huo, Y., Schober, A., Forlow, S.B., Smith, D.F., Hyman, M.C., Jung, S., Littman, D.R., Weber, C., and Ley, K. (2003) Circulating activated platelets exacerbate atherosclerosis in mice deficient in apolipoprotein E. *Nat Med* **9**, pp. 61–67.

51. von Hundelshausen, P., Weber, K.S., Huo, Y., Proudfoot, A.E., Nelson, P.J., Ley, K., and Weber, C. (2001) RANTES deposition by platelets triggers monocyte arrest on inflamed and atherosclerotic endothelium. *Circulation* **103**, pp. 1772–1777.

52. Massberg, S., Brand, K., Grüner, S., Page, S., Müller, E., Müller, I., Bergmeier, W., Richter, T., Lorenz, M., Konrad, I., Nieswandt, B., and Gawaz, M. (2002) A critical role of platelet adhesion in the initiation of atherosclerotic lesion formation. *J Exp Med* **196**, pp. 887–896.

53. Braunersreuther, V., Zernecke, A., Arnaud, C., Liehn, E.A., Steffens, S., Shagdarsuren, E., Bidzhekov, K., Burger, F., Pelli, G., Luckow, B., Mach, F., and Weber, C. (2007) Ccr5 but not Ccr1 deficiency reduces development of diet-induced atherosclerosis in mice. *Arterioscler Thromb Vasc Biol* **27**, pp. 373–379.

54. Ulbrich, H., Eriksson, E.E., and Lindbom, L. (2003) Leukocyte and endothelial cell adhesion molecules as targets for therapeutic interventions in inflammatory disease. *Trends Pharmacol Sci* **24**, pp. 640–647.

55. Koenen, R.R., and Weber, C. (2010) Therapeutic targeting of chemokine interactions in atherosclerosis. *Nat Rev Drug Discov* **9**, pp. 141–153.

56. Bizzarri, C., Beccari, A.R., Bertini, R., Cavicchia, M.R., Giorgini, S., and Allegretti, M. (2006) ELR+ CXC chemokines and their receptors (CXC chemokine receptor 1 and CXC chemokine receptor 2) as new therapeutic targets. *Pharmacol Ther* **112**, pp. 139–149.

57. Abu Nabah, Y.N., Losada, M., Estellés, R., Mateo, T., Company, C., Piqueras, L., Lopez-Gines, C., Sarau, H., Cortijo, J., Morcillo, E.J., Jose, P.J., and Sanz, M.J. (2007) CXCR2 blockade impairs angiotensin II-induced CC chemokine synthesis and mononuclear leukocyte infiltration. *Arterioscler Thromb Vasc Biol* **27**, pp. 2370–2376.

58. Van Wanrooij, E.J., de Jager, S.C., van Es, T., de Vos, P., Birch, H.L., Owen, D.A., Watson, R.J., Biessen, E.A., Chapman, G.A., van Berkel, T.J., and Kuiper, J. (2008) CXCR3 antagonist NBI-74330 attenuates atherosclerotic plaque formation in LDL receptor-deficient mice. *Arterioscler Thromb Vasc Biol* **28**, pp. 251–257.

59. Van Wanrooij, E.J., Happé, H., Hauer, A.D., de Vos, P., Imanishi, T., Fujiwara, H., van Berkel, T.J., and Kuiper, J. (2005) HIV entry inhibitor

TAK-779 attenuates atherogenesis in low-density lipoprotein receptor-deficient mice. *Arterioscler Thromb Vasc Biol* **25**, pp. 2642–2647.

60. Von Hundelshausen, P., Koenen, R.R., Sack, M., Mause, S.F., Adriaens, W., Proudfoot, A.E., Hackeng, T.M., and Weber, C. (2005) Heterophilic interactions of platelet factor 4 and RANTES promote monocyte arrest on endothelium. *Blood* **105**, pp. 924–930.

61. Koenen, R.R., von Hundelshausen, P., Nesmelova, I.V., Zernecke, A., Liehn, E.A., Sarabi, A., Kramp, B.K., Piccinini, A.M., Paludan, S.R., Kowalska, M.A., Kungl, A.J., Hackeng, T.M., Mayo, K.H., and Weber, C. (2009) Disrupting functional interactions between platelet chemokines inhibits atherosclerosis in hyperlipidemic mice. *Nat Med* **15**, pp. 97–103.

62. Nathan C. (2006) Neutrophils and immunity: challenges and opportunities. *Nat Rev Immunol* **6**, pp. 173–182.

63. Yang, D., de la Rosa, G., Tewary, P., and Oppenheim, J.J. (2009) Alarmins link neutrophils and dendritic cells. *Trends Immunol* **30**, pp. 531–537.

64. Soehnlein, O., Weber, C., and Lindbom, L. (2009) Neutrophil granule proteins tune monocytic cell function. *Trends Immunol* **30**, pp. 538–546.

65. Kai-Larsen, Y., and Agerberth, B. (2008) The role of the multifunctional peptide LL-37 in host defense. *Front Biosci* **13**, pp. 3760–3767.

66. Rehaume, L.M., and Hancock, R.E. (2008) Neutrophil-derived defensins as modulators of innate immune function. *Crit Rev Immunol* **28**, pp. 185–200.

67. Soehnlein, O., and Lindbom, L. (2009) Neutrophil-derived azurocidin alarms the immune system. *J Leukoc Biol* **85**, pp. 344–351.

68. Pham, C.T. (2006) Neutrophil serine proteases: specific regulators of inflammation. *Nat Rev Immunol* **6**, pp. 541–550.

69. Lee, T.D., Gonzalez, M.L., Kumar, P., Chary-Reddy, S., Grammas, P., and Pereira, H.A. (2002) CAP37, a novel inflammatory mediator: its expression in endothelial cells and localization to atherosclerotic lesions. *Am J Pathol* **160**, pp. 841–848.

70. Soehnlein, O., Xie, X., Ulbrich, H., Kenne, E., Rotzius, P., Flodgaard, H., Eriksson, E.E., and Lindbom, L. (2005) Neutrophil-derived heparin-binding protein (HBP/CAP37) deposited on endothelium enhances monocyte arrest under flow conditions. *J Immunol* **174**, pp. 6399–6405.

71. Soehnlein, O., Zernecke, A., Eriksson, E.E., Rothfuchs, A.G., Pham, C.T., Herwald, H., Bidzhekov, K., Rottenberg, M.E., Weber, C., and Lindbom, L.

(2008) Neutrophil secretion products pave the way for inflammatory monocytes. *Blood* **112**, pp. 1461–1471.

72. Korkmaz, B., Horwitz, M.S., Jenne, D.E., and Gauthier, F. (2010) Neutrophil elastase, proteinase 3, and cathepsin G as therapeutic targets in human diseases. *Pharmacol Rev* **62**, pp. 726–759.
73. Padrines, M., Wolf, M., Walz, A., and Baggiolini, M. Interleukin-8 processing by neutrophil elastase, cathepsin G and proteinase-3. *FEBS Lett* **352**, pp. 231–235.
74. Nufer, O., Corbett, M., and Walz, A. (1999) Amino-terminal processing of chemokine ENA-78 regulates biological activity. *Biochemistry* **38**, pp. 636–642.
75. Berahovich, R.D., Miao, Z., Wang, Y., Premack, B., Howard, M.C., and Schall, T.J. (2005) Proteolytic activation of alternative CCR1 ligands in inflammation. *J Immunol* **174**, pp. 7341–7351.
76. Wittamer, V., Bondue, B., Guillabert, A., Vassart, G., Parmentier, M., and Communi, D. (2005) Neutrophil-mediated maturation of chemerin: a link between innate and adaptive immunity. *J Immunol* **175**, pp. 487–493.
77. Rao, R.M., Betz, T.V., Lamont, D.J., Kim, M.B., Shaw, S.K., Froio, R.M., Baleux, F., Arenzana-Seisdedos, F., Alon, R., and Luscinskas, F.W. (2004) Elastase release by transmigrating neutrophils deactivates endothelial-bound SDF-1alpha and attenuates subsequent T lymphocyte transendothelial migration. *J Exp Med* **200**, pp. 713–724.
78. Ryu, O.H., Choi, S.J., Firatli, E., Choi, S.W., Hart, P.S., Shen, R.F., Wang, G., Wu, W.W., and Hart, T.C. (2005) Proteolysis of macrophage inflammatory protein-1alpha isoforms LD78beta and LD78alpha by neutrophil-derived serine proteases. *J Biol Chem* **280**, pp. 17415–17421.
79. Soehnlein, O., Kai-Larsen, Y., Frithiof, R., Sorensen, O.E., Kenne, E., Scharffetter-Kochanek, K., Eriksson, E.E., Herwald, H., Agerberth, B., and Lindbom, L. (2008) Neutrophil primary granule proteins HBP and HNP1-3 boost bacterial phagocytosis by human and murine macrophages. *J Clin Invest* **118**, pp. 3491–3502.
80. Påhlman, L.I., Mörgelin, M., Eckert, J., Johansson, L., Russell, W., Riesbeck, K., Soehnlein, O., Lindbom, L., Norrby-Teglund, A., Schumann, R.R., Björck, L., and Herwald, H. (2006) Streptococcal M protein: a multipotent and powerful inducer of inflammation. *J Immunol* **177**, pp. 1221–1228.
81. Cai, T.Q., and Wright, S.D. (1996) Human leukocyte elastase is an endogenous ligand for the integrin CR3 (CD11b/CD18, Mac-1, alpha M

beta 2) and modulates polymorphonuclear leukocyte adhesion. *J Exp Med* **184**, pp. 1213–1223.

82. Ribeiro-Gomes, F.L., Moniz-de-Souza, M.C., Alexandre-Moreira, M.S., Dias, W.B., Lopes, M.F., Nunes, M.P., Lungarella, G., and DosReis, G.A. Neutrophils activate macrophages for intracellular killing of Leishmania major through recruitment of TLR4 by neutrophil elastase. *J Immunol* **179**, pp. 3988–3994.

83. Li, T., Wang, H., and He, S. (2006) Induction of interleukin-6 release from monocytes by serine proteinases and its potential mechanisms. *Scand J Immunol* **64**, pp. 10–16.

84. Michelsen, K.S., Wong, M.H., Shah, P.K., Zhang, W., Yano, J., Doherty, T.M., Akira, S., Rajavashisth, T.B., and Arditi, M. (2004) Lack of Toll-like receptor 4 or myeloid differentiation factor 88 reduces atherosclerosis and alters plaque phenotype in mice deficient in apolipoprotein E. *Proc Natl Acad Sci U S A* **101**, pp. 10679–10684.

85. Soehnlein, O., Lindbom, L., and Weber, C. (2009) Mechanisms underlying neutrophil-mediated monocyte recruitment. *Blood* **114**, pp. 4613–4623.

86. Freer, R.J., Day, A.R., Radding, J.A., Schiffmann, E., Aswanikumar, S., Showell, H.J., and Becker, E.L. Further studies on the structural requirements for synthetic peptide chemoattractants. *Biochemistry* **19**, pp. 2404–2410.

87. Gavins, F.N., Yona, S., Kamal, A.M., Flower, R.J., and Perretti, M. (2003) Leukocyte antiadhesive actions of annexin 1: ALXR- and FPR-related anti-inflammatory mechanisms. *Blood* **101**, pp. 4140–4147.

88. Machado, F.S., Johndrow, J.E., Esper, L., Dias, A., Bafica, A., Serhan, C.N., and Aliberti, J. (2006) Anti-inflammatory actions of lipoxin A4 and aspirin-triggered lipoxin are SOCS-2 dependent. *Nat Med* **12**, pp. 330–334.

89. Stenfeldt, A.L., Karlsson, J., Wennerås, C., Bylund, J., Fu, H., and Dahlgren, C. (2007) Cyclosporin H, Boc-MLF and Boc-FLFLF are antagonists that preferentially inhibit activity triggered through the formyl peptide receptor. *Inflammation* **30**, pp. 224–229.

90. Bae, Y.S., Lee, H.Y., Jo, E.J., Kim, J.I., Kang, H.K., Ye, R.D., Kwak, J.Y., and Ryu, S.H. (2004) Identification of peptides that antagonize formyl peptide receptor-like 1-mediated signaling. *J Immunol* **173**, pp. 607–614.

91. Wenzel-Seifert, K., Grünbaum, L., and Seifert, R. (1991) Differential inhibition of human neutrophil activation by cyclosporins A, D, and

H. Cyclosporin H is a potent and effective inhibitor of formyl peptide-induced superoxide formation. *J Immunol* **147**, pp. 1940–1946.

92. Wenzel-Seifert, K., and Seifert, R. (1993) Cyclosporin H is a potent and selective formyl peptide receptor antagonist. Comparison with N-t-butoxycarbonyl-L-phenylalanyl-L-leucyl-L-phenylalanyl-L- leucyl-L-phenylalanine and cyclosporins A, B, C, D, and E. *J Immunol* **150**, pp. 4591–4599.

93. Yamamoto, Y., Kanazawa, T., Shimamura, M., Ueki, M., and Hazato, T. (1997) Inhibitory effects of spinorphin, a novel endogenous regulator, on chemotaxis, O2- generation, and exocytosis by N-formylmethionyl-leucyl-phenylalanine (FMLP)-stimulated neutrophils. *Biochem Pharmacol* **54**, pp. 695–701.

94. Liang, T.S., Gao, J.L., Fatemi, O., Lavigne, M., Leto, T.L., and Murphy, P.M. (2001) The endogenous opioid spinorphin blocks fMet-Leu-Phe-induced neutrophil chemotaxis by acting as a specific antagonist at the N-formylpeptide receptor subtype FPR. *J Immunol* **167**, pp. 6609–6614.

95. Chen, X., Yang, D., Shen, W., Dong, H.F., Wang, J.M., Oppenheim, J.J., and Howard, M.Z. (2000) Characterization of chenodeoxycholic acid as an endogenous antagonist of the G-coupled formyl peptide receptors. *Inflamm Res* **49**, pp. 744–755.

96. Chen, X., Mellon, R.D., Yang, L., Dong, H., Oppenheim, J.J., and Howard, O.M. (2002) Regulatory effects of deoxycholic acid, a component of the anti-inflammatory traditional Chinese medicine Niuhuang, on human leukocyte response to chemoattractants. *Biochem Pharmacol* **63**, pp. 533–541.

97. Haas, P.J., de Haas, C.J., Kleibeuker, W., Poppelier, M.J., van Kessel, K.P., Kruijtzer, J.A., Liskamp, R.M., and van Strijp, J.A. (2004) N-terminal residues of the chemotaxis inhibitory protein of *Staphylococcus* aureus are essential for blocking formylated peptide receptor but not C5a receptor. *J Immunol* **173**, pp. 5704–5711.

98. Prat, C., Bestebroer, J., de Haas, C.J., van Strijp, J.A., and van Kessel, K.P. (2006) A new staphylococcal anti-inflammatory protein that antagonizes the formyl peptide receptor-like 1. *J Immunol* **177**, pp. 8017–8026.

99. Zhou, C., Zhang, S., Nanamori, M., Zhang, Y., Liu, Q., Li, N., Sun, M., Tian, J., Ye, P.P., Cheng, N., Ye, R.D., and Wang, M.W. (2007) Pharmacological characterization of a novel nonpeptide antagonist for formyl peptide receptor-like 1. *Mol Pharmacol* **72**, pp. 976–983.

100. Steinberg, D. (2009) The LDL modification hypothesis of atherogenesis: an update. *J Lipid Res* **50** Suppl, pp. S376– S381.

101. Cai, H., and Harrison, D.G. (2000) Endothelial dysfunction in cardiovascular diseases: the role of oxidant stress. *Circ Res* **87**, pp. 840–844.

102. Mehta, J.L., Rasouli, N., Sinha, A.K., and Molavi, B. (2006) Oxidative stress in diabetes: a mechanistic overview of its effects on atherogenesis and myocardial dysfunction. *Int J Biochem Cell Biol* **38**, pp. 794–803.

103. Chakravarthy, U., Hayes, R.G., Stitt, A.W., McAuley, E., and Archer, D.B. (1998) Constitutive nitric oxide synthase expression in retinal vascular endothelial cells is suppressed by high glucose and advanced glycation end products. *Diabetes* **47**, pp. 945–952.

104. Madamanchi, N.R., Vendrov, A., and Runge, M.S. (2005) Oxidative stress and vascular disease. *Arterioscler Thromb Vasc Biol* 25, pp. 29–38.

105. Delafontaine, P., and Ku, L. (1997) Reactive oxygen species stimulate insulin-like growth factor I synthesis in vascular smooth muscle cells," *Cardiovasc Res* **33**, pp. 216–222.

106. Stephens, N.G., Parsons, A., Schofield, P.M., Kelly, F., Cheeseman, K., and Mitchinson, M.J. (1996) Randomised controlled trial of vitamin E in patients with coronary disease: cambridge heart antioxidant study (CHAOS). *Lancet* **347**, pp. 781–786.

107. Frasure-Smith, N., Lespérance, F., Prince, R.H., Verrier, P., Garber, R.A., Juneau, M., Wolfson, C., and Bourassa, M.G. (1997) Probucol and multivitamins in the prevention of restenosis after coronary angioplasty. Multivitamins and probucol study group. *N Engl J Med* **337**, pp. 365–372.

108. Kremastinos, D.T. (2008) Olive and oleuropein. *Hellenic J Cardiol* **49**, pp. 295–296.

109. Mehrabian, M., Allayee, H., Wong, J., Shi, W., Wang, X.P., Shaposhnik, Z., Funk, C.D., and Lusis, A.J. (2002) Identification of 5-lipoxygenase mRNA as a major gene contributing to atherosclerosis susceptibility in mice. *Circ Res* **91**, pp. 6959–6963.

110. Dwyer, J.H., Allayee, H., Dwyer, K.M., Fan, J., Wu, H., Mar, R., Lusis, A.J., and Mehrabian, M. (2004) Arachidonate 5-lipoxygenase promoter genotype, dietary arachidonic acid,and atherosclerosis. *N Engl J Med* **350**, pp. 29–37.

111. Rudic, R.D., Shesely, E.G., Maeda, N., Smithies, O., Segal, S.S., and Sessa, W.C. (1998) Direct evidence for the importance of endothelium-derived nitric oxide in vascular remodeling. *J Clin Invest* **101**, pp. 731–736.

112. Suwaidi, J.A., Hamasaki, S., Higano, S.T., Nishimura, R.A., Holmes, D.R. Jr., and Lerman, A. (2000) Long-term followup of patients with mild coronary artery disease and endothelial dysfunction. *Circulation* **101**, pp. 948–954.

113. Lee, J., and Leeson, P.C. (2006) Lipoproteins and the endothelium: past, present and future. *Hellenic J Cardiol* **47**, pp. 158–159.

114. Tousoulis, D., Antoniades, C., and Stefanadis, C. (2006) Statins and anti-oxidant vitamins: should co-administration be avoided? *J Am Coll Cardiol* **47**, p. 1237.

115. Lonn, E.M., Yusuf, S., Dzavik, V., et al. (2001) Effects of ramipril and vitamin E on atherosclerosis: the study to evaluate carotid ultrasound changes in patients treated with Ramipril and vitamin E (SECURE). *Circulation* **103**, pp. 919–925.

116. Dahlöf, B., Devereux, R.B., Kjeldsen, S.E., Julius, S., Beevers, G., de Faire, U., Fyhrquist, F., Ibsen, H., Kristiansson, K., Lederballe-Pedersen, O., Lindholm, L.H., Nieminen, M.S., Omvik, P., Oparil, S., Wedel, H., and LIFE Study Group. (2002) Cardiovascular morbidity and mortality in the Losartan intervention For endpoint study (LIFE): a randomised trial against atenolol. *Lancet* **359**, pp. 995–1003.

117. Taddei, S., Virdis, A., Ghiadoni, L., and Magagna, A., (1998) Salvetti, A. Vitamin C improves endothelium-dependent vasolidation by restoring nitric oxide activity in essential hypertension. *Circulation* **97**, pp. 2222–2229.

118. Tousoulis, D., Antoniades, C., Koumallos, N., Marinou, K., Stefanadi, E., Latsios, G., and Stefanadis, C. (2006) Novel therapies targeting vascular endothelium. *Endothelium* **13**, pp. 411–421.

119. Engler, M.M., Engler, M.B., Malloy, M.J., Chiu, E.Y., Schloetter, M.C., Paul, S.M., Stuehlinger, M., Lin, K.Y., Cooke, J.P., Morrow, J.D., Ridker, P.M., Rifai, N., Miller, E., Witztum, J.L., and Mietus-Snyder, M. (2003) Antioxidant vitamins C and E improve endothelial function in children with hyperlipidemia. *Circulation* **108**, pp. 1059–1063.

120. Carr, A., and Frei, B. (1999) Does vitamin C act as pro-oxidant under physiological conditions? *FASEB J* **13**, pp. 1007–1024.

121. Blankenberg, S., Rupprecht, H.J., Bickel, C., Torzewski, M., Hafner, G., Tiret, L., Smieja, M., Cambien, F., Meyer, J., Lackner, K.J., and AtheroGene Investigators. (2003) Glutathione peroxidase I activity and cardiovascular events in patients with coronary artery disease. *N Engl J Med* **349**, pp. 1605–1613.

122. Nickenig, G., and Harrison, D.G. (2002) The AT1-type angiotensin receptor in oxidative stress and atherogenesis. part i: oxidative stress and atherogenesis. *Circulation* **105**, pp. 393–396.

123. Wassmann, S., Laufs, U., Bäumer, A.T., Müller, K., Ahlbory, K., Linz, W., Itter, G., Rösen, R., Böhm, M., and Nickenig, G. (2001) HMG-CoA reductase inhibitors improve endothelial dysfunction in normocholesterolaemic hypertension via reduced production of reactive oxygen species. *Hypertension* **37**, pp. 1450–1457.

Chapter 14

Platelets as Therapeutic Targets of Atherosclerosis

Dirk Lievens and Philipp von Hundelshausen
Institute for Cardiovascular Prevention, Ludwig-Maximilians-University, Munich, Germany
dirk.lievens@med.uni-muenchen.de

14.1 Introduction

Anti-platelet therapy has become a cornerstone in the treatment and prevention of cardiovascular diseases. These therapies, including aspirin, clopidogrel and integrin IIb3 antagonists all target key pathways of platelet activation and have been shown to reduce platelet aggregation. Although the ability of these drugs to reduce cardiovascular morbidity and mortality has been demonstrated numerous times and appears to be merely driven by the anti-thrombotic properties, the underlying mechanism may be much more intricate than evident at first sight. Since a large body of evidence supports the view that platelets are potent immune cells [1-3], anti-platelet therapies may interfere with the immune system

Atherosclerosis: Treatment and Prevention
Edited by Christian Weber and Oliver Soehnlein

ISBN 978-981-4316-26-2 (Hardcover), ISBN 978-981-4364-26-3 (eBook)
www.panstanford.com

and influence chronic vascular inflammation. Beyond their role in arterial thrombosis we have evidence from experimental research that platelets influence crucially the development of atherosclerotic plaques. Platelets crosstalk with endothelium and leukocytes, thereby triggering autocrine and paracrine activation signals resulting in cell activation and cell recruitment into the vascular wall. Consequently, the present anti-platelet therapies also comprise the potential to modulate platelet immune functions by reducing cellular interactions of platelets with other immune components. In this chapter, we will illuminate the prevailing paradigms of anti-platelet therapies and focus on the capacity of platelets to orchestrate immune responses.

14.2 Mechanisms of Thrombus Formation

Under physiological conditions, platelets circulate in a quiescent state. Vascular injury activates platelets, which leads to platelet aggregation and plug formation. The process of thrombus formation is site dependent. Venous thrombosis is associated with high coagulation activity, producing large amounts of fibrin whereas arterial thrombosis is linked to high platelet activation, leading to platelet rich thrombi [4]. Consequently, anticoagulants (e.g., heparin) will be used for venous thrombosis treatment whereas platelet activation inhibitors will be used for the treatment of arterial thrombosis. In arteries, platelet activation occurs at sites of atherosclerotic plaque rupture where platelets are exposed to the plaque components collagen, von Willebrand factor (VWF), and tissue factor (TF). The mechanism of thrombus formation can be divided in four steps: platelet tethering, activation and firm adhesion, aggregation and platelet recruitment, and, finally, thrombus stabilization [5]. Platelet tethering [1] is mediated by glycoprotein (GP) Ibα, which is a component of the GPIb-V-IX complex. GPIbα is constitutively expressed on platelets and initiates platelet adhesion by binding to collagen bound VWF. Subsequent binding of GPVI to collagen leads to platelet activation [2]. GPVI is the major agonist for initial platelet activation and granule release [6]. In addition, Massberg *et al.* showed that GPVI-collagen interactions are central in all major phases of thrombus formation, i.e., platelet tethering, firm adhesion, and aggregation [7]. The integrin α2β1 plays a supportive role in the interaction between platelets and collagen. Thrombin is rapidly generated at the site of vascular injury and is considered the most potent platelet activator, leading to shape change, integrin activation, and granule secretion. Once firmly adherent, platelets start to spread and release the content of their granules [3]. ADP and thromboxane A2 (TXA2) are released, further promoting activation leading to the conformational change of the integrin αIIbβ3 that increases its affinity for fibrinogen, VWF, and fibronectin. In its active form, αIIbβ3 is the key molecule for platelet aggregation and stabilization [4, 5]. During platelet activation, both growth-arrest-specific gene 6 (GAS6) and CD40 ligand (CD40L) are present in the platelet-platelet synapse and enhance stabilization [8, 9].

14.3 Established Platelet Activation/Aggregation Inhibitors

14.3.1 Aspirin

Aspirin (acetylsalicyl acid, ASA) is well known as the "reference" anti-platelet drug. It acts as an irreversible inhibitor of cyclooxygenase, an enzyme involved in the synthesis of thromboxane A2 (Fig. 14.1), an important amplifier of platelet aggregation [10]. Aspirin is the first discovered member of the class of drugs known as nonsteroidal anti-inflammatory drugs (NSAIDs). Aspirin has been used for over a century to treat fundamental signs of inflammation (heat, redness, swelling, and pain), whereas recently it has been shown to prevent myocardial infarction, stroke, and additionally there is evidence that a daily intake of aspirin reduces the risk of cancer [11]. Other NSAIDs failed to show a protective effect on myocardial infarction in a large observational study [12]. A reason might be that platelets are not able to resynthesize cyclooxygenase causing an inhibition for as long as the platelet circulates, while other NSAIDs bind and inhibit COX-isoenzymes reversible. Numerous large-scale clinical trials and meta-analyses have consistently demonstrated the benefit of low doses of aspirin as a secondary prevention measure for recurrent ischemic events in patients with various manifestations of atherothrombotic disease [13, 14].

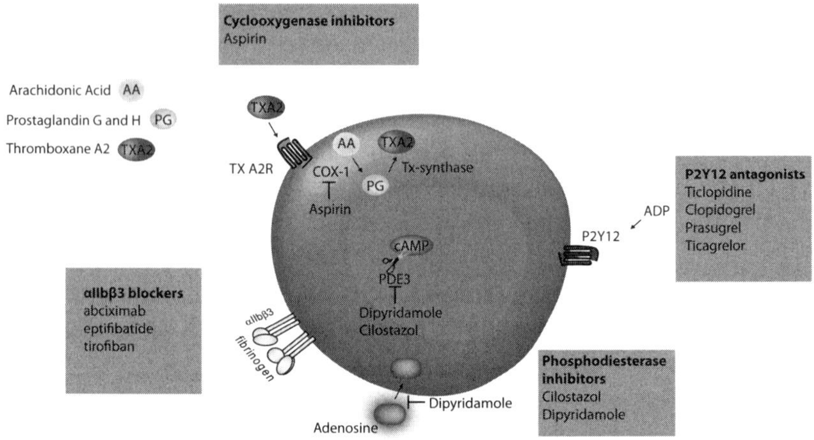

Figure 14.1 Established platelet activation/aggregation inhibitors.

However, the major disadvantage of long-term aspirin therapy is gastrointestinal bleeding that occurs — independent of the range of doses from 75 mg/day to 325 mg/day — at an annual increase of absolute 0.17% [14–16]. In addition, allergic reactions or lack of response of some patients occur. Nevertheless, altogether, low-dose aspirin still represents the best-recognized, nontoxic, and low-cost strategy for secondary prevention of atherothrombotic events.

The role of aspirin in primary prevention, which means that it is used as a prophylactic drug, in persons who have not experienced a cardiovascular event such as stroke or myocardial infarction, is not yet solidly established. Six large studies have been summarized in a meta-analysis, which showed a net benefit of aspirin in subgroups [13]. Mainly the incidence of a first myocardial infarction was prohibited from 0.23% per year to 0.18% per year while serious bleedings increased from 0.07 % per year to 0.10 % per year. Thus, you would need to treat 2000 persons one year to prevent one first myocardial infarction. In the vast majority, these studies included persons with a low cardiovascular risk. Less than 10% had suffered a vascular event in 10 years. Obviously, mainly persons with a considerable cardiovascular risk profit by a prophylactic aspirin therapy. A more recent, large-scale prospective placebo-controlled trial failed to show a protective effect in persons with increased cardiovascular risk as determined by screening for a low ankle-brachial-index [17]. Even in diabetic patients, primary prevention with aspirin is a matter of debate. While early studies in diabetics recommended a prophylactic therapy with aspirin, larger prospective trials resulted in conflicting evidence with no or only a modest benefit of aspirin in diabetics. A position statement of the American diabetes association which included these recent studies led to the recommendation to treat only diabetics with a cardiovascular risk greater than 10% in 10 years to suffer a vascular event [18]. An additional issue is the formulation of aspirin. Enteric-coated (EC) aspirin reduces symptoms resembling gastritis. However, we have hints that EC aspirin may not be equally effective. *In vitro* assays showed that EC-aspirin could lead to activation prone platelets and to more cardiovascular events [19].

An expanding body of evidence designates anti-inflammatory and anti-atherosclerotic properties to the current anti-platelet drugs [20]. Inhibition of platelet activation reduces the release of inflammatory mediators and decreases leukocyte recruitment to sites of injury. Therefore, aspirin administration has been reported to reduce the development and progression of atherosclerotic lesions in hyperlipidemic mice [21–23]. Atherosclerotic lesions contained increased levels of smooth muscle cells, while the number of inflammatory cells was strongly reduced. These plaques are the equivalent of stable plaques in humans. Additionally, aspirin induces the formation of NO-radicals in the body, which decreases inflammation by decreasing leukocyte adhesion [24]. There is also evidence to suggest that aspirin modulates signaling through NF-κB [25, 26]. NF-κB is a transcription factor required for the expression of a plethora of genes-encoding molecules involved in the regulation of inflammation, apoptosis, and cell proliferation. Many of these NF-κB regulated genes have been implicated directly or indirectly in atherosclerosis [27].

14.3.2 ADP Receptor Blockers

ADP plays a pivotal role in platelet activation and aggregation. Consequently, their receptors are potential targets for antithrombotic drugs (Fig. 14.1). Two G protein–coupled P2Y receptors are expressed by platelets. $P2Y_1$ and $P2Y_{12}$, are responsible for the known effects of ADP [28]. Both receptors are needed for a full response towards ADP. Activation of the $P2Y_1$ receptor initiates a rapid platelet shape change and reversible weak aggregation by activation of $G\alpha_q$ and subsequent calcium mobilization. The $P2Y_1$ receptor is distributed in many other tissues, including heart, blood vessels, smooth muscle cells, neural tissue, testis, prostate, and ovary [29]. The activation of $P2Y_{12}$ is more selectively expressed in platelets (the role of its additional expression in the brain remains elusive so far). Activation via $G\alpha_{i2}$ signals through multiple distinct pathways allows for a slow yet progressive platelet aggregation and plays a critical role in the amplification of platelet aggregation induced by other agents, including serotonin, thromboxane A_2, and thrombin [30]. The $P2Y_{12}$ receptor is also involved in platelet secretion [31]. All these features render the $P2Y_{12}$ receptor a pivotal player in sustaining platelet aggregation and, in turn, into thrombus growth and stabilization [32]. Activation of both receptors is, thus, crucial to elicit a normal platelet response. $P2Y_{12}$ is the target of the antithrombotic drugs from the thienopyridine group such as clopidogrel while $P2Y_1$ is a potential target for new anti-platelet compounds. However, since $P2Y_1$ is necessary but not sufficient to support full ADP-induced platelet activation and $P2Y_{12}$ antagonists are broadly investigated, there seems not much interest left to further test $P2Y_1$ antagonists clinically.

Clopidogrel is a selective ADP $P2Y_{12}$ receptor antagonist. It is a prodrug requiring extensive metabolization by cytochrome P450 (CYP) isoenzymes, including CYP2C19 in the intestines and liver, before the active metabolite can bind to platelets. Patients with less functional polymorphisms of this gene generate fewer active metabolites and experience more often atherothrombotic events. The active metabolite irreversible binds to the $P2Y_{12}$ receptor and blocks ADP interactions for the remainder of the platelet's lifespan. The efficiency of thienopyridines was first described for ticlopidine, which showed to have similar effects as aspirin in the treatment of unstable angina [33]. Moreover, ticlopidine showed to have additional benefits in combination with aspirin. However, ticlopidine has been largely driven of the market due to its side effects and has been replaced by clopidogrel, which was first approved by the Food and Drug Administration (FDA) in 1997 [34]. Large randomized studies confirmed the efficiency of clopidogrel, which is today the second and most commonly used prescribed drug worldwide [35]. The use of clopidogrel has also been associated with anti-inflammatory effects. Clopidogrel significantly reduced plaque size and augmented its stability in the atherosclerosis prone Apolipoprotein E (*Apoe*$^{-/-}$)

deficient mice [36]. Clopidogrel is known to decrease the expression of CD40L and P-selectin on platelets and has been associated with reduced CRP levels [20, 37, 38]. Therefore, clopidogrel inhibits platelet–leukocyte interactions and platelet-endothelium adhesion. Moreover, clopidogrel prevents platelet-dependent reactive oxygen species (ROS) production in polymorphonuclear leukocytes (PMN) [39]. It is important to note that not all studies reveal anti-inflammatory effects of anti-platelet therapy. Findings even suggest potential inflammatory effects of clopidogrel in patients with coronary artery disease [40]. In addition, the ability of aspirin to directly lower levels of inflammatory markers is not supported by recent studies in healthy volunteers [20]. Overall, the anti-inflammatory properties of anti-platelet agents are likely to be a result of decreased platelet activation and, therefore, indirect. The clinical relevance of these experimental findings remains to be determined.

When tested clinically in a primary preventive setting in patients with high risk for stroke or myocardial infarction in the CHARISMA trial (Bhatt *et al.* NEJM, 2006), the addition of clopidogrel to aspirin resulted in a tendency to increased bleeding and only marginal improved rate of cardiovascular events compared to aspirin and placebo. Thus, clopidogrel could not be established as a long-term preventive therapy. However, landmark trials in secondary prevention such as the CURE study [41] indicated that dual therapy with clopidogrel and aspirin is more effective than aspirin alone after myocardial infarction [42] and thus has been established as standard therapy for the acute coronary syndrome and after percutaneous coronary interventions (PCI) with stent implantation. Clopidogrel appears to be associated with fewer gastrointestinal bleedings compared with aspirin [43]. Unfortunately, a high inter-patient variability (genetic polymorphisms) in response and its interactions with other drugs (between clopidogrel and proton pump inhibitors (PPIs)) still remain an important issue [44, 45]. Despite its proven antithrombotic activity, clopidogrel has a disadvantage, since it is reliant on hepatic activation of the drug, resulting in a relatively slow onset of action and delayed antithrombotic effect. These drawbacks justify the continuing search for agents that can further improve the clinical outcome of patients with atherosclerosis.

Prasugrel is a third generation thienopyridine that irreversibly binds to the $P2Y_{12}$ receptor to prevent platelet activation (Fig. 14.1). Compared to clopidogrel, prasugrel inhibits ADP-induced platelet aggregation more rapidly and more consistently. Prasugrel is also a prodrug that requires hepatic activation to produce an active metabolite, but it has been shown to be effective in patients that do not respond to clopidogrel [46]. However, the risk of major bleeding episodes and life-threatening hemorrhages is higher for patients taking prasugrel compared with those taking clopidogrel [47]. In late 2009, the FDA approved prasugrel for the treatment of patients with ACS.

Ticagrelor is the first member of a new class of direct acting ADP receptor antagonists called cyclopentyltriazolopyrimidines [48, 49]. Like the thienopyridines, ticagrelor blocks the platelet $P2Y_{12}$ receptor to inhibit ADP-induced platelet aggregation, but in contrast to the thienopyridines, the effect of ticagrelor is reversible, greater, and more rapid [50]. Another advantage of ticagrelor is that it is not a prodrug, thus a metabolic transformation to express its clinical effects is not required [51]. AstraZeneca announced in December 2010 that the European Commission has granted marketing authorization to Brilique® (ticagrelor tablets) for the prevention of atherothrombotic events in patients with acute coronary syndromes and will, therefore, be the first reversibly binding oral ADP receptor antagonist on the European market. However, due to a peculiarly worse outcome only in the subgroup of US patients which differed markedly from the overall study results, the FDA hesitated to approve Ticagrelor.

14.3.3 Integrin αIIbβ3 Inhibitors

The development of αIIbβ3 (GPIIb/IIIa) antagonists (abciximab, eptifibatide, and tirofiban) has become an attractive strategy for anti-platelet therapy with a strong and specific effect. All three drugs are administered intravenously, and clinical trials have demonstrated a clear clinical benefit and good safety profile in high-risk patients, especially those undergoing percutaneous coronary intervention (Lippi, Montagnana *et al.* 2011). αIIbβ3 on resting platelets exhibits very low affinity for its ligands fibrinogen and VWF. Platelet activation leads to conformational changes of αIIbβ3 enhancing its affinity for fibrinogen and VWF. Ligation of αIIbβ3 through fibrinogen and VWF leads to clustering and outside-in signaling, which is important in cytoskeletal rearrangement in the process of aggregation (Buensuceso, de Virgilio *et al.* 2003). Consequently, platelets secrete their α-granules, activate other receptors, promote further aggregation, and retract clots. The primary mechanism of action of the integrin αIIbβ3 antagonists is, therefore, not inhibition of platelet activation but of the final common pathway of platelet-to-platelet aggregation [52]. In addition to restraining platelet aggregation, integrin αIIbβ3 antagonists have a specific anticoagulant action, as evidenced by prolongation of the activated clotting time, inhibition of thrombin generation, and inhibition of platelet procoagulant activity [52]. How αIIbβ3 antagonists influence atherogenesis is not known. Clinically they are applied at PCI and stent implantation in the setting of an acute coronary syndrome with a high risk for an adverse outcome. The formulation is restricted to a parenteral (e.g., intravenous) administration, which prohibits the investigation of the chronic course of atherosclerosis. Orally active αIIbβ3 inhibitors have been developed but never resulted in beneficial effects. In a meta-analysis of four phase III trials [53, 54] oral αIIbβ3 inhibitors brought a higher all cause mortality. The reason for this disappointing result is not entirely clear. Maybe the short lived, reversible inhibition resulted in a prothrombotic effect in the nadir of plasma concentration, but as well other pleiotropic such as proapoptotic effects have been accused. Nevertheless, these results ended the promising future of this particular class of anti-platelet agents. Thus, an assessment of anti-atherosclerotic effects of a permanent αIIbβ3 inhibition remains speculative.

14.3.4 Signaling Inhibitors: The Phodiesterase Inhibitors Cilostazol and Diypridamole

Many signaling pathways in platelets use cyclic adenosine monophosphate (cAMP) and cyclic guanosin monophosphate (cGMP) as second messengers, which are inactivated by cleavage through phosphodiesterases. Phodiesterase III (PDE3) inactivates these second messengers by hydrolyzing the phosphoester bonds, which generates AMP and GMP from the cyclic forms (Fig. 14.1). PDE3 is expressed in two isoforms. While PDE3B is expressed in many tissues, the isoform PDE3A is expressed more selectively in platelets, vascular smooth muscle, and heart muscle. Cilostazol (Pletal®) is a PDE3 inhibitor which results in elevated concentrations of cAMP which increases the activity of protein kinase A (PKA) which in turn leads to the inhibition of platelet aggregation and to direct vasodilatation. Cilostazol has been approved for the medical treatment of symptomatic peripheral artery disease (claudicatio). PDE3A plays an important role for heart muscle contraction; therefore, it is no surprise that interfering with this signaling pathway may create dangerous side effects. Patients with decreased left ventricular pump function experienced a higher mortality in clinical trials. Thus, the application in congestive heart failure is a contra-indication. Although a measurable inhibition of platelet aggregation has been found, no significant elevation of bleedings has been documented. Recent registries and a randomized trial found inconsistent results. A randomized trial compared dual anti-platelet therapy of aspirin and clopidogrel with triple therapy of aspirin, clopidogrel, and cilostazol in patients, which received a coronary intervention after an ACS [55]. After 6 months, a significant reduction of the combined primary endpoint (death, myocardial infarction, stroke) was seen for the triple therapy (15.1% vs 10.3%, $p = 0.011$). Recent registry data (DECREASE registry) of over 3000 patients who had received a drug eluting stent (DES) could not confirm the benefit of the triple therapy for vascular death, but myocardial infarction and stent thrombosis were significantly reduced [56]. These are promising results, as neither minor nor major bleedings differed in both groups. These results will have to be reproduced in large-scale multicenter placebo-controlled trials before a widely used application of cilostazol can be recommended. Another clinically established drug, which inhibits PDE3, is the purin analogon dipyridamole (Persantin®). Dipyridamole not only inhibits platelet aggregation by increasing cAMP/cGMP but also furthermore blocks the enzyme adenosine deaminase and inhibits the uptake of adenosine by erythrocytes, which results in its extracellular accumulation (Fig. 14.1). Adenosine causes vasodilatation and cAMP elevation through the A2-receptor on platelets. More pleiotropic effects of dipyridamole have been reported, including reduced production of ROS and pro-inflammatory mediators, and markers such as MCP-1 and hsCRP. Therefore, the clinical effects cannot be deduced to only one mechanism. Two large multicenter trials, ESPRIT and ESPS-2, have been conducted for secondary prevention in patients with ischemic stroke or TIA. The ESPS-2 trial found a comparable risk reduction after 2 years drug administration for a recurrent stroke by aspirin or dipyridamole monotherapy (relative risk reduction [RR] 16% dipyridamole; 18% aspirin) compared with placebo and an additive effect of the combination of aspirin and dipyridamole (RRR 37%) without influencing significantly the incidence of myocardial infarction [57]. These results were confirmed later by the ESPRIT trial [58] and let to the recommendation to use a combination of aspirin and dipyridamole for secondary prevention of ischemic stroke but not in CAD. Dipyridamole has not been investigated in primary prevention but given its pleiotropic anti-inflammatory effects and low-risk profile could well prove as a valuable strategy to inhibit atherosclerosis.

14.4 New Developments

Despite the proven benefits of the current anti-platelet agents, a substantial limitation of current oral anti-platelet therapies is their associated risk of bleeding. Present anti-platelet therapies target activation pathways that are crucial for normal haemostasis. The challenge is to develop anti-platelet therapies that offer a more sheltered inhibition of platelet activity by targeting other activation pathways or additional platelet functions.

14.4.1 Direct Thromboxane A2 Receptor Antagonists

Since the inhibition of COX-1 through aspirin not only prevents the formation of thromboxane but as well the synthesis of the protective metabolites prostaglandin E2 (PGE2) and prostaglandin I2 (PGI2, prostacyclin) which inhibit platelet aggregation, the development of selective thromboxane synthase inhibitors or thromboxane receptor antagonists seems promising. Already in the 1990s, thromboxane receptor antagonists have been designed but of various reasons never have been tested in the setting of primary prevention of atherosclerosis and were never applied in advanced clinical studies. However, new efforts are currently undertaken to bring two candidates into clinic which have demonstrated in mouse models to be able to reduce atherosclerosis [10]. Terutroban (Fig. 14.2) is a thromboxane receptor antagonist [59] which has entered a phase III trial, the PERFORM study, which compares the effectiveness of aspirin compared to terutroban to prevent the progression of carotid intimal media thickness. The other candidate, picotamide, has been investigated in the DAVID trial 2004. In this double blind multicenter study, aspirin was compared with picotamide in diabetics with peripheral artery disease. Overall mortality was significantly reduced by picotamide but not cardiovascular events [60]. Currently, the results of larger multicenter trials are missing to implement these interesting alternatives to aspirin in a broad clinical routine.

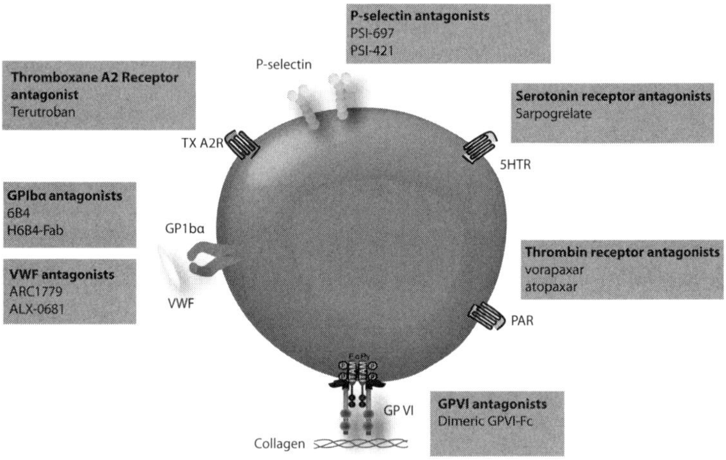

Figure 14.2 Novel potential anti-platelet therapies.

14.4.2 Thrombin Receptor Antagonists

A role of thrombin for the initiation of atherosclerosis is testified by the presence of thrombin-generating activity in early atherosclerotic lesions [61]. Thrombin receptor antagonists represent a novel class of anti-platelet agents that inhibit platelet activation. Thrombin catalyzes the conversion of fibrinogen into fibrin, the final step in the coagulation cascade, and is one of the most potent platelet activators. Thrombin mediated platelet activation occurs via binding to protease-activated receptors (PARs). PARs have been described on platelets, endothelial cells, smooth muscle cells, mononuclear cells and fibroblasts [62]. To date, four PARs have been identified. PAR-1, PAR-3, and PAR-4 are activated by thrombin and PAR-2 by mast cell tryptase. PAR-1 (PAR-4 in mice) acts as the principal thrombin receptor. Thrombin binding to PAR-1 cleaves the aminoterminal end of the receptor, which leads to self-activation causing platelets to release ADP, serotonin, and thromboxane A2. In turn, these agonists activate other platelets, thus amplifying the signals for thrombus formation [6]. Consequently, PAR-1 signaling is important for platelet activation and clot formation but not for the formation of the initial platelet monolayer at sites of injury [63]. PAR-1 antagonists may, therefore, tackle platelet mediated thrombosis rather than platelet haemostasis. Treatment with PAR-1 antagonists in guinea pigs and cynomolgus monkeys significantly prolonged time to thrombotic occlusion after arterial injury, without affecting bleeding times or coagulation parameters [64, 65]. Consistent with these results, PAR-4 deficient mice exhibited normal platelet number and morphology and there was no evidence of spontaneous bleeding. However, after injury, growth of platelet thrombi was markedly diminished in *Par4*$^{-/-}$ mice [66]. The two selective reversible PAR-1 antagonists in most advanced clinical development are *vorapaxar* and *atopaxar*. The latter has been studied in the phase II LANCELOT trials [67–69]. The LANCELOT-ACS trial compared placebo and different doses of atopaxar on top of the standard therapy with aspirin and clopidogrel in 603 patients presenting with non-ST-elevation ACS. While ischemic events as determined by the surrogate parameter continuous ECG monitoring significantly favored atopaxar, neither hard endpoints nor the incidence of bleedings differed significantly. LANCELOT-CAD compared 720 subjects with known stable coronary artery disease placebo and different atopaxar concentrations for 24 weeks. This study was not powered to detect differences in outcome but showed effective platelet inhibition. Another selective PAR-1 antagonist, vorapaxar (SCH 530348), has been shown to be safe and well tolerated and is currently being tested in the phase III trials TRACER and TRA2P in patients with ACS (NCT NCT00527943 and NCT00526474) to answer the question if blocking PAR-1 in secondary prevention after acute coronary syndrome or stroke results in less cardiovascular events.

14.4.3 VWF Antagonists

As described above, VWF is an important molecule for platelet adhesion. Despite the clear association of VWF plasma levels and arterial thrombosis, the causal role of VWF for atherogenesis still remains unclear. The elevated plasma concentration of VWF could primarily mirror endothelial dysfunction but might not necessarily be linked causally to arterial thrombosis [70]. Nevertheless, the pharmaceutical inhibition of VWF is an intriguing field. ARC1779 is an aptamer, which binds the A1 domain of activated VWF and inhibits its interaction with the GPIb receptor on platelets [71]. Aptamers are single-stranded DNA or RNA sequences, usually 15–40 bases long, which bind and inhibit protein targets. The high stability of aptamer-protein complexes combined with high specificity of interaction makes aptamers valued therapeutic tools [72]. ARC1779 is the first antithrombotic drug with anti-VWF action that has reached phase II clinical trials [73]. ARC1779 is a promising new therapeutic for VWF-related platelet disorders, such as thrombotic thrombocytopenia purpura (TTP) [74]. Patients with TTP have a defect in the metalloprotease ADAMTS13, which cleaves VWF. This results in large VWF multimers that bind GPIb and cause widespread and excessive clot formation [74]. Current standard treatment for TTP is plasma exchange. ARC1779 has the prospects to be a treatment for TTP patients by effectively binding and inhibiting the activity of these ultra-large VWF molecules. Additionally, anti-VWF could have therapeutic use in acute coronary care setting by preventing arterial thrombosis [75]. A different strategy is the use of nanobodies, antibody-derived therapeutic proteins that contain the unique structural and functional properties of naturally occurring heavy-chain antibodies [76]. ALX-0681 is a humanized bivalent nanobody, which binds the A1 domain of VWF and is already in clinical evaluation [77]. If successful, ALX-0681 would be the first-ever nano drug to treat thrombosis.

14.4.4 GPIbα Antagonists

Several mutations in the gene for GPIb lead to a rare disorder, the Bernard-Soulier syndrome, which is associated with frequent bleedings and giant platelets. Due to the low number of cases, it is not known whether the inherent lack of GPIb reduces the risk of atherosclerosis. Anyway, patients with Bernard-Soulier syndrome are not fully protected, since relevant coronary artery disease has led to coronary revascularization in the past.

Massberg and colleagues have used anti-GPIbα–treated mice in a ligation-induced injury model of the carotid artery [78]. Inhibition of platelet GPIbα significantly reduced both transient and firm adhesion of platelets to the vascular surface of the common carotid artery. In contrast, inhibition of GPIIb-IIIa (αIIbβ3) had only partial effects on transient platelet adhesion but almost completely prevented firm attachment to endothelial cells *in vivo* [78]. The main ligand of GPIbα is VWF; however platelet GPIbα is also the best-characterized counter receptor for Mac-1, thus mediating platelet–leukocyte interactions. In a mouse model of neointima formation, inhibition of Mac-1-GPIb interactions after wire injury of the femoral artery reduced leukocyte accumulation and neointima thickening [79].

In mouse models, a stronger antithrombotic effect was seen in GPIbα deficient mice than in VWF deficient animals [80], likely because GPIbα binds ligands other than VWF. This implies that the role of GPIbα in arterial thrombosis exceeds that of its main ligand VWF. A murine monoclonal antibody designated as 6B4 that blocks human GPIbα has been developed. This mAb inhibits VWF-dependent platelet adhesion to collagen under high shear-stress conditions [81]. Injection of 6B4-Fab-fragments in baboons had a potent antithrombotic effect and was not accompanied by a prolongation of bleeding times [82]. A recombinant and humanized 6B4-fab fragment, named h6B4-Fab, has been developed and tests in baboons confirmed its antithrombotic effects. H6B4-Fab reduced platelet thrombus formation in flowing blood exposed to atherosclerotic plaques [83, 84]. From these studies, we can speculate that H6B4-Fab is a promising approach, however it needs to be further validated in clinical trials.

14.4.5 Serotonin Receptor Antagonists

Serotonin (5-hydroxytryptamin, 5-HT) is a neurotransmitter involved in sexual behavior, appetite, sleep, and mood [85]. Dysfunction of the 5-HT system can lead to psychiatric diseases, such as depression, schizophrenia, addiction, and autism. At the same time, 5-HT is a peripheral hormone that is transported in high quantities by platelets (stored in dense granules) [86]. To promote haemostasis, activated platelets release 5-HT, which induces vasoconstriction and amplifies platelet activation (Fig. 14.2) at sites of vessel wall injury [87]. Furthermore, release of serotonin and activation of serotonin receptors on platelet surfaces is a potent augmentative stimulus for platelet aggregation [86]. Sarpogrelate (Anplag®) blocks serotonin-induced platelet aggregation by selectively inhibiting the serotonin receptors 5-HT_{2A} and 5-HT_{2B} and may improve coronary microcirculation [88]. However, no large randomized controlled trials (RCT) have been conducted that would prove a benefit for cardiovascular outcomes, the same holds true for APD791 which is a newly developed, potent, and highly selective inverse agonist of the serotonin (5HT2A) receptor [89]. A different modality for reducing peripheral serotonin levels is the chronic use of the antidepressant 5-HT-selective reuptake inhibitor drugs (SSRIs) such as fluoxetine (better known as prozac) [90]. Indeed, chronic treatment with SSRIs was shown to significantly reduce myocardial infarction risk [91]. However, such treatment is not favorable due to side effects (increased bleeding, flattened emotions, reduced libido, and increased aggressiveness). In addition, Dees *et al.* demonstrated recently that platelet-derived serotonin provides an important link between vascular disease and tissue fibrosis [92]. Systemic sclerosis (SSc) patients expose ongoing endothelial cell damage and activation, resulting in activation of platelets. The authors revealed that serotonin induced extracellular matrix synthesis and that inactivation of 5-HT_{2B} effectively prevented the onset of experimental fibrosis and ameliorated established fibrosis. We could, therefore, speculate that 5-HT/5-HT receptor signaling could be a protagonist of atherogenesis as well.

14.4.6 GPVI Antagonists

Glycoprotein VI (GPVI) is expressed uniquely in platelets and megakaryocytes. Although important in the adhesion and aggregation of platelets on collagen [93], a deficiency due to genetic defects in mice and human beings seems not to cause a bleeding diathesis. GPVI is coupled to FcRγII, which associates it to immune processes. GPVI is upregulated on circulating platelets in acute coronary syndrome [94]. Recently, GPVI has been shown to play an important role in atherosclerosis progression [95]. GPVI binds to atherosclerotic endothelium and contributes to platelet-endothelium interactions. Inhibition of this GPVI activity has beneficial effects on the morphology and function of the vessel wall in atherosclerosis. In addition, GPVI has recently been shown to mediate platelet–leukocyte interactions as well. Functional blockade of GPVI on platelets reduced firm adhesion of monocytes to platelets [96], which only occurred at high shear rates. Platelet GPVI triggers interaction with monocytes by binding to the extracellular matrix metalloproteinase inducer (EMMPRIN, CD147), an immunoglobulin-like receptor expressed on monocytes [97]. GPVI blockade did not reduce monocyte adhesion to platelets when venous shear conditions were applied; implying that platelet GPVI has diverse functions according to physiological conditions. Thus, GPVI inhibition has the prospective to become a novel anti-platelet drug. Clinical studies are still in an early stage. A phase I study (NCT 01042964) in Germany has just been terminated where Revacept, a specific GPVI antagonist (dimeric GPVI-Fc), was tested in 30 male volunteers. Revacept inhibited collagen-induced platelet activation without being accompanied by bleeding or significant side effects [98] and has, thus, the potential of a safe and potent platelet inhibitor for the treatment of acute vascular syndromes.

14.5 Platelets in Inflammation

Besides the cell-types present in the plaque, circulating platelets are an important contributor to atherosclerosis. In all relevant stages of atherogenesis, they seem to play a role by initiating and sustaining the chronic inflammatory process, which consists mainly in generating a cellular intramural arterial infiltrate. Platelets facilitate leukocyte recruitment by means of their repertoire of surface molecules and released inflammatory mediators that activate and bridge endothelial cells with immune cells [99]. Platelets mediate inflammation through two distinct ways. First upon activation, platelets produce considerable quantities of cytokines, chemokines, and growth factors [100]. These are released from the dense granules, α-granules, lysosomes, the open canalicular system (OCS), or the cytosol [3]. Proteomic studies indicate that thrombin stimulated platelets released more than 300 proteins [101]. Several of these secreted proteins have been identified in atherosclerotic lesions. Pro-inflammatory mediators such as Regulated on Activation Normal T Expressed and Secreted (RANTES, CCL5), Interleukin-1 beta (IL-1β), monocyte chemoattractant factor 1 (MCP-1, CCL2), platelet factor 4 (PF4, CXCL4), and platelet activating factor (PAF) are secreted by activated platelets. Both CXCL4 and CCL5 are delivered by activated platelets and induce monocyte arrest, thereby inducing atherosclerosis [102, 103]. In addition, CXCL4 and CCL5 have been shown to heterodimerize, which enhances monocyte recruitment. Disruption of this interaction inhibits atherosclerosis in mice [102].

Secondly, activated platelets express a multitude (e.g., P-selectin, GPIbα, CD40L) of receptors on their membrane enabling platelets to interact with different leukocyte subsets and endothelial cells. Activated platelets interact with the endothelium and induce endothelial expression of adhesion molecules, cytokines and chemokines, which in turn mediate leukocyte recruitment to the site of endothelial injury [78]. A complex variety of pathways that control these interactions have been described. P-selectin, VWF, and several glycoproteins (e.g., GPIb and αIIbβ3) mediate platelet interactions with the endothelium [78, 104, 105]. The first step of platelet adhesion to endothelial cells is platelet rolling, which is mediated by P-selectin and GPIbα [106, 107]. Firm adhesion of activated platelets to endothelial cells involves αIIbβ3 and αvβ3 [5].

Moreover, activated platelets promote leukocyte recruitment by direct interactions with leukocyte subsets in the circulation. In particular, platelet-monocyte complexes (PMC) have been observed in clinical inflammatory conditions such as inflammatory bowel disease. Platelets also communicate with neutrophils, dendritic cells, and T cells. The communication between platelets and leukocytes is bidirectional. Platelets stimulate leukocyte differentiation into a proadhesive and promigratory phenotype, and the leukocytes secrete mediators, e.g., PAF and leukotrienes that further activate the platelet. Multiple sets of cell–cell contact molecules mediate the formation of platelet–leukocyte aggregates: P-selectin, CD40L, and αIIbβ3 integrin on the platelet membrane binding respectively to PSGL-1, CD40, and Mac-1 on the leukocyte. Table 14.1 summarizes the potential receptor-ligand pairs on platelets and leukocytes.

14.5.1 Inflammatory Surface Molecules

Platelet activation results in the upregulation of surface expression of P-selectin and CD40L. While P-selectin is restricted to endothleial cells and platelets, CD40L is expressed on multiple cell types present in atherosclerotic lesions [108]. Both are indispensable for the interaction of activated platelets with both endothelium and different leukocyte subsets. Therefore, P-selectin and CD40L expression on platelets is extensively studied in different models of atherosclerosis.

Table 14.1. Candidate receptor-ligand pairs on platelets and leukocytes mediating platelet–leukocyte cross talk

Platelets	**Leukocytes**
P-selectin	PSGL-1
CD40L	CD40
αIIbβ3	Mac-1
ICAM-2	LFA-1, DC-SIGN
JAM-A	LFA-1
JAM-C	LFA-1
GPIb	Mac-1
CX3CR1	CX3CL1

14.5.1.1 P-selectin and PSGL-1

P-selectin and its ligand P-selectin glycoprotein ligand 1 (PSGL-1) are exciting targets to study due to their clear role in both thrombosis and immunity. The selectins are a family of three type-I cell-surface glycoproteins: E-, L-, and P-selectin. P-selectin is an integral membrane glycoprotein expressed by both platelets and endothelial cells. P-selectin is stored in α-granules of platelets and in Weibel-Palade bodies of endothelial cells and is translocated to the cell surface (Fig. 14.2) of activated endothelial cells and platelets [109]. Platelet P-selectin is imperative during the initial "rolling" interactions of platelets on atherosclerotic endothelium [104]. The platelet monolayer formed on the injured vessel provides a platform for leukocyte recruitment to vessel walls [110]. Repeated injections of P-selectin-expressing platelets into *Apoe*$^{-/-}$ mice accelerated the formation of atherosclerotic lesions whereas mice injected with platelets that lacked P-selectin formed smaller lesions [104].

In addition to platelet-endothelium interactions, P-selectin is also important in platelet–leukocyte interactions. Through P-selectin, platelets bind to the P-selectin glycoptrotein ligand 1 (PSGL-1) on leukocytes, and thereby form multicellular conjugates, which promote the release of chemokines (e.g., CCL2 and CCL5) and cytokines (e.g., IL-1β) to further activate leukocytes and promote atherosclerosis [104, 109]. These conjugates tether and roll on ECs with a higher avidity than unconjugated leukocytes, which will improve endothelial cell activation [111]. Platelet-leukocyte aggregates (PLA) have been observed in several clinical conditions and have been described to be efficient markers of acute myocardial infarction [112, 113]. Indeed, P-selectin-blocking antibodies reduced arterial thrombosis, reperfusion injury, and infarct size in mice [114]. Currently, an ongoing clinical trial (phase II) is investigating the efficacy and safety of a P-selectin antagonist (recombinant monoclonal antibody) in preventing atherosclerosis in coronary artery bypass grafts (NCT01245634).

The compound PSI-697 that specifically inhibits P-selectin has been shown to reduce both arterial and venous thrombosis in animal models [115, 116]. PSI-697 has also been shown to reduce *ex vivo* thrombus formation in humans [117]. Unfortunately, in the phase I clinical trial, the desired pharmacokinetic profile was not achieved. A backup compound PSI-421 has been developed that shows remarkable improvement in pharmacokinetics [118]. An alternative strategy is to target the ligand PSGL-1. Recombinant PSGL fusion protein, rPSGL-Ig (YSPSL) enhances thrombolysis in pigs by blocking leukocyte adhesion and, therefore, could be used as a treatment against ischemia reperfusion injury (IRI) in animal models [119]. Additional studies are required; nevertheless, both P-selectin and PSGL-1 harbor the prospective to become novel anti-platelet therapeutics in both arterial and venous thrombosis.

14.5.1.2 CD40-CD40L

CD40 ligand (CD40L), a member of the TNF-family, is a co-stimulatory molecule that, after binding to CD40 on antigen presenting cells (APCs), induces T-cell activation and differentiation [120]. Total inhibition of CD40L in *Apoe*$^{-/-}$ mice resulted in a reduction of atherosclerosis and in the development of a stable, fibrous plaque that was low in inflammation [121]. In 1998, Henn *et al.* reported that besides the T lymphocyte, one of the most important cell types that expresses CD40L is the platelet [122]. Platelet CD40L is expressed upon activation and is found to induce endothelial cells to secrete chemokines (e.g., CCL2) and to express adhesion molecules (e.g., ICAM-1, VCAM-1), thereby directly initiating an inflammatory response of the vessel wall [3]. Platelet CD40L is also important in the formation of platelet leukocyte aggregates and in the recruitment of leukocytes to sites of injury [123]. Platelets deficient in CD40L exhibited a failing adherence to the endothelium. Injection of activated platelets increased atherosclerotic lesion formation, a process that was not observed when activated platelets, deficient in CD40L, were administered [123]. Moreover, injection of activated platelets was able to alter the immune system by affecting T-cell subset distribution. Platelet activation caused an increase in effector T cells in blood and spleen, a T-cell subset generally considered to be proatherogenic, and a decrease in the number of Tregs, a T-cell subset known to be athero-protective [124, 125]. The activated platelet-induced decrease in Tregs was associated with CD40L.

Furthermore, platelets constitutively express the CD40 receptor and the interaction between CD40 and CD40L is needed for the shedding of sCD40L. The role of platelet CD40 is still under debate. However, Danese *et al.* showed that CD40L-positive T cells induced platelet activation through a contact-mediated, CD40-dependent pathway. This resulted in RANTES release, which bound to endothelial cells and mediated T cell recruitment. Furthermore, ligation of platelet CD40 with recombinant soluble CD40L augments P-selectin expression, α-granule and dense granule release and the typical morphological transformations that are associated with platelet activation [126]. This conceives an important role for platelet CD40 in inflammation and indicates a potential function in atherosclerosis.

Taken together, inhibition of CD40-CD40L interactions could be used as a promising therapeutic target to improve plaque stability. However, blockade of CD40L may not be therapeutically feasible, since platelets deficient in CD40L can cause thromboembolic events [123, 127]. A humanized CD40L monoclonal antibody (ABI793) effectively prevented graft rejection in cynomolgus monkeys [128], but all clinical trials were put on hold due to thromboembolic events. Conceivably, platelet aggregation was caused by the antibody-induced crosslinking of platelet FcγRII, similar to the HIT syndrome. Antagonising CD40, the receptor of CD40L, or its signaling intermediates provide a sound alternative providing a number of advantages. In allotransplantation research, two anti-CD40 antibodies were developed: Chi220 in 2002 and 4D11 in 2007 [129, 130]. Both antibodies appear to be encouraging agents for anti-rejection treatment in clinical organ transplantation. Satisfying prolonged allograft survivals in monkeys were obtained without thromboembolic complications. Both antibodies open a new prospective for inhibition of the CD40-CD40L system in atherosclerosis.

14.5.1.3 Toll-like receptors

Toll-like receptors (TLRs) represent an increasingly appreciated class of immune receptors expressed in platelets, contributing to their immune cell function. The initial clearance of pathogens such as bacteria, viruses, fungi, and parasites is initiated by TLRs. Through TLR expression, platelets bind infectious agents and deliver different signals for the secretion of cytokines and chemokines [131]. TLRs recognize common pathogen-associated molecular patterns (PAMPs) such as lipopolysaccharide (LPS), peptidoglycan, bacterial RNA, and mucins. TLRs are expressed on antigen presenting macrophages, dendritic cells, and epithelial cells and have recently been discovered on platelets. TLR2, 4 and 9 are expressed on platelets [132]. The best-known ligand for TLRs is LPS, which binds and activates TLR4. LPS has been shown to induce thrombocytopenia through TLR4-dependent recruitment of platelets to the lung. Platelet activation via TLR4 resulted in increased adhesiveness to fibrinogen but was not associated with increased expression of P-selectin [133]. Further support for the functional activity of platelet TLR4 comes from studies showing an *in vivo* role for LPS-stimulated platelets in triggering TNF-α secretion. Furthermore, platelet TLR4 contributes to thrombocytopenia through neutrophil-dependent pulmonary sequestration in response to LPS [133, 134]. This suggests that platelets could be in part responsible for reactivity against bacterial products. We can speculate that platelets in the circulation could act as a sentinel in the defense against pathogens. Several lines of evidence suggest that TLRs are involved in atherogenesis [131]. TLR1, TLR2, and TLR4 are upregulated in human atheroma with active NF-κB colocalizing with TLR2 and TLR4 in the plaque [135]. Furthermore, we know that genetic polymorphisms leading to a reduced functionality of TLR4 are associated with decreased atherogenesis and diminished reactions on gram-negative infections [136]. ApoE-deficient mice lacking TLR4 displayed reduced aortic atherosclerosis, lower levels of circulatory proinflammatory cytokines, and decreased lipid content in the plaques [137]. Similarly, progression of atherosclerosis in *Ldlr*$^{-/-}$ mice lacking TLR2 is reduced with concomitant decreases in macrophage recruitment and proinflammatory cytokine levels [138]. We can anticipate that there might be a function for platelet TLRs in the progression of atherosclerosis, which has not been reported up to now. Clinical studies that use TLR4 inhibitors are currently focused primarily on acute inflammatory disorders. A lipid A analogue, eritoran, which competes with LPS for the binding to TLR4 has been studied in a phase II trial in septic patients. It reduced inflammatory markers and a trend to an increased survival was reported [139]. Now the large-scale clinical ACCESS trial (NCT00334828) will try to answer the suitability of the compound in severe sepsis. In experimental mouse models of myocardial infarction, eritoran was able to diminish the infarction size in C57B6 mice by limiting ischemia-reperfusion injury. Although promising and intriguing as molecular targets, it seems that Toll like receptors are somewhat far from going to be studied in the treatment and prevention of atherosclerosis in the near future.

14.5.1.4 Chemokine receptors

The first evidence for the functional presence and membrane display of chemokine receptors on platelets was provided for CXCR4. *In vitro* studies revealed its presence on the megakaryocytic lineage from progenitors to platelets and demonstrated that its ligand stromal cell-derived factor-1 (SDF-1, CXCL12) is able to trigger adhesion of megakaryocytes to the endothelium and to induce migration of megakaryocyte precursors. Initially, platelets were reported to be unresponsive to CXCL12, but it was subsequently shown that although CXCL12 is a weak platelet agonist by itself, it has robust activity in conjunction with low doses of ADP or thrombin. Furthermore, the functional expression of the chemokine receptors CCR1, CCR3, CXCR1, and CCR4 has been validated [140]. CCR4 responds to the ligands CCL17 and CCL22 (monocyte-derived chemokine [MDC]) [141]. A comprehensive study showed calcium influx in platelets stimulated by CCL17 and other chemokines, as well as synergistic aggregation with CCL17, CCL22, CCL5, and CXCL12 [140]. Also CX3CR1, the receptor for fractalkine (CX3CL1) is functionally expressed on platelets and promotes the upregulation of P-selectin and platelet adhesion to collagen and fibrinogen [142]. Disruption of CX3CR1 in atherosclerosis prone mice results in a reduced plaque formation and of endothelial fractalkine with platelet CX3CR1 (Table 14.1). The rolling and adhesion mechanism requires the presence of auxiliary adhesive substrates like VWF interacting with platelet GPIb [145]. A recent study observed that aspirin inhibits fractalkine expression in atherosclerotic plaques, thereby reducing atherosclerosis in *Apoe*$^{-/-}$ mice [146]. Blocking platelet CX3CR1 appears advantageous, since it might selectively inhibit platelet activation through atherosclerotic and inflamed endothelium (which is rich in CX3CL1) but would not affect injury-induced bleedings of unaltered endothelium. Up to now, there is only one competitive CX3CR1 receptor antagonist, which has been designed through N-terminal modification of CX3CL1 but not tested in experimental or clinical models of atherosclerosis [147]. The specific functionality and inflammatory potential of singular platelet chemokine receptors will have to be further clarified due to the development of conditional knock-out mouse models using the cre-lox system. Clinical studies to test the available non-peptide antagonists for CCR1 have been conducted in the context of multiple sclerosis, allergy, and Chronic Obstructive Pulmonary Disease (COPD) but not in atherosclerosis. A blocking humanized antibody (KW-0761) to CCR4 is being tested in adult T cell leukemia, and an oral CCR3 antagonist (GW766994) is currently evaluated in a phase II study in asthmatics. Antagonists for CXCR1/2 (SCH 527123) are still in phase I trials (NCT01068145).

The JAM (junctional adhesion molecule) family, a subclass within the Ig superfamily, plays a dual role by mediating leukocyte-endothelial cell contacts and regulates cell polarity [148, 149]. JAM-A and JAM-C have been identified on platelets [150]. JAM-C, so far, appears to be expressed solely on vascular cells and the megakaryocytic lineage. Under conditions of lower shear flow, the selective binding to Mac-1 was found to be responsible for the formation of neutrophil-platelet complexes and adhesion to surface-adherent platelets [151]. JAM-A plays an important role for vascular repair mechanisms after endothelial injury [152]. The role for its presence on activated platelets has to be further elucidated.

14.5.2 Released Inflammatory Mediators

In spite of the recognition of trans-cellular inflammation, only scarce information is present on the interaction mechanisms by which platelets and leukocyte subsets cross talk to produce atherogenic mediators. Also the precise sets of cytokines and chemokines released and how they affect atherosclerosis remain to be fully elucidated. Table 14.2 summarizes the potential inflammatory mediators that could be released from interacting platelet–leukocyte aggregates.

Table 14.2 Candidate inflammatory mediators released by platelet–leukocyte aggregates

Platelets	Leukocytes
RANTES (CCL5)	IFN-γ
TARC (CCL17)	IL-1β
Exodus-2 (CCL21)	IL-6
Gro-γ (CXCL3)	IL-8 (CXCL8)
PF4 (CXCL4)	IL-10
ENA-78 (CXCL5)	IL-12
IL-1β	IL-18
CCL7 (MCP-3)	MCP-1 (CCL2)
PDGF	MIP-1α (CCL3)
sCD40L	TGF-β
TGF-β	TNF-α

14.5.1.5 Junctional adhesion molecules

14.5.2.1 Chemokines

As already defined, platelet activation results in the release of granule contents, which contain several chemokines. These chemokines are stored in the α-granules. Among them, PF4 (CXCL4), RANTES (CCL5), CTAP-III (CXCL7), and SDF-1 (CXCL-12) mediate the adhesion of monocytes, PMN, and even progenitor cells. Among these chemokines are CXCL4 and CXCL7 specific for the megakaryocytic lineage.

RANTES is an extensively characterized platelet chemokine in atherosclerosis. The CC chemokine CCL5 causes the selective migration of human blood monocytes and T cells [153, 154]. In mice, platelets have been demonstrated to deliver CCL5 to the monocyte surface and the endothelium resulting in increased leukocyte adhesion to the vascular wall. The role of CCL5 and its receptors CCR1 and CCR5 in atherosclerosis has been addressed in a number of experimental studies. CCR1 and CCR5 are predominantly expressed on monocytes, macrophages, T cells. As already stated above, injection of activated platelets in atherosclerosis-prone mice lead to the endothelial deposition of CCL5 and CXCL4 [104]. This process is P-selectin dependent. Furthermore, inhibition of CCL5 receptors results in decreased lesion size, both in atherosclerosis and vascular injury [103, 104, 155, 156].

Platelet factor 4 (PF4, CXCL4) was the first chemokine discovered in releasates from platelets [157]. CXCL4 differs from most other chemokines in that it exerts its biological activity at much higher concentrations. CXCL4 is a lysine-rich chemokine belonging to the CXC subfamily, is synthesized mainly by megakaryocytes, and exists as a tetramer in α-granules. Although PF4 has been found in other cell types, it appears to be most relevant in platelets. In the presence of appropriate costimuli, such as TNF-α, CXCL4 induces exocytosis and firm neutrophil adhesion to endothelium [158, 159]. CXCL4 is localized in fatty streaks and atherosclerotic lesion in humans, and CXCL4 expression in the atherosclerotic lesion correlates with histological and clinical severity of disease, indicating its role in human atherosclerosis [160]. As a consequence, a significant decrease in atherosclerotic lesion formation in the absence of CXCL4 has been reported.

A point of great importance is that CCL5 and CXCL4 are found to engage in heterophilic interactions [161]. This heteromeric complex between CCL5 and CXCL4 is a more potent inducer of monocyte arrest onto activated endothelial cells than either chemokine alone, indicating a synergistic enhancement of the monocyte-recruiting function of CCL5 [102]. Immunoprecipitation studies have revealed that these chemokines exist in a preformed complex in platelets, suggesting that platelets carry this heterodimer to specifically promote monocyte arrest under inflammatory conditions [102]. Therapeutic potential may lie in the interference with chemokine heteromerization [162, 163]. Disrupting the CCL5/CXCL4 heterodimer attenuates monocyte accumulation during atherogenesis. A synthetic peptide, termed CKEY2, has been designed that actively competes with CXCL4 for binding to CCL5 [102].

CXCL12 or stromal cell derived factor 1 (SDF-1α) is a well-studied chemokine revealing through its ambivalent role in atherosclerosis the intricate regulation of recruitment of the underlying cellular infiltrate. On the one hand, CXCL12 is expressed in atherosclerotic lesions and has proatherogenic properties by recruiting leukocytes into the subintimal space. CXCL12 plays an essential role in neointima formation after arterial injury as it has been demonstrated to attract bone marrow-derived smooth muscle cell progenitors in *Apoe*$^{-/-}$ mice after wire injury [164]. Recent genome-wide-association studies have further found a relationship with myocardial infarctions by identifying a variation on chromosome 10q11 near the CXCL12 gene as a powerful predictor for the susceptibility of coronary atherosclerosis which is causally linked to the increased expression of CXCL12 [165, 166]. On the other hand, CXCL12 plasma levels have been found to be decreased in the genetic CXCL12 risk variant [167]. The antagonism of the CXCL12 receptor leads to a release of leukocytes from the bone marrow, which has helped implementing CXCR4-antagonists (Plerixafor®) to mobilize and collect hematopoietic stem cells before autologous stem cell transplantation. This leukocytosis may have been the reason why in a murine model of atherosclerosis, the inhibition of the CXCR4-CXCL12 axis led to increased atherosclerosis [168]. Furthermore, platelets contain and release CXCL12 upon activation, which will be displayed on platelets covering the lesion after endothelial injury [169]. The recruitment of progenitors by CXCL12 may lead to neointima formation in case they differentiate to smooth muscle cells but favorably may as well accelerate the healing process and prevent vascular remodeling. Collectively, platelets contain a multitude of chemokines that link platelet activation to the recruitment of immune cells by displaying or depositing chemokines on cell surfaces and activating their cognate receptors, resulting in enhanced integrin activity. The interference with immobilization sites, oligomerization or synergistic heteromerization of chemokines at sites of inflammation will be explored to provide novel avenues for therapeutic targeting. Notably, for pleiotropic chemokines, such as CXCL12, strategies have to be developed enabling antagonists to take effect in a cell specific environment.

14.5.2.2 Cytokines

Platelet-derived CD40L and IL-1β have been shown to play significant roles during vascular inflammation. Upon platelet activation, CD40L is cleaved from the platelet surface over a period of minutes to hours to generate an 18 kDa sCD40L molecule, which is similar to the T cell-released sCD40L [108]. Elevation of sCD40L indicated an increased risk of cardiovascular events [170]. sCD40L is biologically active and can induce TF expression on monocytes, endothelial cells, and VSMCs and is crucial in the stabilization of thrombi, which is mediated via αIIβ3 [9]. It has been reported that αIIbβ3 (GP IIb/IIIa) antagonists inhibit the release of sCD40L from activated platelets. Apart from mediating platelet aggregation, αIIbβ3 also contributes to primary platelet adhesion to endothelial cells. AIIbβ3 mediates arrest of activated platelets via fibrinogen to ICAM-1 and αvβ3 [171, 172]. Although there is still some controversy on the function of sCD40L, we have to consider the potential of sCD40L to mediate inflammatory events within the vasculature.

IL-1β is a prototypic proinflammatory cytokine that induces the production of cytokines and chemokines and increases the expression of adhesion molecules on endothelial cells, thus leading to the recruitment of inflammatory cells. Monocytes, macrophages, and dendritic cells are the primary sources of IL-1β. Additionally, platelets have been recognized as an important IL-1β source, which functions as a principal mediator of platelet-induced endothelial cell activation. An increased expression of IL-1β in arteries was found in hyperlipidemic animals [173, 174]. The IL-1β activity expressed by platelets appears to be associated with the platelet surface, and co-incubation of ECs with thrombin-activated platelets induces IL-1β–dependent secretion of IL-6 and IL-8 from ECs [3, 175]. Furthermore, platelet Il-1β enhances endothelial secretion of the chemokine CCL2 (monocyte chemoattractant protein-1 (MCP-1)) [176]. CCL2 is a chemokine crucial in monocyte recruitment throughout atherogenesis [177, 178] and is also induced by platelet CD40L [123]. Platelets additionally increase the endothelial expression of adhesion molecules. Expression of ICAM-1 and αvβ3 on ECs is significantly enhanced by activated platelets via IL-1β [3, 176]. By enhancing chemokine release and upregulation of ICAM-1 and αvβ3, platelet derived IL-1β promotes leukocyte recruitment towards atherosclerotic lesions. Moreover, adhesion of platelets to the endothelium initiates the activation of NF-κB in ECs. This process was shown to be dependent on platelet IL-1β [179]. We can conclude that platelet IL-1β signaling plays an important role in stimulating endothelial gene expression, promoting atherogenesis as well as plaque progression/destabilization an implicating its therapeutic potential. Currently the antibody canakinumab against IL-1β is tested to prevent cardiovascular events in a large-scale placebo controlled phase III trial (NCT01327846) in patients with stable CAD.

14.6 Conclusion

Prevention and therapy of atherosclerosis is still an unsatisfactorily accomplished challenge. For a long-term follow up of the chronic course of atherosclerosis and to complement and facilitate the planning of clinical outcome studies, imaging techniques are needed that allow the quantification of both plaque burden, and more importantly plaque phenotype. It is well perceivable that, in an individual with increased plaque burden, the actual risk for a cardiovascular event may be reduced if the plaques exhibit a more stable phenotype. Although in animal models histological sections are accessible, current atherosclerosis models cannot replace the research on the "natural" atherogenesis in human beings. For instance, Apoe and Ldl-receptor deficient mice develop atherosclerosis but only seldom plaque rupture. Intravascular ultrasound (IVUS) and optical coherence tomography (OCT) are catheter-based means and suffer from invasiveness, radiation exposure, and high costs. The measurement of the intima media thickness (IMT) of the carotid artery is cost effective but other vascular provinces like the coronary arteries cannot be visualized.

So far only statins have been established for primary prevention of atherosclerosis. Beyond the reduction of cholesterol levels, pleiotropic, and anti-inflammatory effects of statins are thought to be relevant for this success and initiated large trials to investigate anti-inflammatory drugs. Platelets have been evidently identified as main culprits in atherogenesis and atherothrombosis. The efficacy of established anti-platelet therapies differs for each particular vascular bed as inferred from the results of the combination therapy of aspirin/dipyridamole, which was successful in preventing stroke but not myocardial infarction. Aspirin is the best investigated platelet inhibitor, but due to side effects, a careful patient selection is necessary to take advantage of the beneficial effects on cardiovascular mortality and morbidity. Similar to statins, platelet inhibitors owe their preventive effects not only to their primary task, which is to inhibit arterial platelet aggregation and thrombosis, but also to reduce the platelet triggered proinflammatory pathways. In order to identify the best molecular and cellular targets to develop potent antiatherosclerotic drugs, we still have to improve our understanding in the intricated proinflammatory and prothrombotic machinery platelets posses. In dissecting the molecules mediating predominantly inflammation or thrombosis, it would be possible to block them separately and, thus, design a more individualized therapeutic concept. Novel anti-platelet therapies could act at the critical interface between inflammation and thrombosis.

References

1. Galkina, E., and Ley, K. 2009. Immune and inflammatory mechanisms of atherosclerosis. *Annual Review Immunology* 27: 165–197.
2. von Hundelshausen, P., and Weber, C. 2007. Platelets as immune cells: bridging inflammation and cardiovascular disease. *Circulatlion Research* 100: 27–40.
3. Gawaz, M., Langer, H., and May, A.E. 2005. Platelets in inflammation and atherogenesis. *Journalof Clinical Investigation* 115: 3378–3384.
4. Munnix, I.C., Cosemans, J.M., Auger, J.M., and Heemskerk, J.W. 2009. Platelet response heterogeneity in thrombus formation. *Thrombosis and Haemostasis* 102: 1149–1156.
5. Denis, C.V., and Wagner, D.D. 2007. Platelet adhesion receptors and their ligands in mouse models of thrombosis. *Arteriosclerosis Thrombosis Vascular Biology* 27: 728–739.
6. Furie, B., and Furie, B.C. 2008. Mechanisms of thrombus formation. *The New England Journal of Medicine* 359: 938–949.
7. Massberg, S., Gawaz, M., Gruner, S., Schulte, V., Konrad, I., Zohlnhofer, D., Heinzmann, U., and Nieswandt, B. 2003. A crucial role of glycoprotein VI for platelet recruitment to the injured arterial wall *in vivo*. *The Journal of Experimental Medicine* 197: 41–49.
8. Angelillo-Scherrer, A., de Frutos, P., Aparicio, C., Melis, E., Savi, P., Lupu, F., Arnout, J., Dewerchin, M., Hoylaerts, M., Herbert, J., *et al.* 2001. Deficiency or inhibition of Gas6 causes platelet dysfunction and protects mice against thrombosis. *Nature Medicine* 7: 215–221.
9. Andre, P., Prasad, K.S., Denis, C.V., He, M., Papalia, J.M., Hynes, R.O., Phillips, D.R., and Wagner, D.D. 2002. CD40L stabilizes arterial thrombi by a beta3 integrin-dependent mechanism. *Nature Medicine* 8: 247–252.
10. Coccheri, S. 2010. Antiplatelet drugs — do we need new options? With a reappraisal of direct thromboxane inhibitors. *Drugs* 70: 887–908.
11. Rothwell, P.M., Fowkes, F.G., Belch, J.F., Ogawa, H., Warlow, C.P., and Meade, T.W. 2011. Effect of daily aspirin on long-term risk of death due to cancer: analysis of individual patient data from randomised trials. *Lancet* 377: 31–41.

12. Ray, W.A., Stein, C.M., Hall, K., Daugherty, J.R., and Griffin, M.R. 2002. Non-steroidal anti-inflammatory drugs and risk of serious coronary heart disease: an observational cohort study. *Lancet* 359: 118–123.

13. Baigent, C., Blackwell, L., Collins, R., Emberson, J., Godwin, J., Peto, R., Buring, J., Hennekens, C., Kearney, P., Meade, T., *et al.* 2009. Aspirin in the primary and secondary prevention of vascular disease: collaborative meta-analysis of individual participant data from randomised trials. *Lancet* 373: 1849–1860.

14. Serebruany, V.L., Malinin, A.I., Eisert, R.M., and Sane, D.C. 2004. Risk of bleeding complications with antiplatelet agents: META-analysis of 338,191 patients enrolled in 50 randomized controlled trials. *American Journal of Hematology* 75: 40–47.

15. Derry, S., and Loke, Y.K. 2000. Risk of gastrointestinal haemorrhage with long term use of aspirin: meta-analysis. *British Medical Journal* 321: 1183–1187..

16. McQuaid, K.R., and Laine, L. 2006. Systematic review and meta-analysis of adverse events of low-dose aspirin and clopidogrel in randomized controlled trials. *American Journal Medical* 119: 624–638.

17. Fowkes, F.G., Price, J.F., Stewart, M.C., Butcher, I., Leng, G.C., Pell, A.C., Sandercock, P.A., Fox, K.A., Lowe, G.D., and Murray, G.D. 2010. Aspirin for prevention of cardiovascular events in a general population screened for a low ankle brachial index: a randomized controlled trial. *JAMA* 303: 841–848.

18. Pignone, M., Alberts, M.J., Colwell, J.A., Cushman, M., Inzucchi, S.E., Mukherjee, D., Rosenson, R.S., Williams, C.D., Wilson, P.W., and Kirkman, M.S. 2010. Aspirin for primary prevention of cardiovascular events in people with diabetes: a position statement of the American Diabetes Association, a scientific statement of the American Heart Association, and an expert consensus document of the American College of Cardiology Foundation. *Circulation* 121: 2694–2701.

19. Maree, A.O., Curtin, R.J., Dooley, M., Conroy, R.M., Crean, P., Cox, D., and Fitzgerald, D.J. 2005. Platelet response to low-dose enteric-coated aspirin in patients with stable cardiovascular disease. *Journal American College Cardiology* 46: 1258–1263.

20. Steinhubl, S.R., Badimon, J.J., Bhatt, D.L., Herbert, J.M., and Luscher, T.F. 2007. Clinical evidence for anti-inflammatory effects of antiplatelet therapy in patients with atherothrombotic disease. *Vascular Medicine* 12: 113–122.

21. Paul, A., Calleja, L., Camps, J., Osada, J., Vilella, E., Ferre, N., Mayayo, E., and Joven, J. 2000. The continuous administration of aspirin attenuates

atherosclerosis in apolipoprotein E-deficient mice. *Life Sciences* 68: 457–465.

22. Cyrus, T., Sung, S., Zhao, L., Funk, C.D., Tang, S., and Pratico, D. 2002. Effect of low-dose aspirin on vascular inflammation, plaque stability, and atherogenesis in low-density lipoprotein receptor-deficient mice. *Circulation* 106: 1282–1287.
23. Tous, M., Ferre, N., Vilella, E., Riu, F., Camps, J., and Joven, J. 2004. Aspirin attenuates the initiation but not the progression of atherosclerosis in apolipoprotein E-deficient mice fed a high-fat, high-cholesterol diet. *Basic & Clinical Pharmacology & Toxicology* 95: 15–19.
24. Paul-Clark, M.J., Van Cao, T., Moradi-Bidhendi, N., Cooper, D., and Gilroy, D.W. 2004. 15-epi-lipoxin A4-mediated induction of nitric oxide explains how aspirin inhibits acute inflammation. *The Journal of Experimental Medicine* 200: 69–78.
25. McCarty, M.F., and Block, K.I. 2006. Preadministration of high-dose salicylates, suppressors of NF-kappaB activation, may increase the chemosensitivity of many cancers: an example of proapoptotic signal modulation therapy. *Integrative Cancer Therapies* 5: 252–268.
26. Kopp, E., and Ghosh, S. 1994. Inhibition of NF-kappa B by sodium salicylate and aspirin. *Science* 265: 956–959.
27. de Winther, M.P., Kanters, E., Kraal, G., and Hofker, M.H. 2005. Nuclear factor kappaB signaling in atherogenesis. *Arteriosclerosis, Thrombosis, and Vascular Biology* 25: 904–914.
28. Gachet, C. 2006. Regulation of platelet functions by P2 receptors. *Annual Review of Pharmacology and Toxicology* 46: 277–300.
29. Abbracchio, M.P., Burnstock, G., Boeynaems, J.M., Barnard, E.A., Boyer, J.L., Kennedy, C., Knight, G.E., Fumagalli, M., Gachet, C., Jacobson, K.A., *et al.* 2006. International Union of Pharmacology LVIII: update on the P2Y G protein-coupled nucleotide receptors: from molecular mechanisms and pathophysiology to therapy. *Pharmacology Review* 58: 281–341.
30. Offermanns, S. 2006. Activation of platelet function through G protein-coupled receptors. *Circulation Research* 99: 1293–1304.
31. Cattaneo, M., Lecchi, A., Lombardi, R., Gachet, C., and Zighetti, M.L. 2000. Platelets from a patient heterozygous for the defect of P2CYC receptors for ADP have a secretion defect despite normal thromboxane A2 production and normal granule stores: further evidence that some cases of platelet 'primary secretion defect' are heterozygous for a defect of P2CYC receptors. *Arteriosclerosis, Thrombosis, and Vascular Biology* 20:E101–E106.

32. Nergiz-Unal, R., Cosemans, J.M., Feijge, M.A., van der Meijden, P.E., Storey, R.F., van Giezen, J.J., oude Egbrink, M.G., Heemskerk, J.W., and Kuijpers, M.J. 2010. Stabilizing role of platelet P2Y(12) receptors in shear-dependent thrombus formation on ruptured plaques. *PloS One* 5:e10130.

33. Balsano, F., Violi, F., and Cimminiello, C. 1990. Ticlopidine in unstable angina. *Circulation* 82: 2282–2283.

34. Krotz, F., Sohn, H.Y., and Klauss, V. 2008. Antiplatelet drugs in cardiological practice: established strategies and new developments. *Vascular Health and Risk Management* 4: 637–645.

35. Duerschmied, D., Bode, C., and Moser, M. 2010. Clopidogrel in acute coronary syndrome: implications of recent study findings. *Expert Review of Cardiovascular Therapy* 8: 1215–1229.

36. Afek, A., Kogan, E., Maysel-Auslender, S., Mor, A., Regev, E., Rubinstein, A., Keren, G., and George, J. 2009. Clopidogrel attenuates atheroma formation and induces a stable plaque phenotype in apolipoprotein E knockout mice. *Microvascular Research* 77: 364–369.

37. Cha, J.K., Jeong, M.H., Lee, K.M., Bae, H.R., Lim, Y.J., Park, K.W., and Cheon, S.M. 2002. Changes in platelet P-selectin and in plasma C-reactive protein in acute atherosclerotic ischemic stroke treated with a loading dose of clopidogrel. *Journal of Thrombosis and Thrombolysis* 14: 145–150.

38. Hermann, A., Rauch, B.H., Braun, M., Schror, K., and Weber, A.A. 2001. Platelet CD40 ligand (CD40L)–subcellular localization, regulation of expression, and inhibition by clopidogrel. *Platelets* 12: 74–82.

39. Evangelista, V., Manarini, S., Dell'Elba, G., Martelli, N., Napoleone, E., Di Santo, A., and Lorenzet, P.S. 2005. Clopidogrel inhibits platelet-leukocyte adhesion and platelet-dependent leukocyte activation. *Thrombosis Haemostasis* 94: 568–577.

40. Waehre, T., Damas, J.K., Pedersen, T.M., Gullestad, L., Yndestad, A., Andreassen, A.K., Froland, S.S., Semb, A.G., Hansteen, V., Gjertsen, E., *et al.* 2006. Clopidogrel increases expression of chemokines in peripheral blood mononuclear cells in patients with coronary artery disease: results of a double-blind placebo-controlled study. *Journal of Thrombosis and Haemostasis JTH* 4: 2140–2147.

41. Yusuf, S., Zhao, F., Mehta, S.R., Chrolavicius, S., Tognoni, G., and Fox, K.K. 2001. Effects of clopidogrel in addition to aspirin in patients with acute coronary syndromes without ST-segment elevation. The *New England Journal of Medicine* 345: 494–502.

42. Eshaghian, S., Kaul, S., Amin, S., Shah, P.K., and Diamond, G.A. 2007. Role of clopidogrel in managing atherothrombotic cardiovascular disease. *Annals of Internal Medicine* 146: 434–441.

43. Liberopoulos, E.N., Elisaf, M.S., Tselepis, A.D., Archimandritis, A., Kiskinis, D., Cokkinos, D., and Mikhailidis, D.P. 2006. Upper gastrointestinal haemorrhage complicating antiplatelet treatment with aspirin and/or clopidogrel: where we are now? *Platelets* 17: 1–6.

44. Cattaneo, M. 2007. Platelet P2 receptors: old and new targets for antithrombotic drugs. *Expert Review of Cardiovascular Therapy* 5: 45–55.

45. Norgard, N.B., Mathews, K.D., and Wall, G.C. 2009. Drug-drug interaction between clopidogrel and the proton pump inhibitors. *The Annals of Pharmacotherapy* 43: 1266–1274.

46. Mega, J.L., Close, S.L., Wiviott, S.D., Shen, L., Hockett, R.D., Brandt, J.T., Walker, J.R., Antman, E.M., Macias, W.L., Braunwald, E., *et al.* 2009. Cytochrome P450 genetic polymorphisms and the response to prasugrel: relationship to pharmacokinetic, pharmacodynamic, and clinical outcomes. *Circulation* 119: 2553–2560.

47. Wiviott, S.D., Braunwald, E., McCabe, C.H., Montalescot, G., Ruzyllo, W., Gottlieb, S., Neumann, F.J., Ardissino, D., De Servi, S., Murphy, S.A., *et al.* 2007. Prasugrel versus clopidogrel in patients with acute coronary syndromes. *The New England Journal of Medicine* 357: 2001–2015.

48. Siddique, A., Butt, M., Shantsila, E., and Lip, G.Y. 2009. New antiplatelet drugs: beyond aspirin and clopidogrel. *International Journal of Clinical Practice* 63: 776–789.

49. Nawarskas, J.J., and Clark, S.M. 2011. Ticagrelor: a novel reversible oral antiplatelet agent. *Cardiology in Review* 19: 95–100.

50. Hall, R., and Mazer, C.D. 2011. Antiplatelet drugs: a review of their pharmacology and management in the perioperative period. *Anesthesia and Analgesia* 112: 292–318.

51. Husted, S., Emanuelsson, H., Heptinstall, S., Sandset, P.M., Wickens, M., and Peters, G. 2006. Pharmacodynamics, pharmacokinetics, and safety of the oral reversible P2Y(12) antagonist AZD6140 with aspirin in patients with atherosclerosis: a double-blind comparison to clopidogrel with aspirin. *European Heart Journal* 27: 1038–1047.

52. Michelson, A.D. 2010. Antiplatelet therapies for the treatment of cardiovascular disease. *Nature Reviews. Drug Discovery* 9: 154–169.

53. Bhatt, D.L., and Topol, E.J. 2003. Scientific and therapeutic advances in antiplatelet therapy. *Nature Reviews. Drug Discovery* 2: 15–28.

54. Chew, D.P., Bhatt, D.L., Sapp, S., and Topol, E.J. 2001. Increased mortality with oral platelet glycoprotein IIb/IIIa antagonists: a meta-analysis of phase III multicenter randomized trials. *Circulation* 103: 201–206.

55. Han, Y., Li, Y., Wang, S., Jing, Q., Wang, Z., Wang, D., Shu, Q., and Tang, X. 2009. Cilostazol in addition to aspirin and clopidogrel improves long-term outcomes after percutaneous coronary intervention in patients with acute coronary syndromes: a randomized, controlled study. *American Heart Journal* 157: 733–739.

56. Lee, S.W., Park, S.W., Yun, S.C., Kim, Y.H., Park, D.W., Kim, W.J., Lee, J.Y., Lee, C.W., Hong, M.K., Kim, J.J., *et al.* 2010. Triple antiplatelet therapy reduces ischemic events after drug-eluting stent implantation: drug-eluting stenting followed by cilostazol treatment reduces adverse serious cardiac events (DECREASE registry). *American Heart Journal* 159: 284–291 e281.

57. Diener, H.C., Cunha, L., Forbes, C., Sivenius, J., Smets, P., and Lowenthal, A. 1996. European stroke prevention study. 2. dipyridamole and acetylsalicylic acid in the secondary prevention of stroke. *Journal of the Neurological Sciences* 143: 1–13.

58. Halkes, P.H., van Gijn, J., Kappelle, L.J., Koudstaal, P.J., and Algra, A. 2006. Aspirin plus dipyridamole versus aspirin alone after cerebral ischaemia of arterial origin (ESPRIT): randomised controlled trial. *Lancet* 367: 1665–1673.

59. Viles-Gonzalez, J.F., Fuster, V., Corti, R., Valdiviezo, C., Hutter, R., Corda, S., Anand, S.X., and Badimon, J.J. 2005. Atherosclerosis regression and TP receptor inhibition: effect of S18886 on plaque size and composition—a magnetic resonance imaging study. *European Heart Journal* 26: 1557–1561.

60. Neri Serneri, G.G., Coccheri, S., Marubini, E., and Violi, F. 2004. Picotamide, a combined inhibitor of thromboxane A2 synthase and receptor, reduces 2-year mortality in diabetics with peripheral arterial disease: the DAVID study. *European Heart Journal* 25: 1845–1852.

61. Borissoff, J.I., Spronk, H.M., and ten Cate, H. 2011. The hemostatic system as a modulator of atherosclerosis. *The New England Journal of Medicine* 364: 1746–1760.

62. Harker, L.A., Hanson, S.R., and Runge, M.S. 1995. Thrombin hypothesis of thrombus generation and vascular lesion formation. *The American Journal of Cardiology* 75: 12B–17B.

63. Angiolillo, D.J., Capodanno, D., and Goto, S. 2010. Platelet thrombin receptor antagonism and atherothrombosis. *European Heart Journal* 31: 17–28.

64. Kato, Y., Kita, Y., Hirasawa-Taniyama, Y., Nishio, M., Mihara, K., Ito, K., Yamanaka, T., Seki, J., Miyata, S., and Mutoh, S. 2003. Inhibition of arterial thrombosis by a protease-activated receptor 1 antagonist, FR171113, in the guinea pig. *European Journal of Pharmacology* 473: 163–169.

65. Derian, C.K., Damiano, B.P., Addo, M.F., Darrow, A.L., D'Andrea, M.R., Nedelman, M., Zhang, H.C., Maryanoff, B.E., and Andrade-Gordon, P. 2003. Blockade of the thrombin receptor protease-activated receptor-1 with a small-molecule antagonist prevents thrombus formation and vascular occlusion in nonhuman primates. *The Journal of Pharmacology and Experimental Therapeutics* 304: 855–861.

66. Vandendries, E.R., Hamilton, J.R., Coughlin, S.R., Furie, B., and Furie, B.C. 2007. Par4 is required for platelet thrombus propagation but not fibrin generation in a mouse model of thrombosis. *Proceedings of the National Academy of Sciences of the United States of America* 104: 288–292.

67. O'Donoghue, M.L., Bhatt, D.L., Wiviott, S.D., Goodman, S.G., Fitzgerald, D.J., Angiolillo, D.J., Goto, S., Montalescot, G., Zeymer, U., Aylward, P.E., *et al.* 2011. Safety and tolerability of atopaxar in the treatment of patients with acute coronary syndromes: the lessons from antagonizing the cellular effects of thrombin-acute coronary syndromes trial. *Circulation* 123(17):1843–1853.

68. Wiviott, S.D., Flather, M.D., O'Donoghue, M.L., Goto, S., Fitzgerald, D.J., Cura, F., Aylward, P., Guetta, V., Dudek, D., Contant, C.F., *et al.* 2011. Randomized trial of atopaxar in the treatment of patients with coronary artery disease: the lessons from antagonizing the cellular effect of thrombin-coronary artery disease trial. *Circulation* 123: 1854–1863.

69. Van de Werf, F. 2011. Inhibitors of the platelet thrombin receptor: will they live up to their promises? *Circulation* 123: 1833–1835.

70. van Schie, M.C., van Loon, J.E., de Maat, M.P., and Leebeek, F.W. 2011. Genetic determinants of von Willebrand factor levels and activity in relation to the risk of cardiovascular disease. A review. *Journal of Thrombosis and Haemostasis: JTH* 9: 899–908.

71. Spiel, A.O., Mayr, F.B., Ladani, N., Wagner, P.G., Schaub, R.G., Gilbert, J.C., and Jilma, B. 2009. The aptamer ARC1779 is a potent and specific inhibitor of von Willebrand Factor mediated ex vivo platelet function in acute myocardial infarction. *Platelets* 20: 334–340.

72. Syed, M.A., and Pervaiz, S. 2010. Advances in aptamers. *Oligonucleotides* 20: 215–224.

73. Cosmi, B. 2009. ARC-1779, a PEGylated aptamer antagonist of von Willebrand factor for potential use as an anticoagulant or antithrombotic agent. *Current Opinion in Molecular Therapeutics* 11: 322–328.

74. Jilma-Stohlawetz, P., Gorczyca, M.E., Jilma, B., Siller-Matula, J., Gilbert, J.C., and Knobl, P. 2011. Inhibition of von Willebrand factor by ARC1779 in patients with acute thrombotic thrombocytopenic purpura. *Thrombosis and Haemostasis* 105: 545–552.

75. Diener, J.L., Daniel Lagasse, H.A., Duerschmied, D., Merhi, Y., Tanguay, J.F., Hutabarat, R., Gilbert, J., Wagner, D.D., and Schaub, R. 2009. Inhibition of von Willebrand factor-mediated platelet activation and thrombosis by the anti-von Willebrand factor A1-domain aptamer ARC1779. *Journal of Thrombosis and Haemostasis JTH* 7: 1155–1162.

76. Huang, L., Muyldermans, S., and Saerens, D. 2010. Nanobodies(R): proficient tools in diagnostics. *Expert Review of Molecular Diagnostics* 10: 777–785.

77. Firbas, C., Siller-Matula, J.M., and Jilma, B. 2010. Targeting von Willebrand factor and platelet glycoprotein Ib receptor. *Expert Review of Cardiovascular Therapy* 8: 1689–1701.

78. Massberg, S., Brand, K., Gruner, S., Page, S., Muller, E., Muller, I., Bergmeier, W., Richter, T., Lorenz, M., Konrad, I., *et al.* 2002. A critical role of platelet adhesion in the initiation of atherosclerotic lesion formation. *Journal of Experimental Medicine* 196: 887–896.

79. Wang, Y., Sakuma, M., Chen, Z., Ustinov, V., Shi, C., Croce, K., Zago, A.C., Lopez, J., Andre, P., Plow, E., *et al.* 2005. Leukocyte engagement of platelet glycoprotein Ibalpha via the integrin Mac-1 is critical for the biological response to vascular injury. *Circulation* 112: 2993–3000.

80. Bergmeier, W., Piffath, C.L., Goerge, T., Cifuni, S.M., Ruggeri, Z.M., Ware, J., and Wagner, D.D. 2006. The role of platelet adhesion receptor GPIbalpha far exceeds that of its main ligand, von Willebrand factor, in arterial thrombosis. *Proceedings of the National Academy of Sciences of the United States of America* 103: 16900–16905.

81. Cauwenberghs, N., Vanhoorelbeke, K., Vauterin, S., Westra, D.F., Romo, G., Huizinga, E.G., Lopez, J.A., Berndt, M.C., Harsfalvi, J., and Deckmyn, H. 2001. Epitope mapping of inhibitory antibodies against platelet glycoprotein Ibalpha reveals interaction between the leucine-rich repeat N-terminal and C-terminal flanking domains of glycoprotein Ibalpha. *Blood* 98: 652–660.

82. Wu, D., Meiring, M., Kotze, H.F., Deckmyn, H., and Cauwenberghs, N. 2002. Inhibition of platelet glycoprotein Ib, glycoprotein IIb/IIIa,

or both by monoclonal antibodies prevents arterial thrombosis in baboons. *Arteriosclerosis, Thrombosis, and Vascular Biology* 22: 323–328.

83. Fontayne, A., Meiring, M., Lamprecht, S., Roodt, J., Demarsin, E., Barbeaux, P., and Deckmyn, H. 2008. The humanized anti-glycoprotein Ib monoclonal antibody h6B4-Fab is a potent and safe antithrombotic in a high shear arterial thrombosis model in baboons. *Thrombosis and Haemostasis* 100: 670–677.

84. Penz, S.M., Reininger, A.J., Toth, O., Deckmyn, H., Brandl, R., and Siess, W. 2007. Glycoprotein Ibalpha inhibition and ADP receptor antagonists, but not aspirin, reduce platelet thrombus formation in flowing blood exposed to atherosclerotic plaques. *Thrombosis and Haemostasis* 97: 435–443.

85. Anderson, G.M., and Cook, E.H. 2000. Pharmacogenetics. Promise and potential in child and adolescent psychiatry. *Child and Adolescent Psychiatric Clinics of North America* 9: 23–42, viii.

86. Walther, D.J., Peter, J.U., Winter, S., Holtje, M., Paulmann, N., Grohmann, M., Vowinckel, J., Alamo-Bethencourt, V., Wilhelm, C.S., Ahnert-Hilger, G., *et al.* 2003. Serotonylation of small GTPases is a signal transduction pathway that triggers platelet alpha-granule release. *Cell* 115: 851–862.

87. Li, N., Wallen, N.H., Ladjevardi, M., and Hjemdahl, P. 1997. Effects of serotonin on platelet activation in whole blood. *Blood Coagulation & Fibrinolysis: An International Journal in Haemostasis and Thrombosis* 8: 517–523.

88. Satomura, K., Takase, B., Hamabe, A., Ashida, K., Hosaka, H., Ohsuzu, F., and Kurita, A. 2002. Sarpogrelate, a specific 5HT2-receptor antagonist, improves the coronary microcirculation in coronary artery disease. *Clinical Cardiology* 25: 28–32.

89. Przyklenk, K., Frelinger, A.L., 3rd, Linden, M.D., Whittaker, P., Li, Y., Barnard, M.R., Adams, J., Morgan, M., Al-Shamma, H., and Michelson, A.D. 2010. Targeted inhibition of the serotonin 5HT2A receptor improves coronary patency in an *in vivo* model of recurrent thrombosis. *Journal of Thrombosis and Haemostasis: JTH* 8: 331–340.

90. Bampalis, V.G., Khandoga, A.L., and Siess, W. 2010. Fluoxetine inhibition of 5-HT-potentiated platelet aggregation in whole blood. *Thrombosis and Haemostasis* 104: 1272–1274.

91. Andrade, C., Sandarsh, S., Chethan, K.B., and Nagesh, K.S. 2010. Serotonin reuptake inhibitor antidepressants and abnormal bleeding:

a review for clinicians and a reconsideration of mechanisms. *The Journal of Clinical Psychiatry* 71: 1565–1575.

92. Dees, C., Akhmetshina, A., Zerr, P., Reich, N., Palumbo, K., Horn, A., Jungel, A., Beyer, C., Kronke, G., Zwerina, J., *et al.* 2011. Platelet-derived serotonin links vascular disease and tissue fibrosis. *The Journal of Experimental Medicine* 208: 961–972.

93. Bigalke, B., Langer, H., Geisler, T., Lindemann, S., and Gawaz, M. 2007. Platelet glycoprotein VI: a novel marker for acute coronary syndrome. *Seminars in Thrombosis and Hemostasis* 33: 179–184.

94. Bigalke, B., Lindemann, S., Ehlers, R., Seizer, P., Daub, K., Langer, H., Schonberger, T., Kremmer, E., Siegel-Axel, D., May, A.E., *et al.* 2006. Expression of platelet collagen receptor glycoprotein VI is associated with acute coronary syndrome. *European Heart Journal* 27: 2165–2169.

95. Bultmann, A., Li, Z., Wagner, S., Peluso, M., Schonberger, T., Weis, C., Konrad, I., Stellos, K., Massberg, S., Nieswandt, B., *et al.* 2010. Impact of glycoprotein VI and platelet adhesion on atherosclerosis — a possible role of fibronectin. *Journal of Molecular and Cellular Cardiology* 49: 532–542.

96. Schulz, C., von Bruhl, M.L., Barocke, V., Cullen, P., Mayer, K., Okrojek, R., Steinhart, A., Ahmad, Z., Kremmer, E., Nieswandt, B., *et al.* 2011. EMMPRIN (CD147/Basigin) mediates platelet-monocyte interactions *in vivo* and augments monocyte recruitment to the vascular wall. *Journal of Thrombosis and Haemostasis: JTH* 9: 1007–1019.

97. Seizer, P., Borst, O., Langer, H.F., Bultmann, A., Munch, G., Herouy, Y., Stellos, K., Kramer, B., Bigalke, B., Buchele, B., *et al.* 2009. EMMPRIN (CD147) is a novel receptor for platelet GPVI and mediates platelet rolling via GPVI-EMMPRIN interaction. *Thrombosis and Haemostasis* 101: 682–686.

98. Ungerer, M., Rosport, K., Bultmann, A., Piechatzek, R., Uhland, K., Schlieper, P., Gawaz, M., and Munch, G. 2011. Novel antiplatelet drug revacept (Dimeric Glycoprotein VI-Fc) specifically and efficiently inhibited collagen-induced platelet aggregation without affecting general hemostasis in humans. *Circulation* 123: 1891–1899.

99. von Hundelshausen, P., Koenen, R.R., and Weber, C. 2009. Platelet-mediated enhancement of leukocyte adhesion. *Microcirculation* 16: 84–96.

100. Li, Z., Yang, F., Dunn, S., Gross, A.K., and Smyth, S.S. 2010. Platelets as immune mediators: their role in host defense responses and sepsis. *Thrombosis Research* 127: 187–188.

101. Senzel, L., Gnatenko, D.V., and Bahou, W.F. 2009. The platelet proteome. *Current Opinion in Hematology* 16: 329–333.

102. Koenen, R.R., von Hundelshausen, P., Nesmelova, I.V., Zernecke, A., Liehn, E.A., Sarabi, A., Kramp, B.K., Piccinini, A.M., Paludan, S.R., Kowalska, M.A., *et al.* 2009. Disrupting functional interactions between platelet chemokines inhibits atherosclerosis in hyperlipidemic mice. *Nature Medicine* 15: 97–103.

103. von Hundelshausen, P., Weber, K.S., Huo, Y., Proudfoot, A.E., Nelson, P.J., Ley, K., and Weber, C. 2001. RANTES deposition by platelets triggers monocyte arrest on inflamed and atherosclerotic endothelium. *Circulation* 103: 1772–1777.

104. Huo, Y., Schober, A., Forlow, S.B., Smith, D.F., Hyman, M.C., Jung, S., Littman, D.R., Weber, C., and Ley, K. 2003. Circulating activated platelets exacerbate atherosclerosis in mice deficient in apolipoprotein E. *Nature Medicine* 9: 61–67.

105. Theilmeier, G., Michiels, C., Spaepen, E., Vreys, I., Collen, D., Vermylen, J., and Hoylaerts, M.F. 2002. Endothelial von Willebrand factor recruits platelets to atherosclerosis-prone sites in response to hypercholesterolemia. *Blood* 99: 4486–4493.

106. Frenette, P.S., Denis, C.V., Weiss, L., Jurk, K., Subbarao, S., Kehrel, B., Hartwig, J.H., Vestweber, D., and Wagner, D.D. 2000. P-Selectin glycoprotein ligand 1 (PSGL-1) is expressed on platelets and can mediate platelet-endothelial interactions *in vivo*. *The Journal of Experimental Medicine* 191: 1413–1422.

107. Romo, G.M., Dong, J.F., Schade, A.J., Gardiner, E.E., Kansas, G.S., Li, C.Q., McIntire, L.V., Berndt, M.C., and Lopez, J.A. 1999. The glycoprotein Ib-IX-V complex is a platelet counterreceptor for P-selectin. *The Journal of Experimental Medicine* 190: 803–814.

108. Lievens, D., Eijgelaar, W.J., Biessen, E.A., Daemen, M.J., and Lutgens, E. 2009. The multi-functionality of CD40L and its receptor CD40 in atherosclerosis. *Thrombosis and Haemostasis* 102: 206–214.

109. Dole, V.S., Bergmeier, W., Mitchell, H.A., Eichenberger, S.C., and Wagner, D.D. 2005. Activated platelets induce Weibel-Palade-body secretion and leukocyte rolling *in vivo*: role of P-selectin 10.1182/blood-2005-04-1530. *Blood* 106:2334–2339.

110. Huo, Y., and Ley, K.F. 2004. Role of platelets in the development of atherosclerosis. *Trends in Cardiovascular Medicine* 14: 18–22.

111. van Gils, J.M., Zwaginga, J.J., and Hordijk, P.L. 2009. Molecular and functional interactions among monocytes, platelets, and endothelial

cells and their relevance for cardiovascular diseases. *Journal Leukocyte Biology* 85: 195–204.

112. Lippi, G., Montagnana, M., Salvagno, G.L., Cicorella, N., Degan, M., Minuz, P., Lechi, C., and Guidi, G.C. 2007. Risk stratification of patients with acute myocardial infarction by quantification of circulating monocyte-platelet aggregates. *International Journal of Cardiology* 115: 101–102.

113. Furman, M.I., Barnard, M.R., Krueger, L.A., Fox, M.L., Shilale, E.A., Lessard, D.M., Marchese, P., Frelinger, A.L., 3rd, Goldberg, R.J., and Michelson, A.D. 2001. Circulating monocyte-platelet aggregates are an early marker of acute myocardial infarction. *Journal American College of Cardiology* 38: 1002–1006.

114. Oostingh, G.J., Pozgajova, M., Ludwig, R.J., Krahn, T., Boehncke, W.H., Nieswandt, B., and Schon, M.P. 2007. Diminished thrombus formation and alleviation of myocardial infarction and reperfusion injury through antibody- or small-molecule-mediated inhibition of selectin-dependent platelet functions. *Haematologica* 92: 502–512.

115. Myers, D.D., Jr., Wrobleski, S.K., Longo, C., Bedard, P.W., Kaila, N., Shaw, G.D., Londy, F.J., Rohrer, S.E., Fex, B.A., Zajkowski, P.J., *et al.* 2007. Resolution of venous thrombosis using a novel oral small-molecule inhibitor of P-selectin (PSI-697) without anticoagulation. *Thrombosis and Haemostasis* 97: 400–407.

116. Bedard, P.W., Clerin, V., Sushkova, N., Tchernychev, B., Antrilli, T., Resmini, C., Keith, J.C., Jr., Hennan, J.K., Kaila, N., Debernardo, S., *et al.* 2008. Characterization of the novel P-selectin inhibitor PSI-697 [2-(4-chlorobenzyl) 3-hydroxy-7,8,9,10-tetrahydrobenzo[h] quinoline-4-carboxylic acid] *in vitro* and in rodent models of vascular inflammation and thrombosis. *The Journal of Pharmacology and Experimental Therapeutics* 324: 497–506.

117. Chelliah, R., Lucking, A.J., Tattersall, L., Daga, S., Beresford-Cleary, N.J., Cortas, K., Fox, K.A., Feuerstein, G.Z., Connolly, T.M., and Newby, D.E. 2009. P-selectin antagonism reduces thrombus formation in humans. *Journal of Thrombosis and Haemostasis: JTH* 7: 1915–1919.

118. Huang, A., Moretto, A., Janz, K., Lowe, M., Bedard, P.W., Tam, S., Di, L., Clerin, V., Sushkova, N., Tchernychev, B., *et al.* 2010. Discovery of 2-[1-(4-chlorophenyl)cyclopropyl]-3-hydroxy-8-(trifluoromethyl) quinoline-4 -carboxylic acid (PSI-421), a P-selectin inhibitor with improved pharmacokinetic properties and oral efficacy in models of vascular injury. *Journal of Medicinal Chemistry* 53: 6003–6017.

119. Kumar, A., Villani, M.P., Patel, U.K., Keith, J.C., Jr., and Schaub, R.G. 1999. Recombinant soluble form of PSGL-1 accelerates thrombolysis and prevents reocclusion in a porcine model. *Circulation* 99: 1363–1369.

120. Engel, D., Seijkens, T., Poggi, M., Sanati, M., Thevissen, L., Beckers, L., Wijnands, E., Lievens, D., and Lutgens, E. 2009. The immunobiology of CD154-CD40-TRAF interactions in atherosclerosis. *Seminars in Immunology* 21: 308–312.

121. Lutgens, E., Gorelik, L., Daemen, M.J., de Muinck, E.D., Grewal, I.S., Koteliansky, V.E., and Flavell, R.A. 1999. Requirement for CD154 in the progression of atherosclerosis. *Nature Medicine* 5: 1313–1316.

122. Henn, V., Slupsky, J.R., Grafe, M., Anagnostopoulos, I., Forster, R., Muller-Berghaus, G., and Kroczek, R.A. 1998. CD40 ligand on activated platelets triggers an inflammatory reaction of endothelial cells. *Nature* 391: 591–594.

123. Lievens, D., Zernecke, A., Seijkens, T., Soehnlein, O., Beckers, L., Munnix, I.C., Wijnands, E., Goossens, P., van Kruchten, R., Thevissen, L., *et al.* 2010. Platelet CD40L mediates thrombotic and inflammatory processes in atherosclerosis. *Blood* 116: 4317–4327.

124. Zhou, X., Nicoletti, A., Elhage, R., and Hansson, G.K. 2000. Transfer of CD4(+) T cells aggravates atherosclerosis in immunodeficient apolipoprotein E knockout mice. *Circulation* 102: 2919–2922.

125. Ait-Oufella, H., Salomon, B.L., Potteaux, S., Robertson, A.K., Gourdy, P., Zoll, J., Merval, R., Esposito, B., Cohen, J.L., Fisson, S., *et al.* 2006. Natural regulatory T cells control the development of atherosclerosis in mice. *Nature Medicine* 12: 178–180.

126. Inwald, D.P., McDowall, A., Peters, M.J., Callard, R.E., and Klein, N.J. 2003. CD40 is constitutively expressed on platelets and provides a novel mechanism for platelet activation. *Circulation Research* 92: 1041–1048.

127. Kawai, T., Andrews, D., Colvin, R.B., Sachs, D.H., and Cosimi, A.B. 2000. Thromboembolic complications after treatment with monoclonal antibody against CD40 ligand. *Nature Medicine* 6: 114.

128. Schuler, W., Bigaud, M., Brinkmann, V., Di Padova, F., Geisse, S., Gram, H., Hungerford, V., Kleuser, B., Kristofic, C., Menninger, K., *et al.* 2004. Efficacy and safety of ABI793, a novel human anti-human CD154 monoclonal antibody in cynomolgus monkey renal allotransplantation. *Transplantation* 77: 717–726.

129. Pearson, T.C., Trambley, J., Odom, K., Anderson, D.C., Cowan, S., Bray, R., Lin, A., Hollenbaugh, D., Aruffo, A., Siadak, A.W., *et al.* 2002. Anti-

CD40 therapy extends renal allograft survival in rhesus macaques. *Transplantation* 74: 933–940.

130. Imai, A., Suzuki, T., Sugitani, A., Itoh, T., Ueki, S., Aoyagi, T., Yamashita, K., Taniguchi, M., Takahashi, N., Miura, T., *et al.* 2007. A novel fully human anti-CD40 monoclonal antibody, 4D11, for kidney transplantation in cynomolgus monkeys. *Transplantation* 84: 1020–1028.

131. Hodgkinson, C., and Ye, S. 2011. Toll-like receptors, their ligands, and atherosclerosis. *The Scientific World Journal* 11: 437–453.

132. Shiraki, R., Inoue, N., Kawasaki, S., Takei, A., Kadotani, M., Ohnishi, Y., Ejiri, J., Kobayashi, S., Hirata, K., Kawashima, S., *et al.* 2004. Expression of Toll-like receptors on human platelets. *Thrombosis Research* 113: 379–385.

133. Aslam, R., Speck, E.R., Kim, M., Crow, A.R., Bang, K.W., Nestel, F.P., Ni, H., Lazarus, A.H., Freedman, J., and Semple, J.W. 2006. Platelet Toll-like receptor expression modulates lipopolysaccharide-induced thrombocytopenia and tumor necrosis factor-alpha production *in vivo*. *Blood* 107: 637–641.

134. Andonegui, G., Kerfoot, S.M., McNagny, K., Ebbert, K.V., Patel, K.D., and Kubes, P. 2005. Platelets express functional Toll-like receptor-4. *Blood* 106: 2417–2423.

135. Edfeldt, K., Swedenborg, J., Hansson, G.K., and Yan, Z.Q. 2002. Expression of toll-like receptors in human atherosclerotic lesions: a possible pathway for plaque activation. *Circulation* 105: 1158–1161.

136. Kiechl, S., Lorenz, E., Reindl, M., Wiedermann, C.J., Oberhollenzer, F., Bonora, E., Willeit, J., and Schwartz, D.A. 2002. Toll-like receptor 4 polymorphisms and atherogenesis. *The New England Journal of Medicine* 347: 185–192.

137. Michelsen, K.S., Wong, M.H., Shah, P.K., Zhang, W., Yano, J., Doherty, T.M., Akira, S., Rajavashisth, T.B., and Arditi, M. 2004. Lack of Toll-like receptor 4 or myeloid differentiation factor 88 reduces atherosclerosis and alters plaque phenotype in mice deficient in apolipoprotein E. *Proceedings of the National Academy of Sciences of the United States of America* 101: 10679–10684.

138. Mullick, A.E., Tobias, P.S., and Curtiss, L.K. 2005. Modulation of atherosclerosis in mice by Toll-like receptor 2. *The Journal of Clinical Investigation* 115: 3149–3156.

139. Tidswell, M., Tillis, W., Larosa, S.P., Lynn, M., Wittek, A.E., Kao, R., Wheeler, J., Gogate, J., and Opal, S.M. 2010. Phase 2 trial of eritoran tetrasodium (E5564), a toll-like receptor 4 antagonist, in patients with severe sepsis. *Critical Care Medicine* 38: 72–83.

140. Clemetson, K.J., Clemetson, J.M., Proudfoot, A.E., Power, C.A., Baggiolini, M., and Wells, T.N. 2000. Functional expression of CCR1, CCR3, CCR4, and CXCR4 chemokine receptors on human platelets. *Blood* 96: 4046–4054.

141. Fujisawa, T., Fujisawa, R., Kato, Y., Nakayama, T., Morita, A., Katsumata, H., Nishimori, H., Iguchi, K., Kamiya, H., Gray, P.W., *et al.* 2002. Presence of high contents of thymus and activation-regulated chemokine in platelets and elevated plasma levels of thymus and activation-regulated chemokine and macrophage-derived chemokine in patients with atopic dermatitis. *The Journal of Allergy and Clinical Immunology* 110: 139–146.

142. Schafer, A., Schulz, C., Eigenthaler, M., Fraccarollo, D., Kobsar, A., Gawaz, M., Ertl, G., Walter, U., and Bauersachs, J. 2004. Novel role of the membrane-bound chemokine fractalkine in platelet activation and adhesion. *Blood* 103: 407–412.

143. Combadiere, C., Potteaux, S., Gao, J.L., Esposito, B., Casanova, S., Lee, E.J., Debre, P., Tedgui, A., Murphy, P.M., and Mallat, Z. 2003. Decreased atherosclerotic lesion formation in CX3CR1/apolipoprotein E double knockout mice. *Circulation* 107: 1009–1016.

144. Lesnik, P., Haskell, C.A., and Charo, I.F. 2003. Decreased atherosclerosis in CX3CR1-/- mice reveals a role for fractalkine in atherogenesis. *The Journal of Clinical Investigation* 111: 333–340.

145. Meyer Dos Santos, S., Klinkhardt, U., Scholich, K., Nelson, K., Monsefi, N., Deckmyn, H., Kuczka, K., Zorn, A., and Harder, S. 2011. The CX3C chemokine fractalkine mediates platelet adhesion via the von Willebrand receptor glycoprotein Ib. *Blood* 117: 4999–5008.

146. Liu, H., Jiang, D., Zhang, S., and Ou, B. 2010. Aspirin inhibits fractalkine expression in atherosclerotic plaques and reduces atherosclerosis in ApoE gene knockout mice. *Cardiovascular Drugs and Therapy/Sponsored by the International Society of Cardiovascular Pharmacotherapy* 24: 17–24.

147. Dorgham, K., Ghadiri, A., Hermand, P., Rodero, M., Poupel, L., Iga, M., Hartley, O., Gorochov, G., Combadiere, C., and Deterre, P. 2009. An engineered CX3CR1 antagonist endowed with anti-inflammatory activity. *Journal of Leukocyte Biology* 86: 903–911.

148. Ebnet, K., Suzuki, A., Ohno, S., and Vestweber, D. 2004. Junctional adhesion molecules (JAMs): more molecules with dual functions? *Journal of Cell Science* 117: 19–29.

149. Orlova, V.V., and Chavakis, T. 2007. Regulation of vascular endothelial permeability by junctional adhesion molecules (JAM). *Thrombosis and Haemostasis* 98: 327–332.

150. Malergue, F., Galland, F., Martin, F., Mansuelle, P., Aurrand-Lions, M., and Naquet, P. 1998. A novel immunoglobulin superfamily junctional molecule expressed by antigen presenting cells, endothelial cells and platelets. *Molecular Immunology* 35: 1111–1119.

151. Santoso, S., Sachs, U.J., Kroll, H., Linder, M., Ruf, A., Preissner, K.T., and Chavakis, T. 2002. The junctional adhesion molecule 3 (JAM-3) on human platelets is a counterreceptor for the leukocyte integrin Mac-1. *The Journal of Experimental Medicine* 196: 679–691.

152. Zernecke, A., Liehn, E.A., Fraemohs, L., von Hundelshausen, P., Koenen, R.R., Corada, M., Dejana, E., and Weber, C. 2006. Importance of junctional adhesion molecule-A for neointimal lesion formation and infiltration in atherosclerosis-prone mice. *Arteriosclerosis, Thrombosis, and Vascular Biology* 26:e10–13.

153. Schall, T.J., Jongstra, J., Dyer, B.J., Jorgensen, J., Clayberger, C., Davis, M.M., and Krensky, A.M. 1988. A human T cell-specific molecule is a member of a new gene family. *Journal of Immunology* 141: 1018–1025.

154. Schall, T.J., Bacon, K., Toy, K.J., and Goeddel, D.V. 1990. Selective attraction of monocytes and T lymphocytes of the memory phenotype by cytokine RANTES. *Nature* 347: 669–671.

155. Schober, A., Manka, D., von Hundelshausen, P., Huo, Y., Hanrath, P., Sarembock, I.J., Ley, K., and Weber, C. 2002. Deposition of platelet RANTES triggering monocyte recruitment requires P-selectin and Is involved in neointima formation after arterial injury. *Circulation* 106: 1523–1529.

156. Veillard, N.R., Kwak, B., Pelli, G., Mulhaupt, F., James, R.W., Proudfoot, A.E., and Mach, F. 2004. Antagonism of RANTES receptors reduces atherosclerotic plaque formation in mice. *Circulation Research* 94: 253–261.

157. Brandt, E., Ludwig, A., Petersen, F., and Flad, H.D. 2000. Platelet-derived CXC chemokines: old players in new games. *Immunological Reviews* 177: 204–216.

158. Kasper, B., Brandt, E., Bulfone-Paus, S., and Petersen, F. 2004. Platelet factor 4 (PF-4)-induced neutrophil adhesion is controlled by src-kinases, whereas PF-4-mediated exocytosis requires the additional activation of p38 MAP kinase and phosphatidylinositol 3-kinase. *Blood* 103: 1602–1610.

159. Petersen, F., Ludwig, A., Flad, H.D., and Brandt, E. 1996. TNF-alpha renders human neutrophils responsive to platelet factor 4. Comparison of PF-4 and IL-8 reveals different activity profiles of the two chemokines. *Journal of Immunology* 156: 1954–1962.

160. Pitsilos, S., Hunt, J., Mohler, E.R., Prabhakar, A.M., Poncz, M., Dawicki, J., Khalapyan, T.Z., Wolfe, M.L., Fairman, R., Mitchell, M., *et al.* 2003. Platelet factor 4 localization in carotid atherosclerotic plaques: correlation with clinical parameters. *Thrombosis and Haemostasis* 90: 1112–1120.

161. von Hundelshausen, P., Koenen, R.R., Sack, M., Mause, S.F., Adriaens, W., Proudfoot, A.E., Hackeng, T.M., and Weber, C. 2005. Heterophilic interactions of platelet factor 4 and RANTES promote monocyte arrest on endothelium. *Blood* 105: 924–930.

162. Kramp, B.K., Sarabi, A., Koenen, R.R., and Weber, C. 2010. Heterophilic chemokine receptor interactions in chemokine signaling and biology. *Experimental Cell Research*.

163. Koenen, R.R., and Weber, C. 2010. Therapeutic targeting of chemokine interactions in atherosclerosis. *Nature Reviews. Drug Discovery* 9: 141–153.

164. Karshovska, E., Zernecke, A., Sevilmis, G., Millet, A., Hristov, M., Cohen, C.D., Schmid, H., Krotz, F., Sohn, H.Y., Klauss, V., *et al.* 2007. Expression of HIF-1alpha in injured arteries controls SDF-1alpha mediated neointima formation in apolipoprotein E deficient mice. *Arteriosclerosis, Thrombosis, and Vascular Biology* 27: 2540–2547.

165. Kathiresan, S., Voight, B.F., Purcell, S., Musunuru, K., Ardissino, D., Mannucci, P.M., Anand, S., Engert, J.C., Samani, N.J., Schunkert, H., *et al.* 2009. Genome-wide association of early-onset myocardial infarction with single nucleotide polymorphisms and copy number variants. *Nature Genetics* 41: 334–341.

166. Mehta, N.N., Li, M., William, D., Khera, A.V., Derohannessian, S., Qu, L., Ferguson, J.F., McLaughlin, C., Shaikh, L.H., Shah, R., *et al.* 2011. The novel atherosclerosis locus at 10q11 regulates plasma CXCL12 levels. *European Heart Journal* 32: 963–971.

167. Kiechl, S., Laxton, R.C., Xiao, Q., Hernesniemi, J.A., Raitakari, O.T., Kahonen, M., Mayosi, B.M., Jula, A., Moilanen, L., Willeit, J., *et al.* 2010. Coronary artery disease-related genetic variant on chromosome 10q11 is associated with carotid intima-media thickness and atherosclerosis. *Arteriosclerosis, Thrombosis, and Vascular Biology* 30: 2678–2683.

168. Zernecke, A., Bot, I., Djalali-Talab, Y., Shagdarsuren, E., Bidzhekov, K., Meiler, S., Krohn, R., Schober, A., Sperandio, M., Soehnlein, O., *et al.* 2008.

Protective role of CXC receptor 4/CXC ligand 12 unveils the importance of neutrophils in atherosclerosis. *Circulation Research* 102: 209–217.

169. Massberg, S., Konrad, I., Schurzinger, K., Lorenz, M., Schneider, S., Zohlnhoefer, D., Hoppe, K., Schiemann, M., Kennerknecht, E., Sauer, S., *et al.* 2006. Platelets secrete stromal cell-derived factor 1alpha and recruit bone marrow-derived progenitor cells to arterial thrombi *in vivo*. *The Journal of Experimental Medicine* 203: 1221–1233.

170. Heeschen, C., Dimmeler, S., Hamm, C.W., van den Brand, M.J., Boersma, E., Zeiher, A.M., and Simoons, M.L. 2003. Soluble CD40 ligand in acute coronary syndromes. *New England Journal of Medicine* 348: 1104–1111.

171. Massberg, S., Schurzinger, K., Lorenz, M., Konrad, I., Schulz, C., Plesnila, N., Kennerknecht, E., Rudelius, M., Sauer, S., Braun, S., *et al.* 2005. Platelet adhesion via glycoprotein IIb integrin is critical for atheroprogression and focal cerebral ischemia: an *in vivo* study in mice lacking glycoprotein IIb. *Circulation* 112: 1180–1188.

172. Massberg, S., Enders, G., Matos, F.C., Tomic, L.I., Leiderer, R., Eisenmenger, S., Messmer, K., and Krombach, F. 1999. Fibrinogen deposition at the postischemic vessel wall promotes platelet adhesion during ischemia-reperfusion *in vivo*. *Blood* 94: 3829–3838.

173. Merhi-Soussi, F., Kwak, B.R., Magne, D., Chadjichristos, C., Berti, M., Pelli, G., James, R.W., Mach, F., and Gabay, C. 2005. Interleukin-1 plays a major role in vascular inflammation and atherosclerosis in male apolipoprotein E-knockout mice. *Cardiovascular Research* 66: 583–593.

174. Brody, J.I., Pickering, N.J., Capuzzi, D.M., Fink, G.B., Can, C.A., and Gomez, F. 1992. Interleukin-1 alpha as a factor in occlusive vascular disease. *American Journal of Clinical Pathology* 97: 8–13.

175. Kaplanski, G., Farnarier, C., Kaplanski, S., Porat, R., Shapiro, L., Bongrand, P., and Dinarello, C.A. 1994. Interleukin-1 induces interleukin-8 secretion from endothelial cells by a juxtacrine mechanism. *Blood* 84: 4242–4248.

176. Gawaz, M., Brand, K., Dickfeld, T., Pogatsa-Murray, G., Page, S., Bogner, C., Koch, W., Schomig, A., and Neumann, F.-J. 2000. Platelets induce alterations of chemotactic and adhesive properties of endothelial cells mediated through an interleukin-1-dependent mechanism. Implications for atherogenesis. *Atherosclerosis* 148: 75.

177. Boring, L., Gosling, J., Cleary, M., and Charo, I.F. 1998. Decreased lesion formation in CCR2-/- mice reveals a role for chemokines in the initiation of atherosclerosis. *Nature* 394: 894–897.

178. Lutgens, E., Faber, B., Schapira, K., Evelo, C.T., van Haaften, R., Heeneman, S., Cleutjens, K.B., Bijnens, A.P., Beckers, L., Porter, J.G., *et al.* 2005. Gene profiling in atherosclerosis reveals a key role for small inducible cytokines: validation using a novel monocyte chemoattractant protein monoclonal antibody. *Circulation* 111: 3443–3452.

179. Gawaz, M., Page, S., Massberg, S., Nothdurfter, C., Weber, M., Fisher, C., Ungerer, M., and Brand, K. 2002. Transient platelet interaction induces MCP-1 production by endothelial cells via I kappa B kinase complex activation. *Thrombosis and Haemostasis* 88: 307–314.

Chapter 15

Co-stimulatory Molecules in Atherosclerosis

Norbert Gerdes[a,b] **and Esther Lutgens**[a,b]
[a]*Institute for Cardiovascular Prevention (IPEK), Pettenkoferstr 9, Ludwig-Maximilians University Munich, 80336 Munich, Germany*
[b]*Department of Medical Biochemistry, Experiment Vascular Biology, Academic Medical Center(AMC), University of Amsterdam, M05 AZ, Amsterdam, The Netherlands*
norbert.gerdes@med.uni-muenchen.de, e.lutgens@amc.uva.uc

15.1 Introduction

Atherosclerosis is a chronic inflammatory disease of the large arteries that is characterized by the accumulation of immune cells, lipids, and calcification in the artery wall. Although it starts out as an asymptomatic disease, atherosclerosis is the most common underlying cause of cardiovascular diseases, including myocardial infarction, stroke, and peripheral arterial disease.[1,2]

In histology, the initial stages of atherosclerosis are characterized by accumulations of lipid-loaded macrophages, foam cells that form the so-called intimal xanthoma. Later, more inflammatory cells infiltrate in the arterial wall, cells start dying, and extracellular matrix is formed. A so called "fibrous cap atheroma" has formed.

Atherosclerosis: Treatment and Prevention
Edited by Christian Weber and Oliver Soehnlein

ISBN 978-981-4316-26-2 (Hardcover), ISBN 978-981-4364-26-3 (eBook)
www.panstanford.com

Atherosclerotic plaques have a propensity to become symptomatic when they contain a high amount of inflammatory cells and have low levels of extracellular matrix, the "thin fibrous cap atheromas". This plaque-stage is prone to "plaque rupture". Rupture of an atherosclerotic plaque exposes its thrombogenic components to the blood and results in thrombosis and often in acute occlusion of the respective artery.[3]

From an immunologic point of view, atherosclerosis starts with the retention and modification of low-density lipoproteins in the artery wall. These lipids activate endothelial cells and attract monocytes and macrophages that produce adhesion molecules and chemokines. In parallel, intimal DCs become activated and T-, B-, NK-, NKT-, and mast cells become attracted to the lesion, resulting in activation of both the innate and adaptive immune system.[2] Recent insights have shown that the immune reaction in atherosclerosis is a cause of autoreactivity against apoB100, a component of LDL. ApoB-reactive T-cell clones that escape thymic education are kept non-reactive by peripheral tolerance mechanisms. However, when LDL accumulates in the arterial wall, it undergoes modifications that cause inflammation and presentation of apoB100 epitopes by APCs, resulting in the activation of ApoB100 reactive T cells and thereby initiating the chronic inflammatory response that contributes to atherogenesis.[4]

Within the plaque, the interactions between different immune cells and their bidirectional signaling define the inflammatory activity.[5] These interactions also mediate the fate and function of different T-lymphocyte subsets, such as Th1 (producing TNFα, IL-1, IFNγ, IL-12), Th2 (producing IL-4, IL-5, IL-10), Tregs (regulatory T cells; producing TGFβ, IL-10), and Th17 (producing IL-17, IL-6, IL-23), which were shown to minutely regulate immune responses in the plaque. The Th1 response is generally pro-atherogenic, while Th2 and Th17 responses were reported to have either pro- or anti-atherogenic effects, whereas regulatory T cells exert clear anti-atherogenic functions.[6] Polarization of naïve T cells into effector T cells is regulated by interaction with antigen presenting cells (APCs: DCs, macrophages, B-lymphocytes), both in the plaque and in lymphoid organs. Upon interaction with APCs, naïve T cells undergo clonal expansion and differentiate into effector T cells. Moreover, APCs undergo maturation and start producing cytokines such as IL-10, IL-12, and TGFβ.[5]

Antigen-dependent activation of naïve T cells and their differentiation into pro-atherogenic effector T cells are strongly induced by *co-stimulation* and regulated by *co-inhibition*. Most of the co-stimulatory and co-inhibitory molecules belong to either the B7[7] or TNF[8] superfamilies. Not surprisingly, many of the known co-stimulatory and co-inhibitory receptor-ligand pairs are expressed in atherosclerotic lesions,[9,10] and all affect atherogenesis in various ways. In the next section, we will provide an overview of the different co-stimulatory receptor-ligand dyads and their role in the pathogenesis of atherosclerosis.

15.2 The B7-Family

The B7-CD28 superfamily is the primary group of co-stimulatory molecules involved in T cell co-stimulatory and coinhibitory processes. The B7 superfamily comprises the following receptor-ligand pairs: CD28/CTLA-4:CD80/CD86, ICOS:ICOSL, and PD:PDL1/PDL2. In addition, there are two members of the B7 superfamily of which no human receptors have been identified: B7-H3 and B7-H4. Pathways that are initiated by the B7:CD28 family play key roles in regulating T cell activation and tolerance. These pathways not only provide critical positive second signals that promote and sustain T cell responses but also contribute critical negative second signals that downregulate T cell responses. These negative signals function to limit, terminate, and/or attenuate T cell responses, and they appear to be especially important for regulating T cell tolerance and autoimmunity, and consequently, also in atherosclerosis.[7]

15.2.1 B7.1/2- CD28/CTLA4

The first co-stimulatory molecules ever described were B7.1 (CD80) and B7.2 (CD86). When binding to their receptor CD28, T-cell activation and survival is promoted, whereas binding to the co-inhibitory receptor cytotoxic T-lymphocyte-associated antigen CTLA-4 inhibits T-cell responses and regulates peripheral T-cell tolerance.[11] CTLA-4 constitutes a T cell-intrinsic control mechanism as it competes with CD28 for the ligands B7.1/2 without activating the T cells.

Interestingly, monocyte-derived DCs of patients suffering from cardiovascular disease displayed an increased expression of B7.1 and B7.2.[12] Moreover, in the human atherosclerotic plaque, B7.1 and B7.2 were found to be present on a small proportion of T cells, macrophages, and other APCs and were associated with plaque inflammation.[9,10] In hypercholesterolemic mice, expression of B7.1/2 was increased in the spleen and B7.1/2 and CD28 were found in T cells, DCs, and macrophages in the atherosclerotic plaque, irrespective of plaque stage.[13,14]

Deficiency of B7-1 and B7-2 resulted in a protection against graft arterial disease in MHCII-mismatched allograft hearts.[15] In an experimental model for atherosclerosis, *B7.1/2*$^{-/-}$*Ldlr*$^{-/-}$ mice developed less atherosclerosis when studied after 8 or 20 weeks of high fat/cholesterol diet. At both time points, the amount of MHCII^{-} expressing cells in their atherosclerotic plaques was reduced, and CD4^{+} effector T cells of spleen and lymph nodes of *B7.1/2*$^{-/-}$*Ldlr*$^{-/-}$ mice produced less IFNγ,[14] suggesting that the B7.1/2-CD28 system regulates atherosclerosis by priming T cells.

Surprisingly, different results were obtained when *B7-1/2*$^{-/-}$ bone marrow was given to irradiated *Ldlr*$^{-/-}$ mice. Chimeric *B7-1/2*$^{-/-}$*Ldlr*$^{-/-}$ mice developed more atherosclerosis, a discrepancy potentially explained by several phenomena. Upon bone marrow transplantation, there is lymphopenia, and T cell proliferation is less dependent on co-stimulation.[16] In addition, Treg development relies on the B7.1/2-CD28 axis.[16] Consequently, the *B7-1/2*$^{-/-}$*Ldlr*$^{-/-}$ chimeras hardly had any Tregs, thereby promoting inflammation and atherosclerosis.

For CD28 and CTLA4, less data are available. In human atherosclerotic plaques, both CD28 and CTLA4 can be detected on a small amount of T cells.[9] Gene expression analysis of human atherosclerotic plaques revealed that both CD28 and CTLA4 are part of the indoleamine 2,3-dioxygenase (IDO)-related gene pathway, a pathway known to be involved in T cell suppression.[17]

Similar to the *B7-1/2*$^{-/-}$*Ldlr*$^{-/-}$ chimeras, *Cd28*$^{-/-}$*Ldlr*$^{-/-}$ chimeras developed more atherosclerosis, most likely due to the lack of regulatory T cells.[16] Long-term blocking of CTLA4 in an allograft rejection model prevented intimal thickening.[18] Furthermore, administration of recombinant CTLA4, which disrupts B7/CD28 signaling and is commonly used to treat rheumatoid arthritis, also prevents experimental hypertension.[19] However, no data are currently available on the functional role of CTLA4 in atherosclerosis.

15.2.2 ICOS-ICOSL

Another member of the CD28/B7-co-stimulatory molecule family is the inducible co-stimulatory molecule (ICOS) and its ligand ICOS-L. ICOS is not present on naïve $CD4^+$ cells but is induced upon T-cell activation on $CD4^+$ effector T cells[20] where it supports T-cell proliferation and Th2 polarization.[21–23] ICOS is also constitutively expressed on Tregs, thereby exerting a dual role in immune-modulation.[24] In human and murine atherosclerotic plaques, ICOS and ICOS-L are abundantly present on T cells, macrophages, and APCs.[9,10,25] Remarkably, monocyte-derived DCs of patients suffering from coronary artery disease displayed enhanced expression of ICOS.[17] In the spleen, constitutive expression of ICOS decreased in atherosclerotic mice. However, ICOS expression of splenocytes increased dose-dependently after priming with oxLDL.[25] In atherosclerosis *in vivo*, reducing ICOS activity by either immunization against ICOS in *Apoe*$^{-/-}$ mice or by transplanting bone marrow of *Icos*$^{-/-}$ mice into *Ldlr*$^{-/-}$ mice aggravated atherosclerosis.[25,26] Inhibition of ICOS in atherosclerosis resulted in increased activation of $CD4^+$ T cells, which produced high amounts of Th1 and Th2 cytokines, which could be due to the decrease in Tregs in absence of ICOS.[26] Accordingly, promoting ICOS activity could provide a useful strategy for prevention of atherosclerosis.

15.2.3 PD-PDL1/2

Programmed death-ligand 1 (PD-L1) and 2 (PD-L2) are co-inhibitory molecules of the B7 family.[27] They are expressed on several cell types, such as T cells, B cells, DCs, and macrophages, and their interaction with the PD-receptor on T cells suppresses activation.[28] As expected, deficiency of PD-L1 and PD-L2 in mice aggravated atherosclerotic plaque formation. Plaques contained increased numbers of $CD4^+$ and $CD8^+$ T cells. In lymphoid organs of *Pdl1/2*$^{-/-}$*Ldlr*$^{-/-}$ mice, $CD4^+$ T cells were abundantly present, and *in vitro*, PD-L1/2 deficient APCs showed in increased capability to activate $CD4^+$ T cells.[29]

In patients suffering from coronary artery disease, the expression of PD-1 and PD-L1 on circulating T cells and myeloid DCs was significantly decreased and was correlated to increased T cell immune responses in these patients.[30]

PD-L1 and PD-L2 seem to play a crucial role in controlling the immune response in atherosclerosis, thereby exerting a protective effect.

Experimental work verified a role for the B7 superfamily in atherosclerosis. However, the different members of this family affect atherosclerosis in opposite ways. Inhibition of the co-stimulatory molecule B7 and CD28 can aggravate or reduce atherosclerosis in different settings, and ICOS deficiency, unexpectedly, induces atherosclerosis, although it is involved in T cell activation. In addition, the role of several of the B7 superfamily members like CTLA4, B7-H3, and B7-H4 in atherosclerosis is not addressed yet.

Nonetheless, the data that are available illustrates the complex interplay of the co-stimulatory molecules of the B7 superfamily with the different immune cells. How members of the B7 superfamily interact, how they affect the immune system, and which signal transduction cascades are key in atherosclerosis still need to be elucidated.

15.3 The TNF-TNF-Receptor Superfamily

The TNF-TNFR superfamily is the second largest family of co-stimulatory molecules. To date, the family contains 19 ligands and 30 receptors of which OX40L:OX40; CD40L:CD40; CD137:CD137L; CD27:CD70; glucocorticoid-induced TNF-R like protein (GITR):GITRL and LIGHT;LTβR are the most common.

Although the primary function of the TNF(R) superfamily is to regulate cell survival, members of this family have also proven to positively regulate T cell responses and cross-talk of T cells with other cell-types, thereby inducing activation of the immune system.[8] Many of the family members have an important role in atherosclerosis.[31]

15.3.1 OX40L-OX40

OX40 ligand (TNFSF4) was first discovered in 1987 and was found to be expressed on activated $CD4^+$ T cells.[32] Now, Ox40(L) is known to strongly regulate conventional $CD4^+$ and $CD8^+$ T cells and is also able to modulate NK and NKT cell function and mediate crosstalk between APCs, mast cells, smooth muscle cells, and endothelial cells.[33]

Its association with cardiovascular disease was first discovered in the 1980s when a study determined the susceptibility to atherosclerosis of 10 different inbred mouse strains.[34] Genetic mapping identified the first atherosclerosis susceptibility locus *ath1*, which was later refined to a 0.66 cM region on chromosome 1.[35] One of the genes present in this locus was Ox40L.

Interestingly, in humans, a single nucleotide polymorphism (SNP) in the first intron of Ox40L and haplotypes consisting of a SNP upstream of exon 1 and two SNPs in the intron of Ox40L were associated with risk of myocardial infarction and coronary artery disease.[36] In addition, T-lymphocytes of patients suffering from acute coronary syndromes have increased expression of the Ox40-OX40L system,[37] and elevation of soluble OX40 ligand in serum was a prognostic indicator for recurrent cardiovascular events.[38]

OX40L appeared to be abundantly expressed in immune cells of mouse atherosclerotic lesions. Deficiency of Ox40L made C57Bl6 mice less susceptible for atherosclerosis, while mice over-expressing OX40L have accelerated atherosclerosis.[35,36] In an additional study, inhibition of OX40L in atherosclerotic Ldlr$^{-/-}$ mice using a blocking antibody also resulted in a 53% decrease in plaque area, which was associated with inhibition of IL4-induced Th2 isotype switching and an increased level of anti-oxLDL IgM.[39] OX40L and OX40 are not only promising biomarkers for the occurrence of cardiovascular disease, they are also potential therapeutic targets to reduce atherosclerosis.

15.3.2 CD40L-CD40

CD40 (TNFRSF5) and CD40L (TNFSF5) show homology to Ox40L and Ox40 and were discovered around the same time. The CD40L (CD154)-CD40 pathway is a special co-stimulatory dyad. It is not strictly a mediator of T-cell co-stimulation but functions mainly to activate APCs by T cells. Then, CD40 signaling in the APC induces the expression of other co-stimulatory molecules and, thus, also activates T cells.[37,40] Interestingly, the expression of CD40L is not restricted to T cells and the expression of CD40 is not confined to the APC, suggesting functions of the CD40L-CD40 dyad other than mere co-stimulation.[41,42]

The CD40L-CD40 dyad is one of the best-described co-stimulatory molecule pair in the pathogenesis of atherosclerosis. In the mid 1990s, it was found that both CD40L and CD40 are expressed on the vast majority of immune cells (T- and B-lymphocytes, macrophages, DCs, neutrophils, and mast cells) and non-immune cells (e.g., ECs and VSMCs) present in the plaque, as well as on monocytes and platelets in the circulation.[42–44] Both CD40L and CD40 are already expressed in early stages of atherosclerosis, in fatty streak lesions. Their expression increases with plaque progression and is highest in the "thin fibrous cap atheroma" and "ruptured plaque".[44]

In the late 1990s, the functional importance of CD40L in atherosclerosis became clear. In 1998, Mach et al. showed in hyperlipidemic *Ldlr*$^{-/-}$ mice that treatment with an anti-CD40L antibody significantly reduced the size and lipid content of aortic atherosclerotic lesions.[45] In 1999, it was shown that *Cd40l*$^{-/-}$*Apoe*$^{-/-}$ mice exhibited a 5.5-fold decrease in plaque area[46] and that these mice displayed a remarkable plaque phenotype. Advanced atherosclerotic plaques of *Cd40l*$^{-/-}$*Apoe*$^{-/-}$ mice contained increased amounts of collagen and SMC, while plaque lipid levels and the number of inflammatory cells were strongly reduced.[46] These plaques resemble clinically favorable, stable plaques in humans. In a follow-up study, an antagonizing anti-CD40L antibody was administered to *Apoe*$^{-/-}$ mice on normal chow diet, either at the onset of atherosclerosis or when established atherosclerotic lesions were present, as the equivalent for the situation in patients. In both treatment groups, anti-CD40L antibody treatment did not result in a decrease in plaque area but resulted in the development of lipid-poor, collagen-rich, stable plaques.[47] Schonbeck et al. showed similar results with a different anti-CD40L antibody (M158, Immunex) in *Ldlr*$^{-/-}$ mice that consumed a high fat diet.[48] Transplantation of *Cd40l*$^{-/-}$ bone marrow into *Ldlr*$^{-/-}$ mice did not significantly alter atherosclerosis.[49,50] Interestingly, repeated administration of *Cd40L*$^{-/-}$ platelets in *Apoe*$^{-/-}$ mice did prevent the accelerated atherosclerosis that is induced by administration of wild type plateletsz.[51]

Besides the membrane-associated form, CD40L also exists in a truncated soluble form, sCD40L, which is cleaved from the CD40L protein upon activation, especially in platelets.[52] Numerous studies have proven sCD40L to be a useful biomarker for cardiovascular disease severity. Elevated levels of sCD40L have been associated with hypercholesterolemia, diabetes, ischemic stroke, and acute coronary syndromes and predict increased restenosis after percutaneous coronary and carotid interventions.[53–58]

For CD40, the receptor for CD40L, the results are contradictory. In *Cd40$^{-/-}$Apoe$^{-/-}$* mice, atherosclerosis was decreased, and plaques that contained only few inflammatory cells and an increased level of fibrosis were observed. The phenotype was due to CD40 expressing haematopoietic cells, since bone marrow transplantation of *Cd40$^{-/-}$* bone marrow into irradiated *Ldlr$^{/-}$* recipients resulted in similar results.[59] Zirlik et al. reported that *Cd40$^{-/-}$Ldlr$^{-/-}$* mice do not have any changes in atherosclerosis and claims that CD40 is not the only receptor for CD40L, but that CD40L can interact with the integrin Mac-1.[60]

The mechanisms and pathways as well as the interacting cell-types that modulate CD40L-CD40 signaling in vascular biology are still under investigation, but many *in vitro* studies have provided insights into how CD40L-CD40 interactions affect atherosclerosis.[61] CD40L-CD40 endothelial-leukocyte interactions mediate expression of chemokines and adhesion molecules, thereby affecting leukocyte adhesion and diapedesis.[62,63] Platelet-monocyte CD40L-CD40 interactions facilitate leukocyte recruitment and induce the expression of cytokines, whereas platelet CD40L affects platelet aggregation.[51] Activation of CD40-CD40L interactions seems to polarize T cells towards the pro-atherogenic Th1 phenotype, and CD40 is an important player in the activation of classically activated macrophages and DCs, which upon activation release a plethora of pro-atherogenic chemokines and cytokines.[59]

CD40-CD40L interactions, thus, play a crucial role in the development and progression of atherosclerosis, are involved in the many different aspects of the disease, and constitute promising biomarkers for cardiovascular disease.

15.3.3 CD137-CD137L

CD137, also known as TNFRSF9 or 4-1BB, is mainly expressed by activated CD8$^+$ and to a lesser degree CD4$^+$ T cells.[64] In addition, CD137 is found on DC, NK cells, and granulocytes. Engagement of CD137 by CD137 ligand (CD137L), which is constitutively expressed by monocytes, DC, and B cells, leads to signaling through TRAF2 and activation of NFκB.[65] In T cells, such signaling enhances proliferation, IL-2 secretion, and cytolytic activity.

Olofsson and coworkers recently demonstrated expression of CD137 not only on immune cells of atherosclerotic lesions but also in vascular EC and SMC.[66] *In vitro*, these cells responded to ligation of CD137 by enhanced expression of adhesion molecules and decreased proliferation, respectively.

Although treatment of *Apoe*$^{-/-}$ mice with a CD137-activating antibody increased atherosclerotic lesion size only marginally, plaque phenotype changed substantially. Indeed, T cell infiltration, mainly of CD8^{+} cells, and aortic expression of inflammatory mediators such as adhesion molecules and cytokines increased dramatically.[66] Genetic deficiency of CD137 in both *Apoe*$^{-/-}$ and *Ldlr*$^{-/-}$ mice confirmed its pro-atherogenic role.[67] Interestingly, administration of recombinant soluble CD137 to hyperlipidemic, *Cd137*$^{-/-}$ mice resulted in enhanced inflammatory response within the aorta suggesting reverse signaling through CD137L, although such mechanisms are controversial.[67] Notably, patients with ACS or UA have higher levels of soluble and leukocyte-bound CD137, corroborating a pro-atherogenic function of this co-stimulatory molecule.[68]

15.3.4 CD70-CD27

While CD70 (TNFSF7) is transiently expressed on activated T cells, B cells, and DCs, its receptor CD27 (TNFRSF7) is mainly found on T cells, although regulated rather dynamically.[69] Functional interaction of this co-stimulatory pair is required for generation and long-term maintenance of T cell immune responses.[64] Continuous stimulation of CD27 through over-expression of CD70 on B cells leads to an expansion of Th1-polarized T cells in mice. Unexpectedly, despite the potentially pro-atherogenic phenotype, this experimental setup led to protection from atherosclerosis.[70] This discrepancy may be explained through a decreased survival of monocytic cells in these mice, although further research is certainly needed to clarify the relevance of CD27-CD70 interaction in atherosclerosis.

15.3.5 GITR/GITRL

Glucocorticoid-induced TNF receptor-related protein (GITR; TNFRSF 18) and its ligand, GITRL (TNFSF18), are also members of the TNF (R) superfamily.[71] GITR is expressed by several cells and tissues, including T- and NK cells, and is activated by its ligand, GITRL, which is mainly expressed on APCs and ECs.[72] The GITR-GITRL axis affects both innate and adaptive immunity and is pivotal in mediating inflammatory responses. Upon activation of GITR-GITRL interactions several concurrent processes are initiated, including co-activation of effector T cells and NK cells, inhibition of Tregs, activation of macrophages, and modulation of DC function.[73]

GITR co-stimulation induces expression of IFNγ and IL-2 and T cell activation markers.[73] Interestingly, GITR triggering also inhibits Treg suppression and mediates their expansion.[72] Remarkably, GITR also modulates DC activity, for example, by regulating IL-12 production.[74]

In *in vivo* models, deficiency of GITR prevents pancreatitis,[75] diabetes,[76] shock,[77] arthritis[78] and inflammatory bowel disease, pleurisy, and bleomycin-induced lung fibrosis.[79]

Until now, the role of GITR in cardiovascular disease is poorly characterized. GITR is known to stimulate macrophages to produce NFκB, TNFα, and MMP9 and is, therefore, considered pro-atherogenic.[80] Moreover, $GITR^+$ (regulatory) T cells and $GITR^+$ macrophages were found to be present in human atherosclerotic plaques.[10]

Consideringtheabovedescribedeffectsof GITR-GITRLinteractions in inflammation, particularly on T cell and macrophage activation, a profound role for the GITR-GITRL system in atherosclerosis is fairly conceivable.

15.3.6 LIGHT

LIGHT (TNFSF14) is, after lymphotoxin β, the second ligand for HVEM (TNFRSF14).[81] Human carotid atherosclerotic plaques express high levels of LIGHT in regions rich in macrophages and foam cells.[82] In atheroma-associated cell types such as ECs and macrophages, LIGHT leads to expression of pro-inflammatory factors, including adhesion molecules, chemokines, and matrix metalloproteinases.[82,83] These mechanisms are partly mediated by proteinase-activated receptor (PAR)-2, suggesting a link between inflammatory cells and the hemostatic system.[84] In addition, LIGHT and lymphotoxin β seem to be critical factors in regulating lipid metabolism in liver.[85] Supporting this notion, LIGHT is released from activated platelets and concentrations are elevated in the serum of patients with ACS.[84] Nonetheless, no studies have directly addressed the role of LIGHT in experimental models of atherosclerosis using either gene-deficiency or specific inhibition *in vivo*.

15.4 TRAF Signaling

The members of the TNF-R family use the TNF-R associated factor (TRAF) adaptor proteins to exert signaling, which mostly results in activation of the canonical and/or non-canonical NFκB pathway. TRAF adaptor molecules are also known to be crucial in TLR and IL-1 signaling. There are six different TRAF family members, of which five can bind to the TNFR family members. The TRAF-protein family is composed of six members and is characterized by a conserved 180 amino acid fold, the TRAF domain (TD), which supports the interaction between the TNF-receptor and its downstream signaling intermediates. The C-terminus of the TRAF-domain mediates homo- and hetero-dimerization with other TRAF-proteins and the receptor that recruits them.[86]

In cardiovascular diseases, TRAF proteins play a significant role. TRAF1, 2, 3, 5, and 6 can be detected in primary ECs, SMCs, and macrophages upon stimulation with inflammatory cytokines.[87] In the human non-diseased arterial wall, TRAF-1, -2, -3, -5, and -6 are barely detectable, whereas in atherosclerotic plaques of humans and mice, all TRAFS are clearly observed, especially in macrophages, SMCs, and ECs.[87] Interestingly, TRAF1, 2, 3, 5, and 6 are differentially modulated in the different cell types and upon the different stimuli. In ECs, TRAF1 deficiency enhances CD40L or TNFα-induced IL6 and MCP-1 expression, whereas TRAF2 and TRAF5 deficiency inhibit IL6, but not MCP-1 expression. Interestingly, in macrophages, TRAF2 and/or TRAF5 deficiency did not affect CD40L or TNFα-induced expression at all.[87]

In blood of patients suffering from coronary artery disease, mRNA levels of TRAF1 were significantly elevated, whereas TRAF5 had decreased in the blood of patients with acute coronary syndromes and TRAF6 levels were not affected.[88–90]

Not surprisingly, the different TRAF molecules have differential effects on atherogenesis. Deficiency of TRAF1 in atherosclerotic mice strongly reduces atherosclerosis, particularly by inhibiting monocyte recruitment into the arterial wall.[88] Deficiency of TRAF5 aggravated atherosclerosis, especially by enhancing monocyte migration into the arterial wall and by reducing the number of regulatory T cells.[89] Surprisingly, deficiency of TRAF2 or TRAF6 did not affect atherosclerosis.[90]

Since the different TRAF molecules can not only bind TNFR1 family members but also mediate TLR signaling and IL1 signaling, a more detailed analysis of TNFR-family member-TRAF interactions is needed.

15.4.1 CD40-TRAF Signaling in Cardiovascular Disease

So far, the only TNF-R family member for which the effects of the different TRAF interactions on vascular disease have been described is CD40. Like the other TNF-R family members, CD40 lacks intrinsic signaling activity and recruits TRAFs upon activation. The cytoplasmic domain of CD40 has a proximal TRAF-6 binding site and a more distal TRAF-2/3/5 binding site. The TRAF-2/3/5 binding site is most often occupied by TRAF-2 and TRAF-3. TRAF-1 only binds to CD40 when CD40-signaling is already active. It can bind to the TRAF-2/3/5 binding site and replaces or hetero-dimerizes with TRAF-2 and acts as a regulator rather than an activator of CD40 signaling.[91] Whether TRAF-5 directly or indirectly binds to the TRAF-2/3/5 binding domain is still under debate. TRAF5 was found to bind CD40 directly in a yeast 2⁻ hybrid study.[92] However, more recent studies state that TRAF-5 is only able to bind to CD40 via TRAF-3/TRAF-5 heterodimers.[86] Recently, a second TRAF-2 binding site on CD40 was identified, that appeared functional in mediating B cell activation, proliferation, and differentiation.[93] Until now, TRAF-6 is the only protein able to bind the TRAF-6 binding site of CD40.[86]

When TRAF proteins bind to the cytoplasmic tail of CD40, multiple signaling cascades, including NFκB, C-Jun N-terminal kinase (JNK), and p38 mitogen-activated protein (MAP) kinase pathways, can be activated.[86] Which one that will be, depends on the TRAF family member that binds, on the cell-type that is activated, and on the conditions that are present.

For example, in B-lymphocytes, CD40-TRAF-6 interactions are required for CD40-mediated IgM production, IL-6 secretion, and isotype switching, whereas the TRAF-2/3/5 binding site is required for CD40-mediated upregulation of B7 and protection from B cell antigen-receptor mediated growth arrest.[94] Moreover, both binding domains also seem to exert cell type⁻ specific actions.

This is also true for the cell-types present in atherosclerotic plaques. In monocytes and macrophages, the interaction between CD40 and TRAF-6 is crucial for the activation of Src/ERK1/2 and IKK/NFκB pro-inflammatory pathways, while CD40-TRAF2/3/5 interactions are not required for induction of inflammation.[95] However, in ECs and SMCs, TRAF-2 mediates the activation of pro-inflammatory pathways.[96] Interestingly, during shear stress, TRAF-3 inhibits CD40-signaling, thereby preventing recruitment of inflammatory cells into the arterial wall.[97]

To obtain insights which CD40-TRAF interactions are required in vascular biology, we used mice carrying a CD40 transgene with targeted mutations at the CD40-TRAF2/3/5, CD40-TRAF6, or CD40-TRAF2/3/5/6 recognition site. In a model of carotid neointima formation, we found that deficiency in CD40-TRAF6 and CD40-TRAF2/3/5/6 signaling, but not CD40-TRAF2/3/5 signaling, resulted in a strong decrease in neointima formation, indicating that CD40-TRAF6 signaling is specifically required for arterial neointima formation.[98] CD40-TRAF6 signaling was required for inflammatory cell infiltration and collagen turnover in the neointima. In a subsequent study, we examined the role of the different CD40-TRAF interactions in atherosclerosis. Here, we observed that deficiency of CD40-TRAF6 signaling, but not of CD40-TRAF2/3/5 signaling, almost prevented the development of atherosclerosis. This was particularly due to a decrease in the Ly6C^{high} monocyte population, which did not migrate into the arterial wall. The CD40-TRAF2/3/5/6$^{-/-}$ mice had an intermediated phenotype.[59] These data unveil a clear bifurcation of CD40-signaling in vascular biology with a role for CD40-TRAF6 but not CD40-TRAF2/3/5 interactions in vascular biology and establish that targeting specific components of the CD40L-CD40 pathway *in vivo* harbors the potential to achieve therapeutic effects in atherosclerosis.

15.5 Conclusion

As for the B7 superfamily, there is a clear role for members of the TNF and TNF-R superfamily in atherosclerosis. Again, the different members of this family affect atherosclerosis in opposite ways, and there seems to be an intricate interplay between the different members of this family. However, inhibition of the TNF(-R) superfamily members mostly results in a decrease of atherosclerosis, unless regulatory T-cell function is diminished.

15.6 Perspectives

Co-stimulatory molecules are powerful agents that modulate the immune system towards either pro- or anti-inflammatory actions. In cardiovascular disease, numerous clinical and laboratory studies have provided evidence that co-stimulatory molecules can be used as biomarkers and play a crucial role in the pathogenesis of neointima formation and atherosclerosis. Since total inhibition of respective co-stimulatory molecule family members is likely to induce immune suppression or over-activation of the immune system, the use of co-stimulatory molecules as therapeutic targets should be considered with care. Interestingly, signal transduction cascades initiated by the different co-stimulatory molecules seem rather cell-type specific and also depend on the pathology involved. Although most of these specific signal transduction pathways still need to be revealed, they provide strong therapeutic targets. One imminent example is the CD40-TRAF pathway. While CD40-TRAF2/3/5 signaling in $MHCII^-$ expressing cell types seems not to affect atherosclerosis, disruption of CD40-TRAF6 interactions in $MHCII^+$ cells results in a strong reduction of atherosclerosis in a laboratory model.[59] On the other hand, disruption of all TRAF6 signaling has no effect on atherosclerosis whatsoever.[90] This nicely illustrates the requirement for further research for the cell- and disease type-specific signal transduction cascades of the co-stimulatory molecules. When revealed, these signal transduction molecules will prove to be excellent and specific therapeutic targets for inflammatory diseases, including atherosclerosis. Ideally, they will modulate the immune system without causing massive side effects, since most of the immune system will remain intact. However, although intervening in this co-stimulatory pathway yields interesting opportunities for treatment of atherosclerosis, caution should be applied and unexpected, potential pro-inflammatory side effects should be monitored carefully.

References

1. Hansson GK, Libby P. The immune response in atherosclerosis: a double-edged sword. *Nat Rev Immunol* 2006;6(7): 508–519.
2. Hansson GK, Hermansson A. The immune system in atherosclerosis. *Nat Immunol* 2011;12(3): 204–212.
3. Virmani R, Kolodgie FD, Burke AP, Farb A, Schwartz SM. Lessons from sudden coronary death: a comprehensive morphological classification scheme for atherosclerotic lesions. *Arterioscler Thromb Vasc Biol* 2000;20(5): 1262–1275.
4. Hermansson A, Ketelhuth DF, Strodthoff D, Wurm M, Hansson EM, Nicoletti A, Paulsson-Berne G, Hansson GK. Inhibition of T cell response to native low-density lipoprotein reduces atherosclerosis. *J Exp Med* 2010; 207(5): 1081–1093.
5. Galkina E, Ley K. Immune and inflammatory mechanisms of atherosclerosis. *Annu Rev Immunol* 2009;27: 165–197.
6. Kuiper J, van Puijvelde GH, van Wanrooij EJ, van Es T, Habets K, Hauer AD, van den Berkel TJ. Immunomodulation of the inflammatory response in atherosclerosis. *Curr Opin Lipidol* 2007;18(5): 521–526.
7. Leitner J, Grabmeier-Pfistershammer K, Steinberger P. Receptors and ligands implicated in human T cell costimulatory processes. *Immunol Lett* 2010;128(2): 89–97.
8. Croft M. The role of TNF superfamily members in T-cell function and diseases. *Nat Rev Immunol* 2009;9(4): 271–285.
9. de Boer OJ, Hirsch F, van der Wal AC, van der Loos CM, Das PK, Becker AE. Costimulatory molecules in human atherosclerotic plaques: an indication of antigen specific T lymphocyte activation. *Atherosclerosis* 1997;133(2): 227–234.
10. Kim WJ, Kang YJ, Suk K, Park JE, Kwon BS, Lee WH. Comparative analysis of the expression patterns of various TNFSF/TNFRSF in atherosclerotic plaques. *Immunol Invest* 2008;37(4): 359–373.
11. Zang X, Allison JP. The B7 family and cancer therapy: costimulation and coinhibition. *Clin Cancer Res* 2007;13(18 Pt 1): 5271–5279.
12. Dopheide JF, Sester U, Schlitt A, Horstick G, Rupprecht HJ, Munzel T, Blankenberg S. Monocyte-derived dendritic cells of patients with coronary artery disease show an increased expression of costimulatory molecules CD40, CD80 and CD86 *in vitro*. *Coron Artery Dis* 2007;18(7): 523–531.

13. Lee TS, Yen HC, Pan CC, Chau LY. The role of interleukin 12 in the development of atherosclerosis in ApoE-deficient mice. *Arterioscler Thromb Vasc Biol* 1999;19(3): 734–742.

14. Buono C, Pang H, Uchida Y, Libby P, Sharpe AH, Lichtman AH. B7-1/B7-2 costimulation regulates plaque antigen-specific T-cell responses and atherogenesis in low-density lipoprotein receptor-deficient mice. *Circulation* 2004;109(16): 2009–2015.

15. Furukawa Y, Mandelbrot DA, Libby P, Sharpe AH, Mitchell RN. Association of B7-1 co-stimulation with the development of graft arterial disease. Studies using mice lacking B7-1, B7-2, or B7-1/B7-2. *Am J Pathol* 2000;157(2): 473–484.

16. Ait-Oufella H, Salomon BL, Potteaux S, Robertson AK, Gourdy P, Zoll J, Merval R, Esposito B, Cohen JL, Fisson S, Flavell RA, Hansson GK, Klatzmann D, Tedgui A, Mallat Z. Natural regulatory T cells control the development of atherosclerosis in mice. *Nat Med* 2006;12(2): 178–180.

17. Niinisalo P, Oksala N, Levula M, Pelto-Huikko M, Jarvinen O, Salenius JP, Kytomaki L, Soini JT, Kahonen M, Laaksonen R, Hurme M, Lehtimaki T. Activation of indoleamine 2,3-dioxygenase-induced tryptophan degradation in advanced atherosclerotic plaques: tampere vascular study. *Ann Med* 2010;42(1): 55–63.

18. Yan S, Zhang Q, Cai M, Yu D, Chen J, Yu P, Zhao Q, Zhou L, Hoffmann M, Zheng S. A novel model of portal vein transplantation in mice using two-cuff technique. *Microsurgery* 2007;27(6): 569–574.

19. Vinh A, Chen W, Blinder Y, Weiss D, Taylor WR, Goronzy JJ, Weyand CM, Harrison DG, Guzik TJ. Inhibition and genetic ablation of the B7/CD28 T-cell costimulation axis prevents experimental hypertension *Circulation* 2010;122(24): 2529–2537.

20. Dong C, Juedes AE, Temann UA, Shresta S, Allison JP, Ruddle NH, Flavell RA. ICOS co-stimulatory receptor is essential for T-cell activation and function. *Nature* 2001;409(6816): 97–101.

21. Vieira PL, Wassink L, Smith LM, Nam S, Kingsbury GA, Gutierrez-Ramos JC, Coyle AJ, Kapsenberg ML, Wierenga EA. ICOS-mediated signaling regulates cytokine production by human T cells and provides a unique signal to selectively control the clonal expansion of Th2 helper cells. *Eur J Immunol* 2004;34(5): 1282–1290.

22. Nurieva RI, Duong J, Kishikawa H, Dianzani U, Rojo JM, Ho I, Flavell RA, Dong C. Transcriptional regulation of th2 differentiation by inducible costimulator. *Immunity* 2003;18(6): 801–811.

23. Lohning M, Hutloff A, Kallinich T, Mages HW, Bonhagen K, Radbruch A, Hamelmann E, Kroczek RA. Expression of ICOS *in vivo* defines CD4+ effector T cells with high inflammatory potential and a strong bias for secretion of interleukin 10. *J Exp Med* 2003;197(2): 181–193.
24. Herman AE, Freeman GJ, Mathis D, Benoist C. CD4+CD25+ T regulatory cells dependent on ICOS promote regulation of effector cells in the prediabetic lesion. *J Exp Med* 2004;199(11): 1479–1489.
25. Afek A, Harats D, Roth A, Keren G, George J. A functional role for inducible costimulator (ICOS) in atherosclerosis. *Atherosclerosis* 2005;183(1): 57–63.
26. Gotsman I, Grabie N, Gupta R, Dacosta R, MacConmara M, Lederer J, Sukhova G, Witztum JL, Sharpe AH, Lichtman AH. Impaired regulatory T-cell response and enhanced atherosclerosis in the absence of inducible costimulatory molecule. *Circulation* 2006;114(19): 2047–2055.
27. Greenwald RJ, Freeman GJ, Sharpe AH. The B7 family revisited. *Annu Rev Immunol* 2005;23: 515–548.
28. Latchman Y, Wood CR, Chernova T, Chaudhary D, Borde M, Chernova I, Iwai Y, Long AJ, Brown JA, Nunes R, Greenfield EA, Bourque K, Boussiotis VA, Carter LL, Carreno BM, Malenkovich N, Nishimura H, Okazaki T, Honjo T, Sharpe AH, Freeman GJ. PD-L2 is a second ligand for PD-1 and inhibits T cell activation. *Nat Immunol* 2001;2(3): 261–268.
29. Gotsman I, Grabie N, Dacosta R, Sukhova G, Sharpe A, Lichtman AH. Proatherogenic immune responses are regulated by the PD-1/PD-L pathway in mice. *J Clin Invest* 2007;117(10): 2974–2982.
30. Lee J, Zhuang Y, Wei X, Shang F, Wang J, Zhang Y, Liu X, Yang Y, Liu L, Zheng Q. Contributions of PD-1/PD-L1 pathway to interactions of myeloid DCs with T cells in atherosclerosis. *J Mol Cell Cardiol* 2009;46(2): 169–176.
31. Aukrust P, Sandberg WJ, Otterdal K, Vinge LE, Gullestad L, Yndestad A, Halvorsen B, Ueland T. Tumor necrosis factor superfamily molecules in acute coronary syndromes. *Ann Med* 2011: 43(2): 90–103.
32. Paterson DJ, Jefferies WA, Green JR, Brandon MR, Corthesy P, Puklavec M, Williams AF. Antigens of activated rat T lymphocytes including a molecule of 50,000 Mr detected only on CD4 positive T blasts. *Mol Immunol* 1987;24(12): 1281–1290.
33. Croft M. Control of immunity by the TNFR-related molecule OX40 (CD134). *Annu Rev Immunol*2010;28: 57–78.

34. Paigen B, Morrow A, Brandon C, Mitchell D, Holmes P. Variation in susceptibility to atherosclerosis among inbred strains of mice. *Atherosclerosis* 1985;57(1): 65–73.

35. Paigen B, Mitchell D, Reue K, Morrow A, Lusis AJ, LeBoeuf RC. Ath-1, a gene determining atherosclerosis susceptibility and high density lipoprotein levels in mice. *Proc Natl Acad Sci U S A* 1987;84(11): 3763–3767.

36. Wang X, Ria M, Kelmenson PM, Eriksson P, Higgins DC, Samnegard A, Petros C, Rollins J, Bennet AM, Wiman B, de Faire U, Wennberg C, Olsson PG, Ishii N, Sugamura K, Hamsten A, Forsman-Semb K, Lagercrantz J, Paigen B. Positional identification of TNFSF4, encoding OX40 ligand, as a gene that influences atherosclerosis susceptibility. *Nat Genet* 2005;37(4): 365–372.

37. Yan J, Chen G, Gong J, Wang C, Du R. Upregulation of OX40-OX40 ligand system on T lymphocytes in patients with acute coronary syndromes. *J Cardiovasc Pharmacol* 2009;54(5): 451–455.

38. Yan J, Gong J, Chen G, Liu P, Wang C, Yang P. Evaluation of serum soluble OX40 ligand as a prognostic indicator in acute coronary syndrome patients. *Clin Chim Acta* 2010;411(21–22): 1662–1665.

39. van Wanrooij EJ, van Puijvelde GH, de Vos P, Yagita H, van Berkel TJ, Kuiper J. Interruption of the Tnfrsf4/Tnfsf4 (OX40/OX40L) pathway attenuates atherogenesis in low-density lipoprotein receptor-deficient mice. *Arterioscler Thromb Vasc Biol* 2007;27(1): 204–210.

40. Grewal IS, Flavell RA. CD40 and CD154 in cell-mediated immunity. *Annu Rev Immunol* 1998;16: 111–135.

41. Lutgens E, Lievens D, Beckers L, Donners M, Daemen M. CD40 and its ligand in atherosclerosis. *Trends Cardiovasc Med* 2007;17(4): 118–123.

42. Engel D, Seijkens T, Poggi M, Sanati M, Thevissen L, Beckers L, Wijnands E, Lievens D, Lutgens E. The immunobiology of CD154-CD40-TRAF interactions in atherosclerosis. *Semin Immunol* 2009;21(5): 308–312.

43. Schonbeck U, Libby P. CD40 signaling and plaque instability. *Circ Res* 2001;89(12): 1092–1103.

44. Lutgens E, Daemen MJ. CD40-CD40L Interactions in Atherosclerosis. *Trends Cardiovasc Med* 2002;12(1): 27–32.

45. Mach F, Schonbeck U, Sukhova GK, Atkinson E, Libby P. Reduction of atherosclerosis in mice by inhibition of CD40 signalling. *Nature* 1998;394(6689):200–203.

46. Lutgens E, Gorelik L, Daemen MJ, de Muinck ED, Grewal IS, Koteliansky VE, Flavell RA. Requirement for CD154 in the progression of atherosclerosis. *Nat Med* 1999;5(11): 1313–1316.

47. Lutgens E, Cleutjens KB, Heeneman S, Koteliansky VE, Burkly LC, Daemen MJ. Both early and delayed anti-CD40L antibody treatment induces a stable plaque phenotype. *Proc Natl Acad Sci U S A* 2000;97(13): 7464–7469.

48. Schonbeck U, Sukhova GK, Shimizu K, Mach F, Libby P. Inhibition of CD40 signaling limits evolution of established atherosclerosis in mice. *Proc Natl Acad Sci U S A* 2000;97(13): 7458–7463.

49. Smook ML, Heeringa P, Damoiseaux JG, Daemen MJ, de Winther MP, Gijbels MJ, Beckers L, Lutgens E, Cohen Tervaert JW. Leukocyte CD40L deficiency affects the CD25(+) CD4 T cell population but does not affect atherosclerosis. *Atherosclerosis* 2005;183(2): 275–282.

50. Bavendiek U, Zirlik A, LaClair S, MacFarlane L, Libby P, Schonbeck U. Atherogenesis in mice does not require CD40 ligand from bone marrow-derived cells. *Arterioscler Thromb Vasc Biol* 2005;25(6): 1244–1249.

51. Lievens D, Zernecke A, Seijkens T, Soehnlein O, Beckers L, Munnix IC, Wijnands E, Goossens P, van Kruchten R, Thevissen L, Boon L, Flavell RA, Noelle RJ, Gerdes N, Biessen EA, Daemen MJ, Heemskerk JW, Weber C, Lutgens E. Platelet CD40L mediates thrombotic and inflammatory processes in atherosclerosis. *Blood* 2010;116(20): 4317–4327.

52. Foy TM, Aruffo A, Bajorath J, Buhlmann JE, Noelle RJ. Immune regulation by CD40 and its ligand GP39. *Annu Rev Immunol* 1996;14: 591–617.

53. Garlichs CD, John S, Schmeisser A, Eskafi S, Stumpf C, Karl M, Goppelt-Struebe M, Schmieder R, Daniel WG. Upregulation of CD40 and CD40 ligand (CD154) in patients with moderate hypercholesterolemia. *Circulation* 2001;104(20): 2395–2400.

54. Kopp CW, Steiner S, Nasel C, Seidinger D, Mlekusch I, Lang W, Bartok A, Ahmadi R, Minar E. Abciximab reduces monocyte tissue factor in carotid angioplasty and stenting. *Stroke* 2003;34(11): 2560–2567.

55. Sanguigni V, Pignatelli P, Lenti L, Ferro D, Bellia A, Carnevale R, Tesauro M, Sorge R, Lauro R, Violi F. Short-term treatment with atorvastatin reduces platelet CD40 ligand and thrombin generation in hypercholesterolemic patients. *Circulation* 2005;111(4): 412–419.

56. Cipollone F, Chiarelli F, Davi G, Ferri C, Desideri G, Fazia M, Iezzi A, Santilli F, Pini B, Cuccurullo C, Tumini S, Del Ponte A, Santucci A, Cuccurullo F, Mezzetti A. Enhanced soluble CD40 ligand contributes

to endothelial cell dysfunction in vitro and monocyte activation in patients with diabetes mellitus: effect of improved metabolic control. *Diabetologia* 2005;48(6): 1216–1224.

57. Heeschen C, Dimmeler S, Hamm CW, van den Brand MJ, Boersma E, Zeiher AM, Simoons ML. Soluble CD40 ligand in acute coronary syndromes. *N Engl J Med* 2003;348(12): 1104–1111.

58. Cipollone F, Ferri C, Desideri G, Paloscia L, Materazzo G, Mascellanti M, Fazia M, Iezzi A, Cuccurullo C, Pini B, Bucci M, Santucci A, Cuccurullo F, Mezzetti A. Preprocedural level of soluble CD40L is predictive of enhanced inflammatory response and restenosis after coronary angioplasty. *Circulation* 2003;108(22): 2776–2782.

59. Lutgens E, Lievens D, Beckers L, Wijnands E, Soehnlein O, Zernecke A, Seijkens T, Engel D, Cleutjens J, Keller AM, Naik SH, Boon L, Oufella HA, Mallat Z, Ahonen CL, Noelle RJ, de Winther MP, Daemen MJ, Biessen EA, Weber C. Deficient CD40-TRAF6 signaling in leukocytes prevents atherosclerosis by skewing the immune response toward an antiinflammatory profile. *J Exp Med*2010;207(2): 391–404.

60. Zirlik A, Maier C, Gerdes N, MacFarlane L, Soosairajah J, Bavendiek U, Ahrens I, Ernst S, Bassler N, Missiou A, Patko Z, Aikawa M, Schonbeck U, Bode C, Libby P, Peter K. CD40 ligand mediates inflammation independently of CD40 by interaction with Mac-1. *Circulation* 2007;115(12): 1571–1580.

61. Lievens D, Eijgelaar WJ, Biessen EA, Daemen MJ, Lutgens E. The multi-functionality of CD40L and its receptor CD40 in atherosclerosis *Thromb Haemost* 2009;102(2): 206–214.

62. Wagner AH, Guldenzoph B, Lienenluke B, Hecker M. CD154/CD40-mediated expression of CD154 in endothelial cells: consequences for endothelial cell-monocyte interaction. *Arterioscler Thromb Vasc Biol* 2004;24(4): 715–720.

63. Mach F, Schonbeck U, Bonnefoy JY, Pober JS, Libby P. Activation of monocyte/macrophage functions related to acute atheroma complication by ligation of CD40: induction of collagenase, stromelysin, and tissue factor. *Circulation* 1997;96(2): 396–399.

64. Watts TH. TNF/TNFR family members in costimulation of T cell responses. *Annu Rev Immunol* 2005;23: 23–68.

65. Vinay DS, Kwon BS. Role of 4-1BB in immune responses. *Semin Immunol* 1998;10(6): 481–489.

66. Olofsson PS, Soderstrom LA, Wagsater D, Sheikine Y, Ocaya P, Lang F, Rabu C, Chen L, Rudling M, Aukrust P, Hedin U, Paulsson-Berne G, Sirsjo

A, Hansson GK. CD137 is expressed in human atherosclerosis and promotes development of plaque inflammation in hypercholesterolemic mice. *Circulation* 2008;117(10): 1292–1301.

67. Jeon HJ, Choi JH, Jung IH, Park JG, Lee MR, Lee MN, Kim B, Yoo JY, Jeong SJ, Kim DY, Park JE, Park HY, Kwack K, Choi BK, Kwon BS, Oh GT. CD137 (4-1BB) deficiency reduces atherosclerosis in hyperlipidemic mice. *Circulation*121(9): 1124–1133.

68. Dongming L, Zuxun L, Liangjie X, Biao W, Ping Y. Enhanced levels of soluble and membrane-bound CD137 levels in patients with acute coronary syndromes. *Clin Chim Acta*411(5–6): 406–410.

69. Nolte MA, van Olffen RW, van Gisbergen KP, van Lier RA. Timing and tuning of CD27-CD70 interactions: the impact of signal strength in setting the balance between adaptive responses and immunopathology. *Immunol Rev* 2009;229(1): 216–231.

70. van Olffen RW, de Bruin AM, Vos M, Staniszewska AD, Hamann J, van Lier RA, de Vries CJ, Nolte MA. CD70-driven chronic immune activation is protective against atherosclerosis. *J Innate Immun* 2010;2(4): 344–352.

71. Croft M. Co-stimulatory members of the TNFR family: keys to effective T-cell immunity? *Nat Rev Immunol* 2003;3(8): 609–620.

72. Azuma M. Role of the glucocorticoid-induced TNFR-related protein (GITR)-GITR ligand pathway in innate and adaptive immunity. *Crit Rev Immunol* 2010;30(6): 547–557.

73. Nocentini G, Riccardi C. GITR: a modulator of immune response and inflammation. *Adv Exp Med Biol* 2009;647: 156–173.

74. Ronchetti S, Nocentini G, Petrillo MG, Bianchini R, Sportoletti P, Bastianelli A, Ayroldi EM, Riccardi C. Glucocorticoid-Induced TNFR family Related gene (GITR) enhances dendritic cell activity. *Immunol Lett* 2010;135(1–2): 24–33.

75. Galuppo M, Nocentini G, Mazzon E, Ronchetti S, Esposito E, Riccardi L, Sportoletti P, Di Paola R, Bruscoli S, Riccardi C, Cuzzocrea S. The glucocorticoid-induced TNF receptor family-related protein (GITR) is critical to the development of acute pancreatitis in mice. *Br J Pharmacol* 2011;162(5): 1186–1201.

76. You S, Poulton L, Cobbold S, Liu CP, Rosenzweig M, Ringler D, Lee WH, Segovia B, Bach JF, Waldmann H, Chatenoud L. Key role of the GITR/GITRLigand pathway in the development of murine autoimmune diabetes: a potential therapeutic target. *PLoS One* 2009;4(11): e7848, doi: 10.1371/journal.pone.0007848.

77. Cuzzocrea S, Nocentini G, Di Paola R, Mazzon E, Ronchetti S, Genovese T, Muia C, Caputi AP, Riccardi C. Glucocorticoid-induced TNF receptor family gene (GITR) knockout mice exhibit a resistance to splanchnic artery occlusion (SAO) shock. *J Leukoc Biol* 2004;76(5): 933–940.

78. Cuzzocrea S, Ayroldi E, Di Paola R, Agostini M, Mazzon E, Bruscoli S, Genovese T, Ronchetti S, Caputi AP, Riccardi C. Role of glucocorticoid-induced TNF receptor family gene (GITR) in collagen-induced arthritis. *FASEB J* 2005;19(10): 1253–1265.

79. Nocentini G, Cuzzocrea S, Bianchini R, Mazzon E, Riccardi C. Modulation of acute and chronic inflammation of the lung by GITR and its ligand. *Ann N Y Acad Sci* 2007;1107: 380–391.

80. Kim WJ, Bae EM, Kang YJ, Bae HU, Hong SH, Lee JY, Park JE, Kwon BS, Suk K, Lee WH. Glucocorticoid-induced tumour necrosis factor receptor family related protein (GITR) mediates inflammatory activation of macrophages that can destabilize atherosclerotic plaques. *Immunology* 2006;119(3): 421–429.

81. Mauri DN, Ebner R, Montgomery RI, Kochel KD, Cheung TC, Yu GL, Ruben S, Murphy M, Eisenberg RJ, Cohen GH, Spear PG, Ware CF. LIGHT, a new member of the TNF superfamily, and lymphotoxin alpha are ligands for herpesvirus entry mediator. *Immunity* 1998;8(1): 21–30.

82. Lee WH, Kim SH, Lee Y, Lee BB, Kwon B, Song H, Kwon BS, Park JE. Tumor necrosis factor receptor superfamily 14 is involved in atherogenesis by inducing proinflammatory cytokines and matrix metalloproteinases. *Arterioscler Thromb Vasc Biol* 2001;21(12): 2004–2010.

83. Otterdal K, Smith C, Oie E, Pedersen TM, Yndestad A, Stang E, Endresen K, Solum NO, Aukrust P, Damas JK. Platelet-derived LIGHT induces inflammatory responses in endothelial cells and monocytes. *Blood* 2006;108(3): 928–935.

84. Sandberg WJ, Halvorsen B, Yndestad A, Smith C, Otterdal K, Brosstad FR, Froland SS, Olofsson PS, Damas JK, Gullestad L, Hansson GK, Oie E, Aukrust P. Inflammatory interaction between LIGHT and proteinase-activated receptor-2 in endothelial cells: potential role in atherogenesis. *Circ Res* 2009;104(1): 60–68.

85. Lo JC, Wang Y, Tumanov AV, Bamji M, Yao Z, Reardon CA, Getz GS, Fu YX. Lymphotoxin beta receptor-dependent control of lipid homeostasis. *Science* 2007;316(5822): 285–288.

86. Zapata JM. TNF-receptor-associated factors as targets for drug development. *Expert Opin Ther Targets* 2003;7(3): 411–425.

87. Zirlik A, Bavendiek U, Libby P, Macfarlane L, Gerdes N, Jagielska J, Ernst S, Aikawa M, Nakano H, Tsitsikov E, Schonbeck U. TRAF-1, -2, -3, -5, and

-6 Are Induced in atherosclerotic plaques and differentially mediate proinflammatory functions of CD40L in endothelial cells. *Arterioscler Thromb Vasc Biol* 2007;27(5): 1101–1107.

88. Missiou A, Kostlin N, Varo N, Rudolf P, Aichele P, Ernst S, Munkel C, Walter C, Stachon P, Sommer B, Pfeifer D, Zirlik K, MacFarlane L, Wolf D, Tsitsikov E, Bode C, Libby P, Zirlik A. Tumor necrosis factor receptor-associated factor 1 (TRAF1) deficiency attenuates atherosclerosis in mice by impairing monocyte recruitment to the vessel wall. *Circulation* 2010;121(18): 2033–2044.
89. Missiou A, Rudolf P, Stachon P, Wolf D, Varo N, Aichele P, Colberg C, Hoppe N, Ernst S, Munkel C, Walter C, Sommer B, Hilgendorf I, Nakano H, Bode C, Zirlik A. TRAF5 deficiency accelerates atherogenesis in mice by increasing inflammatory cell recruitment and foam cell formation. *Circ Res* 2010;107(6): 757–766.
90. Stachon P, Missiou A, Walter C, Varo N, Colberg C, Wolf D, Buchner M, von Zur Muhlen C, Zirlik K, Bode C, Zirlik A. Tumor necrosis factor receptor associated factor 6 is not required for atherogenesis in mice and does not associate with atherosclerosis in humans. *PLoS One* 2010;5(7): e11589. doi:10.1371/journal.pone.0011589.
91. Arron JR, Pewzner-Jung Y, Walsh MC, Kobayashi T, Choi Y. Regulation of the subcellular localization of tumor necrosis factor receptor-associated factor (TRAF)2 by TRAF1 reveals mechanisms of TRAF2 signaling. *J Exp Med* 2002;196(7): 923–934.
92. Ishida TK, Tojo T, Aoki T, Kobayashi N, Ohishi T, Watanabe T, Yamamoto T, Inoue J. TRAF5, a novel tumor necrosis factor receptor-associated factor family protein, mediates CD40 signaling. *Proc Natl Acad Sci U S A* 1996;93(18): 9437–9442.
93. Lu LF, Ahonen CL, Lind EF, Raman VS, Cook WJ, Lin LL, Noelle RJ. The in vivo function of a noncanonical TRAF2-binding domain in the C-terminus of CD40 in driving B-cell growth and differentiation. *Blood* 2007;110(1): 193–200.
94. Ahonen C, Manning E, Erickson LD, O'Connor B, Lind EF, Pullen SS, Kehry MR, Noelle RJ. The CD40-TRAF6 axis controls affinity maturation and the generation of long-lived plasma cells. *Nat Immunol* 2002;3(5): 451–456.
95. Mukundan L, Bishop GA, Head KZ, Zhang L, Wahl LM, Suttles J. TNF receptor-associated factor 6 is an essential mediator of CD40-activated proinflammatory pathways in monocytes and macrophages. *J Immunol* 2005;174(2): 1081–1090.

96. Mukundan L, Milhorn DM, Matta B, Suttles J. CD40-mediated activation of vascular smooth muscle cell chemokine production through a Src-initiated, MAPK-dependent pathway. *Cell Signal* 2004;16(3): 375–384.

97. Urbich C, Mallat Z, Tedgui A, Clauss M, Zeiher AM, Dimmeler S. Upregulation of TRAF-3 by shear stress blocks CD40-mediated endothelial activation. *J Clin Invest* 2001;108(10): 1451–1458.

98. Donners MM, Beckers L, Lievens D, Munnix I, Heemskerk J, Janssen BJ, Wijnands E, Cleutjens J, Zernecke A, Weber C, Ahonen CL, Benbow U, Newby AC, Noelle RJ, Daemen MJ, Lutgens E. The CD40-TRAF6 axis is the key regulator of the CD40/CD40L system in neointima formation and arterial remodeling. *Blood* 2008;111(9): 4596–4604.

Index